CONTEMPORARY ENDOCRINOLOGY

Series Editor:
P. Michael Conn, PhD
Oregon Health & Science University
Beaverton, OR

For other titles published in this series, go to
www.springer.com/series/7680

Immunoendocrinology: Scientific and Clinical Aspects

Edited by

George S. Eisenbarth

*University of Colorado Health Sciences Center, Barbara Davis Center
for Childhood Diabetes, Aurora, CO, USA*

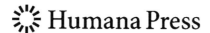

Editor
George S. Eisenbarth
University of Colorado Health Sciences Center
Barbara Davis Center for Childhood Diabetes
Aurora, CO
USA
george.eisenbarth@UCHSC.edu

ISBN 978-1-60327-477-7   e-ISBN 978-1-60327-478-4
DOI 10.1007/978-1-60327-478-4
Springer New York Dordrecht Heidelberg London

© Springer Science+Business Media, LLC 2011
All rights reserved. This work may not be translated or copied in whole or in part without the written permission of the publisher (Humana Press, c/o Springer Science+Business Media, LLC, 233 Spring Street, New York, NY 10013, USA), except for brief excerpts in connection with reviews or scholarly analysis. Use in connection with any form of information storage and retrieval, electronic adaptation, computer software, or by similar or dissimilar methodology now known or hereafter developed is forbidden.
The use in this publication of trade names, trademarks, service marks, and similar terms, even if they are not identified as such, is not to be taken as an expression of opinion as to whether or not they are subject to proprietary rights.
While the advice and information in this book are believed to be true and accurate at the date of going to press, neither the authors nor the editors nor the publisher can accept any legal responsibility for any errors or omissions that may be made. The publisher makes no warranty, express or implied, with respect to the material contained herein.

Printed on acid-free paper

Humana Press is part of Springer Science+Business Media (www.springer.com)

Dedication

This book is dedicated to the millions of families affected by autoimmunity who have partnered in research to prevent these disorders and have created Centers and Programs for Care and Research through gifts large and small.

Preface

As illustrated by the chapters in this book, autoimmune disorders are diverse and the same. At the heart of these diseases are specific alleles of genes of the major histocompatibility complex favoring the targeting of specific antigens, with diseases differing in the specific alleles favoring or preventing autoimmunity. The fine balance between self tolerance and autoimmunity is upset by major mutations in a few families, and multiple polymorphisms in most families. Large scale genetic (research involving the screening of hundreds of thousands of newborns) and then immunologic prediction of many autoimmune disorders is now a reality for both families and the general population. With the exception of celiac disease, environmental factors essential for disease and contributing to the marked increase in many of these disorders are undefined. Despite our lack of comprehensive knowledge, multiple immunotherapeutic clinical trials are underway. It is my hope that our current knowledge base for Immunoendocrinology presented here will prove sufficient to design and test preventive paradigms. Nevertheless, it is my belief that our current basic research knowledge, also presented here, is insufficient to be assured of disease prevention with current trials. Contained within each of the chapters are incomplete drafts of maps that should eventually lead to disease prevention for specific disorders that in combination provide a comprehensive draft of our knowledge and ignorance of the continent of autoimmunity.

Contents

Preface... *vii*
Contributors... *xi*

PART I IMMUNOENDOCRINOLOGY: SCIENTIFIC AND CLINICAL ASPECTS

1. Primer on Immunoendocrinology.. 3
   Jean Jasinski and George S. Eisenbarth
2. Discovering Novel Antigens... 15
   Janet M. Wenzlau, Leah Sheridan, and John C. Hutton
3. Developing and Validating High Sensitivity/Specificity
   Autoantibody Assays... 41
   Ezio Bonifacio, Anne Eugster, and Vito Lampasona
4. Characterizing T-Cell Autoimmunity..................................... 53
   Ivana Durinovic-Belló and Gerald T. Nepom
5. Metabolic Syndrome and Inflammation.................................. 69
   Rodica Pop-Busui and Massimo Pietropaolo

PART II SYNDROMES

6. The Mouse Model of Autoimmune Polyglandular Syndrome Type 1.......... 95
   James Gardner and Mark Anderson
7. Autoimmune Polyendocrine Syndrome Type I: Man....................... 115
   Eystein S. Husebye and Olle Kämpe
8. IPEX Syndrome: Clinical Profile, Biological Features,
   and Current Treatment.. 129
   Rosa Bacchetta, Laura Passerini, and Maria Grazia Roncarolo
9. Autoimmune Polyendocrine Syndrome Type 2: Pathophysiology,
   Natural History, and Clinical Manifestations........................... 143
   Jennifer M. Barker
10. Drug-Induced Endocrine Autoimmunity................................. 157
    Paolo Pozzilli, Rocky Strollo, and Nicola Napoli

PART III SPECIFIC DISEASES

11. The BB Rat.. 183
    *Ulla Nøhr Dalberg, Claus Haase, Lars Hornum,
    and Helle Markholst*
12. Immunopathogenesis of the NOD Mouse................................. 199
    Li Zhang and George S. Eisenbarth

13	Virus-Induced Type 1 Diabetes in the Rat	215
	Travis R. Wolter and Danny Zipris	
14	Autoimmune Pathology of Type 1 Diabetes	231
	Roberto Gianani and Mark Atkinson	
15	Genetics of Type 1 Diabetes	251
	Aaron Michels, Joy Jeffrey, and George S. Eisenbarth	
16	Epidemiology of Type 1 Diabetes	267
	Molly M. Lamb and Jill M. Norris	
17	Natural History of Type 1 Diabetes	279
	Spiros Fourlanos, Leonard C. Harrison, and Peter G. Colman	
18	Immunotherapy of Type-1 Diabetes: Immunoprevention and Immunoreversal	293
	Frank Waldron-Lynch and Kevan C. Herold	
19	Latent Autoimmune Diabetes in Adults	315
	Barbara M. Brooks-Worrell and Jerry P. Palmer	
20	Fulminant Type 1 Diabetes Mellitus	331
	Akihisa Imagawa and Toshiaki Hanafusa	
21	Insulin Autoimmune Syndrome (Hirata Disease)	343
	Yasuko Uchigata and Yukimasa Hirata	
22	Lessons from Patients with Anti-Insulin Receptor Autoantibodies	369
	Angeline Y. Chong and Phillip Gorden	
23	Islet and Pancreas Transplantation	385
	Gaetano Ciancio, Alberto Pugliese, George W. Burke, and Camillo Ricordi	
24	Addison's Disease	399
	Alberto Falorni	
25	Animal Models of Autoimmune Thyroid Disease	415
	Yuji Nagayama and Norio Abiru	
26	Genetics of Thyroid Autoimmunity	427
	Yaron Tomer	
27	Immunopathogenesis of Thyroiditis	443
	Su He Wang and James R. Baker	
28	Immunopathogenesis of Graves' Disease	457
	Syed A. Morshed, Rauf Latif, and Terry F. Davies	
29	Graves' Ophthalmopathy	483
	Wilmar M. Wiersinga	
30	Hypoparathyroidism	501
	Ogo I. Egbuna and Edward M. Brown	
31	Premature Gonadal Insufficiency	519
	Janice Huang, Micol S. Rothman, and Margaret E. Wierman	
32	Celiac Disease and Intestinal Endocrine Autoimmunity	535
	Leonardo Mereiles, Marcella Li, Danielle Loo, and Edwin Liu	
33	Pituitary Autoimmunity	547
	Annamaria De Bellis, Antonio Bizzarro, and Antonio Bellastella	

Index *569*

Contributors

NORIO ABIRU • *Department of Medical and Dental Sciences, Nagasaki University Hospital, Nagasaki, Japan*

MARK ANDERSON • *Diabetes Center, University of California San Francisco, San Franciso, CA, USA*

MARK ATKINSON • *The Department of Pathology, University of Florida, Gainesville, FL, USA*

ROSA BACCHETTA • *Division of Regenerative Medicine, Stems Cells and Gene Therapy, San Raffaele Scientific Institute, San Raffaele Telethon Institute for Gene Therapy (HSR-TIGET), Milan, Italy*

JAMES R. BAKER • *Michigan Nanotechnology Institute for Medicine and the Biological Sciences, University of Michigan, Ann Arbor, MI, USA*

JENNIFER M. BARKER • *Pediatric Endocrinology, The Children's Hospital, Aurora, CO, USA*

ANTONIO BELLASTELLA • *Department of Clinical and Experimental Medicine and Surgery, "F. Magrassi, A. Lanzara", Second University of Naples, Naples, Italy*

ANTONIO BIZZARRO • *Department of Clinical and Experimental Medicine and Surgery, "F. Magrassi, A. Lanzara", Second University of Naples, Naples, Italy*

EZIO BONIFACIO • *Center for Regenerative Therapies Dresden, Dresden University of Technology, Dresden, Germany*

EDWARD M. BROWN • *Division of Endocrinology, Diabetes and Hypertension, Department of Medicine, Brigham and Women's Hospital and Harvard Medical School, Boston, MA, USA*

BARBARA M. BROOKS-WORRELL • *DVA Medical Center Puget Sound Health Care System, University of Washington, Seattle, WA, USA*

GEORGE W. BURKE • *Surgery, Division of Transplantation, Jackson Memorial Hospital, University of Miami Hospital, Miami, FL, USA*

GAETANO CIANCIO • *Surgery, Division of Transplantation, Jackson Memorial Hospital, University of Miami Hospital, Miami, FL, USA*

ANGELINE Y. CHONG • *NIDDK/Clinical Endocrinology Branch, Clinical Research Center, National Institutes of Health, Bethesda, MD, USA*

PETER G. COLMAN • *Diabetes and Endocrinology, Royal Melbourne Hospital, Melbourne, VIC, Australia*

ULLA NØHR DALBERG • *Department of Immunopharmacology, Novo Nordisk Park, Måløv, Denmark*

TERRY F. DAVIES • *Mount Sinai Medical Center and James J Peters VA Medical Center, New York, NY, USA*

ANNAMARIA DE BELLIS • *Endocrinology and Metabolism, Second University of Naples, Naples, Italy*

IVANA DURINOVIC-BELLÓ • *Benaroya Research Institute at Virginia Mason, Seattle, WA, USA*

OGO I. EGBUNA • *Endocrinology Department, Brigham and Women's Hospital, Boston, MA, USA*

GEORGE S. EISENBARTH • *Barbara Davis Center for Childhood Diabetes, School of Medicine, University of Colorado Denver, Aurora, CO, USA*

ANNE EUGSTER • *Center for Regenerative Therapies Dresden, Dresden University of Technology, Dresden, Germany*

ALBERTO FALORNI • *Department of Internal Medicine, Section of Internal Medicine and Endocrine & Metabolic Sciences, University of Perugia, Perugia, Italy*

SPIROS FOURLANOS • *Department of Diabetes & Endocrinology, Royal Melbourne Hospital, Melbourne, VIC, Australia*

JAMES GARDNER • *Diabetes Center, University of California San Francisco, San Francisco, CA, USA*

ROBERTO GIANANI • *Barbara Davis Center for Childhood Diabetes, University of Colorado Denver, Aurora, CO, USA*

PHILLIP GORDEN • *NIDDK/Clinical Endocrinology Branch, Clinical Research Center, National Institutes of Health, Bethesda, MD, USA*

MARIA GRAZIA RONCAROLO • *Division of Regenerative Medicine, Stems Cells and Gene Therapy, San Raffaele Scientific Institute, San Raffaele Telethon Institute for Gene Therapy (HSR-TIGET), Milan, Italy*

CLAUS HAASE • *Department of Immunopharmacology, Novo Nordisk Park, Måløv, Denmark*

TOSHIAKI HANAFUSA • *First Department of Internal Medicine, Osaka Medial College, Takatsuki, Japan*

LEONARD C. HARRISON • *Walter and Eliza Hall Institute of Medical Research and Burnet Clinical Research Unit, Melbourne, VIC, Australia*

KEVAN C. HEROLD • *Departments of Immunobiology and Internal Medicine, Yale University, New Haven, CT, USA*

LARS HORNUM • *Department of Immunopharmacology, Novo Nordisk Park, Måløv, Denmark*

JANICE HUANG • *Departments of Medicine, University of Colorado at Denver, Aurora, CO, USA*

EYSTEIN S. HUSEBYE • *Department of Medicine, Institute of Medicine, Haukeland University Hospital, University of Bergen, Bergen, Norway*

JOHN C. HUTTON • *Barbara Davis Center for Childhood Diabetes, School of Medicine, University of Colorado Denver, Aurora, CO, USA*

AKIHISA IMAGAWA • *Graduate School of Medicine, Osaka University, Suita, Japan*

JEAN JASINSKI • *Strand Life Sciences Pvt. Ltd, Fort Collins, CO, USA*

JOY JEFFREY • *Barbara Davis Center for Childhood Diabetes, University of Colorado Denver, Aurora, CO, USA*

OLLE KÄMPE • *Department of Medical Sciences, Uppsala University Hospital, Uppsala, Sweden*

Molly M. Lamb • *Department of Epidemiology, Colorado School of Public Health, University of Colorado Denver, Aurora, CO, USA*
Vito Lampasona • *Center for Genomics, Bioinformatics and Biostatistics, San Raffaele Scientific Institute, Milan, Italy*
Rauf Latif • *Endocrinology & Metabolism, James J Peter's VA Medical Center & Mount Sinai School of Medicine, Bronx, NY, USA*
Marcella Li • *The Children's Hospital, Aurora, CO, USA*
Edwin Liu • *Section of Gastroenterology, Hepatology and Nutrition, The Children's Hospital, Aurora, CO, USA*
Danielle Loo • *The Children's Hospital, Aurora, CO, USA*
Helle Markholst • *Department of Immunopharmacology, Novo Nordisk a/s, Måløv, Denmark*
Leonardo Mereiles • *The Children's Hospital, Aurora, CO, USA*
Aaron Michels • *Barbara Davis Center for Childhood Diabetes, School of Medicine, University of Colorado Denver, Aurora, CO, USA*
Syed A. Morshed • *Endocrinology Department, James J Peters VA Medical Center and Mount Sinai School of Medicine, Bronx, NY, USA*
Yuji Nagayama • *Department of Medical Gene Technology, Atomic Bomb Disease Institute, Nagasaki University Graduate School of Biomedical Sciences, Nagasaki, Japan*
Nicola Napoli • *Endocrinology & Diabetes, University Campus Bio-Medico, Rome, Italy*
Gerald T. Nepom • *Benaroya Research Institute at Virginia Mason, Seattle, WA, USA*
Jill M. Norris • *Epidemiology Department, Colorado School of Public Health, University of Colorado Denver, Aurora, CO, USA*
Jerry P. Palmer • *Department of Medicine, DVA Puget Sound Health Care System, University of Washington, Seattle, WA, USA*
Laura Passerini • *Division of Regenerative Medicine, Stems Cells and Gene Therapy, San Raffaele Scientific Institute, San Raffaele Telethon Institute for Gene Therapy (HSR-TIGET), Milan, Italy*
Massimo Pietropaolo • *Division of Metabolism, Department of Internal Medicine, Laboratory of Immunogenetics, The Brehm Center for Type 1 Diabetes Research and Analysis, Endocrinology & Diabetes, University of Michigan Medical School, Ann Arbor, MI, USA*
Rodica Pop-Busui • *Division of Metabolism, Endocrinology & Diabetes, Department of Internal Medicine, University of Michigan Medical School, Ann Arbor, MI, USA*
Paolo Pozzilli • *Department of Endocrinology and Diabetes, University Campus Bio-Medico, Rome, Italy*
Alberto Pugliese • *Miller School of Medicine, Diabetes Research Institute, University of Miami, Miami, FL, USA*
Camillo Ricordi • *Diabetes Research Institute, University of Miami, Miami, FL, USA*

MICOL S. ROTHMAN • *Departments of Medicine, University of Colorado at Denver, Aurora, CO, USA*

LEAH SHERIDAN • *Barbara Davis Center for Childhood Diabetes, School of Medicine, University of Colorado Denver, Aurora, CO, USA*

ROCKY STROLLO • *Endocrinology & Diabetes, University Campus Bio-Medico, Rome, Italy*

YARON TOMER • *Division of Endocrinology, Cincinnati VA Medical Center, University of Cincinnati College of Medicine, Cincinnati, OH, USA*

YASUKO UCHIGATA • *Diabetes Center, Tokyo Women's Medical University School of Medicine, Tokyo, Japan*

FRANK WALDRON-LYNCH • *Departments of Immunobiology and Internal Medicine, Yale University, New Haven, CT, USA*

SU HE WANG • *Michigan Nanotechnology Institute for Medicine and the Biological Sciences, University of Michigan, Ann Arbor, MI, USA*

JANET M. WENZLAU • *Barbara Davis Center for Childhood Diabetes, School of Medicine, University of Colorado Denver, Aurora, CO, USA*

MARGARET E. WIERMAN • *Physiology and Biophysics Hospital, University of Colorado, Denver, CO, USA*

WILMAR M. WIERSINGA • *Department of Endocrinology & Metabolism, Academic Medical Center, University of Amsterdam, The Netherlands*

TRAVIS R. WOLTER • *Barbara Davis Center for Childhood Diabetes, University of Colorado Denver, Aurora, CO, USA*

LI ZHANG • *Barbara Davis Center for Childhood Diabetes, University of Colorado Denver, Aurora, CO, USA*

DANNY ZIPRIS • *Davis Center for Childhood Diabetes, University of Colorado Denver, Aurora, CO, USA*

Part I

Immunoendocrinology: Scientific and Clinical Aspects

Chapter 1

Primer on Immunoendocrinology

Jean Jasinski and George S. Eisenbarth

Key Words: Autoimmunity, Tolerance, T-cell receptor, Major histocompatibility complex, Autoimmune polyendocrine syndromes, Regulatory T cells

INTRODUCTION

This book on immunoendocrinology deals primarily with autoimmune disorders. The study of endocrine autoimmune diseases has played a prominent role in advancing the understanding of autoimmunity including creation of the first models of induced autoimmune disease (*1*), demonstration that autoimmunity can cause human pathology (*2*), and characterization of remarkable syndromes linking multiple autoimmune diseases, as well as the first discovery of genes contributing to multiple diseases such mutations of the *AIRE* (Autoimmune Regulator) gene (*3*) of APS-1 (Autoimmune Polyendocrine Syndrome) and a specific polymorphism (R620W) of the *PTPN22* gene associated with type 1 diabetes and rheumatoid arthritis (*4, 5*). Autoimmunity can be driven primarily by autoantibodies (e.g., targeting of the TSH-receptor by antibodies in Graves' disease) or predominantly by T cells (e.g., Type 1A diabetes), but in general, both humoral and cellular autoimmunity occur together. Autoimmune endocrine disorders may affect single organs, a few organs, or many organs. Regardless of the number of organs affected, the underlying autoimmune disease mechanisms are similar with potential variation in the probability of loss of tolerance. In general, persons suffering from rare single organ-specific autoimmune diseases tend to develop multi-organ autoimmunity over time.

Immunologists typically divide the immune system into two branches, the innate immune system and the adaptive immune system.

The fundamental characteristic of the innate immune system is programmed "nonadaptive" (germ-line encoded) (6) responses mediated by PRRs (pattern-recognition receptors) that recognize specific molecules called PAMPS (pathogen-associated molecular patterns) (7). Components of the innate immune system including Toll-like receptors and the inflammasome target a wide variety of specific PAMPS (8). In contrast to the innate immune system, the adaptive immune system evidences "memory" with clonal expansion of cells with specific receptors [T-cell receptors (TCR) or B-cell receptors (BCR)]. The divisions between these branches are becoming somewhat blurred with greater molecular understanding. In particular, activation of the innate immune system is important for activation of the adaptive immune system, even for the function of commonly used adjuvants such as alum (9). In addition, specific TCR rearrangements, such as the TCR of NKT cells, produce cytokine-secreting cells that respond to glycosphingolipids in a manner analogous to the PRRs of the innate immune system (10).

The cell-mediated and humoral (antibody) branches of the adaptive immune system are both diverse with receptors that can recognize billions of different epitopes by virtue of the specificity of TCRs and BCRs, with each clone having a unique amino sequence. These receptors can recognize minute differences in antigens and respond differentially. TCRs usually react with antigenic peptides (but not always) that are presented by specialized MHC (major histocompatibility complex) molecules on antigen-presenting cells (APCs). The MHC-presenting molecule, peptide (or other molecule) bound in its groove, and the TCR comprise a trimolecular complex, the essential determinant of T-cell-mediated organ-specific autoimmunity (Fig. 1.1 inset). TCRs recognize molecules presented in the binding groove of class I and class II MHC molecules whereas B lymphocyte receptors can react with intact molecules. However, few rules of immunology are invariant; the TCR of NKT cells recognizes a glycolipid (rather than a peptide) presented by a class I-like molecule (CD1d), and γδ T cells can recognize antigen in the absence of a classical MHC-presenting molecule (11).

The innate and adaptive immune systems are linked by specialized phagocytic and endocytic cells, also known as APCs (dendritic cells, macrophages, and B lymphocytes) that can internalize and process pathogens, cells or molecules. Once inside an APC, the engulfed targets are digested into peptides by a redundant system of endopeptidases, exopeptidases, and an interferon-γ-induced lysosomal thiol reductase (12) and this results in a pool of peptides for binding to MHC class II molecules. Component peptides are bound to class II receptors of the MHC in the endocytic pathway, and the peptide-MHC molecules are exported to the cell surface to "present" the antigen for immune surveillance. A simplified schematic shows the interaction between a CD4+ T cell and an APC (Fig. 1.1). In reality, the interaction is complex

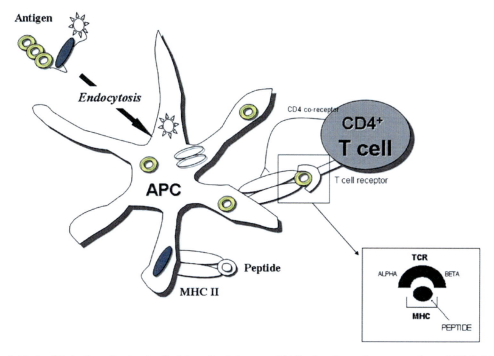

Fig. 1.1 A simplified schematic showing the interaction between a CD4 T cell and an antigen-presenting cell (APC). APCs can ingest pathogens or dead/dying cells via endocytosis. Once inside an APC, the engulfed targets are lysed. Component proteins are digested and are bound to class II receptors of the MHC in the endocytic pathway, and the peptide-MHC molecules are exported to the cell surface to "present" the antigen for immune surveillance. *Inset* shows the trimolecular complex formed by the binding of a peptide, an MHC molecule, and a T-cell receptor. Modified from Eisenbarth (65) teaching slides at http://www.uchsc.edu/misc/diabetes/Chapter1.ppt.

involving multiple costimulatory molecules, signaling cascades, cytoskeleton rearrangements, etc. The term "immunological synapse" has been coined to describe the physical structure of interaction (13) that leads to activation of T lymphocytes. An important property of T- and B-cell cooperation is linked to stimulation by which a CD4 T cell recognizes a peptide derived from a molecule bound to the BCR which leads to activation of the B cell by the T cell.

HUMAN AND MURINE MHC GENES

The MHC is the genetic locus that includes the genes that encode the class I and class II MHC molecules that present antigens to T cells and many other genes important in the immune response (14). The MHC is a gene-dense, highly variable region with low recombination rates (15). In man, this complex is called HLA (human leukocyte antigen) and is located on chromosome 6p. In mouse, this complex is called H-2 and is located on chromosome 17. The MHC complex was first identified for its role in tissue transplantation (*16*), and HLA alleles were associated with T1DM in 1974 (*17, 18*). MHC molecules are expressed codominantly on most cell surfaces. Class I MHC molecules, which are recognized by CD8 T cells, are found on all nucleated cells of the body whereas Class II MHC molecules, which are recognized by CD4 T cells, are found on APCs of the mouse but can also be induced in T lymphocytes of man. Rather than presenting exogenous peptides, the class I MHC molecules usually load and present to CD8 T-cell peptides that were produced inside the cell.

The MHC genes involved in peptide presentation are called "classical" MHC genes. The classical class I genes in man include HLA-A, HLA-B, and HLA-C. In the mouse, class I genes are K, D, and L. Class II (classical) genes in man include DP, DQ, and DR; in the mouse, they are I-A and I-E. The class III region includes genes important for immune function [e.g., complement, TNF-α, and TNF-β (tissue necrosis factor)] as well as genes that do not have immune function (hemochromatosis and 21-hydroxylase genes).

The recognition of any specific peptide by the immune system is influenced by these highly polymorphic class II genes that must bind peptide for presentation to TCRs (*19, 20*). The specific amino acids lining the groove of the class II molecule determine which peptides can be bound and the specific "register" of binding. This in turn influences specific TCR recognition in the trimolecular complex (e.g., DR molecule + peptide + TCR). One theory is that class II molecules implicated in autoimmune diseases bind their antigens less efficiently leading to incomplete tolerance (*21*) although this has been disputed (*22*) and seems unlikely as a general rule since the same HLA molecules can be associated with an increase or decrease in different autoimmune disorders. An autoimmune disease, such as type 1 diabetes, is not only dependent on the class II-specific alleles, but is also associated with polymorphisms of genes that influence development and maintenance of tolerance. Polymorphisms and mutations of many genes influencing immune function are associated with risk of organ-specific autoimmunity as suggested by candidates genes discovered by genetic association, linkage, and, most recently by large genome-wide association studies (*23–31*).

The nomenclature for defining MHC molecules and genes of man and mouse differ. The mouse nomenclature is simpler with all class I and class II MHC alleles of standard strains assigned a single letter designation. For example, alleles of BALB/c mice are denoted with a superscript "d" following the gene name (I-A^d I-E^d K^d D^d) while C57BL/6 mice have the superscript "b" (I-A^b I-E^b K^b D^b). As new strains of mice are discovered or created, they can have different mixtures of alleles, such as the NOD mouse that is I-A^{g7} I-E null K^d and D^b. Mouse strains are usually inbred and are not diallelic at any locus (always homozygous).

For man, each unique sequence is assigned a four-digit number that follows the gene designation (e.g., DRB1*0401). A fifth digit may be added to denote nucleotide differences that do not alter an amino acid. Class II DQ MHC molecules are composed of two chains (A and B), and both chains can be polymorphic and thus need to be defined (e.g., DQA1*0301-DQB1*0302). In contrast, DR molecules are predominantly polymorphic for DRB only but not for the DRA chain, and thus one usually just denotes the DRB chain (e.g., DRB1*0301). For class I MHC molecules, the second chain is invariant and is coded for by a gene outside of the MHC (β-2 microglobulin). Risk of autoimmunity is usually not determined by a single MHC allele, but rather by a combination of polymorphisms of multiple MHC genes on the same chromosome, called a haplotype. For instance, DRB1*0401, DQA1*0301-DQB1*0302 is high-risk haplotype for type 1 diabetes, whereas both DRB1*0403 with DQA1*0301-DQB1*0302 and DRB1*0401 with DQA1*0301-DQB1*0301 are much lower risk. In addition to the "proper" naming of these MHC molecules, certain shorthand designations are extant such as DR3 (for DRB1*0301-DQA1*0501-DQB1*0201) which is strongly associated with multiple autoimmune endocrine diseases (Type 1A diabetes, Addison's disease, Graves' disease). It is the combination of the allelic variants on both chromosomes (genotype) that ultimately determines disease risk; there are both protective and pathogenic MHC genotypes.

TCR GENE REARRANGEMENT

While MHC molecules of the trimolecular complex are "static" with only allelic variation inherited in a standard Mendelian manner and expressed codominantly, TCRs are created by DNA rearrangements of multiple component genetic segments. The creation of T cells is primarily a function of the thymus. TCRs are classified structurally according to their heterodimeric chains, either αβ or γδ. In mice and man, the majority of T cells are αβ T cells. Gamma-delta T cells (*32*) have a similar structure to αβ TCRs but function in a different context (*33*). Alpha-beta TCRs are composed of two different chains, TCRα and TCRβ (*34–36*). As shown in Fig. 1.2, the TCRα chain is composed of three domains: Variable, Joining, and Constant (VJC). The TCRβ chain is more complex and is composed of four domains: Variable, Diversity, Joining, and Constant (VDJC).

T cell and BCRs are unique genetically and violate the axiom that every nucleated cell contains the same genomic DNA. Rather than each T- and B-cell receptor being encoded by individual genes, the genes for T (and B) receptors are assembled by cutting

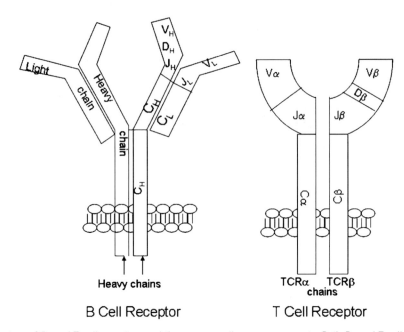

Fig. 1.2 Structure of B- and T-cell receptors and the corresponding gene segments. Both B- and T-cell receptors are multimers; the B-cell receptor is comprised of two identical heavy chains and two identical light chains whereas the T-cell receptor is composed of TCRα and TCRβ chains. Each individual chain consists of multiple segments (VDJC or VJC) encoded by separate gene segments. Chains are joined by disulfide bonds (not shown).

and pasting individual germ-line gene segments. Germ-line genomic DNA for the TCR α/β genes is composed of cassettes of multiple V, J, D, and C regions (Fig. 1.3). One segment from each region is randomly selected from the cassette and is assembled into a functional TCR chain. Germ-line (genomic) DNA is excised and spliced somatically with the aid of two nonredundant enzymes, recombinase-activating genes 1 and 2 (RAG1 and RAG2) (*37*). Mice deficient in either RAG1 or RAG2 cannot produce B or T lymphocytes (*38*).

The TCRβ chain is assembled first followed by the TCRα chain. Once a functional TCRβ chain is expressed (a successful translation), further rearrangement of the TCRβ chain genes is suppressed so that only one TCRβ chain is expressed on a T cell (allelic exclusion) (*39*). Further rearrangements are suppressed by controlling DNA accessibility and availability of DNA cutting/repair enzymes. A similar process occurs for TCRα chains albeit less efficiently (*40, 41*). This random pairing of variable, diversity, joining, and constant domains (combinatorial joining) can potentially generate at least three million different TCRs in the mouse (*42*). Additional diversity is provided by stochastic events such as the insertion of palindromic or random base insertions at some of the V–J, V–D, and D–J junctions that increases the potential TCR repertoire to greater than ten 10^{11} on one hundred billion. In general, each T and B cell will express multiple copies of a single (clonal) rearranged receptor (*41, 43, 44*).

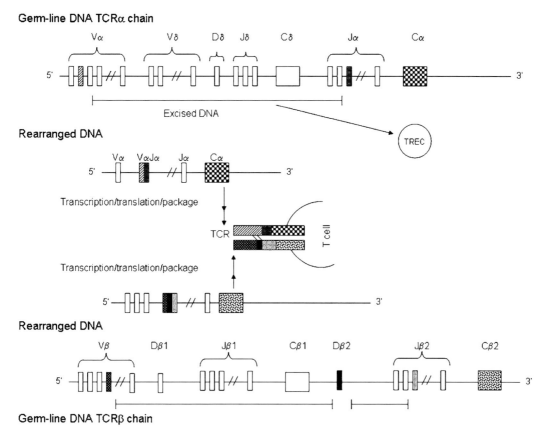

Fig. 1.3 Genetic rearrangements form a T-cell receptor. Rather than encoding each T- and B-cell receptor as a separate gene, the genes for T (and B)-cell receptors are assembled by cutting and splicing individual germ-line gene segments. Germ-line genomic DNA for the TCR α/β genes is composed of cassettes of multiple V, D, J, and C regions. One segment from each region is randomly selected from the cassette and is assembled with the other gene segments into a complete TCR gene. Excised DNA forms TRECs (T-cell receptor excision circles), extrachromosomal DNA which may be used to identify recent thymic emigrants. The rearrangement process, including the addition and deletion of nucleotides at junctions during the process, generates a much larger diversity of T-cell receptors than can be encoded in genomic DNA. Patterned segments within each cassette highlight which gene was selected to produce the TCR in the middle of the figure. A similar rearrangement process occurs for B-cell receptors.

CENTRAL AND PERIPHERAL TOLERANCE

It is generally thought that control of autoimmunity rests with T lymphocytes despite the higher propensity for autoimmunity in B lymphocytes. B lymphocytes not only create their BCR with a similar combinatorial process, but also "hypermutate" to edit BCRs after formation. Such mutations, in combination with clonal expansion of the B cells with the best binding BCRs, enhance the binding affinity of antibodies. Because B-cell clones require T cell help to expand and function, T cells provide a "brake" for humoral autoimmunity.

T cells are produced primarily in the bone marrow but migrate to the thymus where TCR α/β gene rearrangement occurs.

The random genetic rearrangement and introduction of non-germ-line encoded nucleotides might result in TCRs that cannot be translated, in TCRs that cannot be positively selected, or in TCRs that are autoreactive. Positive and negative selection processes in the thymus select T cells that can weakly bind "self" (MHC+peptide) but do not bind autoreactive antigens with high affinity/avidity (central tolerance). Cells that survive thymic selection are allowed to exit the thymus; failures either die of neglect or are actively signaled to undergo apoptosis. This repertoire shaping (central tolerance) is not perfect since self-reactive T cells can be detected in the periphery of all individuals (45).

T cells exit the thymus as naïve T cells. If autoreactive T (or B) cells never encounter their cognate antigen, they will not be activated and will not become effector cells. If a self-reactive T or B cell does encounter antigen, the context (e.g., presence of additional signals often dependent upon innate immunity) and peripheral tolerance mechanisms usually prevent autoimmune disease. Regulatory T cells (46) may actively suppress pathogenic T cells (47, 48). T cells that see antigen without a danger signal (i.e., a costimulatory signal on an activated APC caused by inflammation, tissue damage, etc.) or with a suppressive signal may become anergic (49) and may undergo apoptosis due to active cytokine signaling or cytokine withdrawal (50). T cells that receive strong signals may undergo activation-induced cell death (AICD) (51). The importance of regulatory T cells is now well recognized with multiple forms of such cells being defined. Perhaps that most dramatic example of the importance of one set of regulatory cells (termed "natural") is associated with mutations of the gene *FOXP3*. Patients with mutations of this gene may die from overwhelming autoimmunity but can be treated with bone marrow transplantation (52, 53).

The development of an autoimmune disease, therefore, requires circumventing several tolerance mechanisms. This requires a set of genetic variants in MHC and TCR alleles, but also defects in either central or peripheral tolerance. Multiple different environmental factors can play a role in inducing some autoimmune endocrine disorders given genetic susceptibility (54). For instance, treatment with IFN-α (interferon alpha) for hepatitis C infection can induce islet autoantibodies, thyroiditis, and can accelerate diabetes development (55, 56).

CONCLUSIONS

As applied specifically to the autoimmune disorders encompassing immunoendocrinology, an important subset of "answered" questions and many unanswered questions exist. In general, endocrine autoimmune disorders are characterized by a prodromal phase that increasingly allows assessment of risk with a combination of genetic factors, detection of autoantibodies, specific immunologic abnormalities, and progressive abnormalities of physiologic function (*57*). This has perhaps been most intensively studied for type 1A diabetes, with large preventive trials now underway, but most disorders of tissue destruction appear to follow the same paradigm. HLA alleles are the most important current genetic predictors, and many autoimmune disorders share similar risk alleles (*58, 59*). Highly sensitive and specific prediction for type 1A diabetes is possible. The presence of two or more of a series of biochemically defined islet autoantibodies (GA65, insulin, IA-2, and ZnT8) measured with fluid phase radioassays is associated with progression to overt diabetes both for relatives and the general population (*60–62*). Prediction is primarily achieved by utilizing the assays in combination and is difficult to achieve with noncompetitive ELISA autoantibody assays (*63*). At present, T-cell assays of autoreactivity are at a formative stage, perhaps similar to autoantibody assays two decades ago, but we believe as relevant autoantigenic peptides are discovered and improved assays are developed, T-cell assays may also contribute to disease prediction.

Multiple immune therapies are being introduced into clinical practice for diseases such as multiple sclerosis and rheumatoid arthritis and are being studied for prevention of type 1A diabetes. Most of these therapies lack sufficient disease-specificity and may not be safe enough for widespread treatment of endocrine disorders since improvements in physiologic hormone replacements are being successfully pursued (*64*). In this vein, we believe that antigen-specific immunotherapy will be the key to ultimate safe prevention of endocrine autoimmunity, but better understanding of the trimolecular complex underlying disease targeting is needed. Antigen-specific therapies targeting components of this complex are not available currently for any autoimmune disease in man. Thus the shared knowledge and expertise that crosses all immunologic disciplines (and certainly the diseases covered in this book) will likely be necessary for the ultimate development of safe and effective immunologic therapies for the field of immunoendocrinology.

ACKNOWLEDGMENTS

This work was supported by the National Institutes of Health (DK32083, DK32493, DK057538), Autoimmunity Prevention Center (AI50964), Diabetes Endocrine Research Center

(P30 DK57516), Clinical Research Centers (MO1 RR00069, MO1 RR00051), the Immune Tolerance Network (AI15416), the American Diabetes Association, the Juvenile Diabetes Research Foundation, the Brehm Coalition, and the Children's Diabetes Foundation.

REFERENCES

1. Rose NR, Witebsky E. Studies on organ specificity. V. Changes in the thyroid glands of rabbits following active immunization with rabbit thyroid extracts. J Immunol 1956;76: 417–427.
2. Doniach D, Roitt IM. Human organ specific autoimmunity: personal memories. Autoimmunity 1988;1:11–13.
3. Mathis D, Benoist C. A decade of AIRE. Nat Rev Immunol 2007;7:645–650.
4. Bottini N, Musumeci L, Alonso A, et al. A functional variant of lymphoid tyrosine phosphatase is associated with type I diabetes. Nat Genet 2004;36:337–338.
5. Lee YH, Rho YH, Choi SJ, et al. The PTPN22 C1858T functional polymorphism and autoimmune diseases – a meta-analysis. Rheumatology (Oxford) 2007;46:49–56.
6. Medzhitov R, Janeway CA, Jr. On the semantics of immune recognition. Res Immunol 1996;147:208–214.
7. Medzhitov R, Preston-Hurlburt P, Janeway CA, Jr. A human homologue of the Drosophila Toll protein signals activation of adaptive immunity. Nature 1997;388:394–397.
8. Medzhitov R. Recognition of microorganisms and activation of the immune response. Nature 2007;449:819–826.
9. Eisenbarth SC, Colegio OR, O'Connor W, Sutterwala FS, Flavell RA. Crucial role for the Nalp3 inflammasome in the immunostimulatory properties of aluminium adjuvants. Nature 2008;453:1122–1126.
10. MacDonald HR. NKT cells: In the beginning. Eur J Immunol 2007;37(Suppl 1):111–115.
11. Chien YH, Konigshofer Y. Antigen recognition by gamma delta T cells. Immunol Rev 2007;215:46–58.
12. Watts C. The exogenous pathway for antigen presentation on major histocompatibility complex class II and CD1 molecules. Nat Immunol 2004;5:685–692.
13. Dustin ML. T-cell activation through immunological synapses and kinapses. Immunol Rev 2008;221:77–89.
14. Benacerraf B, McDevitt H. Histocompatibility-linked immune response genes. Science 1972;175:273–279.
15. Traherne JA. Human MHC architecture and evolution: implications for disease association studies. Int J Immunogenet 2008;35:179–192.
16. Lengerova A. Immunogenetics of Tissue Transplantation. New York: Wiley Interscience, 1969.
17. Nerup J, Platz P, Anderson OO, et al. HLA antigens and diabetes mellitus. Lancet 1974;2:864–866.
18. Nerup J, Anderson O, Ortved C, Platz P. HLA, autoimmunity, virus and the pathogenesis of juvenile diabetes mellitus. Acta Endocrinol Suppl 1976;205:167–173.
19. Gardiner A, Richards KA, Sant AJ, Arneson LS. Conformation of MHC class II-A(g7) is sensitive to the P9 anchor amino acid in bound peptide. Int Immunol 2007;19:1103–1113.
20. Logunova NN, Viret C, Pobezinsky LA, et al. Restricted MHC-peptide repertoire predisposes to autoimmunity. J Exp Med 2005; 202:73–84.
21. Ounissi-Benkalha H, Polychronakos C. The molecular genetics of type 1 diabetes: new genes and emerging mechanisms. Trends Mol Med 2008;14:268–275.
22. Wucherpfennig KW. MHC-linked susceptibility to type 1 diabetes a structural perspective. Ann NY Acad Sci 2003;1005:119–127.
23. Lowe CE, Cooper JD, Brusko T, et al. Large-scale genetic fine mapping and genotype-phenotype associations implicate polymorphism in the IL2RA region in type 1 diabetes. Nat Genet 2007;39:1074–1082.
24. Todd JA, Walker NM, Cooper JD, et al. Robust associations of four new chromosome regions from genome-wide analyses of type 1 diabetes. Nat Genet 2007;39:857–864.
25. WTCCC. Genome-wide association study of 14,000 cases of seven common diseases and 3,000 shared controls. Nature 2007;447: 661–678.
26. Nistico L, Buzzetti R, Pritchard LE, et al. The CTLA-4 gene region of chromosome 2q33 is linked to, and associated with, type 1 diabetes. Hum Mol Genet 1996;5:1075–1080.
27. Smyth DJ, Cooper JD, Bailey R, et al. A genome-wide association study of nonsynonymous SNPs identifies a type 1 diabetes locus

in the interferon-induced helicase (IFIH1) region. Nat Genet 2006;38:617–619.
28. Ueda H, Howson JM, Esposito L, et al. Association of the T-cell regulatory gene CTLA4 with susceptibility to autoimmune disease. Nature 2003;423:506–511.
29. Hakonarson H, Grant SF, Bradfield JP, et al. A genome-wide association study identifies KIAA0350 as a type 1 diabetes gene. Nature 2007;448:591–594.
30. Nejentsev S, Smink LJ, Smyth D, et al. Sequencing and association analysis of the type 1 diabetes-linked region on chromosome 10p12-q11. BMC Genet 2007;8:24.
31. Vella A, Cooper JD, Lowe CE, et al. Localization of a type 1 diabetes locus in the IL2RA/CD25 region by use of tag single-nucleotide polymorphisms. Am J Hum Genet 2005;76:773–779.
32. Brenner MB, McLean J, Dialynas DP, et al. Identification of a putative second T-cell receptor. Nature 1986;322:145–149.
33. Carding SR, Kyes S, Jenkinson EJ, et al. Developmentally regulated fetal thymic and extrathymic T-cell receptor gamma delta gene expression. Genes Dev 1990;4:1304–1315.
34. Kappler J, Kubo R, Haskins K, White J, Marrack P. The mouse T cell receptor: comparison of MHC-restricted receptors on two T cell hybridomas. Cell 1983;34:727.
35. McIntyre BW, Allison JP. The mouse T cell receptor: structural heterogeneity of molecules of normal T cells defined by xenoantiserum. Cell 1983;34:739–746.
36. Oettgen HC, Kappler J, Tax WJ, Terhorst C. Characterization of the two heavy chains of the T3 complex on the surface of human T lymphocytes. J Biol Chem 1984;259: 12039–12048.
37. Schatz DG, Baltimore D. Stable expression of immunoglobulin gene V(D)J recombinase activity by gene transfer into 3T3 fibroblasts. Cell 1988;53:107–115.
38. Shultz LD, Lang PA, Christianson SW, et al. NOD/LtSz-Rag1null mice: an immunodeficient and radioresistant model for engraftment of human hematolymphoid cells, HIV infection, and adoptive transfer of NOD mouse diabetogenic T cells. J Immunol 2000;164:2496–2507.
39. Sieh P, Chen J. Distinct control of the frequency and allelic exclusion of the V beta gene rearrangement at the TCR beta locus. J Immunol 2001;167:2121–2129.
40. Corthay A, Nandakumar KS, Holmdahl R. Evaluation of the percentage of peripheral T cells with two different T cell receptor alpha-chains and of their potential role in autoimmunity. J Autoimmun 2001;16:423–429.
41. Lacorazza HD, Nikolich-Zugich J. Exclusion and inclusion of TCR alpha proteins during T cell development in TCR-transgenic and normal mice. J Immunol 2004;173:5591–5600.
42. Goldsby RA, Kindt TJ, Osborne BA, Kuby J. T Cell Receptor. In: Kuby Immunology. 4th ed. New York: W. H. Freeman and Company, 2003:215–238.
43. Legrand N, Freitas AA. CD8(+) T lymphocytes in double alpha beta TCR transgenic mice. I. TCR expression and thymus selection in the absence or in the presence of self-antigen. J Immunol 2001;167:6150–6157.
44. Hah C, Kim M, Kim M. Induction of peripheral tolerance in dual TCR T cells: an evidence for non-dominant signaling by one TCR. J Biochem Mol Biol 2005;38:334–342.
45. Hsieh CS, Zheng Y, Liang Y, Fontenot JD, Rudensky AY. An intersection between the self-reactive regulatory and nonregulatory T cell receptor repertoires. Nat Immunol 2006;7:401–410.
46. Yi H, Zhen Y, Jiang L, Zheng J, Zhao Y. The phenotypic characterization of naturally occurring regulatory CD4+CD25+ T cells. Cell Mol Immunol 2006;3:189–195.
47. Sakaguchi S, Sakaguchi N, Asano M, Itoh M, Toda M. Immunologic self-tolerance maintained by activated T cells expressing IL-2 receptor alpha-chains (CD25). Breakdown of a single mechanism of self-tolerance causes various autoimmune diseases. J Immunol 1995;155:1151–1164.
48. Sakaguchi S, Toda M, Asano M, Itoh M, Morse SS, Sakaguchi N. T cell-mediated maintenance of natural self-tolerance: its breakdown as a possible cause of various autoimmune diseases. J Autoimmun 1996;9:211–220.
49. Powell JD. The induction and maintenance of T cell anergy. Clin Immunol 2006;120:239–246.
50. Lohr J, Knoechel B, Nagabhushanam V, Abbas AK. T-cell tolerance and autoimmunity to systemic and tissue-restricted self-antigens. Immunol Rev 2005;204:116–127.
51. Lenardo M, Chan KM, Hornung F, et al. Mature T lymphocyte apoptosis – immune regulation in a dynamic and unpredictable antigenic environment. Annu Rev Immunol 1999;17:221–253.
52. Zhan H, Sinclair J, Adams S, et al. Immune reconstitution and recovery of FOXP3 (forkhead box P3)-expressing T cells after transplantation for IPEX (immune dysregulation, polyendocrinopathy, enteropathy, X-linked) syndrome. Pediatrics 2008;121:e998–e1002.

53. Fuchizawa T, Adachi Y, Ito Y, et al. Developmental changes of FOXP3-expressing CD4(+)CD25(+) regulatory T cells and their impairment in patients with FOXP3 gene mutations. Clin Immunol 2007;125:237–246.
54. Bailey R, Cooper JD, Zeitels L, et al. Association of the vitamin D metabolism gene CYP27B1 with type 1 diabetes. Diabetes 2007;56:2616–2621.
55. Fabris P, Floreani A, Tositti G, Vergani D, De Lalla F, Betterle C. Type 1 diabetes mellitus in patients with chronic hepatitis C before and after interferon therapy. Aliment Pharmacol Ther 2003;18:549–558.
56. Schreuder TC, Gelderblom HC, Weegink CJ, et al. High incidence of type 1 diabetes mellitus during or shortly after treatment with pegylated interferon alpha for chronic hepatitis C virus infection. Liver Int 2008; 28:39–46.
57. Coco G, Dal Pra C, Presotto F, et al. Estimated risk for developing autoimmune Addison's disease in patients with adrenal cortex autoantibodies. J Clin Endocrinol Metab 2006; 91:1637–1645.
58. Erlich H, Valdes AM, Noble J, et al. HLA DR-DQ haplotypes and genotypes and type 1 diabetes risk: analysis of the type 1 diabetes genetics consortium families. Diabetes 2008; 57:1084–1092.
59. Aly TA, Ide A, Jahromi MM, et al. Extreme genetic risk for type 1A diabetes. Proc Natl Acad Sci USA 2006;103:14074–14079.
60. Verge CF, Gianani R, Kawasaki E, et al. Prediction of type I diabetes in first-degree relatives using a combination of insulin, GAD, and ICA512bdc/IA-2 autoantibodies. Diabetes 1996;45:926–933.
61. Wenzlau JM, Juhl K, Yu L, et al. The cation efflux transporter ZnT8 (Slc30A8) is a major autoantigen in human type 1 diabetes. Proc Natl Acad Sci USA 2007;104:17040–17045.
62. Achenbach P, Bonifacio E, Williams AJ, Ziegler AG, Gale EA, Bingley PJ. Autoantibodies to IA-2beta improve diabetes risk assessment in high-risk relatives. Diabetologia 2008;51:488–492.
63. Liu E, Eisenbarth GS. Accepting clocks that tell time poorly: fluid-phase versus standard ELISA autoantibody assays. Clin Immunol 2007;125:120–126.
64. Eisenbarth GS. Update in type 1 diabetes. J Clin Endocrinol Metab 2007;92:2403–2407.
65. Teaching Slides: Type 1 Diabetes: Cellular, Molecular and Clinical Immunology. http://www.uchsc.edu/misc/diabetes/books.html.

Chapter 2

Discovering Novel Antigens

Janet M. Wenzlau, Leah Sheridan, and John C. Hutton

Summary

This chapter aims to highlight the importance of autoantigen discovery for the development of immunological interventions following diagnosis and/or progression of type 1 diabetes, an autoimmune disease that specifically targets and destroys pancreatic β cells within the Islets of Langerhans. Both humoral (B-cell) and cell-mediated (T-cell) autoimmunity will be discussed, specifically focusing on the experimental models through which novel autoantigens have been discovered, characterized, and exploited for diagnostic purposes.

Key Words: ZnT8 zinc transporter 8, GAD65 glutamic acid decarboxylase, Insulin autoantibody, Proteomics, Expression library

INTRODUCTION

Type 1 autoimmune diabetes (T1D) is a progressive disease characterized by the targeted destruction of the insulin-secreting β-cells within the islets of Langerhans of the pancreas (*1*). It is generally accepted that T1D is a T-cell mediated disease and results from immune dysregulation with consequential loss of tolerance to β-cell antigens and ultimately insulitis, the infiltration of CD4+ and CD8+ lymphocytes into the islets. The major antigenic targets of autoimmunity have been defined via analysis of circulating autoantibodies, although they are not believed to be intrinsically diabetogenic. However, there is increasing evidence that autoantigen-specific B-cells play a significant role in the pathogenesis of T1D, as they are critical mediators of antigen presentation and comprise a large proportion of the mononuclear cells in the insulitic lesions of the pancreas (*2*). As the disease progresses and β-cell deterioration ensues, the disease manifests as impaired glucose tolerance and ultimately proceeds to symptomatic hyperglycemia (*2*).

Despite the prevalence of sporadic disease (greater than 80%), there is a clear genetic predisposition associated with the development of β-cell autoimmunity. The majority of genetic determinants reside in the major histocompatibility loci, particularly HLA-DR and DQ, which account for greater than 40% of inheritability (*3, 4*). Furthermore, first-degree relatives of T1D individuals carry a significantly greater risk of developing T1D (6%) than individuals in the general population (0.4%) (*5, 6*). Thus, the disease presumably arises from failure to tolerate β-cell antigens in individuals with intrinsic (genetic) defects in critical immunomodulatory mechanisms (*7*). This underlying genetic predisposition combined with potential environmental triggers such as viral infections or dietary customs may initiate the process of autoimmune β-cell destruction, which can proceed for years without symptoms prior to overt clinical disease.

The prediction of T1D can be based on genetic susceptibility (*8, 9*), metabolic tests (*10–12*), or the detection of autoantibodies. A risk score based on a metabolic model including BMI, age, fasting C-peptide measurement, and post-challenge glucose and C-peptide levels from 2-hr oral glucose tolerance tests was indeed predictive of T1D; however, the subjects in the study were preselected as ICA positive (*11*). Currently, the measure of autoantibodies in circulation provides the most reliable preclinical indicator for diabetic autoimmunity, as their appearance can precede disease onset for years. Furthermore, the presence of multiple autoantibodies rather than their individual titer has the highest predictive value for progression to disease. The molecules recognized by autoantibodies generated in B-cells should likewise be targets for autoreactive diabetogenic T-cells as has been demonstrated for the established T1D antigens insulin, phogrin, and GAD65 (*13, 14*). Since the underlying mechanism required to generate antibodies requires the participation of T-cells, it is logical that B-and T-cells recognize the same antigens.

Identification of the autoantigens in T1D provides potential development of antigen-specific B-cell and T-cell therapies. Individual autoantibody profiling is vital to evaluate antigen-specific therapeutic interventions to prevent or delay clinical onset. Autoantibodies typically appear sequentially rather than concurrently during the course of the disease, and the prevalence and titer of autoantibodies varies with age (*15–17*). For instance, the titer and prevalence of insulin autoantibodies (IAA) display dramatic age dependency, as they are present in 90% of children who progress to disease onset prior to age 5, and from then on display an inverse correlation with age as disease develops (*18*). In adults, insulinoma autoantigen-2/protein tyrosine phosphatase autoantibodies (IA2A) and the 65-kD form of glutamate decarboxylase GAD65 autoantibodies (GADA) are most prevalent (*19, 20*). Prevalence of ZnT8A is low in young individuals, increases significantly after the age of 3, and peaks in late adolescence (*21*). It is crucial to evaluate and discriminate potential antigen-based administration therapies. Given the long phase of asymptomatic autoimmunity characteristic of T1D, comprehensive autoantibody detection would allow identification of susceptible individuals at an earlier stage of disease when β-cell mass is still relatively high and when immunological-based therapies are most effective (as has been documented in animal models and clinical trials (*22, 23*)). This time-sensitive opportunity for treatment may be tailored to the autoantibody repertoire of the patient to prevent or delay T1D onset.

Given the ability to profile circulating autoantibodies in subjects, immunosuppression and immunomodulation therapy for T1D has potential. The development of the B cell depletion drug Rituximab as a lymphoma therapy has been useful for evaluating its success for other immune disorders. Rituximab is a humanized anti-CD20 monoclonal antibody that can induce B cell depletion for more than a year in peripheral blood lymphocytes and is generally well tolerated (*24*). In new onset diabetic non-obese (NOD) mice, anti-CD20 therapy reversed and prevented T1D diabetes, confirming the rationale for clinical trials (*25*). TrialNet, conducting the study "The effects of Rituximab on the progression of type 1 diabetes in new onset subjects," administers Rituximab within 3 months of diagnosis to individuals displaying residual β-cell function as measured by C-peptide levels.

Preliminary results imply that Rituximab may preserve C-peptide and thus β-cell mass (*26*). Similarly, a T-cell depletion immunosuppressive drug, Teplizumab, comprised of anti-CD3 monoclonal antibodies (mAbs), was initially shown to inhibit β-cell destruction in T1D subjects in the first year post onset and for another year thereafter when administered at diagnosis (*27*). Subsequent trials suggested β cells may be conserved for up to 5 years in drug-treated patients (*28*). These initial studies indicate that both B and T cells are appropriate targets for altering the immunologic course of T1D, and advances in immunomodulatory drugs will likely include targeting of B and T cell specific populations.

To date, the detection of circulating autoantibodies is the most reliable preclinical indicator and diagnostic test for diabetic autoimmunity. Currently, three established autoantibody assays based on fluid phase (radioimmunoassay, RIAs) are employed for IAA, GADA, and IA2A. Immune complexes are formed with ^{125}I-labeled insulin and ^{35}S-labeled GAD and IA-2, the latter generated by recombinant DNA production of antigen and subsequent incubation with antibodies (*29*). The combined biochemical detection of these autoantibodies reveals 80% of at-risk individuals or patients at disease onset. Measurement of these autoantibodies has been critical for identifying genetically at-risk individuals who have progressed to autoimmunity and their recruitment to therapeutic trials aimed at preventing a slow progression to T1D.

However, the assays fail to achieve the high sensitivity and specificity essential for detection of prediabetes in the general population, where only one in 300 individuals are identified even with additional consideration of genetic predisposition (HLA).

Combining the relatively new ZnT8 RIA with the established autoantibody assays for IAA, GADA, and IA2A significantly enhances prediction of T1D development (90% of newly diagnosed individuals) (21), but may not be adequate to determine risk in the general population, where specificity and sensitivity ideally demand 99 and 99%, respectively. The validity of a measure for prediction or diagnosis of disease is determined by its sensitivity (the number of individuals who are diabetic, possessing autoantibodies) divided by the number of individuals who develop the disease, specificity (the number of individuals without autoantibodies who do not develop T1D) divided by the number of subjects who do not progress to disease and finally is positive predictive value. Autoantibody detection has proven to be a valuable biomarker for T1D owing to the long prodromal phase between initial autoantibody detection and clinical onset and their high predictive indication. Comprehensive population screening also requires reliable, efficient, cost-effective, high-throughput protocols for corroboration among labs. Such improvements in disease prediction will hopefully be accompanied by advances in disease prevention. Antigen-specific immune therapy offers potential evasion or delay of disease onset, and may be further strengthened by the identification of novel autoantigens.

Islet Cell Autoantibody

Despite earlier speculation, it was not until the 1970s that T1D was generally accepted as an autoimmune disease (30). This realization stemmed largely from two sets of observations. First, insulin-dependent diabetes (IDD) was more frequently associated with other autoimmune conditions, such as Hashimoto's thyroiditis, pernicious anemia, and Addison's disease, than would be expected by chance (31). Second, lymphocytic infiltration of the islets of Langerhans was evident in some juveniles who had died shortly after onset of clinical disease (32–34). The presence of insulitis in subjects with functional islet abnormalities suggested that cell-mediated immunity might contribute to disease. Consistent with this hypothesis, two independent reports subsequently showed that some patients with IDD showed evidence of cellular hypersensitivity to islet extracts (35, 36).

Although it was evident that the serum of some IDD patients contained autoantibodies to the cytoplasm of thyroid gastric parietal and adrenal cortical cells, these individuals being clinically asymptomatic for the associated autoimmune diseases (37–39), initial attempts to demonstrate the presence of antibodies that recognized islet cells in the serum of IDD patients by indirect immunofluorescence were unsuccessful (40). However, a combination of technical improvements in microscopy and serendipity finally enabled

Bottazzo (*41*) and subsequently MacCuish (*42*) to confirm the predicted existence of disease-associated islet cell antibodies (ICAs). The breakthrough advanced from the use of frozen sections of human pancreas from blood group O donors, which provided a lower background, and sera from subjects with autoimmune polyendocrinopathies, which in retrospect were shown typically to have relatively high titers of ICAs. Both of these initial reports concluded that ICAs were rare and confined to only a small subset of patients with multiple autoimmune diseases (*36, 41*). However, it later became evident that this conclusion was erroneous, stemming mainly from the use of a relatively insensitive assay, and a failure to appreciate the transient nature of ICAs post-onset (*30*). It is now accepted that at least 70–80% of all T1D patients have ICAs at onset (*42*). Moreover, elevated ICAs are predictive of progression to T1D in at least a subset of asymptomatic genetically at risk individuals.

Although the identification of ICAs represented a major advance in understanding T1D, the assay has proved difficult to standardize and requires specifically trained personnel for accurate interpretation. Consequently, considerable effort has been devoted towards identifying the molecular targets of the autoantibodies and designing robust high-throughput biochemical assays for their measurement. Initial studies suggested that sialic acid-containing glycolipids were a major target of ICAs (*43*), although doubt was later cast on this conclusion by the observation that recombinant GAD65 could at least partially quench ICAs in many individuals (*44*). Indeed, it is now appreciated that ICAs are highly heterogeneous and react both with antigens common to all islet endocrine cell types, as well as to multiple cytoplasmic and membrane-associated epitopes restricted to particular cell types (*45*). Moreover, it is highly likely that a number of the targets of ICAs have yet to be characterized, evidenced by the presence of individuals with ICAs that do not react with any of currently defined T1D autoantigens. Consequently, the search for novel targets of ICAs is an ongoing area of significant research interest, especially since in addition to their value as diagnostic and predictive markers, autoantibodies can in most cases also identify the targets of disease causing autoreactive T-cells.

In the following sections, we survey both B cell and T-cell autoantigen discovery. The methods employed typically adhere to a "candidate gene" approach where knowledge of the molecular and cellular biology of the disease is exploited. These include: biochemical analyses of the constituents of T1D sera or β cells, RNA expression profiling of β cells, and microarray analysis of tissue-specific gene expression and splicing. However, the results from recent genome-wide association studies (GWAS) (*46*) and advances in epigenetics have highlighted the degree of interindividual variation, suggesting the need to develop novel strategies for biomarker discovery. To illustrate the utility of such approaches, we discuss the technologies that permitted the demonstration that ZnT8, a zinc transporter localized to islet cell secretory granules, is a major target of humoral autoimmunity in T1D.

B CELL AUTOANTIGEN DISCOVERY

Many T1D autoantigens have been identified by screening genes via various expression scenarios with sera derived from T1D subjects (*47–53*). An assortment of successful expression systems have included: λ gt-11 expression libraries, recombinant fusion protein libraries, and Western blotting of islet lysates with T1D sera. We will consider each system separately below.

Screening λ gt-11 Expression Libraries

Protein expression libraries constructed from RNA specifically derived from human islets and screened with T1D sera have served as a rich resource for antigen discovery. Selection of clone ICA512 from a λ gt-11 human islet expression library using sera from T1D subjects revealed the ICA512 antigen (*47*). It encodes a neuroendocrine-specific transmembrane protein that contains a cryptic protein tyrosine phosphatase (PTP) catalytic domain and displays near identical amino acid sequence to the insulinoma antigen (IA-2), which was independently cloned from a human insulinoma library (*48*). IA-2/ICA512 was the second component of ICA to be identified, and was found to bind 70% of T1D sera in Western blots. Ongoing characterization of the GAD molecule revealed that tryptic peptides of the 64 kD molecule yielded the 50 kD GAD product as well as 37 and 40 kD peptides, the latter of which was identified as IA-2. Like preabsorption with recombinant GAD65, prebinding of recombinant IA-2 diminished ICA autoreactivity. However, as stated above, since not all of the ICA reaction can be accounted for with preabsorption to both molecules, other unidentified autoantigens contribute to the ICA reaction.

Like IA-2, ICA69 was identified as an autoantigen by screening a human islet λ gt-11 expression library with ICA-positive sera (*49*). Interestingly, ICA69 is the human counterpart to the cow's milk-related protein p69, and data exists to demonstrate the presence of circulating antibodies in a subset of T1D subjects to bovine serum albumin (BSA) (*50*). However, it should be noted that ICA69 and BSA share modest regions (five amino acids) of homology one of which is the "ABBOS" albumin peptide T-cell epitope. The relationship of ICA69 with T1D is apparent, however not exclusive, as such antibodies are also present in the sera of rheumatoid arthritis patients (*55*). The association of albumin (as an immunogen) and T1D is controversial.

Phogrin (phosphatase of granules of rat insulinoma), also referred to as IA-2β, was likewise cloned from an expression library screened with sera raised against a secretory-granule membrane fraction from insulinoma cells (*51*). Subsequently, mouse IA-2β was cloned using degenerate PCR primers to amplify PTP family members (Lu 1998). Phogrin shares 80% amino acid identity with IA-2 in the PTP domain and was named the target for autoantibodies directed to the 37 kD tryptic peptide described above. Nearly all autoantibodies reacting with phogrin likewise react with IA-2 (typically in the PTP domain), although ~10% of T1D patients show autoreactivity only to IA-2 and not phogrin. In light of this, assays designed to detect IA-2 autoantibodies are sufficient to capture autoantibodies directed to the phogrin antigen. However, Achenbach (*56*) has shown that in ICA+IA2A+ individuals, autoantibodies to phogrin is associated with a very high risk for T1D.

The primary screen of the human islet λ gt-11 expression library that disclosed ICA512 as a T1D-associated antigen also revealed molecule ICA12, now identified as SOX13, a transcription factor. In enzyme linked immuno-absorption assays (ELISA) assays to SOX13, 18% T1D subjects display autoantibodies to ICA12, although it is uncertain whether a relationship with T1D exists, as these antibodies are also present (6.9%) in patients with other autoimmune disorders (lupus and rheumatoid arthritis). It is possible that these autoantibodies are the result of a common mechanism for development of autoimmunity to endocrine tissues. SOX13 autoantibodies tend to be more prevalent among older subjects (>20 years) and seem to persist after diagnosis. Its utility as a T1D marker would be specialized for detection of ICA+, GAD−, and IA2− adults. The low frequency of SOX13 autoantibodies in healthy control sera (2.5%) and T2D sera (3.4%) may be misleading, as it is not clear if these are age and HLA-matched controls. However, sera from 7.6% newly diagnosed T1D subjects were exclusively positive for SOX13 autoantibodies, but not IA-2, GAD65, or ICA, thus possibly representing a distinct autoantibody positive population (*57*).

Some sera from T1D individuals that contains autoantibodies to GAD65 was found to immunoprecipitate a 38 kD protein from pancreatic islets (*58*). Screening a cDNA expression library with high titer sera for the 38 kD protein and GAD65 identified clones encoding JunB, a nuclear transcription factor. T cells exhibit a pronounced response in proliferation assays challenged with JunB recombinant protein containing amino acids 1–180 in 71% of new-onset diabetic subjects and in 50% ICA+ first-degree relatives. However, 25% of sera derived from individuals with other autoimmune diseases also contain autoantibodies to JunB implying their presence may be related to a more general defect in the immune response rather than specifically to T1D (*58*).

Screening of islet λ gt-11 expression libraries with prediabetic sera disclosed carboxypeptidase H(E) as an autoantigen in T1D (*59*). Carboxypeptidase E is not islet specific, as it has been localized to both neuroendocrine cells and islet secretory granules.

Abundant in islet granules, it functions in processing proinsulin to insulin. Detection among newly diagnosed T1D individuals ranges from 5 to 10% and 25% in ICA+ sera. Assays for high-throughput screening for carboxypeptidase E have not been pursued yet.

Screening Fusion-Peptide Libraries

A random peptide library screened with sera from T1D subjects identified autoantigens osteopontin, expressed in the somatostatin producing δ islet cells, and importin β, in neuroendocrine cells. RIAs did not detect binding of antibodies to either of the recombinant protein probes, whereas ELISA assays revealed 60% T1D sera and 30% of sera derived from subjects with other autoimmune diseases was positive for the importin β antigen probe (53). Similarly, the osteopontin recombinant protein could detect autoantibodies in T1D sera only by ELISA. Often ELISA assays are deemed less sensitive than RIAs, albeit antigen dependent (60).

Western Blotting of Human Islet Extracts with T1D Sera

CD38 (ADP-ribosyl cyclase/cADPR hydrolase) autoantibodies have been reported at modest prevalence in T1D patients via Western blot with T1D sera against islet extracts (61). A 52 kD β cell-specific granule antigen sharing an epitope with the PC2 protein of the rubella virus has likewise been identified by the same strategy. It is notable that congenital rubella virus infection has been correlated to the development of T1D, and may suggest that the rubella virus capsid protein mimics a β-cell antigen that may sensitize at-risk individuals for an autoimmune response (62).

Immunoprecipitation of Islet Antigens with T1D Patient Sera

Immunoprecipitation of IgG autoantibodies from the sera of T1D subjects has identified a heavily glycosylated islet cell membrane-associated (GLIMA) protein of apparent molecular weight 38 kD, which is present in 38% of T1D patients and 35% of prediabetics. The discovery of GLIMA-38 illustrates the contribution of posttranslational modification as a criterion for some cases of immunoreactivity. GLIMA-38 displays the neuroendocrine tissue-specific expression pattern in islets and neuronal cell lines and is strongly associated (and possibly redundant) with the presence of IA-2 autoantibodies (63, 64).

Glycolipid Preabsorption of the ICA Reaction

Although peptide antigens are more abundant, lipid antigens are also apparent epitopes in autoimmune diabetes. Substantial effort to purify potential lipid antigens to test for autoantigenicity has been achieved using biochemical fractionation (65). Glycolipids extracted from pancreas tissue and separated from protein and lipid fractions have been shown to competitively inhibit the ICA reaction. Chromatographic separation of gangliosides indicated monosialoganglioside, GM-2, the major ganglioside from pancreatic islets, could effectively inhibit the ICA reaction (65). Circulating autoantibodies specifically to GM-2, in lieu of the other abundant pancreatic gangliosides, GD-3 and GM-3, have been demonstrated in new onset and prediabetic subject sera (*66*) through an indirect immunoperoxidase assay on thin layer chromatography plates.

Screening Ganglioside ELISAs with T1D Sera

Binding of sera from new-onset T1D subjects to pancreatic gangliosides immobilized for ELISA analysis indicated that ganglioside GT3 is a target antigen for autoantibodies (~35%) (*67*). Human ganglioside GT3 also readily binds mouse mAbs reactive to polysialgangliosides and an anti-β cell-specific mouse monoclonal antibody (*67*). Although ganglioside autoantibodies are apparent, their mode of detection has not yet been standardized. More recently, the relationship between T1D, neuropathy, and ganglioside autoantibodies has been explored, as gangliosides are expressed in both peripheral nerves and the pancreas (*68*). Twelve of 16 diabetic individuals with neuropathy were found to have autoantibodies to ganglioside. Sera from subjects having other autoimmune diseases served as controls and was 10% positive for ganglioside antibodies. The prevalence of ganglioside autoantibodies among T1D patients versus controls might reflect similar criteria for antigens in peripheral nerve and pancreatic islet cells (*68*). However, nondisease, age-, and genotype-matched control sera was not monitored.

Once a contribution of antigenic lipids to the ICA was established (*65, 69*), a family of four lysophospholipids was identified as a component of the ICA (*70*). Using purified lipids in a chemiluminescent dot blot immunoassay, autoantibodies were identified in 61% of new-onset T1D sera. Interestingly, 65% of ICA new-onset sera was positive for lysophospholipid antigen. One member of the family of four lysophospholipids has been identified as lysophosphatidylmyoinositol (*70*).

Generation of Hybridomas of Islet Infiltrating B Lymphocytes and Identification of Their Cognate Antigen

To determine the antigenic array of islet-infiltrating B cells, hybridoma cell lines were generated from NOD mice developing insulitis. The majority of such hybridomas generated mAbs to the peripheral nervous system (PNS) components. The autoantigens recognized by the mAbs was determined to reside in a cytoskeletal fraction by biochemical fractionation of neuroblastoma cell extracts. Western blot analysis of neuroblastoma, insulinoma, and pancreatic islet extracts with the mAbs detected a 58 kD protein. Further characterization by two-dimensional gel electrophoresis and ultimately mass spectroscopy identified the antigen as peripherin. Most mAbs were found to recognize a major eptiope in the C-terminal domain of two peripherin isoforms (*71*).

Screening Nucleic Acid Programmable Protein Arrays

Nucleic Acid Programmable Protein Arrays (NAAPAs) have been employed to identify novel candidate autoantigens related to T1D. The arrays are constructed by depositing candidate recombinant DNAs encoding an affinity tag onto glass slides and subjecting the slides to an *in vitro* translation cocktail to generate affinity-tagged and immobilized protein probes *in situ*. An array of 6,000 human proteins has been screened in a "proof of principle" study using three independent sera from T1D individuals. The initial "training" screen reduced the candidate antigens to 750, while a third screen narrowed the putative antigens to a set of 19, which could discriminate between T1D sera and healthy control sera. Among the unidentified antigens were the characterized autoantigens GAD65, IA-2, and insulin (*72*).

Candidate B Cell Gene Approach

Candidate genes for autoantigens have often been deduced from their association with T1D itself or other autoimmune disorders and their various afflictions. Insulin was the first T1D autoantigen characterized at the molecular level (*73*) and is predominantly a β cell-specific autoantigen, although modestly present in parts of the brain and thymus. Although an obvious autoantigen candidate, the potential development of antibodies to insulin within 2 weeks of treatment (a consequence of exogenous insulin therapy) deemed autoantibody measurement difficult. However, as sensitive assays developed, serum from T1D individuals was found to contain antibodies that bound insulin prior to the initiation of an insulin therapy regime. Currently, the autoantibody epitopes developed as a result of insulin treatment differ from those present prior to treatment and can be distinguished by their lower affinity to antigen (*74*). Methodologies have been explored to discriminate the epitope populations derived from these two antigen sources (*75*).

T1D is often associated with other endocrinopathies or autoimmune disorders. DNA topoisomerase I (TOPI) and II (TOPII) autoantibodies have been found to be associated with systemic sclerosis (TOPI) (*76*) and lupus juvenile rheumatoid arthritis, cryogenic fibrosing alveolitis, and arcoidosis (TOPII) (*77–79*). To determine whether TOPII is an autoantigen in T1D, overlapping DNA fragments spanning the gene were expressed as recombinant antigens to screen sera from T1D subjects. The redundant TOPII peptides were capable of detecting antibodies in 49.2% of T1D individuals. Interestingly, the reactive TOPII epitopes mimicked those of previously identified autoantigens (insulin, HSP65, and GAD) (*80*).

Expression of nephrin (*81*), densin, and filtrin have been localized to the kidney and pancreatic islets, thus elevating their candidacy as autoantigens. Recombinant autoantigen probes of densin and filtrin were employed in RIAs to evaluate their reactivity to sera from T1D patients. Indeed, autoantibodies were detected in 33 and 11% of sera screened with the densin and filtrin probes, respectively (*82*). Similarly, a recombinant nephrin antigen probe was found to be immunoprecipitated by 24% of sera from newly diagnosed T1D individuals (*83*).

Patients afflicted with autoimmune disease often develop an autoantibody response against molecular mediators of these diseases

(*84*). Recently, the chemokines have been shown to be inducers of the inflammatory process in various inflammatory autoimmune diseases. Specifically, CCL3 was recently reported to be a major antigen target for T1D. Ninety-five percent of first-degree relatives positive for at least one of the gold standard autoantibodies (insulin, ICA, GAD) were also positive for CCL3 autoantibodies (*85*).

Some of T1D autoantigens are not expressed solely in β cells, but are also prevalent in neuroendocrine tissues (GAD65, IA-2). Islet β cells and neurons share several phenotypic similarities, and there appears to be some link between islet and nervous system autoimmunity. Immunohistochemistry of pancreatic islets has shown that the peri-islet Schwann cells (pSCs), which form a mantle that envelops the endocrine islet tissue, are an autoimmune target among individuals at risk for T1D as well as NOD mice (*86*). The predominant proteins expressed in pSCs are glial fibrillary acidic protein (GFAP), a cytoskeletal element, and S100β, both of which are antigenic targets for CD8+ T cells and B cells in NOD mice. In humans, a component of the ICA reaction is assigned to autoantibodies that localize to pSCs. This autoimmune targeting of the pancreatic nervous system could conceivably precede β-cell destruction (*86*).

Stress proteins are often associated with autoimmune diseases (*87*); thus, HSP60 and HSP70, identified as autoantigens in lupus and multiple sclerosis, were similarly named as antigens in the sera of NOD mice via solid-phase RIA prior to the onset of diabetes (*88*). In NOD mice, anti-HSP60 T cells mediate the manifestations of T1D, and inhibition of the anti-HSP60 T-cell response can reduce the rate of β-cell destruction. The major epitope target, peptide 277 (p277), has been shown to elicit human T-cell proliferative responses (*89*), and T-cell proliferative responses to human HSP70 have likewise been confirmed (*90*). Furthermore, autoantibodies specific for human HSP60 (45%) and HSP70 (30%) have been described in the sera of T1D individuals by ELISAs.

Glutamic acid decarboxylase autoantibodies (GADA) were discovered by their clinical association with disease and were originally defined as a 65 kD protein in patients with a rare neurological disorder involving GABAergic neurons resulting in muscle spasms or rigidity (stiff-man syndrome, exhibits a high coincidence with T1D). GAD catalyzes gamma-aminobutyric acid synthesis in the nervous system and the islets. Sera from patients with stiff-man syndrome contain antibodies that cross-react with islet cells, and the same autoantibodies were subsequently identified in T1D patients. Anti-GAD autoantibodies were shown to account for a portion of the ICA reaction via preabsorption of sera with recombinant GAD65. Two highly homologous GAD isoforms are expressed in β cells and brain (GAD65 and GAD67), although autoantibodies against GAD65 are significantly more prevalent (80 vs. 16%, respectively) in T1D patient sera (*81*).

The association of T1D with stiffman syndrome and possibly Guillain–Barré syndrome (*91*) imply common antigens between endocrine pancreas and nervous tissue. Sulfatide, a glycosphingolipid, has been localized to the secretory granules of α and β cells of rat pancreatic islets as well as the neural system, specifically in association with myelin (*92*), but not exocrine tissue (*69*). Antisulfatide antibodies have been identified in both prediabetic and new-onset T1D individuals (88%) using ELISAs. Of those T1D patients positive for sulfatide autoantibodies, the majority (68%) were also ICA+ at diagnosis; however, sulfatide autoantibodies appear to be independent of ICA. Although none of the control group measured positive for sulfatide autoantibodies, the subjects were not age or HLA-matched. Bouchard (*69*) did not indicate if a subset of the individuals in the study also suffered from Guillain–Barré syndrome, where 65% are positive for the same sulfatide antigen. When mouse spleen cells are challenged with sulfatide *in vitro*, they exhibit a robust proliferative response (*93*). The appearance of sulfatide autoantibodies further illustrates the importance of modification of molecules as antigenic targets, as sulfatide displays both carbohydrate and sulfate moieties (*94*).

Recently, an extensive gene candidate screening of mostly secretory vesicle-associated proteins (37 of 56) was conducted to determine their capacity for autoreactivity in T1D using RIAs. For initial assays, a panel of 50 T1D sera that were previously determined to be positive for IA-2 or GAD65 was employed. A panel of 200 sera that were triple positive (IA2A, GADA, IAA) was used for validation assays with 200 age-matched controls. Two new minor autoantigens were identified through this study, vesicle-associated membrane protein 2 (VAMP2) and neuropeptide Y (NPY), detecting 23 and 25%, of sera respectively. Importantly, the previously identified antigens Sox13, JunB, Imogen38, IGRP, and S100β were shown to have autoantibody counterparts in sera derived from triple-positive individuals. However, several putative minor autoantigens reported to have autoantibody counterparts were not confirmed in this study (CPE, GFAP, HSP70, ICA69, or TOPII) (*95*). Since the sera employed in this study was preselected to be autoantibody positive, it is impossible to determine if these new autoantigens contribute to the power of detection. Screening a panel of sera negative for the current four major autoantibodies, IAA, IA-2, GADA, and ZnT8A, is necessary to evaluate the utility of new autoantigens to enhance detection. This study corroborates the hypothesis that secretory vesicle-associated proteins are vital, yet not exclusive antigenic targets in T1D.

Displaced Binding of mAbs by T1D Sera

A panel of mouse mAbs reacting with a rat insulinoma cell line was assembled to define novel autoantigens by their displacement of monoclonal antibody binding to insulinoma cells. T1D sera specifically competed for binding of one monoclonal antibody (IA-2) in membrane extracts from rat insulinoma cells and the islets of various mammals including humans. The antibody was found to detect the 150 kD diabetes-associated protein 1 (DAP1), which is heavily glycosylated as determined by Western analysis. The autoantibodies are directed against the protein versus the glycosylation as measured with immunoprecipitation of *in vitro* translated probes. Similarly, sera from T1D subjects detects a 150 kD protein in Western analysis of rat brain lysates (*96*). Although autoantibodies to the human protein (138 kD) are present in a large proportion of T1D sera (87 vs. 4% control sera), they are likewise present in sera from first-degree relatives of T1D individuals (38%), and thus are either not specific or represent an early marker for T1D. Although there appeared to be no correlation for positive immunoreactivity to the 138 kD antigen and HLA genotype, the control subjects were not HLA-matched, albeit age-matched. Autoantibodies to DAP1 appeared prior to clinical onset in 17/20 subjects. Although the competitive displacement assay for this antigen appears promising, with 86.9% sensitivity and 95.6% specificity, the characterization has not been reproduced.

Proteomics

An attribute of proteomics is its capacity to survey large numbers of proteins for quantitative differences in concentration in an unbiased fashion to ultimately identify candidate biomarkers. A pilot proteomic study of human plasma and sera from control and T1D individuals was conducted to evaluate the use of capillary liquid chromatography (LC) coupled with mass spectrometry (MS) to identify novel biomarkers in T1D (*97*). Initially, MC–MS/MS was performed on control plasma to establish a comprehensive peptide database. Subsequently, high-throughput and quantitative LC–MS analysis identified significant differences in the levels of five proteins in the sera of T1D individuals: α-2-glycoprotein 1 (zinc), corticosteroid-binding globulin, and lumican were twofold upregulated in T1D sera relative to control sera, while clusterin and serotransferrin were twofold upregulated in control samples relative to T1D sera (*97*). Further confirmation of these candidate biomarkers for T1D is required to determine their predictive and/or diagnostic value.

T CELL AUTOANTIGEN DISCOVERY

The targets for autoreactive diabetogenic T cells typically parallel the same antigens recognized by B cells. This hypothesis has been demonstrated in humans and animal models for insulin (*98*), GAD65 (*13*), phogrin (*14*), and IA-2 (*99*). However, not all T cell antigens have demonstrated B cell autoantibody-producing counterparts. T cell "orphan" clones isolated from T1D patients that do not respond to the current collection of antigens do exist. These orphan clones were generated from lymphocytes isolated from pancreatic lymph nodes or islet infiltrates of spontaneous diabetes and then restimulated with whole islets or insulin granule membrane preparations. Presumably, their target antigens have yet to be defined.

T Cell Responses to Epitope Libraries

After sequential stimulation of T cells isolated from a T1D patient with a membrane fraction derived from extracts of rat insulinoma cells, a cytotoxic CD4+ mouse T-cell clone was isolated and determined to react to a 38 kD protein. The epitope of the 38 kD antigen was mapped by screening a subtracted cDNA expression library. Ultimately, the full-length human cDNA clone was isolated and determined to encode a mitochondrial protein, imogen 38; however, the human protein did not stimulate the mouse T-cell clone. Imogen 38 is highly, but not specifically, expressed in β cells. Its immunoreactivity may represent a bystander effect (*100*). Clones generated in the same study identified several ICA components and indicated that the PBMCs of T1D do indeed recognize β-cell proteins.

IGRP

The ligand for the NOD mouse T-cell clone, NY8.3 CD8+, was identified through a proteomic approach as islet-specific glucose-6-phosphatase-related protein (IGRP) (*101*). Specifically, H-2K^d class I MHC molecules from the NOD-derived pancreatic β-cell line were purified by immunoaffinity chromatography, fractionated by reverse-phase HPLC multiple times, and coupled to tandem mass spectrometry to define eluted peptides. Candidate peptides were tested in epitope reconstitution assays, and IGRP, identified in the NCBI database, was found to cause a response to clone 8.3.

IGRP was originally cloned by screening a cDNA library created by subtractive hybridization of mouse insulinoma β-cell cDNAs from mouse glucagonoma (α) cDNAs with a probe homologous to the mouse liver glucose-6-phosphatase (G-6-P). Two alternatively spliced isoforms distinguished by the presence of exon IV (118 bp) were characterized and found to be specifically expressed in pancreatic β cells, but not in cells or cell lines of nonislet neuroendocrine origin. In addition to being a major β cell-specific antigen targeted by an abundant, pathological population of CD8+ T cells of NOD mice, data has recently emerged identifying IGRP is also a CD8+ T-cell antigen in humans. Using interferon-gamma (IFN-γ) ELISPOT assays with four peptides to IGRP, 65% of T1D patients were found to be positive to at least one peptide. However, no IGRP autoantibodies have been detected either in NOD mice or in humans (*101, 102*).

Dystrophia Myotonica Kinase

Another orphan CD8+ T cell clone, AI4, was isolated from the earliest detectable infiltrates of the islets. By screening a recombinant peptide library in positional scanning format with subsequent pattern searches of the mouse protein database, the target antigen was determined to be a widely expressed ligand from dystrophia myotonica kinase (*103*).

ZnT8 AS A TARGET OF T1D AUTOIMMUNITY

The advent of technologies to compare differences in expression patterns of genes across multiple tissues, species, and conditions has advanced disease biomarker discovery. In particular, utilizing microarray expression analysis has allowed the survey and comparison of vast amounts of gene expression data, permitting the identification of novel disease-specific autoantigens in T1D. Discovery of such molecular targets is essential for the induction of antigen-specific immune tolerance therapies that may modulate or eliminate T and B cell populations of the immune system, and may eventually delay onset or prevent T1D altogether.

ZnT8 was originally identified as a candidate autoantigen using a combination of multidimensional analysis of microarray expression profiling data coupled with the premise that established β-cell autoantigens display a series of common features. T1D autoantigens typically display β cell-specific gene expression at moderate to high levels and are often localized to the insulin secretory granule itself, or play a role in the regulated secretory pathway. With the exception of insulin, most autoantigens are transmembrane proteins and contain at least one major cytoplasmic domain. Moreover, they often display tissue-specific alternative splicing.

Originally, our screen for novel candidate antigens interrogated the public domain multitissue custom array (*104, 105*) using Shannon entropy plots that impart an index of tissue specificity based on tissue distribution and relative abundance. Once pancreas and islet specificity was established, our criteria focused on β cell-specific expression by comparison of microarray expression profiles among β TC3 insulinoma, α TC1–6 glucagonoma, and mPAC ductal cell lines as well as embryonic neurogenin 3 knockout mouse pancreas (lacking islets) (*106*), which permitted refinement of our candidate list from 300 to 68 antigens. Affirming the predictive value of our ranking algorithm was the appearance of all the major known T1D autoantigens: insulin (*106*), GAD65 (GAD2) (*81*), IA-2 (*107*), and phogrin (PTPRN2) (*108*), as well as the more peripheral autoantigens such as heat shock protein 90B (*109*), carboxypeptidase C (*59*), islet glucose-6-phosphatase catalytic subunit-related protein (IGRP) (*100*), pancreas associated protein

(Reg3a) (*110*), islet amyloid polypeptide (IAPP) (*111*), Imogen 38 (MRPS31) (*99*), ICA69 (*49*), peripherin (*112*), GAD67 (GAD1) (*113*), and SOX13 (*47*). Among the many genes that had not yet been proposed as autoantigens, the highest ranking was ZnT8 (*21*), a member of a family of genes that function in cation diffusion efflux from the secretory granule (Fig. 2.1).

ZnT8 Autoantibody Detection

RIAs for detection of ZnT8 autoantibodies were developed using ^{35}S-labeled protein derivatives of the ZnT8 gene generated in a coupled *in vitro* transcription/translation system followed by fluid-phase assays. Immune complexes were captured by protein A Sepharose beads followed by a series of washes in a 96-well filter plate format. Radioactive antigen probe trapped by sera bound to beads was then assessed by scintillation counting.

Nearly half of the ZnT8 molecule is confined to six putative hydrophobic transmembrane regions, which are inaccessible to antibodies and may interfere with proper protein folding in an *in vitro* translation system. The N-terminal and C-terminal domains, however, are believed to reside on the cytosolic face of the membrane, predicted to be hydrophilic, and they do indeed contain autoantibody epitopes. The C-terminal domain, when employed as an antigen probe, displays a striking 70% sensitivity at 99.5% specificity with new-onset T1D sera. Further optimization

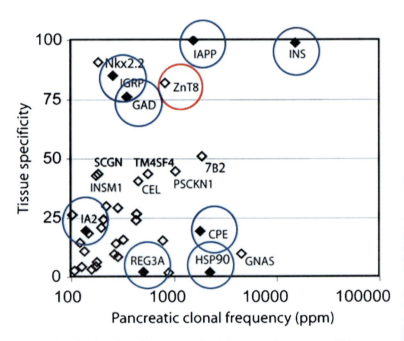

Fig. 2.1 Identification of candidate autoantigens in mouse. Pancreas specificity versus pancreatic abundance (number of pancreatic EST clones per all tissues). Approximate positions are shown for known autoantigens (*blue circles*) and ZnT8 (*red circle*).

of the probe design has extended the sensitivity of the assay to nearly 80% without conceding specificity. The sensitivity realized with the ZnT8 C-terminal probe is comparable to that achieved with the gold standard autoantibody of IA2A and exceeds that of IAA. ZnT8A measurement provides an independent measure of autoreactivity, as 25–30% of individuals classified as autoantibody negative possess ZnT8 autoantibodies. The ZnT8 measurement, when used in combination with classic assays, advances autoreactivity detection to greater than 90% (*21*). Consequently, individuals classified as single antibody positive can now be identified as double antibody positive, and are thus at increased risk for developing the disease.

Immunodominant Epitopes

Characterization of the epitopes recognized by autoantibodies is essential for the design of antigen-specific therapeutic agents as well as probe optimization. Alignment of the mouse and human ZnT8 C-terminal domains indicate that they are highly conserved (80% identical), differing only at 21 out of 102 amino acids. Although the spontaneous model of T1D, the NOD mouse, mimics many aspects of the human disease, they do not appear to harbor ZnT8 autoantibodies (Wenzlau and Hutton, unpublished data). The mouse C-terminal domain used as an antigenic probe in RIAs with sera that is highly reactive to the human C-terminal domain fails to immunoprecipitate despite its conservation with the human protein (Wenzlau and Hutton, unpublished data).

The crystal structure of the bacterial iron transporter Yiip has been solved and has been employed to model, via molecular threading of the human ZnT8 C-terminal domain (*114*). Noteworthy is that the amino acid differences between human and mouse lie at the predicted surface of the molecule. In fact, the nonsynonymous SNP that has been associated with susceptibility to T2D in GWAS (*46*) encodes residue 325, which is conspicuously positioned in a readily accessible amino-acid cluster. The single nucleotide polymorphism encodes either Arg (R_{325}) or Trp (W_{325}). The former, which confers risk of T2D, is present in 75% of European Caucasians, 98% African Americans, and 50% Asians.

A second nonsynonymous SNP exists in the second nucleotide of the same codon and encodes a Gln (Q_{325}), the residue existing in mZnT8, and occurs in less than 1% of Europeans, 9% of African Americans, and 1–2% of Asian populations (*115*). Substitution of the mZnT8 Q_{325} by the human R_{325} residue restored 12.5% autoreactivity (Wenzlau and Hutton, unpublished data).

Evaluation of autoreactivity of sera derived from newly diagnosed T1D to the three allelic variant forms of the ZnT8 antigen (R_{325}, W_{325}, and Q_{325}) indicated three epitopes residing in the C-terminal domain: one defined by R_{325} (30%), one for which

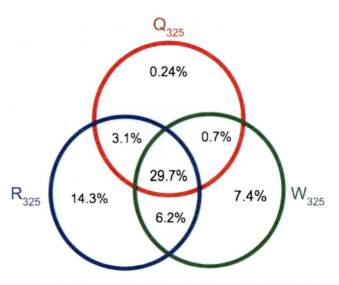

Fig. 2.2 Relationship between autoreactivity to R_{325}, W_{325}, and Q_{325} ZnT8 variants. Venn diagram illustrating the intersection of autoantibody reactivity with three polymorphic variant probes in a population of new-onset T1D individuals ($n=420$). The percent of the total population reacting with each antigenic probe is indicated in the sectors.

W_{325} is essential (15%), and a third epitope at a topologically distinct location independent of the residue at position 325 (30%) (Fig. 2.2). Generally, 70% of new-onset T1D subjects react to one of the ZnT8 variant forms. The epitopes are conformational as recombinant epitope-specific protein, but not peptides, competitively inhibit binding to antigen probes. There is a strict correlation between genotype frequencies and autoreactivity to a given ZnT8 variant form (*116*) (Table 2.1). However, the functional relevance of the polymorphism to the β cell remains elusive.

Humoral responses to an antigen expressing a particular amino acid implies an oligoclonal response to self, and thus a restricted B-cell repertoire in T1D individuals. Within an oligoclonal response, it is probable that the surviving immunodominant clones will have arisen from a limited number of parental cells. This feature may enhance its suitability for therapeutic targeting, since a limited set of peptides or ligands may be administered to tolerize individuals to ZnT8 antigen. Furthermore, since ZnT8 expression is highly β cell specific, protocols to induce tolerance by effector or regulatory T cells will suffer fewer off-target effects than those directed to GAD65 or IA-2, which are more widely expressed in neuroendocrine cells. The presence of high-affinity, class-switched B cells specific for ZnT8 implies the likely presence of ZnT8-reactive T cells. Preliminary results from an ongoing study suggest that this is indeed the case (*117*).

Table 2.1
Levels of Autoreactivity Associated with rs13266634 SNP Genotype

Response	XX (351) Mean ± SEM	rs13266634 CC (194) Mean ± SEM	CT (127) Mean ± SEM	TT (30) Mean ± SEM	P
Q probe	0.108 ± 0.011	0.111 ± 0.016	0.100 ± 0.019	0.047 ± 0.018	ns
R probe	0.214 ± 0.018	0.269 ± 0.027	0.170 ± 0.026	0.050 ± 0.022	**[*]**
W probe	0.145 ± 0.014	0.100 ± 0.015	0.187 ± 0.028	0.253 ± 0.063	*[ns]**
Insulin	0.058 ± 0.010	0.057 ± 0.013	0.047 ± 0.011	0.110 ± 0.054	ns
GAD65	0.210 ± 0.018	0.202 ± 0.024	0.224 ± 0.033	0.205 ± 0.059	ns
IA2	0.585 ± 0.024	0.608 ± 0.031	0.539 ± 0.041	0.628 ± 0.088	ns

Sera from T1D individuals was measured by RIA with ZnT8 C-terminal polymorphic variant probes containing R_{325}, W_{325}, or Q_{325} or insulin, GAD65, or IA2 probes
P values between CC and CT/CT and TT/CC and TT genotypes were calculated by a Mann–Whitney nonparametric test
*P = 0.01–0.05; **P = 0.01–0.001; ***P < 0.001

CONCLUSIONS

The ability to predict ZnT8 as a major autoantigen in T1D can be attributed to advances in molecular engineering. Its discovery has enhanced the predictive value of autoantibodies for individuals' progression to disease and is an independent biomarker for β-cell mass and/or function in its own right. The uniqueness of a single amino acid determinant for specificity of antibodies is remarkable and speaks to the oligoclonality of the B-cell response. It is probable that some polymorphic variants may not be antigenic, further confirming reactivity to self. The circumstance of a nonsynonymous SNP conferring risk for T2D at the precise residue defining autoantibody specificity for T1D might appear to connect the diseases at the molecular level. However, T2D at least in part, involves β-cell dysfunction, whereas T1D arises following autoimmune attack on the β cell. Thus, while GWAS and autoantibody studies have linked the two distinct diseases via ZnT8 (21, 46), their association likely merely reflects the common target of the diseases, the pancreatic β cell.

The currently identified T1D autoantigens discussed above appear to sort into distinct associations, those that are specific to T1D and thus provide predictive value for disease, and those that are more broadly polyendocrine-related. Antigens with T1D disease association (or complications thereof) may be further distinguished by their tissue-specific, β-cell expression pattern (IAA,

ZnT8A) contrasted with wide tissue distribution (GADA, IA2A). As not all autoantigens define unique or significant groups of individuals at risk for T1D, their utility for detection and prediction of T1D is negligible, and they are thus classified as minor. Antigens reacting with less than 20% of new-onset T1D sera or whose specificity in a given assay is less than 95% are relatively insignificant. Such assays require optimization or alternate modes of autoantibody measurement. Yet, the existing set of antigens does not completely account for ICA, indicating that other autoantigens have yet to be defined.

The application of proteomics and molecular modification is in its infancy as applied to identification of novel antigens. The citrunillated autoantibodies associated with rheumatoid arthritis sets the precedent for the role of posttranslational modifications in autoimmune disease (118). Furthermore, the identity of the antigenic ligand for the BDC 2.5 T-cell clone is believed to be a modified peptide (119). It is possible that alternatively spliced variants of common genes or specific modifications of characterized proteins will contribute to the expanding list of autoantigens in T1D. As the pursuit of autoantigens proceeds, the "candidate" approach will excel as the technology for proteomics and genomics, epigenetics and posttranslational modification have yet to be rigorously applied. We will continue to identify novel autoantigens possibly among obvious, previously characterized, but slightly altered proteins.

REFERENCES

1. Rosmalen JG, van Ewijk W, Leenen PJ. T-cell education in autoimmune diabetes: teachers and students. Trends Immunol 2002;23(1):40–46.
2. Pihoker C, Gilliam L, Hampe C, Lernmark A. Autoantibodies in diabetes. Diabetes 2005;54:S52–S61.
3. Concannon P, Erlich HA, Julier C, Morahan G, Nerup J, Pociot F, Todd JA, Rich SS. Type 1 diabetes: evidence for susceptibility loci from four genome-wide linkage scans in 1,435 multiplex families. Type 1 Diabetes Genetics Consortium. Diabetes 2005;54(10):2995–3001.
4. Nerup J, Platz P, Andersen OO, Christy M, Lyngsoe J, Poulsen JE, Ryder LP, Nielsen LS, Thomsen M, Svejgaard A. HL-A antigens and diabetes mellitus. Lancet 1974;122(7885):864–866.
5. Kyvik KO, Green A, Beck-Nielsen H. Concordance rates of insulin dependent diabetes mellitus: a population based study of young Danish twins. BMJ 1995;311(7010):913–917.
6. Redondo MJ, Gottlieb PA, Motheral T, Mulgrew C, Rewers M, Babu S, Stephens E, Wegmann DR, Eisenbarth GS. Heterophile anti-mouse immunoglobulin antibodies may interfere with cytokine measurements in patients with HLA alleles protective for type 1A diabetes. Diabetes 1999;48(11):2166–2170.
7. Kukreja A, Cost G, Marker J, Zhang C, Sun Z, Lin-Su K, Ten S, Sanz M, Exley M, Wilson B, Porcelli S, Maclaren N. Multiple immunoregulatory defects in type-1 diabetes. J. Clin. Invest 2002;109(1):131–140.
8. Redondo MJ, Babu S, Zeidler A, Orban T, Yu L, Greenbaum C, Palmer JP, Cuthbertson D, Eisenbarth GS, Krischer JP, Schatz D. Specific human leukocyte antigen DQ influence on expression of antiislet autoantibodies and progression to type 1 diabetes. J Clin Endocrinol Metab 2006;91:1705–1713.
9. Kulmala P, Rahko J, Savola K, Vahasalo P, Veijola R, Sjoroos M, Reunanen A, Ilonen J, Knip M. Stability of autoantibodies and their relation to genetic and metabolic markers of type I diabetes in initially unaffected schoolchildren. Diabetologia 2000;43:457–464.

10. Bingley PJ. Interactions of age, islet cell antibodies, insulin autoantibodies, and first-phase insulin response in predicting risk of progression to IDDM in ICA+ relatives: the ICARUS data set. Islet cell antibody register users study. Diabetes 1996;45:1720–1728.

11. Sosenko JM, Palmer JP, Greenbaum CJ, Mahon J, Cowie C, Krischer JP, Chase HP, White NH, Buckingham B, Herold KC, Cuthbertson D, Skyler JS. Increasing the accuracy of oral glucose tolerance testing and extending its application to individuals with normal glucose tolerance for the prediction of type 1 diabetes: the Diabetes Prevention Trial-Type 1. Diabetes Care 2007;30:38–42.

12. Stene LC, Thorsby PM, Berg JP, Ronningen KS, Undlien DE, Joner G. The relation between size at birth and risk of type 1 diabetes is not influenced by adjustment for the insulin gene (-23HphI) polymorphism or HLA-DQ genotype. Diabetologia 2006;49:2068–2073.

13. Oling V, Marttila J, Ilonen J, Kwok WW, Nepom G, Knip M, Simell O, Reijonen H. GAD65- and proinsulin-specific CD4+ T-cells detected by MHC class II tetramers in peripheral blood of type 1 diabetes patients and at-risk subjects. J Autoimmun 2005; 25(3):235–243. Epub 2005 Nov 2. Erratum in: J Autoimmun 2006;27(1):69.

14. Kelemen K, Gottlieb PA, Putnam AL, Davidson HW, Wegmann DR, Hutton JC. HLA-DQ8-associated T cell responses to the diabetes autoantigen phogrin (IA-2 beta) in human prediabetes. J Immunol 2004;172(6): 3955–3962.

15. Verge CF, Gianani R, Kawasaki E, Yu L, Pietropaolo M, Jackson RA, Chase HP, Eisenbarth GS. Prediction of type 1 diabetes in first-degree relatives using a combination of insulin, GAD, and ICA512bdc/IA-2 autoantibodies. Diabetes 1996;45:926–933.

16. Bingley PJ, Bonifacio E, Williams AJ, Genovese S, Bottazzo GF, Gale EA. Prediction of IDDM in the general population: strategies based on combinations of autoantibody markers. Diabetes 1997;46(11):1701–1710.

17. Gardner SG, Gale EA, Williams AJ, Gillespie KM, Lawrence KE, Bottazzo GF, Bingley PJ. Progression to diabetes in relatives with islet autoantibodies. Is it inevitable? Diabetes Care 1999;22(12):2049–2054.

18. Miao D, Yu L, Eisenbarth GS. Role of autoantibodies in type 1 diabetes. Front Biosci 2007;12:1889–1898.

19. Kulmala P, Savola K, Petersen JS, Vähäsalo P, Karjalainen J, Löpponen T, Dyrberg T, Akerblom HK, Knip M. Prediction of insulin-dependent diabetes mellitus in siblings of children with diabetes. A population-based study. The Childhood Diabetes in Finland Study Group. J Clin Invest 1998;101(2):327–336.

20. Decochez K, De Leeuw IH, Keymeulen B, Mathieu C, Rottiers R, Weets I, Vandemeulebroucke E, Truyen I, Kaufman L, Schuit FC, Pipeleers DG, Gorus FK. IA-2 autoantibodies predict impending type I diabetes in siblings of patients. Belgian Diabetes Registry. Diabetologia 2002;45(12):1658–1666.

21. Wenzlau JM, Juhl K, Yu L, Moua O, Sarkar S, Gottlieb P, Rewers M, Eisenbarth GS, Jensen J, Davidson HW, and Hutton JC. The cation efflux transporter ZnT8 (Slc30A8) is a major autoantigen in human type 1 diabetes. Proc Natl Acad Sci U S A 2007;104:17040–17045.

22. Roep BO. Immune markers of disease and therapeutic intervention in type 1 diabetes. Novartis Found Symp 2008;292:159–171. Discussion 171–173, 202–203.

23. Waldron-Lynch F, von Herrath M, Herold KC. Towards a curative therapy in type 1 diabetes: remission of autoimmunity, maintenance and augmentation of beta cell mass. Novartis Found Symp 2008;292:146–155. Discussion 155–158, 202–203.

24. Bour-Jordan H, Bluestone JA. B cell depletion: a novel therapy for autoimmune diabetes? J Clin Invest 2007;117(12):3642–3645.

25. Hu CY, Rodriguez-Pinto D, Du W, Ahuja A, Henegariu O, Wong FS, Shlomchik MJ, Wen L. Treatment with CD20-specific antibody prevents and reverses autoimmune diabetes in mice. Clin Investig 2007;117(12): 3642–3645.

26. O'Neill SK, Liu E, Cambier JC. Change you can B(cell)live in: recent progress confirms a critical role for B cells in type 1 diabetes. Curr Opin Endocrinol Diabetes Obes 2009;16:293–298.

27. Herold KC, Gitelman SE, Masharani U, Hagopian W, Bisikirska B, Donaldson D, Rother K, Diamond B, Harlan DM, Bluestone JA. A single course of anti-CD3 monoclonal antibody hOKT3gamma1(Ala–Ala) results in improvement in C-peptide responses and clinical parameters for at least 2 years after onset of type 1 diabetes. Diabetes 2005;54(6):1763–1769.

28. Herold KC, Gitelman S, Greenbaum C, Puck J, Hagopian W, Gottlieb P, Sayre P, Bianchine P, Wong E, Seyfert-Margolis V, Bourcier K, Bluestone JA, Immune Tolerance Network ITN007AI Study Group. Treatment of patients with new onset type 1 diabetes with a single course of anti-CD3 mAb Teplizumab preserves insulin production for up to 5 years. Clin Immunol 2009;132(2):166–173.

29. Yu L, Robles D, Rewers M, Kaur P, Keleman K, Eisenbarth GS. High-throughput insulin autoantibody assay: 96 well filtration plate format. Diabetes 1999;48(Suppl 1):A213.
30. Gale EAM. The discovery of type 1 diabetes. Diabetes 2001;50:217–226.
31. Nerup J, Binder C. Thryroid, gastric and adrenal auto-immunity in diabetes mellitus. Acta Endocrinol 1970;72(2):279–286.
32. Warren S. The pathology of diabetes in children. Lancet 1927;88(2);99–101.
33. LeCompte PM. "Insulitis" in early juvenile diabetes. Arch Pathol 1958;66:450–457.
34. Gepts W. Pathologic anatomy of the pancreas in juvenile diabetes mellitus. Diabetes 1965;14:619–633.
35. Nerup J, Andersen OO, Bendixen G, Egeberg J, Gunnarsson R, Kromann H, Poulsen JE. Cell-mediated immunity in diabetes mellitus. Proc R Soc Med 1974;67: 506–513.
36. MacCuish AC, Irvine WJ, Barnes EW, Duncan LJ. Antibodies to pancreatic islet cells in insulin-dependent diabetics with coexistent autoimmune disease. Lancet 1974;2(7896):1529–1531.
37. Goldstein DE, Drash A, Biggs J, Blizzard RM. Diabetes mellitus: the incidence of circulating antibodies against thyroid, gastric, and adrenal tissue. J Pediatr 1970;77(2):304–306.
38. Irvine WJ, Scarth L, Clarke BF, Cullen DR. Thyroid and gastric autoimmunity in patients with diabetes mellitus. Lancet 1970;296: 163–168.
39. Nerup J, Platz P, Andersen OO, Christy M, Lyngsoe J, Poulsen JE, Ryder LP, Nielsen LS, Thomsen M, Svejgaard A. HL-A antigens and diabetes mellitus. Lancet 1974;2(7885): 864–866.
40. Nerup J, Binder C. Thyroid, gastric and adrenal auto-immunity in diabetes mellitus. Acta Endocrinol 1973;72(2):279–286.
41. Bottazzo GF, Florin-Christensen A, Doniach D. Islet-cell antibodies in diabetes mellitus with autoimmune polyendocrine deficiencies. Lancet 1974;2(7892):1279–1283.
42. Atkinson MA, Maclaren NK, Riley WJ, Winter WE, Fisk DD, Spillar RP. Are insulin autoantibodies markers for insulin-dependent diabetes mellitus? Diabetes 1986;35(8): 894–898.
43. Nayak RC, Omar MA, Rabizadeh A, Srikanta S, Eisenbarth GS. Cytoplasmic islet cell antibodies. Evidence that the target antigen is a sialoglycoconjugate. Diabetes 1985;34(6): 617–619.
44. Marshall MO, Hoyer PE, Petersen JS, Hejnaes KR, Genoves S, Dyrberg T, Bottazzo GF. Contribution of glutamate decarboxylase antibodies to the reactivity of islet cell cytoplasmic antibodies. J Autoimmun 1994;7:497–508.
45. Tsirogianni A, Pipi E, Soufleros K. Specificity of islet cell autoantibodies and coexistence with other organ specific autoantibodies in type 1 diabetes mellitus. Autoimmun Rev 2009;8:687–691.
46. Sladek R, Rocheleau G, Rung J, Dina C, Shen L, Serre D, Boutin P, Vincent D, Belisle A, Hadjadj S, Bilkau B, Haude B, Charpentier G, Hudson TJ, Montpetit A, Pshezhetsky AV, Prentki M, Posner BI, Balding DJ, Meyre D, Ploychronakos C, Froguel P. A genome-wide association study identifies novel risk loci for type 2 diabetes. Nature 2007;445:881–885.
47. Rabin DU, Pleasic SM, Palmer-Crocker R, Shapiro JA. Cloning and expression of IDDM-specific human autoantigens. Diabetes 1992;41(2):183–186.
48. Lan MS, Lu J, Goto Y, Notkins AL. Molecular cloning and identification of a receptor-type protein tyrosine phosphatase, IA-2, from human insulinoma. DNA Cell Biol 1994;13(5):505–514.
49. Pietropaolo M, Castano L, Babu S, Buelow R, Martin S, Martin A, et al. Islet cell autoantigen 69 kDa (ICA69): molecular cloning and characterization of a novel diabetes associated autoantigen. J Clin Invest 1993;92:359–371.
50. Füchtenbusch M, Karges W, Standl E, Dosch HM, Ziegler AG. Antibodies to bovine serum albumin (BSA) in type 1 diabetes and other autoimmune disorders. Exp Clin Endocrinol Diabetes 1997;105(2):86–91.
51. Wasmeier C, Hutton JC. Molecular cloning of phogrin, a protein-tyrosine phosphatase homologue localized to insulin secretory granule membranes. J Biol Chem 1996;271(30):18161–18170.
52. Daaboul J, Schatz D. Overview of prevention and intervention trials for type 1 diabetes. Rev Endocr Metab Disord 2003;4(4):317–323.
53. Ola TO, Biro PA, Hawa MI, Ludvigsson J, Locatelli M, Puglisi MA, Bottazzo GF, Fierabracci A. Importin beta: a novel autoantigen in human autoimmunity identified by screening random peptide libraries on phage. J Autoimmun 2006;26(3):197–207.
54. Pietropaolo M, Castano L, Babu S, Buelow R, Kuo YL, Martin S, Martin A, Powers AC, Prochazka M, Naggert J, et al. Islet cell autoantigen 69 kDa(CA69). Molecular cloning and characterization of a novel diabetes-associated autoantigen. J Clin Invest 1996;97:172–176.
55. Martin S, Kardorf J, Schulte B, Lampeter EF, Gries FA, Melchers I. Autoantibodies to the

islet antigen ICA69 occur in IDDM and in rheumatoid arthritis. Diabetologia 1995;38(3): 351–355.
56. Achenbach P, Bonifacio E, Williams AJ, Ziegler AG, Gale EA, Bingley PJ, ENDIT Group. Autoantibodies to IA-2beta (β) improve diabetes risk assessment in high-risk relatives. Diabetologia 2008;51(3):488–492.
57. Kasimiotis H, Fida S, Rowley MJ, Mackay IR, Zimmet PZ, Gleason S, Rabin DU, Myers MA. Antibodies to SOX13 (ICA12) are associated with type l diabetes. Autoimmunity 2001;33(2): 95–101.
58. Honeyman MC, Cram DS, Harrison LC. Transcription factor jun-B is target of autoreactive T-cells in IDDS. Diabetes 1993;42(4):626–630.
59. Castano L, Russo E, Zhou L, Lipes MA, Eisenbarth GS. Identification and cloning of a granule autoantigen (carboxypeptidase-H) associated with type I diabetes. J Clin Endocrinol Metab 1991;7:1197–1201.
60. Greenbaum CJ, Palmer JP, Nagataki S, Yamaguchi Y, Molenaar JL, Van Beers WAM, et al. Improved specificity of ICA assays in the Fourth International Immunology of Diabetes Exchange Workshop. Diabetes 1992;41:1570–1574.
61. Mallone R, Perin PC. Anti-CD38 autoantibodies in type 1 diabetes. Diabetes Metab Res Rev 2006;22(4):284–294.
62. Karounos DG, Wolinsky JS, Thomas JW. Monoclonal antibody to rubella virus capsid protein recognizes a beta-cell antigen. J Immunol 1993;150(7):3080–3085.
63. Aanstoot HJ, Kang SM, Kim J, Lindsay LA, Roll U, Knip M, Atkinson M, Mose-Larsen P, Fey S, Ludvigsson J, Landin L, Bruining J, Maclaren N, Akerblom HK, Baekkeskov S. Identification and characterization of glima 38, a glycosylated islet cell membrane antigen, which together with GAD65 and IA2 marks the early phases of autoimmune response in type l diabetes. J Clin Invest 1996;97(12):2772–2783.
64. Winnock F, Christie MR, Batstra MR, Aanstoot HJ, Weets I, Decochez K, Jopart P, Nicolaij D, Gorus FK. Autoantibodies to a 38-kDa glycosylated islet cell membrane-associated antigen in (pre)type 1 diabetes: association with IA-2 and islet cell autoantibodies. Diabetes Care 2001;24(7):1181–1186.
65. Colman PG, Nayak RC, Campbell IL, Eisenbarth GS. Binding of cytoplasmic islet cell antibodies is blocked by human pancreatic glycolipid extracts. Diabetes 1988;37(5):645–652.
66. Dotta F, Gianani R, Previti M, Lenti L, Dionisi S, D'Erme M, Eisenbarth GS, Di Mario U. Autoimmunity to the GM2-1 islet ganglioside before and at the onset of type I diabetes. Diabetes 1996;45(9):1193–1196.
67. Gillard BK, Thomas JW, Nell LJ, Marcus DM. Antibodies against ganglioside GT3 in the sera of patients with type I diabetes mellitus. J Immunol 1989;142(11):3826–3832.
68. Lucchetta M, Rudilosso S, Costa S, Bruttomesso D, Ruggero S, Toffanin E, Faggian D, Plebani M, Battistin L, Alaedini A, Briani C. Anti-ganglioside autoantibodies in type 1 diabetes. Muscle Nerve 2010;41(1): 50–53.
69. Buschard K, Josefsen K, Horn T, Fredman P. Sulphatide and sulphatide antibodies in insulin-dependent diabetes mellitus. Lancet 1993;342:840.
70. Bleich D, Polak M, Chen S, Swiderek SM, Levey-Marchal C. Sera from children with type 1 diabetes mellitus react against a new group of antigen composed of lysophospholipids. Horm Res 1999;52:86–94.
71. Puertas MC, Carrillo J, Pastor X, Ampudia RM, Planas R, Alba A, Bruno R, Pujol-Borrell R, Estanyol JM, Vives-Pi M, Verdaguer J. Peripherin is a relevant neuroendocrine autoantigen recognized by islet-infiltrating B lymphocytes. J Immunol 2007;178(10):6533–6539.
72. Miersch S, Sibani S, Logvinenko T, Atkinson M, Schatz D, LaBaer J. Serological screening for novel autoantibodies associated with type 1 diabetes using nuclei acid programmable protein arrays. Immunology of Diabetes Society 10th International Congress. Malmo, Sweden, May 17–20, 2009.
73. Palmer JP, Asplin CM, Clemons P, Lyen K, Tatpati O, Raghu PK, et al. Insulin antibodies in insulin-dependent diabetics before insulin treatment. Science 1983;222(4630): 1337–1339.
74. Franke B, Galloway TS, Wilkin TJ. Developments in the prediction of type diabetes mellitus, with special reference to insulin autoantibodies. Diabetes Metab Res Rev 2005;21(5):395–415.
75. Brooks-Worrell BM, Nielson D, Palmer JP. Insulin autoantibodies and insulin antibodies have similar binding characteristics. Proc Assoc Am Physicians 1999;111(1):92–96.
76. Tan PL, Wigley RD, Borman GB. Clinical criteria for systemic sclerosis. Arthritis Rheum 1981;24(12):1589–1590.
77. Hoffmann A, Heck MMS, Bordwell BJ, Rothfiedls NF, Earnshaw WC. Human autoantibody to topoisomerase II. Exp Cell Res 1989;180:409–418.
78. Meliconci R, Bestagno M, Sturani C, Begri C, Galavotti V, Sala C, Facchini A, Ciarrocchi G,

Gasvarrini G, Astaldi Ricotti GCB. Autoantibodies to DNA 418 topoisomerase II in cryptogenic fibrosing alveolitis and connective tissue disease. Clin Exp Immunol 1989;76:184–189.
79. Zuklys KL, Szer IAS, Szer W. Autoantibodies to DNA topoisomerase II in juvenile rheumatoid arthritis. Clin Exp Immunol 1991;84:245–249.
80. Chang YH, Hwang J, Shang HF, Tsai ST. Characterization of human DNA topoisomerase II as an autoantigen recognized by patients with IDDM. Diabetes 1996;45(4):408–414.
81. Baekkeskov S, Aanstoot HJ, Christgau S, Reetz A, Solimena M, Cascalho M, et al. Identification of the 64K autoantigen in insulin-dependent diabetes as the GABA-synthesizing enzyme glutamic acid decarboxylase. Nature 1990;347(6289):151–156.
82. Rinta-Valkama J, Aaltonen P, Lassila M, Palmén T, Tossavainen P, Knip M, Holthöfer H. Densin and filtrin in the pancreas and in the kidney, targets for humoral autoimmunity in patients with type 1 diabetes. Diabetes Metab Res Rev 2007;23(2):119–126.
83. Aaltonen P, Rinta-Valkama J, Pätäri A, Tossavainen P, Palmén T, Kulmala P, Knip M, Holthöfer H. Circulating antibodies to nephrin in patients with type 1 diabetes. Nephrol Dial Transplant 2007;22(1):146–153.
84. Wildbaum G, Youssef S, Karin N. A targeted DNA vaccine augments the natural immune response to self TNF-alpha and suppresses ongoing adjuvant arthritis. J Immunol 2000;165:5860–5866.
85. Shehadeh N, Pollack A, Wildbaum G, Zohar Y, Shafat I, Makhoul R, Daod E, Hakikm R, Perlman R, Karin N. Selective autoantibody production against CCL3 is associated with human type 1 diabetes mellitus and serves as a novel biomarker for its diagnosis. J Immunol 2009;182(12):8104–8109.
86. Winer S, Tsui H, Lau A, Song A, Li X, Cheung RK, Sampson A, Afifiyan F, Elford A, Jackowski G, Becker DJ, Santamaria P, Ohashi P, Dosch HM. Autoimmune islet destruction in spontaneous type 1 diabetes is not beta-cell exclusive. Nat Med 2003;9(2):198–205.
87. van Eden W, Thole JE, van der Zee R, Noordzij A, van Embden JD, Hensen EJ, Cohen IR. Cloning of the mycobacterial epitope recognized by T lymphocytes in adjuvant arthritis. Nature 1988;331(6152): 171–173.
88. Elias D, Reshef T, Birk OS, van der Zee R, Walker MD, Cohen IR. Vaccination against autoimmune mouse diabetes with a T-cell epitope of the human 65-kDa heat shock protein. Proc Natl Acad Sci U S A 1991;88(8): 3088–3091.
89. Abulafia-Lapid R, Elias D, Raz I, Keren-Zur Y, Atlan H, Cohen IR. T cell proliferative responses of type 1 diabetes patients and healthy individuals to human hsp60 and its peptides. J Autoimmun 1999;12(2):121–129.
90. Abulafia-Lapid R, Gillis D, Yosef O, Atlan H, Cohen IR. T cells and autoantibodies to human HSP70 in type 1 diabetes in children. J Autoimmun 2003;20(4):313–321.
91. Rabinowe SL. Immunology of diabetic and polyglandular neuropathy. Diabetes Metab Rev 1990;6:169–188.
92. Norton ET, Autilio LA. The lipid composition of purifies bovine brain myelin. J Neurochem 1966;13:1213–1222.
93. Buschard K, Hanspers, K, Fredman P, Reich EP. Treatment with sulfatide or its prescursor, galactosylceramide, prevents diabetes in NOD mice. Autoimmunity 2001;34(1): 9–17.
94. Blomqvist M, Kaas A, Mansson J-E, Formby B, Rynmark B-M, Buschard K, Fredman P. Developmental expression of the type I diabetes related antigen sulfatide and sulfated lactosylceramide in mammalian pancreas. J Cell Biochem 2003;89:301–310.
95. Hirai H, Miura J, Hu Y, Larsson H, Larsson K, Lernmark A, Ivarsson SA, Wu T, Kingman A, Tzioufas AG, Notkins AL. Selective screening of secretory vesicle-associated proteins for autoantigens in type 1 diabetes: VAMP2 and NPY are new minor autoantigens. Clin Immunol 2008;127(3):366–374.
96. McEvoy RC, Thomas NM, Greig F, Larson S, Vargas-Rodriguez I, Felix I, Wallach E, Rubinstein P, Goetz FC, Ginsberg-Fellner F. Anti-islet autoantibodies detected by monoclonal antibody IA2: further studies suggesting a role in the pathogenesis of IDDM. Diabetologia 1996;39(11):1365–1371.
97. Metz TO, Qian WJ, Jacobs JM, Gritsenko MA, Moore RJ, Polypitiya AD, Monroe ME, Cam II DG, Mueller PW, Smith RD. Application of proteomics in the discovery of candidate protein biomarkers in a Diabetes Autoantibody Standardization Program (DASP) sample subset. J Proteome Res 2008;7(2):698–707.
98. Peakman M. CD8 and cytotoxic T cells in type 1 diabetes. Novartis Found Symp. 2008;292:113–119. Discussion 119–129, 202–203.
99. Dromey JA, Weenink SM, Peters GH, Endl J, Tighe PJ, Todd I, Christie MR. Mapping of epitopes for autoantibodies to the type 1 diabetes autoantigen IA-2 by peptide phage display and molecular modeling: overlap of

antibody and T cell determinants. J Immunol 2004;172(7):4084–4090.
100. Arden SD, Roep BO, Neophytou PI, Usac EF, Duinkerken G, De Vries RRP, Hutton JC. Imogen 38: a novel 38-kD islet mitochondrial autoantigen recognized by T cells from a newly diagnosed type I diabetic patient. J Clin Invest 1996;97(2):551–561.
101. Lieberman SM, Evans AM, Han B, Takaki T, Vinnitskaya Y, Caldwell JA, Serreze DV, Shabanowitz J, Hunt DF, Nathenson SG, Santamaria P, DiLorenzo TP. Identification of the beta cell antigen targeted by a prevalent population of pathogenic CD8+ T cells in autoimmune diabetes. Proc Natl Acad Sci U S A 2003;100(14):8384–8388.
102. Hutton JC, Eisenbarth GS. A pancreatic {beta}-cell-specific homolog of glucose-6-phosphatase emerges as a major target of cell-mediated autoimmunity in diabetes. Proc Natl Acad Sci U S A 2003;100: 8626–8628.
103. Lieberman SM, Takaki T, Han B, Santamaria P, Serreze DV, DiLorenzo TP. Individual nonobese diabetic mice exhibit unique patterns of CD8+ T cell reactivity to three islet antigens, including the newly identified widely expressed dystrophia myotonica kinase. J Immunol 2004;173(11): 6727–6734.
104. Novartis Gene Atlas V.2. http://www.symatlas.gnf.org.
105. Su A, Wiltshire T, Batalov S, et al. A gene atlas of the mouse and human protein-encoding transcriptomes. Proc Natl Acad Sci U S A 2004;101:6062–6067.
106. Juhl K, Sarkar SA, Wong R, Jensen J, Hutton JC. Mouse pancreatic endocrine cell transcriptome defined in the embryonic Ngn-3-null mouse. Diabetes 2008;57:2755–2761.
107. Bonifacio E, Lampasona V, Genovese S, Ferrari M, Bosi E. Identification of protein tyrosine phosphatase-like IA2 (islet cell antigen 512) as the insulin-dependent diabetes-related 37/40K autoantigen and a target of islet-cell antibodies. J Immunol 1995;155(11): 5419–5426.
108. Hawkes CJ, Wasmeier C, Christie MR, Hutton JC. Identification of the 37-kDa antigen in IDDM as a tyrosine phosphatase-like protein (phogrin) related to IA-2. Diabetes 1996;45:1187–1192.
109. Qin JY, Mahon JL, Atkinson MA, Chaturvedi P, Lee-Chan E, Singh B. Type 1 diabetes alters antihsp90 autoantigen (carboxypeptidase-H) associated with type 1 diabetes. J Autoimmun 2003;20:237–245.
110. Gurr W, Shaw M, Li Y, Sherwin R. RegII is a beta-cell protein and autoantigen in diabetes of NOD mice. Diabetes 2007;56:34–40.
111. Clark A, Yon SM, de Koning EJ, Homan RR. Autoantibodies to islet amyloid polypeptide in diabetes. Diabet Med 1991;8:668–673.
112. Boitard C, Villa MA, Becourt C, Gia HP, Huc C, Sempe P, Portier MM, Bach JF. Peripherin: an islet antigen that is cross-reactive with nonobese diabetic mouse class II gene products. Proc Natl Acad Sci U S A 1992;89:172–176.
113. Lühder F, Schlosser M, Mauch L, Haubruck H, Rjasanowski I, Michaelis D, Kohnert KD, Ziegler M. Autoantibodies against GAD65 rather than GAD67 precede the onset of type 1 diabetes. Autoimmunity 1994;19(2):71–80.
114. Lu M, Fu D. Structure of the zinc transporter YiiP. Science 2007;317:1746–1748.
115. Wenzlau JM, Frisch L, Gardner T, Sarkar S, Hutton JC, and Davidson, HW. Novel antigens in type 1 diabetes: the importance of ZnT8. Curr Diab Rep 2009;8(2):109–112.
116. Wenzlau JM, Liu Y, Yu L, Moua O, Fowler KT, Rangasamy S, Walters J, Eisenbarth GS, Davidson HW, Hutton JC. A common nonsynonymous single nucleotide polymorphism in the SLC30A8 gene determines ZnT8 autoantibody specificity in type 1 diabetes. Diabetes 2008;57(10):2693–2697.
117. Davidson HW, Rockell J, Wagner R, Wenzlau JM, Zipris D, Hutton JC, Gottlieb PT. CD4 T cell reactivity to the major diabetes autoantigen Slc30A8 in newly diabetic subjects. Diabetologia 2008;51(S1):S103 (Oral presentation, EASD annual meeting, Rome, Italy).
118. Szodoray P, Szabó Z, Kapitány A, Gyetvai A, Lakos G, Szántó S, Szücs G, Szekanecz Z. Anti-citrullinated protein/peptide autoantibodies in association with genetic and environmental factors as indicators of disease outcome in rheumatoid arthritis. Autoimmun Rev 2010;9(3):140–143.
119. Delong T, Barbour G, Bradley B, Reisdorph N, Standinski B, Kappler J, Haskins K. A new antigen for autoreactive T cells in type 1 diabetes. 10th International Congress of the Immunology of Diabetes Society. Malmo, Sweden, May 17–20, 2009.

Chapter 3

Developing and Validating High Sensitivity/Specificity Autoantibody Assays

Ezio Bonifacio, Anne Eugster, and Vito Lampasona

Summary

Endocrine autoimmune diseases are frequently characterised by the presence of autoantibodies to the affected target organ. These autoantibodies appear prior to clinical disease and can be used as markers to identify individuals with preclinical disease, track disease pathogenesis and in some cases to classify disease. Autoantibodies to a multitude of antigens have been described, and in many diseases there are multiple target autoantigens reported. Some, but not all reported autoantibodies are valid disease markers. Here we discuss the process of identifying bona fide disease-relevant autoantibody markers and how to achieve highly sensitive and specific standardised assays for their measurement.

Key Words: Autoantibodies, Immunoassay, Type 1 diabetes, Autoantigen

Endocrine autoantibodies were first identified in 1954 (*1*, *2*). Measurement was by a functional assay in which immunoglobulin from a patient with Graves disease was found to stimulate thyroid cells (*1*) and by a crude immuno-precipitation assay in which a thyroid extract overlaid with patient's serum gave a precipitate of immune complexes at the interface (*2*). These were pivotal findings from opposite sides of the globe that confirmed the existence of autoantibodies and autoimmune disease. The experiments also told us that autoantibodies could cause disease and provided us with a general rule that disease-relevant autoantibodies can (and probably should) bind to native antigen. After these first findings, autoantibodies to almost every organ or tissue in the body have been described. A minority of these are directly responsible for disease pathology, others contribute indirectly to the disease, and the majority are simply markers of the disease or non-specifically associated with disease. The better autoantibody markers can be used to predict future disease (*3*), classify disease (*4*), and monitor disease (*5*). However, their ability to predict, classify, and monitor disease depends very much on the quality of the assays used to measure autoantibodies and the sensitivity and specificity of these assays.

Autoantibody requirements

Autoantibody should bind to native antigen or antigen conformation found *in vivo*.

Autoantibody binding to antigen can be <u>specifically</u> competed with excess antigen.

Autoantibody-antigen binding can be detected in fluid phase assay.

Autoantigen requirements

Are polymorphic forms relevant to autoantibody binding?

Expression of antigen in a form that is expected *in vivo*.

Disease relevance

A threshold for positivity that identifies <1% of control subjects.

More disease subjects identified than control subjects.

Fig. 3.1

In designing highly sensitive and specific assays, we need to first answer some basic questions about the autoantibody and have an understanding of the diversity of autoantibodies and what could influence their binding to antigen (Fig. 3.1).

AUTOANTIBODIES AS HETERO-GENEOUS ANALYTES

Many biomarkers may be polymorphic and therefore potentially heterogeneous between individuals, but few compare to the heterogeneity found in the autoantibody as an analyte. In any single B-cell response to antigen, it is the purpose to develop high-affinity multivalent antibodies through a selection and edit process that gives rise to multiple B-cell clones that can persist throughout life (6). Clearly, evolution of the humoral immune system did not have our ability to predict or classify disease in mind, but to develop an efficient and versatile means to neutralise and opsonise invading organisms and their toxins which themselves have a profound capacity to mutate and present diversity. Almost every B-cell clone that is generated in the immune response to an organism or antigen produces a different antibody. This holds also for autoantibodies. The vast majority of autoantibodies are of IgG isotype. For type 1 diabetes, the major subclass is IgG1, although the distribution of islet autoantibody subclasses can vary between individuals and antigens (7). The unique feature of an (auto)antibody is the antigen-binding site, and this varies between each B-cell clone in an individual. The specificity of every antibody is determined by a unique sequence of amino acids in its variable region (*8*). At correct conformation and conditions, the antibody should bind tightly and specifically and only to its cognate antigen. The cognate antigen itself is often a complex structure, which presents itself in its tertiary or quaternary conformational form. As such, the antigen, although comprising preferred antigenic sites, is riddled with sites to which autoantibodies could bind. These sites are characterised by their shape as well as physical interactions that will occur between their exposed amino acids and those in the binding region of the autoantibody (*9*). It should also be considered that autoantigens can themselves vary due to polymorphism within coding regions and therefore the same antigenic site could differ between individuals (*10*). Thus when we talk about autoantibodies to even a single antigen, we are talking about highly diverse analytes. Perhaps the most important consequence of this when speaking of disease-relevant autoantibodies, is that it may not be surprising to find that under certain conditions antibodies can potentially bind to structures that are not cognate antigen. It is therefore important that the conditions used for antibody–antigen binding should exclude detection of imperfect antibody–antigen fits.

CONSIDERATIONS ON THE TARGET OR COGNATE AUTOANTIGEN

In considering how the cognate antigen should be seen by the autoantibodies, one has to remember that the autoantibodies arise in vivo. While we do not know the exact form and conformation of cognate antigen that the B cells see, we do have some clues that point us to the likelihood that endocrine disease-relevant autoreactive B cells see native or near native antigen in vivo. For type 1 diabetes, the original description of autoantibodies used frozen sections of human pancreas as substrate (*11*). Fixation of the pancreas abolished binding of some islet cell autoantibodies suggesting that even minimal manipulation of the antigen would render it unrecognisable by autoantibodies (Bottazzo, personal communication). Detailed study of the autoantibody epitopes of known autoantigens shows that the majority need to be conformational for binding, i.e. require tertiary shape (*12*). Thus when trying to identify disease-relevant autoantibodies, it is perhaps wise not to tamper with antigen, and avoid the use of denatured proteins. Some will argue that the destructive process of autoimmunity will also destroy antigen and uncover hidden epitopes (*13*). However, we are not yet able to mimic these potential in vivo processes in our in vitro assays. Sometimes, as in the case of insulin autoantibodies in man, even the attachment of antigen to a solid phase is sufficient to disturb antibody–antigen binding and result in low sensitivity and low specificity (*14*). Along similar reasoning, it also seems unwise to randomly chop whole proteins in order to unveil or identify epitopes. A more sensible approach would be to consider conformational domains of the antigen, natural processing, and potential degradation products of the antigen that may occur in vivo when designing antigens for autoantibody detection. One must also consider that a number of autoantigens are transmembrane proteins and that the transmembrane region is difficult to express in its native form except in high concentration detergents and it is easier to obtain correctly folded protein when the domains either side of the transmembrane regions are expressed separately (*15*). As a useful rule of thumb, try to use antigen in a form that is likely to have a conformation closely resembling native antigen or native antigen products when first establishing an autoantibody detection assay.

CHARACTERISTICS OF THE AUTOANTIBODY DETECTION ASSAY

Since we are measuring autoantibody we are more or less forced to use immuno assay for its detection. Immuno assays come in various forms. We believe that the immuno assays of choice for the identification and validation of autoantibodies should be those in which antigen is not constrained, i.e. liquid phase immuno assays where free antibodies and free antigen are allowed to bind. One notes that each of the major autoantigens identified in type 1 diabetes were first detected in liquid phase binding assays. Both GAD and IA2/IA2b were immuno precipitated from labelled islet membrane extracts (*16, 17*), autoantibodies to insulin were detected using iodinated monovalin injectable insulin in liquid phase (*18*), and autoantibodies to the zinc-transporter eight protein were first detected using recombinant cytoplasmic domains in liquid phase (*15*). A number of other proteins have been suggested to be autoantigens in type 1 diabetes on the basis of binding that was originally described in solid phase assays or using denatured antigen. These include proteins such as ICA69, CD38, and others. The majority of these, however, could not be confirmed to have diabetes specificity (*19*).

Despite all the precautions one can take, it is always possible that the antibody–antigen binding that is detected has little to do with autoimmune disease and is simply artefact. This could occur from change of protein shape so that it resembles that of the cognate epitope of the antibodies detected, and of course when conditions favour binding of low affinity or imperfect fitting antibody–antigen pairs. A useful approach to reduce the likelihood of detecting artefact is to show that the antibody binding to antigen can be specifically competed with excess antigen and importantly not with an excess amount of unrelated antigens (*14, 20, 21*). Further confidence in true autoantibody would be obtained through competition with increasing amounts of target and unrelated antigens so that competition curves confirming high-affinity target antigen-specific binding can be obtained (*22, 23*). Finding a panel of autoantibodies against the antigen in question with different or slightly different epitopes binding to different antigenic sites (within one patient or within a group of patients) would also strongly support a true interaction (*24*).

We consider the above to be very first steps before considering the development of highly specific and sensitive assays of autoantibodies, i.e. demonstrate binding to native or close to native antigen, show that binding is specific to the antigen in question and not against unrelated antigens, and show a convincing competition curve to the antigen in question and not to unrelated antigen. Of course, fulfilling these requisites is likely to define true autoantibodies, but disease relevance and utility would not yet be established.

ASSAY SPECIFICITY AND DISEASE RELEVANCE

Bayes' theory forms the basis of clinical diagnosis and describes the relationship between three parameters fundamental to diagnostic tests. These are the sensitivity for disease, the specificity in health or confounding disease, and the a priori probability of disease in the subject being tested. When applying autoantibodies in tests for autoimmune disease, we therefore need to know these fundamental parameters of the test that is being applied. In situations where the a priori probability of disease is low, the specificity of the test has a profound effect on the diagnostic utility. Indeed, one of the limitations of autoantibodies with respect to disease diagnosis or prediction is that the majority of individuals with single autoantibodies do not have autoimmune disease (*25–27*). The detection of autoantibodies, therefore, can rarely diagnose disease in the absence of corroborating clinical or laboratory evidence.

While an idea of sensitivity and specificity can be obtained by testing relatively few patient and control subjects, the establishment of assays for wide spread use, requires that large cohorts, and potentially several large cohorts are tested. In general, assays will be most helpful if they have high specificity. An assay with specificity of 95% is likely to be a poor predictor of diabetes in most circumstances. A specificity of 99% or higher will improve our predictive power and to determine 99% specificity with precision, a large number, e.g. >1,000 of control subjects are required. We are not saying that autoantibodies do not exist or should not exist in controls, but for the assay to be effective in prediction and classification of diabetes, we must be able to set a threshold of positivity providing high specificity or alternatively use the antibody measurement in combination with other markers for example other autoantibodies or characteristics, e.g. affinity, that may discriminate diabetes' relevance.

HIGH QUALITY STANDARDISED ASSAYS

Typically, once assays have been validated, one or more laboratories develop their own high quality assays. For the scientific and clinical community as a whole, an appreciation of which assays can achieve high sensitivity and specificity is important so that findings with respect to pathophysiology and prognostic value are not blurred by reports from low quality assays. The type 1 diabetes community recognised this and developed standardisation programmes in the mid-1980s (*14, 28, 29*). From these programmes it was possible to identify assays in laboratories that could achieve highest sensitivity with high specificity (*30*). Other laboratories could learn from this and mimic the assays, but perfect concordance between laboratories was difficult to achieve (*31*). Other autoantibodies are undergoing similar processes (*32*).

Islet autoantibodies have become important markers for large cohort studies. Thus, international funding agencies demanded that standardisation was further improved such that autoantibody prevalences and even quantification could be compared between studies. This led to a harmonisation programme (*33*). The programme envisaged three phases (Fig. 3.2) that started with the development

Phase 1: Working calibrators

Pooled disease sera – should represent the diversity of disease related autoantibodies.

Multiple concentrations covering a wide range of measurement – dilutions in negative serum.

Large volumes of calibrators for daily use in multiple laboratories over a long time frame.

Phase 2: Selection and improvement of assays

Identification of high performance assays (at least 2) from workshops.

Harmonization of methods into common protocol.

Phase 3: Concordance and threshold selection

Measurement of large numbers of control and disease sera with harmonized assays in multiple laboratories.

Fig. 3.2

of common working calibrators. Several qualities of these calibrators were deemed necessary. First the calibrators should be representative of the vast majority of autoantibodies that will be measured. Since we know that autoantibodies were heterogeneous and that individuals differed in their islet autoantibody profiles even to single antigens, calibrators should be made from pooling serum obtained from multiple patients. Large volumes are required since the calibrators are to be used daily. Calibrators should cover a range of measurement from negative across expected thresholds of positivity to autoantibody concentrations that reached upper limits of linearity in most assays. The second phase requires selection of laboratories with high quality assays as determined by standardisation programmes followed by harmonisation of their methods so that common reagents, buffers, and procedures could be used as much as possible. After showing concordance in a small number of samples, the last phase requires that the selected laboratories perform measurements with the working calibrators and harmonised assays in a respectable number of control and patient samples in order to establish the degree of concordance and determine thresholds for positivity that would render the harmonised assays useful in disease classification and prediction. This process has recently been completed for autoantibodies to GAD and IA-2 and has now been reported.

THRESHOLDS FOR POSITIVITY

How to select thresholds of positivity remains an area of debate. There are different objectives that need to be considered. One is the identity of true autoantibody regardless of disease status, and on the other side we wish to select thresholds with maximum specificity so that true disease relevance can be ascertained. We also need to understand that whatever assay is used and how much care we take to identify only antigen-specific high-affinity autoantibodies, ultimately we see a quantified signal and not the autoantibody itself. Looking in a cohort of healthy subjects we will find that these signals will vary, i.e. even within negative samples there will be a range of signals. We expect that the range of signals of truly negative samples are made up of a number of factors that include matrix effects and random variation due to counting or signal precision, and that such truly negative signals should be normally distributed. We also know that truly positive autoantibody signals have a range of titre or concentration, and we expect that these signals will have a different distribution to those of truly negative samples. Thus we believe that it is possible to identify signals, which have a high probability of representing true autoantibody. We have used these concepts and applied

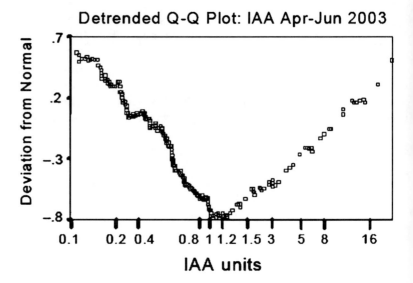

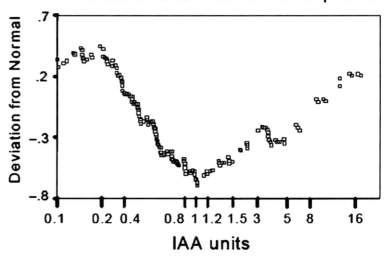

Fig. 3.3

distribution plots such as the QQ-plot to cohort data in order to define the thresholds for distinguishing positive from negative antibody signals (*34*). In the example shown (Fig. 3.3), which are pooled date from control and samples measured over two consecutive 3-month periods, one can visualise a straight line representing a normal distribution between values of 0.2 and 1 unit, a point of inflexion at around 1–1.1, followed by another line in a different direction. We interpret these to represent the true negative signals, the upper limit of true negative signals and the positive signals, respectively. This sort of selection of a threshold may be effective to study natural history and pathogenesis since we are looking for a time point when signals move from the negative distribution to the positive distribution and remain there. However, the same thresholds may not be appropriate for prediction or diagnosis. Here again we need to consider Bayes' theorem and determine what level of false positivity the purpose of testing will allow in order to select the appropriate threshold. The use of methods such as receiver operating characteristic (ROC) plots is useful to investigate if a marker can discriminate disease from non-disease and can be used to identify a threshold, but the investigator should not simply take the point of greatest discrimination (*35*), but consider a target specificity. Again, erring on the conservative side sacrificing sensitivity for the sake of high specificity is likely to provide higher quality measurement. The use of thresholds with substantially lower specificity is possible, if the autoantibodies are used together with other markers. For example, the likelihood that two islet autoantibodies against two different islet autoantigens are present in non-disease-relevant samples will be extremely low such that it may be possible to use strategies whereby disease is identified by the presence of two autoantibodies above the 97.5th percentile of controls or by the presence of one antibody above the 99.5th percentile. Creating binomial distributions with multiple markers is challenging, but may be the ideal approach to get the best from multiple validated autoantibodies.

FUTURE PERSPECTIVES

Advances in technology are likely to change the way we measure autoantibodies. Detection systems will improve with advances in the quality and range of labels (*36, 37*). Array-based measurement of antibodies to multiple targets (*38–41*), or examining single B-cell characteristics (*42, 43*) are novel advances that are likely to find their way into research laboratories. Particularly interesting would be an ability to rapidly identify autoreactive B cells by their immunoglobulin genes using DNA-sequencing technology. It is hoped that such advances will improve the measurement and unearth novel true targets of autoimmunity and that with proper validation, the expansion of a list of autoantibodies with minimal or no disease relevance can be avoided.

ACKNOWLEDGMENTS

EB and AE are supported by grants from the European Union (EP7-HEALTH-2007, DIAPREPP N202013), the Federal Ministry of Education and Research of Germany (Kompetenznetz

Diabetes mellitus, FKZ 01GI0805-07), and the DFG-Center for Regenerative Therapies Dresden, Cluster of Excellence (FZ 111).

REFERENCES

1. Adams DD. The presence of an abnormal thyroid-stimulating hormone in the serum of some thyrotoxic patients. J Clin Endocrinol Metab 1958;18:699–712.
2. Campbell, PN, Doniach D, Hudson RV, Roitt IM. Auto-antibodies in Hashimoto's disease (lymphadenoid goitre). Lancet 1956;271:820–821.
3. Rose NR. Prediction and prevention of autoimmune disease. Ann NY Acad Sci 2007;1109: 117–128.
4. Koenig M, Joyal F, Fritzler MJ, Roussin A, Abrahamowicz M, Boire G, Goulet J, Rich E, Grodzicky T, Raymond Y, Senécal J. Autoantibodies and microvascular damage are independent predictive factors for the progression of Raynaud's phenomenon to systemic sclerosis: a twenty-year prospective study of 586 patients, with validation of proposed criteria for early systemic sclerosis. Arthritis Rheum 2008;58:3902–3912.
5. Wiik AS. Anti-nuclear autoantibodies: clinical utility for diagnosis, prognosis, monitoring, and planning of treatment strategy in systemic immunoinflammatory diseases. Scand J Rheumatol 2005;34:260–268.
6. Lanzavecchia A, Sallusto F. Human B cell memory. Curr Opin Immunol 2009;21:298–304.
7. Bonifacio E, Scirpoli M, Kredel K, Füchtenbusch, M, Ziegler, AG. Early autoantibody responses in prediabetes are IgG1 dominated and suggest antigen-specific regulation. J Immunol 1999;163:525–532.
8. Chitarra V, Alzari PM, Bentley GA, Bhat TN, Eiselé JL, Houdusse A, Lescar J, Souchon H, Poljak RJ. Three-dimensional structure of a heteroclitic antigen-antibody cross-reaction complex. Proc Natl Acad Sci USA 1993;90:7711–7715.
9. Benjamin DC, Berzofsky JA, East IJ, Gurd FRN, Hannum C, Leach SJ, Margoliash E, Michael JG, Miller A, Prager EM, Reichlin M, Sercarz EE, Smith-Gill SJ, Todd PE, Wilson AC. The antigenic structure of proteins: a reappraisal. Annu Rev Immunol 1984;2:67–101.
10. Wenzlau JM, Liu Y, Yu, L, Moua O, Fowler KT, Rangasamy S, Walters J, Eisenbarth, GS, Davidson HW, Hutton JC. A common nonsynonymous single nucleotide polymorphism in the SLC30A8 gene determines ZnT8 autoantibody specificity in type 1 diabetes. Diabetes 2008;57:2693–2697
11. Bottazzo G F, Florin-Christensen, A, Doniach D. Islet-cell antibodies in diabetes mellitus with autoimmune polyendocrine deficiencies. Lancet 1974;2:1279–1283.
12. Binder KA, Banga JP, Madec A, Ortqvist E, Luo D, Hampe, CS. Epitope analysis of GAD65Ab using fusion proteins and rFab. J Immunol Methods 2004;295:101–109.
13. Vanderlugt CL, Miller SD. Epitope spreading in immune-mediated diseases: implications for immunotherapy. Nat Rev Immunol 2002;2: 85–95.
14. Greenbaum C, Palmer J, Kuglin B, Kolb H. Insulin autoantibodies measured by radioimmunoassay methodology are more related to insulin-dependent diabetes mellitus than those measured by enzyme-linked immunosorbent assay: results of the Fourth International Workshop on the Standardization of Insulin Autoantibody Measurement. J Clin Endocrinol Metab 1992;74:1040–1044.
15. Wenzlau JM, Juhl K, Yu L, Moua O, Sarkar SA, Gottlieb P, Rewers M, Eisenbarth GS, Jensen J, Davidson HW, Hutton, JC. The cation efflux transporter ZnT8 (Slc30A8) is a major autoantigen in human type 1 diabetes. Proc Natl Acad Sci USA 2007;104:17040–17045.
16. Baekkeskov S, Nielsen JH, Marner B, Bilde T, Ludvigsson J, Lernmark A. Autoantibodies in newly diagnosed diabetic children immunoprecipitate human pancreatic islet cell proteins. Nature 1982;298:167–169.
17. Christie MR, Vohra G, Champagne P, Daneman D, Delovitch TL. Distinct antibody specificities to a 64-kD islet cell antigen in type 1 diabetes as revealed by trypsin treatment. J Exp Med 1990;172:789–794.
18. Palmer J, Asplin C, Clemons P, Lyen K, Tatpati O, Raghu P, Paquette T. Insulin antibodies in insulin-dependent diabetics before insulin treatment. Science 1983;222: 1337–1339.
19. Lampasona V, Ferrari M, Bosi E, Pastore MR, Bingley PJ, Bonifacio E. Sera from patients with IDDM and healthy individuals have antibodies to ICA69 on western blots but do not immunoprecipitate liquid phase antigen. J Autoimmun 1994;7:665–674.

20. Bonifacio E, Atkinson M, Eisenbarth G, Serreze D, Kay TW, Lee-Chan E, Singh B. International workshop on lessons from animal models for human type 1 diabetes: identification of insulin but not glutamic acid decarboxylase or IA-2 as specific autoantigens of humoral autoimmunity in nonobese diabetic mice. Diabetes 2001;50:2451–2458.

21. Schwab C, Bosshard HR. Caveats for the use of surface-adsorbed protein antigen to test the specificity of antibodies. J Immunol Methods 1992;147:125–134.

22. Achenbach P, Schlosser M, Williams AJK, Yu L, Mueller PW, Bingley PJ, Bonifacio E. Combined testing of antibody titer and affinity improves insulin autoantibody measurement: Diabetes Antibody Standardization Program. Clin Immunol 2007;122:85–90.

23. Mayr A, Schlosser M, Grober N, Kenk H, Ziegler AG, Bonifacio E, Achenbach, P. GAD autoantibody affinity and epitope specificity identify distinct immunization profiles in children at risk for type 1 diabetes. Diabetes 2007;56:1527–1533.

24. Bearzatto M, Lampasona V, Belloni C, Bonifacio E. Fine mapping of diabetes-associated IA-2 specific autoantibodies. J Autoimmun 2003;21:377–382.

25. Bingley PJ, Bonifacio E, Shattock M, Gillmor HA, Sawtell PA, Dunger DB, Scott RD, Bottazzo GF, Gale EA. Can islet cell antibodies predict IDDM in the general population? Diabetes Care 1993;16:45–50.

26. Bingley PJ, Bonifacio E, Williams AJ, Genovese S., Bottazzo GF, Gale EA. Prediction of IDDM in the general population: strategies based on combinations of autoantibody markers. Diabetes 1997;46:1701–1710.

27. Hagopian WA, Sanjeevi CB, Kockum I, Landin-Olsson M, Karlsen AE, Sundkvist G, Dahlquist G, Palmer J, Lernmark A. Glutamate decarboxylase-, insulin-, and islet cell-antibodies and HLA typing to detect diabetes in a general population-based study of Swedish children. J Clin Invest 1995;95:1505–1511.

28. Gleichmann H, Bottazzo GF. Progress toward standardization of cytoplasmic islet cell-antibody assay. Diabetes 1987;36:578–584.

29. Bingley PJ, Williams AJK. Validation of autoantibody assays in type 1 diabetes: Workshop Programme. Autoimmunity 2004;37:257.

30. Verge CF, Stenger D, Bonifacio E, Colman PG, Pilcher C, Bingley PJ, Eisenbarth, GS. Combined use of autoantibodies (IA-2 autoantibody, GAD autoantibody, insulin autoantibody, cytoplasmic islet cell antibodies) in type 1 diabetes: Combinatorial Islet Autoantibody Workshop. Diabetes 1998;47:1857–1866.

31. Törn C, Mueller P, Schlosser M, Bonifacio E, Bingley P. Participating Laboratories. Diabetes Antibody Standardization Program: evaluation of assays for autoantibodies to glutamic acid decarboxylase and islet antigen-2. Diabetologia 2008;51:846–852.

32. Li M, Yu L, Tiberti C, Bonamico M, Taki I, Miao D, Murray JA, Rewers MJ, Hoffenberg EJ, Agardh D, Mueller P, Stern M, Bonifacio E, Liu E. A report on the International Transglutaminase Autoantibody Workshop for Celiac Disease. Am J Gastroenterol 2009;104:154–163.

33. Bonifacio E, Yu L, Williams A, Eisenbarth G, Bingley P, Koczwara K, Mueller P, Schatz D, Krischer J, Steffes M, Akolkar B. Harmonization of GAD and IA.2 autoantibody assays for NIDDK Consortia. Immunology of Diabetes Society 10th International Congress 2009;Abs 135.

34. Ziegler AG, Hummel M, Schenker M, Bonifacio E. Autoantibody appearance and risk for development of childhood diabetes in offspring of parents with type 1 diabetes: the 2-year analysis of the German BABYDIAB Study. Diabetes 1999;48:460–468.

35. Grubin CE, Daniels T, Toivola B, Landin-Olsson M, Hagopian WA, Li L, Karlsen AE, Boel E, Michelsen B, Lernmark A. A novel radioligand binding assay to determine diagnostic accuracy of isoform-specific glutamic acid decarboxylase antibodies in childhood IDDM. Diabetologia 1994;37:344–350.

36. Burbelo PD, Groot S, Dalakas MC, Iadarola MJ. High definition profiling of autoantibodies to glutamic acid decarboxylases GAD65/GAD67 in stiff-person syndrome. Biochem Biophys Res Commun 2008;366:1–7.

37. Burbelo PD, Hirai H, Leahy H, Lernmark A, Ivarsson S, Iadarola MJ, Notkins AL. A new luminescence assay for autoantibodies to mammalian cell-prepared IA-2. Diabetes Care 2008;31:1824–1826

38. Joos TO, Schrenk M, Höpfl P, Kröger K, Chowdhury U, Stoll D, Schörner D, Dürr M, Herick K, Rupp S, Sohn K, Hämmerle H. A microarray enzyme-linked immunosorbent assay for autoimmune diagnostics. Electrophoresis 2000;21:2641–2650.

39. Quintana FJ, Hagedorn PH, Elizur G, Merbl Y, Domany E, Cohen IR. Functional immunomics: microarray analysis of IgG autoantibody repertoires predicts the future response of mice to induced diabetes. Proc Natl Acad Sci USA 2004;101(Suppl 2):14615–14621.

40. Qin S, Qiu W, Ehrlich JR, Ferdinand AS, Richie JP, O'leary MP, Lee MT, Liu BC. Development of a "reverse capture" autoantibody microarray for studies of antigen-autoantibody profiling. Proteomics 2006;6:3199–3209.
41. Hueber W, Utz PJ, Steinman L, Robinson WH. Autoantibody profiling for the study and treatment of autoimmune disease. Arthritis Res 2002;4:290–295.
42. Tiller T, Meffre E, Yurasov S, Tsuiji M, Nussenzweig MC, Wardemann H. Efficient generation of monoclonal antibodies from single human B cells by single cell RT-PCR and expression vector cloning. J Immunol Methods 2008;329:112–124.
43. Wrammert J, Smith K, Miller J, Langley T, Kokko K, Larsen C, Zheng N, Mays I, Garman L, Helms C, James J, Air GM, Capra JD, Ahmed R, Wilson PC. Rapid cloning of high affinity human monoclonal antibodies against influenza virus. Nature 2008;453:667–671.

Chapter 4

Characterizing T-Cell Autoimmunity

Ivana Durinovic-Belló and Gerald T. Nepom

Summary

Immunological mechanisms which precipitate autoimmune diabetes involve the influence of a genetic footprint on the phenotype of the T-cell response to self-antigens, and on development of pathological outcomes in immune responses resulting in T1D. For one of the human diabetes antigens, proinsulin, recent findings allow the emergence of a model in which elements of genetically biased T-cell development and peptide epitope-specific T-cell avidity result in expression of autoimmune disease. Understanding such self-reactive T-cell responses is key to implementation of specific immunotherapies for modulating disease risk and progression.

Key Words: Autoimmunity, Proinsulin, Type 1 diabetes, T lymphocytes

The immune system is delicately balanced between self-antigen-driven tolerance and pathogen-driven immunity, an equilibrium achieved by regulatory mechanisms controlled centrally, during lymphocyte development, and peripherally, during immune activation. Both mechanisms constrain the T-cell functional repertoire by eliminating, silencing, or reprogramming T cells, and are capable of accomplishing this control in an antigen-specific fashion.

MAINTENANCE OF TOLERANCE TO SELF-ANTIGENS

In humans, T cells specific for tissue-restricted antigens are part of a natural T-cell receptor (TCR) repertoire in the periphery of both autoimmune patients and healthy individuals (*1–5*). This raises the fundamental question of whether T-cell selection during development or subsequent T-cell activation in the periphery is the key determinant of autoimmune pathogenesis. In both cases, the interaction of the antigen-specific TCR with self-peptides presented in the context of self-MHC molecules is sufficient to induce a functional program, which is influenced by a host of genetic and environmental factors mediated in large part through cytokines and costimulatory molecules. The strength of the TCR–peptide–MHC interaction itself is probably the most influential of all these factors, however. Defined as functional T-cell avidity, this term represents a measure of T-cell sensitivity to activation by its peptide/MHC (p/MHC) ligand and subsequent induction of signaling and biological function upon interaction with antigen-presenting cell (APC) (*6–9*).

The importance of avidity-based T-cell selection for central tolerance has been demonstrated in animal studies showing that low expression of a strong agonist peptide in the thymus mediates positive selection, while high expression of the same peptide causes clonal deletion of self-reactive thymocytes (*10, 11*). Tolerance induction to self-protein is mediated in the thymus through specialized medullary thymic epithelial cells (mTEC) located in Hassall's corpuscles (*12*), regions of the human thymus containing apoptotic T cells consistent with their role as a site of negative selection (*13*). mTECs promiscuously express antigens which, in later life, are mainly tissue-restricted in expression unique to peripheral organs or expressed during puberty or pregnancy (*14, 15*). They synthesize and directly present self-antigens to CD4+ and CD8+ T cells, resulting in deletion of most high avidity cells, but also lead to selection of regulatory self-specific nTregs for the purpose of tolerance induction (*16, 17*).

Similar mechanisms exist in the periphery to control or eliminate high avidity T cells primed with endogenous amounts of self-antigen. Somewhat analogous to the mTEC lineage, similar nonhematopoietic cells that promiscuously express self-antigens have recently also been found in peripheral lymph nodes, termed lymph node stromal cells (*18*). Both mTECs and lymph node stromal cells express AIRE (and possibly other related genes), a broad-spectrum transcription factor regulator which has been shown to influence the expression level of multiple tissue-restricted antigens (*19–21*). In addition, a secondary network to reinforce tolerance induction may exist, in which immature dendritic cells cross-present self-antigens to T cells by either transporting them from peripheral organs (*22*) or by up-taking them from apoptotic mTECs or stromal lymph node cells (*17, 23*).

Mutations in the AIRE gene cause autoimmune polyendocrine syndrome type I (APS-1) which mostly starts with infection (candidiasis) followed by hypoparathyroidism, Addison's disease and over time multiple autoimmune diseases like T1D, hypothyroidism, pernicious anemia, alopecia, vitiligo, hepatitis, ovarian atrophy, keratitis, and destruction of gastrointestinal endocrine cells (*24, 25*). As autoimmunity spreads, patients successively develop tissue-restricted autoantibodies and T cells which are used as clinical markers of disease progression (*25*). Knockout of the AIRE gene in mouse models produces similar widespread autoimmunity with relatively mild phenotype (*24*). Interestingly, only 18% of APS-1 patients develop T1D (*25*), as well as also only a portion of AIRE knockout mice (*19, 26*) implying that the relative dependence on AIRE for intrathymic transcription of self-antigens is not the only mechanism for targeting a particular organ. Patients with T1D commonly also have appearance of thyroid autoimmunity in 8–50% of the subjects and 21-OH autoimmunity in 1–2% of the subjects, suggesting the possibility that similar shared tolerance mechanisms may interconnect these autoimmune conditions.

Detailed studies of genes expressed by mTECs which are controlled by AIRE have shown that some diabetes-associated autoantigens, but not all, are regulated in this fashion. In particular, insulin, but not GAD or IA-2, show differential expression patterns depending on AIRE expression, which suggests that understanding the autoantigen-specific response to insulin may help clarify the relationship between central and peripheral tolerance mechanisms in autoimmune disease. In mice, there are two forms of insulin encoded by separate genes; both Insulin 1 and Insulin 2 are expressed in the pancreatic beta cells, but Insulin 2 is expressed at a much higher level than Insulin 1 in the thymus. To examine what effect thymic insulin levels may have on the selection or deletion of insulin reactive T cells, the group of C. Polychronakos has produced mice carrying different numbers of insulin gene alleles (*27*). They have observed a decrease in thymic insulin expression levels corresponding to a decrease in the number of insulin gene alleles while pancreatic insulin levels remained constant. Interestingly, mice with low thymic insulin expression showed a spontaneous T-cell reactivity to proinsulin when compared to control animals, consistent with selection of more autoreactive cells. Moreover, defective tolerance to insulin is transferable by thymus transplants (*28*), and in the diabetes prone NOD mice low expression of insulin in the thymus has also been reported and may play a role in disease pathophysiology of this mouse strain (*29*). NOD mice deficient in Insulin 2 gene (NOD-Ins-2KO) have reduced insulin expression levels in the thymus and accelerated T1D development (*30*), and immunization with insulin B-chain APL (alanine substitution in P16) shown to prevent T1D in NOD mice (*31*), could not prevent the disease in NOD-Ins-2KO mice showing that thymic insulin levels play a critical role in T-cell tolerance and disease development of NOD mice (*32*). Furthermore, in the NOD mouse, diabetes development is suppressed either by expressing proinsulin through intranasal vaccination or in tolerogenic dendritic cells (*33–35*); indeed, tolerance to proinsulin abrogated the development of cytotoxic T cells specific for another islet autoantigen, IGRP, indicating that proinsulin autoimmunity is likely an early event during pathogenesis of diabetes in the NOD model (*36*).

In humans, expression levels of insulin are also differentially regulated, due to the direct transcriptional influence of a polymorphic genetic element associated with the proinsulin gene promoter region. Both insulin and the acetylcholine receptor are examples of tissue-restricted self-antigens in autoimmune diseases like T1D and myasthenia gravis (MG), respectively, for which polymorphisms in the promoter regions influence modest (two to fourfold) variations in their thymic expression levels (*37–39*). These moderate differences in the level of self-antigen transcription in mTECs in both diseases have been shown to influence differences in the disease susceptibility (*39–41*). Alleles of proinsulin at the INS-VNTR locus have been classified depending on the number of repeats of the 14 bp long consensus motif as class I (26–63 repeats), class II (63–140 repeats), and class III (141–209 repeats) (*42, 43*), but only class I and class III alleles are present in Caucasian populations. The expression level of both INS and CHRNA1 (acetylcholine receptor) in humans are additive with AIRE expression in that, at a given level of AIRE, insulin transcription is higher in the protective VNTR I/III than in the susceptible I/I haplotype (*15, 44*). The protective class III allele confers three to fourfold higher expression level of insulin in the thymus and is associated with protection from diabetes, whereas class I alleles in homozygous form are associated with lower level of insulin in thymus and an increased relative risk (RR) to T1D that ranges between 1.9 and 5 (*40*). In MG patients the expression level of the protective CHRNA1 allele also shows a clear correlation with AIRE expression in mTECs, while for the susceptible allele this correlation is abolished due to lack of the binding site for the interferon response regulatory factor-8 (IRF-8) in this allele. While the INS-VNTR genotype correlates with incidence of the disease the effect of the CHRNA1 in MG is more subtle and correlates only with the disease onset (*39*).

The INS-VNTR expression pattern in the thymus has been proposed to influence the level of self-tolerance to proinsulin and therefore the pattern and phenotype of the response to proinsulin in the periphery. Mechanisms proposed for this effect are summarized in Table 4.1. Studies in our group and others have demonstrated associations at the functional level of the protective INS-VNTR class III genotype with the protective phenotype of the immune responses to proinsulin in the periphery. Increased IL-10 secretion and regulatory phenotype of T-cell responses to proinsulin epitope, PI73–90, has been associated with this protective VNTR genotype in high risk DRB1*0401 subjects (*45*) as well as the lower frequency of PI73–90 specific CD4+ T cells detected by DRB1*0401-PI73–90 tetramers (*46*). Furthermore, subjects with the protective VNTR genotype have been found to produce lower frequency of anti-insulin antibodies of lower titer (*47*), and recent-onset T1D patients with the protective VNTR allele had more preserved beta cell function (*48*). Also, in identical twins a lower disease concordance rate has been found in subjects with the protective VNTR allele (*49*).

Table 4.1
Associations Between Immunologic Function and Presence of Two *INS-VNTR* Genotypes, the Susceptible Class I/I and the Protective Class III (I/III or III/III), Suggest the Possibility of Stratification of Autoreactive Phenotype Based on *INS-VNTR* Genotype

	INS-VNTR I/I	*INS-VNTR* I/III or III/III
Proinsulin gene expression level in thymus (*37, 38*)	Low	High
Frequency and avidity of proinsulin-specific T cells in the periphery[a]	High	Low
IL-10 secretion (*45*)	Low	High
Frequency and titer of anti-insulin antibodies (*46*)	High	Low
T1D concordance rate of identical twins (*48*)	High	Low
T1D disease association (*40, 41*)	High	Low

Interestingly, genotype variation at INS-VNTR significantly influences disease susceptibility in all HLA genotype risk categories but the distribution of VNTR genotypes varies significantly dependent on HLA genotype (*50*). The VNTR predisposing genotype is significantly less-frequent in high risk HLA genotype-positive patients than in those with intermediate- and low-risk categories (*47, 51, 52*). This stronger association of INS-VNTR with T1D in subjects who do not carry the strong HLA susceptibility genes, compared to subjects with HLA-DR3 and DR4 haplotypes, likely reflects a gradation of cumulative genetic load, in which strong HLA susceptibility overrides the relative predispositional effect of the weaker INS susceptibility genotype. Nonetheless, there is also an interaction between HLA and INS. As shown by Eisenbarth et al. the likelihood that HLA DR3/4 subjects will express early islet-specific autoantibodies is greatest in children who also carry INS susceptibility alleles (*53*).

This type of interaction between the major HLA susceptibility genes and other genes, like INS, which modify disease risk, may be a general phenomenon. For example, protein tyrosine phosphatase N22 (PTPN22) and its gene variant 1858 with single nucleotide change from C to T resulting in single amino acid substitution from arginine to tryptophan at position 620 of the Lyp protein has also been associated with increased risk for the development of T1D (*54–56*) as well as multiple other autoimmune diseases including rheumatoid arthritis (*57*), systemic lupus erythematosus (*58*) and Graves disease (*59*). As with INS-VNTR, however, the PTPN22 effect is more pronounced in subjects with lower-risk HLA haplotypes.

These observations fit models which suggest that additive effects of minor immunologic variations, or perhaps specific combinations of such variations, are sufficient to confer disease risk through mechanisms of failed immunological tolerance. In the case of INS, perhaps the avidity of HLA molecules for proinsulin peptides and the level of these peptides in thymus act as key regulators of T1D autoimmunity through their effects on T-cell selection (50). For genes such as PTPN22, which influence the strength of T-cell activation, perhaps allelic variation is sufficient to modify thresholds for deletional tolerance. Cumulatively, these types of effects can determine the selection of the TCR repertoire by influencing the extent and avidity spectrum of the deleted self-reactive effector cell repertoire, the selection and skewing of the regulatory T-cell repertoire, and ultimately manifestation of autoimmunity (60).

PERIPHERAL AUTOREACTIVITY IN T1D

While central tolerance mechanisms are key regulators of autoreactive T-cell repertoire, T cells with self-antigen specificity nevertheless routinely survive, and populate the periphery (61, 62). In many cases, these are low avidity cells which represent the potential for autoimmunity when peripheral conditions, such as activation by higher nonphysiological levels of self-antigen or by a mimic of the self-antigen and proinflammatory conditions, lead to loss of tolerance (17, 63). When this occurs, T cells with self-antigen specificity are found in the periphery which carry phenotypic markers of memory, chronic activation, and high avidity, indicating their in vivo reactivation in association with pathogenic responses in patients (3, 5).

Insulin is an important antigen in T1D autoimmunity, most likely the primary causative antigen in the NOD mouse, and a target autoantigen in many human T1D subjects. T-cell reactivity to a major proinsulin epitope, PI73–90, occurs as early marker of disease progression in the prediabetic stage of high risk DRB1*0401 subjects, followed by intra- and intermolecular spreading of T-cell response to other epitopes of proinsulin as well as to the additional self-proteins (64, 65). In addition, high titer insulin autoantibodies may appear as a first marker of the disease initiation in early childhood (6–12 months of age) (66–68), consistent with an important role of proinsulin in T1D autoimmunity.

In subjects with T1D, numerous proinsulin T-cell epitopes have been identified; in addition to epitopes identified within the insulin A and B chains (2, 65, 69), earlier studies have also identified several dominant epitopes within the C peptide and

B–C chain junction (*70*) and the C–A chain junction region of proinsulin (*71–73*). The later include preproinsulin (PPI) 73–90 (PI C17-A1), PPI 74–90 (PI C18-A1), PPI 69–88 (PI C13-C32), PPI 75–92 (PI C19-A3), and PPI 77–94 (PI C21-A5) (*1, 2, 65, 69, 74*). The PPI 69–88, PPI 75–92, and PPI 77–94 peptides are found on the cell surface of antigen-presenting cells that express HLA-DR0401 after pulsing these cells with preproinsulin (*1*), and the core region PPI 76–90 (PI C20-A1) SLQPLALEGSLQKR↓G, contains a DR0401-binding motif (this epitope is not a conventional product of endopeptidase II cleavage [↓ indicates the endopeptidase II cleavage site for the conversion of preproinsulin to insulin]). In our previous studies we have shown that in young DRB1*0401 subjects with islet-cell autoimmunity, CD4+ T-cell responses to PPI 73–90 are a marker of disease progression (*2, 65*). The cytokines seen in the mixed PBMC response to PPI 73–90 were predominantly of down-regulatory T helper (Th) 2 phenotype (IL-4, IL-5 and IL-10) (*2*). However, even within a single individual, PPI 73–90 specific responses demonstrated various cytokine output profiles. The same PPI 73–90 epitope was also found as immunodominant in humanized HLA-DR4/CD4 double-transgenic mice immunized with human proinsulin (*69*). Although functional differences distinguishing pathogenic from beneficial T-cell responses in T1D autoimmunity are still under active investigation, there are strong implications that they might be caused by variations in their frequency, cytokine phenotype, and ratio of major cell subsets, i.e., Th1 and Th17 (*1–5, 75*) vs. Th2 and Th10 (*76*) vs. Treg and Th35 (*77–79*), which may also differ in their avidity for antigen-MHC ligands (*80–82*).

In human autoimmune diseases many epitopes recognized by autoreactive T cells are of moderate or low avidity, which may allow these cells to escape deletional tolerance mechanisms and promote their survival in the periphery. To improve the detection of low avidity CD4+ self-reactive T cells in T1D, HLA class II tetramer reagents have been developed with agonist peptides where a single amino acid substitution was exchanged to improve the binding of the tetramer to the antigen-specific TCR (*83, 84*). Recently, using the immunodominant proinsulin epitope (PI76–90) of DRB1*0401 subjects with diabetes autoimmunity (*1, 65, 74*), with substitution of lysine to serine at peptide position p9 (super-agonist), a tetramer positive CD4 T-cell population could be readily detected in T1D patients but not in healthy subjects (*5*). This indicates that T cells of T1D patients (similar to T cells of NOD mice) likely have undergone avidity maturation in the course of disease progression, whereas T cells of healthy control subjects remained of low avidity. Figure 4.1 is an example of the detection of insulin-specific CD4+ T cells using human class II tetramers representing the PI76–90 epitope.

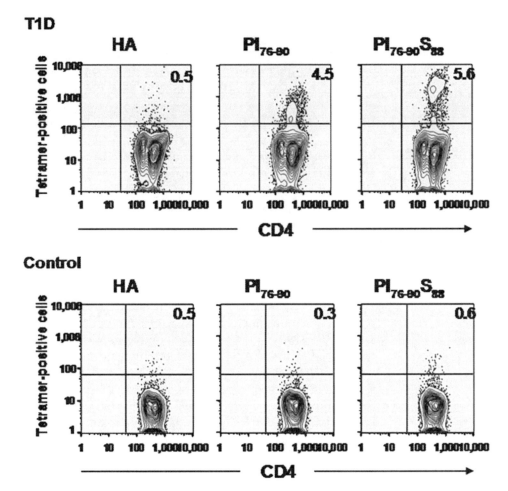

Fig. 4.1 HLA class II tetramer analysis of proinsulin-specific CD4+ T cells from two HLA-DRB1*0401/*INS-VNTR* I/I subjects. CD4+ T cells specific for the proinsulin epitope, PI76–90 are present in the peripheral lymphocyte population. CD4+ T cells were enriched from peripheral blood lymphocytes of HLA-DRB1*0401 subjects by no-touch microbead selection (Miltenyi Biotec) followed by depletion of CD4+CD25+ T cells. Purified CD4+CD25– T cells were stimulated for 14 days with 10 μg/ml of the immunodominant PI76–90 peptide (*1, 65, 74*) or its substituted superagonist variant PI76–90S88, which contains a lysine to serine substitution at peptide position p9. Autologous CD4– cells were plated in microwells, and the adherent population used as antigen-presenting cells; on days 6, 9, and 11, IL-2 (10 IU/ml) was added to the cultures. Tetramer-binding analyses were performed on day 14 using either PI76–90, PI76–90S88 peptides, or irrelevant control (HA306–318), each loaded into DRB1*0401 Tetramers. Binding was evaluated by flow cytometry on a gated CD4+ T-cell population and frequency of CD4+ TMr positive cells is shown on the upper right quadrant. In these representative examples, proinsulin tetramer positive cells were readily detected in a T1D patient but not in the healthy control (*5, 83, 84*).

Apart from T-cell avidity maturation, a number of additional mechanisms have been proposed to contribute to leaky tolerance by quantitative and qualitative alterations of self-antigen in peripheral tissues. They include posttranslational modification through mechanisms like glycosylation (*85, 86*), transglutamination (*87*), or citrullination (*88*), perhaps happening preferentially in an inflammatory environment which creates T-cell epitopes unique to peripheral tissues which are absent from mTEC lineages (*89*). Insulin-specific T cells have been described in subjects with islet-cell autoimmunity which recognize a CD4+ T-cell epitope of insulin A-chain, A1–13 which has been posttranslationally modified (*72*). T-cell recognition was dependent on the formation of a vicinal disulfide bond between adjacent cysteine residues A6 and A7 which occurs during refolding of insulin and its oxidation in vitro, and after presentation of recombinant and native proinsulin (*90*).

Another intriguing possibility for the generation of peripheral neoepitopes is differential splicing of autoantigens. In particular, tyrosine phosphatase-like protein (IA-2), another autoantigen in T1D, was found to be enriched in the secretory granules of pancreatic islet cells and neuroendocrine cells but also in the thymus and peripheral lymphoid organs (*91*). Unlike insulin transcription polymorphisms in the thymus associated with T1D susceptibility, no association of IA-2 or GAD65 expression in thymus has been associated with T1D. Interestingly, however, pancreatic islets express full length IA-2 mRNA, whereas thymus and spleen exclusively express an alternatively spliced transcript lacking exon 13 (*92*). Since the protein region deleted in this IA-2 splice variant comprises several epitopes implicated in T1D autoimmunity, this finding supports the possibility that tolerance to these epitopes may not been achieved in the thymus, allowing for a peripheral mechanism breaking self-tolerance which may play a permissive role in T1D autoimmunity.

THERAPEUTIC TARGETING OF ANTIGEN-SPECIFIC AUTOREACTIVE T CELLS

In most human autoimmune disorders, as in T1D, an evolving and expanding immune response to self-antigens occurs during the course of disease progression. Autoreactive T cells recognize large numbers of diverse epitopes within the same autoantigen (epitope spreading) as well as increasing numbers of autoantigens (intermolecular spreading) (*64, 65, 93, 94*). Most likely, continuous tissue damage in the target organ under proinflammatory conditions liberates sufficient autoantigen to prime these cumulative immune responses. In spite of this daunting complexity, however, it appears that single dominant antigenic responses can have major impact, both in the initiation and in the regulation of disease. In experimental models it has been shown that loss of tolerance to a single autoantigen can be sufficient to cause organ-specific autoimmune disease, even in otherwise self-tolerant organism (*95*). And with respect to therapy, regulatory responses can be invoked by single peptide epitopes which, through a mechanism known as bystander suppression or "infectious tolerance," can modulate tissue-specific polyclonal responses (*96–99*).

In animal models, numerous peptide approaches have been described which have successfully delayed or prevented autoimmunity, using different protocols varying route, timing or dose of soluble peptide injection as well as different adjuvants. Successful mechanisms of pathogenic effector T cells inactivation include activation-induced cell death (AICD) and apoptosis (*100, 101*), anergy defined as unresponsive state in which T cell cannot proliferate or produce IL-2 after TCR stimulation (*102*) and regulation through either naturally occurring Treg (*103*) or cytokine-secreting Treg which do not necessarily express Foxp3 but secrete IL-10 or TGFβ (*104, 105*). Peptide dose is an important determining factor which influences the outcome of immunization (*106*), high dose of peptide administered either orally or intravenously can induce deletion (*107*), anergy (*108*), or apoptosis (*109*), and low dose of peptide on the other hand administered orally can induce cells of Th3 (TR1) subtype which produce TGFβ and IL-10 (*107, 110*). Induction of bystander suppression for therapeutic intervention by generating potent regulatory populations that inhibit other activated immune cells in the affected organ are especially promising. This may have broad therapeutic potential, as there is evidence that nTreg cells not only suppress adaptive T-cell responses, but are also able to down-modulate antigen-presenting cells and may also control pathology mediated by innate immunity. As shown recently in the mouse model of bacterially triggered intestinal inflammation, T-cell independent intestinal pathology caused by activation of the innate immune system appeared to be inhibited by Treg cells (*111*).

These examples illustrate the potential for translation of antigen-specific therapeutics to human disease, and several peptide- or protein-therapy approaches are currently under development or in clinical trials. Recently a human phase 1 safety study has been performed with a natural peptide sequence of proinsulin PI76–92 tested in long standing T1D patients in two doses, low (30 μg) and high (300 μg) with the goal to evaluate two major risks of peptide therapy, induction of hypersensitivity (*112, 113*) and exacerbation of the proinflammatory autoimmune response (*114*). Lower doses of peptide have been well tolerated and have induced transitory IL-10 secreting peptide-specific T cells, thus encouraging progression to phase II clinical trials. In another set of clinical trials, an altered peptide ligand of insulin B-chain, amino acid region B9–23, which can be recognized by IFNg producing Th1 lymphocytes in T1D patients, was administered subcutaneously to T1D subjects early after diagnosis. No therapeutic benefit on metabolic control was achieved, although in vitro studies suggested the possibility of shifting Th1 responses to a Th2 phenotype (*115*). An alternate route of administration, via the nasal mucosa, has also been evaluated in a pilot safety study in subjects at risk for T1D (*116*). The results suggest that intranasal insulin does not accelerate loss of beta-cell function in individuals at risk for T1D and may induce immune changes consistent with mucosal tolerance to insulin. A similar study was recently undertaken with alum-formulated human recombinant GAD65, administered subcutaneously in Latent Autoimmune Diabetes in Adults (LADA) patients (*117*) and in recent-onset T1D subjects (*118*), also documenting safety in humans, with some preliminary evidence of potential immune deviation.

Looking forward, there are new opportunities to strategically evaluate the function of various candidate peptides in triggering the cascade of pathological vs. protective events before going into human clinical trials. For example, if human genetic variation in the INS-VNTR influences the character of the autoreactive T-cell response to INS, it is possible that response to therapy with differing doses or routes of insulin peptide administration may lead to differential outcomes. Using humanized animal models with inserted portions of the human genome consisting of various combinations of genes shown to be associated with the disease is one such approach: For this purpose NOD mice with complete gene knock-outs for murine insulin and rescued by the human INS gene knock-in have been generated in the laboratory of C. Polychronakos (human and mouse proinsulin differ in 17 amino acids) (*119, 120*). Two strains of these mice have been generated by now, one containing the INS promoter with T1D predisposing VNTR class I allele and the other with the protective class III allele. The allelic VNTR transgenes recapitulate the human transcriptional effect, in that the VNTR class III human proinsulin expression is threefold higher in thymus and lower in pancreas, relative to the VNTR class I expression (*38, 45*). Importantly, both strains develop diabetes, VNTR class I mice with higher frequency than class III mice. These animals are being intercrossed with HLA-DRB1*0401 mice and will be used to reconstitute proinsulin peptide responses of pathogenic vs. protective T cells through transgenic or retrogenic (*121*) insertion of TCR genes. This model, and others like it, will be necessary to address questions of human genetic variation and phenotypic heterogeneity in the character of the autoreactive T-cell response, particularly for antigen-specific approaches to modify the functional phenotype of the autoimmune response in vivo.

REFERENCES

1. Arif S, Tree TI, Astill TP, et al. Autoreactive T cell responses show proinflammatory polarization in diabetes but a regulatory phenotype in health. J Clin Invest 2004;113(3):451–463.
2. Durinovic-Belló I, Schlosser M, Riedl M, et al. Pro- and anti-inflammatory cytokine production by autoimmune T cells against preproinsulin in HLA-DRB1*04, DQ8 type 1 diabetes. Diabetologia 2004;47:439–450.
3. Monti P, Scirpoli M, Rigamonti A, et al. Evidence for in vivo primed and expanded autoreactive T cells as a specific feature of patients with type 1 diabetes. J Immunol 2007;179(9):5785–5792.
4. Viglietta V, Kent SC, Orban T, Hafler DA. GAD65-reactive T cells are activated in patients with autoimmune type 1a diabetes. J Clin Invest 2002;109(7):895–903.

5. Yang J, Danke N, Roti M, et al. CD4+ T cells from type 1 diabetic and healthy subjects exhibit different thresholds of activation to a naturally processed proinsulin epitope. J Autoimmun 2008;31:30–41.
6. Alegre ML, Frauwirth KA, Thompson CB. T-cell regulation by CD28 and CTLA-4. Nat Rev Immunol 2001;1(3):220–228.
7. Nikolich-Zugich J, Slifka MK, Messaoudi I. The many important facets of T-cell repertoire diversity. Nat Rev Immunol 2004;4(2):123–132.
8. Friedl P, den Boer AT, Gunzer M. Tuning immune responses: diversity and adaptation of the immunological synapse. Nat Rev Immunol 2005;5(7):532–545.
9. Huppa JB, Gleimer M, Sumen C, Davis MM. Continuous T cell receptor signaling required for synapse maintenance and full effector potential. Nat Immunol 2003;4(8):749–755.
10. Sebzda E, Wallace VA, Mayer J, Yeung RS, Mak TW, Ohashi PS. Positive and negative thymocyte selection induced by different concentrations of a single peptide. Science 1994;263(5153):1615–1618.
11. Laurie KL, La Gruta NL, Koch N, van Driel IR, Gleeson PA. Thymic expression of a gastritogenic epitope results in positive selection of self-reactive pathogenic T cells. J Immunol 2004;172(10):5994–6002.
12. Chentoufi AA, Palumbo M, Polychronakos C. Proinsulin expression by Hassall's corpuscles in the mouse thymus. Diabetes 2004;53(2):354–359.
13. Douek DC, Altmann DM. T-cell apoptosis and differential human leucocyte antigen class II expression in human thymus. Immunology 2000;99(2):249–256.
14. Derbinski J, Schulte A, Kyewski B, Klein L. Promiscuous gene expression in medullary thymic epithelial cells mirrors the peripheral self. Nat Immunol 2001;2(11):1032–1039.
15. Kyewski B, Klein L. A central role for central tolerance. Annu Rev Immunol 2006;24:571–606.
16. Aschenbrenner K, D'Cruz LM, Vollmann EH, et al. Selection of Foxp3+ regulatory T cells specific for self antigen expressed and presented by Aire+ medullary thymic epithelial cells. Nat Immunol 2007;8(4):351–358.
17. Zehn D, Bevan MJ. More promiscuity resulting in more tolerance. Nat Immunol 2007;8:120–122.
18. Lee J. Nat Immunol 2007;8:181–190.
19. Anderson MS, Venanzi ES, Klein L, et al. Projection of an immunological self shadow within the thymus by the aire protein. Science 2002;298(5597):1395–1401.
20. Liston A, Lesage S, Wilson J, Peltonen L, Goodnow CC. Aire regulates negative selection of organ-specific T cells. Nat Immunol 2003;4(4):350–354.
21. Gardner JM, Devoss JJ, Friedman RS, et al. Deletional tolerance mediated by extrathymic Aire-expressing cells. Science 2008;321(5890):843–847.
22. Bonasio R, Scimone ML, Schaerli P, Grabie N, Lichtman AH, von Andrian UH. Clonal deletion of thymocytes by circulating dendritic cells homing to the thymus. Nat Immunol 2006;7(10):1092–1100.
23. Bonasio R, von Andrian UH. Generation, migration and function of circulating dendritic cells. Curr Opin Immunol 2006;18(4):503–511.
24. Cheng MH, Shum AK, Anderson MS. What's new in the Aire? Trends Immunol 2007;28(7):321–327.
25. Eisenbarth GS. Autoimmune polyendocrine syndromes. Adv Exp Med Biol 2004;552:204–218.
26. Jiang W, Anderson MS, Bronson R, Mathis D, Benoist C. Modifier loci condition autoimmunity provoked by Aire deficiency. J Exp Med 2005;202(6):805–815.
27. Chentoufi AA, Polychronakos C. Insulin expression levels in the thymus modulate insulin-specific autoreactive T-cell tolerance: the mechanism by which the IDDM2 locus may predispose to diabetes. Diabetes 2002;51(5):1383–1390.
28. Faideau B, Lotton C, Lucas B, et al. Tolerance to proinsulin-2 is due to radioresistant thymic cells. J Immunol 2006;177(1):53–60.
29. Brimnes MK, Jensen T, Jorgensen TN, Michelsen BK, Troelsen J, Werdelin O. Low expression of insulin in the thymus of non-obese diabetic mice. J Autoimmun 2002;19(4):203–213.
30. Thebault-Baumont K, Dubois-Laforgue D, Krief P, et al. Acceleration of type 1 diabetes mellitus in proinsulin 2-deficient NOD mice. J Clin Invest 2003;111(6):851–857.
31. Nakayama M, Babaya N, Miao D, et al. Long-term prevention of diabetes and marked suppression of insulin autoantibodies and insulitis in mice lacking native insulin B9-23 sequence. Ann N Y Acad Sci 2006;1079:122–129.
32. Nakayama M, Abiru N, Marlyama H, et al. Prime role for an insulin epitope in the development of type 1 diabetes in NOD mice. Nature 2005;435:220–223.
33. Every AL, Kramer DR, Mannering SI, Lew AM, Harrison LC. Intranasal vaccination

with proinsulin DNA induces regulatory CD4+ T cells that prevent experimental autoimmune diabetes. J Immunol 2006; 176(8):4608–4615.
34. Fernando MM, Stevens CR, Sabeti PC, et al. Identification of two independent risk factors for lupus within the MHC in United Kingdom families. PLoS Genet 2007; 3(11):e192.
35. Steptoe RJ, Ritchie JM, Jones LK, Harrison LC. Autoimmune diabetes is suppressed by transfer of proinsulin-encoding Gr-1+ myeloid progenitor cells that differentiate in vivo into resting dendritic cells. Diabetes 2005;54(2):434–442.
36. Krishnamurthy B, Dudek NL, McKenzie MD, et al. Responses against islet antigens in NOD mice are prevented by tolerance to proinsulin but not IGRP. J Clin Invest 2006; 116(12):3258–3265.
37. Pugliese A, Zeller M, Fernandez A, et al. The insulin gene is transcribed in the human thymus and transcription levels correlated with allelic variation at the INS VNTR-IDDM2 susceptibility locus for type 1 diabetes. Nat Genet 1997;15(3):293–297.
38. Vafiadis P, Bennett ST, Todd JA, et al. Insulin expression in human thymus is modulated by INS VNTR alleles at the IDDM2 locus. Nat Genet 1997;15(3):289–292.
39. Giraud M, Taubert R, Vandiedonck C, et al. An IRF8-binding promoter variant and AIRE control CHRNA1 promiscuous expression in thymus. Nature 2007;448(7156):934–937.
40. Undlien DE, Bennett ST, Todd JA, et al. Insulin gene region-encoded susceptibility to IDDM maps upstream of the insulin gene. Diabetes 1995;44(6):620–625.
41. Liston A, Lesage S, Gray DH, Boyd RL, Goodnow CC. Genetic lesions in T-cell tolerance and thresholds for autoimmunity. Immunol Rev 2005;204:87–101.
42. Bennett ST, Lucassen AM, Gough SC, et al. Susceptibility to human type 1 diabetes at IDDM2 is determined by tandem repeat variation at the insulin gene minisatellite locus. Nat Genet 1995;9(3):284–292.
43. Lucassen AM, Julier C, Beressi JP, et al. Susceptibility to insulin dependent diabetes mellitus maps to a 4.1 kb segment of DNA spanning the insulin gene and associated VNTR. Nat Genet 1993;4(3):305–310.
44. Sabater L, Ferrer-Francesch X, Sospedra M, Caro P, Juan M, Pujol-Borrell R. Insulin alleles and autoimmune regulator (AIRE) gene expression both influence insulin expression in the thymus. J Autoimmun 2005;25(4):312–318.

45. Durinovic-Belló I, Jelinek E, Eiermann T, et al. Class III alleles at the insulin VNTR polymorphism are associated with regulatory T-cell responses to proinsulin epitopes in HLA-DR4, DQ8 individuals. Diabetes 2005;54(Suppl 2):S18–S24.
46. Durinovic-Belló I, Wu R, Gersuk V, Sanda S, Shiling H and Nepom GT, Genetic control of the autoimmune response to proinsulin, Genes and Immunity 2010;11:188–193.
47. Walter M, Albert E, Conrad M, et al. IDDM2/insulin VNTR modifies risk conferred by IDDM1/HLA for development of type 1 diabetes and associated autoimmunity. Diabetologia 2003;46(5):712–720.
48. Nielsen LB, Mortensen HB, Chiarelli F, et al. Impact of IDDM2 on disease pathogenesis and progression in children with newly diagnosed type 1 diabetes: reduced insulin antibody titres and preserved beta cell function. Diabetologia 2006;49(1):71–74.
49. Hermann R, Laine AP, Veijola R, et al. The effect of HLA class II, insulin and CTLA4 gene regions on the development of humoral beta cell autoimmunity. Diabetologia 2005;48(9):1766–1775.
50. Motzo C, Contu D, Cordell HJ, et al. Heterogeneity in the magnitude of the insulin gene effect on HLA risk in type 1 diabetes. Diabetes 2004;53(12):3286–3291.
51. Bain SC, Prins JB, Hearne CM, et al. Insulin gene region-encoded susceptibility to type 1 diabetes is not restricted to HLA-DR4-positive individuals. Nat Genet 1992;2(3): 212–215.
52. Laine AP, Hermann R, Knip M, Simell O, Akerblom HK, Ilonen J. The human leukocyte antigen genotype has a modest effect on the insulin gene polymorphism-associated susceptibility to type 1 diabetes in the Finnish population. Tissue Antigens 2004;63(1):72–74.
53. Lamb MM, Myers MA, Barriga K, Zimmet PZ, Rewers M, Norris JM. Maternal diet during pregnancy and islet autoimmunity in offspring. Pediatr Diabetes 2008;9(2):135–141.
54. Bottini N, Musumeci L, Alonso A, et al. A functional variant of lymphoid tyrosine phosphatase is associated with type I diabetes. Nat Genet 2004;36(4):337–338.
55. Bottini N, Vang T, Cucca F, Mustelin T. Role of PTPN22 in type 1 diabetes and other autoimmune diseases. Semin Immunol 2006;18(4):207–213.
56. Smyth D, Cooper JD, Collins JE, et al. Replication of an association between the lymphoid tyrosine phosphatase locus (LYP/PTPN22) with type 1 diabetes, and evidence

for its role as a general autoimmunity locus. Diabetes 2004;53(11):3020–3023.
57. Begovich AB, Carlton VE, Honigberg LA, et al. A missense single-nucleotide polymorphism in a gene encoding a protein tyrosine phosphatase (PTPN22) is associated with rheumatoid arthritis. Am J Hum Genet 2004;75(2):330–337.
58. Kyogoku C, Langefeld CD, Ortmann WA, et al. Genetic association of the R620W polymorphism of protein tyrosine phosphatase PTPN22 with human SLE. Am J Hum Genet 2004;75(3):504–507.
59. Velaga MR, Wilson V, Jennings CE, et al. The codon 620 tryptophan allele of the lymphoid tyrosine phosphatase (LYP) gene is a major determinant of Graves' disease. J Clin Endocrinol Metab 2004;89(11):5862–5865.
60. Kyewski B, Taubert R. How promiscuity promotes tolerance: the case of myasthenia gravis. Ann N Y Acad Sci 2008;1132: 157–162.
61. Reijonen H, Novak EJ, Kochik S, et al. Detection of GAD65-specific T-cells by major histocompatibility complex class II tetramers in type 1 diabetic patients and at-risk subjects. Diabetes 2002;51(5):1375–1382.
62. Zehn D, Bevan MJ. T cells with low avidity for a tissue-restricted antigen routinely evade central and peripheral tolerance and cause autoimmunity. Immunity 2006;25:261–270.
63. van den Boorn JG, Le Poole IC, Luiten RM. T-cell avidity and tuning: the flexible connection between tolerance and autoimmunity. Int Rev Immunol 2006;25(3–4):235–258.
64. Durinovic-Belló I, Hummel M, Ziegler AG. Cellular immune response to diverse islet cell antigens in IDDM. Diabetes 1996;45(6): 795–800.
65. Durinovic-Belló I, Boehm BO, Ziegler AG. Predominantly recognized proinsulin T helper cell epitopes in individuals with and without islet cell autoimmunity. J Autoimmun 2002;18(1):55–66.
66. Barker JM, Barriga KJ, Yu L, et al. Prediction of autoantibody positivity and progression to type 1 diabetes: diabetes autoimmunity study in the young (DAISY). J Clin Endocrinol Metab 2004;89(8):3896–3902.
67. Hummel M, Williams AJ, Norcross A, et al. Proinsulin-specific autoantibodies are relatively infrequent in young offspring with pre-type 1 diabetes. Diabetes Care 2001;24(10): 1843–1844.
68. Ziegler AG, Hummel M, Schenker M, Bonifacio E. Autoantibody appearance and risk for development of childhood diabetes in offspring of parents with type 1 diabetes: the 2-year analysis of the German BABYDIAB study. Diabetes 1999;48(3):460–468.
69. Congia M, Patel S, Cope AP, De Virgiliis S, Sonderstrup G. T cell epitopes of insulin defined in HLA-DR4 transgenic mice are derived from preproinsulin and proinsulin. Proc Natl Acad Sci U S A 1998;95(7): 3833–3838.
70. Semana G, Gausling R, Jackson RA, Hafler DA. T cell autoreactivity to proinsulin epitopes in diabetic patients and healthy subjects. J Autoimmun 1999;12(4):259–267.
71. Mannering SI, Morris JS, Stone NL, Jensen KP, van Endert PM, Harrison LC. CD4+ T cell proliferation in response to GAD and proinsulin in healthy, pre-diabetic, and diabetic donors. Ann N Y Acad Sci 2004;1037: 16–21.
72. Mannering SI, Harrison LC, Williamson NA, et al. The insulin A-chain epitope recognized by human T cells is posttranslationally modified. J Exp Med 2005;202(9):1191–1197.
73. Kent CS, Chen Y, Bregoli L, et al. Expended T cells from pancreatic lymph nodes of type 1 diabetic subjects recognize an insulin epitope. Nature 2005;435:224–228.
74. Durinovic-Belló I, Rosinger S, Olson J, et al. DRB1*0401-restricted human T-cell clone, specific for the major proinsulin73–90 epitope expresses a down regulatory T helper 2 phenotype. Proc Natl Acad Sci U S A 2006;103(31):11683–11688.
75. Acosta-Rodriguez EV, Rivino L, Geginat J, et al. Surface phenotype and antigenic specificity of human interleukin 17-producing T helper memory cells. Nat Immunol 2007;8(6):639–646.
76. Trinchieri G. Interleukin-10 production by effector T cells: Th1 cells show self control. J Exp Med 2007;204(2):239–243.
77. Collison LW, Workman CJ, Kuo TT, et al. The inhibitory cytokine IL-35 contributes to regulatory T-cell function. Nature 2007; 450(7169):566–569.
78. Fontenot JD, Gavin MA, Rudensky AY. Foxp3 programs the development and function of CD4+CD25+ regulatory T cells. Nat Immunol 2003;4(4):330–336.
79. Sakaguchi S, Sakaguchi N, Asano M, Itoh M, Toda M. Immunologic self-tolerance maintained by activated T cells expressing IL-2 receptor alpha-chains (CD25). Breakdown of a single mechanism of self-tolerance causes various autoimmune diseases. J Immunol 1995;155(3):1151–1164.
80. Amrani A, Verdaguer J, Serra P, Tafuro S, Tan R, Santamaria P. Progression of autoimmune

80. diabetes driven by avidity maturation of a T-cell population. Nature 2000;406(6797):739–742.
81. Mallone R, Kochik SA, Laughlin EM, et al. Differential recognition and activation thresholds in human autoreactive GAD-specific T-cells. Diabetes 2004;53(4):971–977.
82. Mallone R, Kochik SA, Reijonen H, et al. Functional avidity directs T-cell fate in autoreactive CD4+ T cells. Blood 2005;106(8):2798–2805.
83. Danke NA, Yang J, Greenbaum C, Kwok WW. Comparative study of GAD65-specific CD4+ T cells in healthy and type 1 diabetic subjects. J Autoimmun 2005;25(4):303–311.
84. Yang J, Danke NA, Berger D, et al. Islet-specific glucose-6-phosphatase catalytic subunit-related protein-reactive CD4+ T cells in human subjects. J Immunol 2006;176(5):2781–2789.
85. Backlund J, Carlsen S, Hoger T, et al. Predominant selection of T cells specific for the glycosylated collagen type II epitope (263–270) in humanized transgenic mice and in rheumatoid arthritis. Proc Natl Acad Sci U S A 2002;99(15):9960–9965.
86. Savage PA, Boniface JJ, Davis MM. A kinetic basis for T cell receptor repertoire selection during an immune response. Immunity 1999;10(4):485–492.
87. Molberg O, McAdam SN, Korner R, et al. Tissue transglutaminase selectively modifies gliadin peptides that are recognized by gut-derived T cells in celiac disease. Nat Med 1998;4(6):713–717.
88. Hill JA, Southwood S, Sette A, Jevnikar AM, Bell DA, Cairns E. Cutting edge: the conversion of arginine to citrulline allows for a high-affinity peptide interaction with the rheumatoid arthritis-associated HLA-DRB1*0401 MHC class II molecule. J Immunol 2003;171(2):538–541.
89. Holmdahl R. Aire-ing self antigen variability and tolerance. Eur J Immunol 2007;37(3):598–601.
90. Hua QX, Jia W, Frank BH, Phillips NF, Weiss MA. A protein caught in a kinetic trap: structures and stabilities of insulin disulfide isomers. Biochemistry 2002;41(50):14700–14715.
91. Solimena M, Dirkx R Jr, Hermel JM, et al. ICA 512, an autoantigen of type I diabetes, is an intrinsic membrane protein of neurosecretory granules. EMBO J 1996;15(9):2102–2114.
92. Diez J, Park Y, Zeller M, et al. Differential splicing of the IA-2 mRNA in pancreas and lymphoid organs as a permissive genetic mechanism for autoimmunity against the IA-2 type 1 diabetes autoantigen. Diabetes 2001;50(4):895–900.
93. Lehmann PV, Forsthuber T, Miller A, Sercarz EE. Spreading of T-cell autoimmunity to cryptic determinants of an autoantigen. Nature 1992;358(6382):155–157.
94. Vanderlugt CL, Miller SD. Epitope spreading in immune-mediated diseases: implications for immunotherapy. Nat Rev Immunol 2002;2(2):85–95.
95. DeVoss J, Hou Y, Johannes K, et al. Spontaneous autoimmunity prevented by thymic expression of a single self-antigen. J Exp Med 2006;203(12):2727–2735.
96. Brusko TM, Putnam AL, Bluestone JA. Human regulatory T cells: role in autoimmune disease and therapeutic opportunities. Immunol Rev 2008;223:371–390.
97. Qin S, Cobbold SP, Pope H, et al. "Infectious" transplantation tolerance. Science 1993;259(5097):974–977.
98. Cobbold S, Waldmann H. Infectious tolerance. Curr Opin Immunol 1998;10(5):518–524.
99. Waldmann H, Adams E, Fairchild P, Cobbold S. Regulation and privilege in transplantation tolerance. J Clin Immunol 2008;28(6):716–725.
100. Green DR. Apoptotic pathways: paper wraps stone blunts scissors. Cell 2000;102(1):1–4.
101. Lenardo M, Chan KM, Hornung F, et al. Mature T lymphocyte apoptosis-immune regulation in a dynamic and unpredictable antigenic environment. Annu Rev Immunol 1999;17:221–253.
102. Singh NJ, Schwartz RH. The strength of persistent antigenic stimulation modulates adaptive tolerance in peripheral CD4+ T cells. J Exp Med 2003;198(7):1107–1117.
103. Fontenot JD, Rasmussen JP, Williams LM, Dooley JL, Farr AG, Rudensky AY. Regulatory T cell lineage specification by the forkhead transcription factor Foxp3. Immunity 2005;22:329–341.
104. Vieira PL, Christensen JR, Minaee S, et al. IL-10-secreting regulatory T cells do not express Foxp3 but have comparable regulatory function to naturally occurring CD4+CD25+ regulatory T cells. J Immunol 2004;172(10):5986–5993.
105. Anderson PO, Sundstedt A, Yazici Z, et al. IL-2 overcomes the unresponsiveness but fails to reverse the regulatory function of antigen-induced T regulatory cells. J Immunol 2005;174(1):310–319.
106. Mitchison NA. The dosage requirements for immunological paralysis by soluble proteins. Immunology 1968;15(4):509–530.
107. Chen Y, Inobe J, Marks R, Gonnella P, Kuchroo VK, Weiner HL. Peripheral dele-

108. Liblau RS, Pearson CI, Shokat K, Tisch R, Yang XD, McDevitt HO. High-dose soluble antigen: peripheral T-cell proliferation or apoptosis. Immunol Rev 1994;142:193–208.
109. Friedman A, Weiner HL. Induction of anergy or active suppression following oral tolerance is determined by antigen dosage. Proc Natl Acad Sci U S A 1994;91(14):6688–6692.
110. Kearney ER, Pape KA, Loh DY, Jenkins MK. Visualization of peptide-specific T cell immunity and peripheral tolerance induction in vivo. Immunity 1994;1(4):327–339.
111. Maloy KJ, Salaun L, Cahill R, Dougan G, Saunders NJ, Powrie F. CD4+CD25+ T(R) cells suppress innate immune pathology through cytokine-dependent mechanisms. J Exp Med 2003;197(1):111–119.
112. McDevitt H. Specific antigen vaccination to treat autoimmune disease. Proc Natl Acad Sci U S A 2004;101:14627–14630.
113. Pedotti R, Sanna M, Tsai M, et al. Severe anaphylactic reactions to glutamic acid decarboxylase (GAD) self peptides in NOD mice that spontaneously develop autoimmune type 1 diabetes mellitus. BMC Immunol 2003;4:2.
114. Thrower SL, James L, Hall W, et al. Proinsulin peptide immunotherapy in type 1 diabetes: report of a first-in-man phase I safety study. Clin Exp Immunol 2009;155:156–165.
115. Alleva DG, Maki RA, Putnam AL, et al. Immunomodulation in type 1 diabetes by NBI-6024, an altered peptide ligand of the insulin B epitope. Scand J Immunol 2006;63(1):59–69.
116. Harrison LC, Honeyman MC, Steele CE, et al. Pancreatic beta-cell function and immune responses to insulin after administration of intranasal insulin to humans at risk for type 1 diabetes. Diabetes Care 2004;27(10):2348–2355.
117. Agardh CD, Cilio CM, Lethagen A, et al. Clinical evidence for the safety of GAD65 immunomodulation in adult-onset autoimmune diabetes. J Diabetes Complications 2005;19(4):238–246.
118. Ludvigsson J, Faresjo M, Hjorth M, et al. GAD treatment and insulin secretion in recent-onset type 1 diabetes. N Engl J Med 2008;359(18):1909–1920.
119. Ounissi-Benkalha H, Polychronakos C. The molecular genetics of type 1 diabetes: new genes and emerging mechanisms. Trends Mol Med 2008;14(6):268–275.
120. Ounissi-Benkalha H, Polychronakos C. Transcriptional effects of the insulin variable number of tandem repeats (VNTR) polymorphism. Diabetes 2005;54(Suppl 2):S159. Ref Type: Generic
121. Chaparro RJ, Burton AR, Serreze DV, Vignali DA, DiLorenzo TP. Rapid identification of MHC class I-restricted antigens relevant to autoimmune diabetes using retrogenic T cells. J Immunol Methods 2008;335:106–115.

Chapter 5

Metabolic Syndrome and Inflammation

Rodica Pop-Busui and Massimo Pietropaolo

Summary

The "metabolic syndrome" is a cluster of cardiovascular disease (CVD) risk factors including abdominal obesity, hyperlipidemia, hypertension, insulin resistance, and hyperglycemia. These components reflecting overnutrition, sedentary lifestyles, and resultant excess adiposity may associate with various conditions and therefore multiple definitions were developed over time.

The prevalence of metabolic syndrome is increasing at rates paralleling the epidemic prevalence of type 2 diabetes in the USA as well as in the rest of the world including the developing nations. Unlike autoimmune diabetes, accumulating evidence suggests that metabolic syndrome is strongly linked to chronic systemic inflammation. The presence of metabolic syndrome is associated with an approximate doubling of cardiovascular disease risk and a fivefold increased risk for incident type 2 diabetes. Although it is unclear whether a unifying pathophysiological mechanism results in the presence of the specific clinical clusters of the metabolic syndrome, abdominal adiposity with subsequent chronic inflammation and increased oxidative stress and insulin resistance appear to play a central role.

Landmark investigations of the inflammasome activity provide great potential for insights into the molecular basis for the inflammatory nature of metabolic syndrome beginning a story that continues to unfold. The evolving concept of insulin resistance, type 2 diabetes and hypertension as having common inflammatory components provides new opportunities for developing strategies, currently underway, to correct the metabolic consequences of metabolic syndrome and chronic inflammation.

Key Words: Type 2 diabetes, Inflammasome, Cardiovascular disease, Obesity, Insulin resistance, C-reactive protein

INTRODUCTION

Metabolic syndrome was originally described by Reaven (1) and is also known as the "insulin resistance syndrome," "syndrome X" or "pre-diabetes." It is well accepted that the majority of individuals who develop cardiovascular disease (CVD) events present with multiple risk factors including hyperlipidemia, hypertension, obesity, and hyperglycemia. Reaven proposed that the common pathway linking the occurrence of these risk factors in a given individual is the presence of insulin resistance, which mediates the downstream effects in deterioration of glucose and lipids metabolism and of blood pressure (*1*). Subsequently, the term metabolic syndrome was, in general, accepted by most researchers, given that, arguably, insulin resistance is not the sole cause for this clustering of metabolic risk factors. The National Cholesterol Education Program's Adult Treatment Panel III report (ATP III) used this denomination and identified six components of the metabolic syndrome that relate to CVD deserving more clinical attention (*2*). These components are abdominal obesity, insulin resistance ± glucose intolerance, atherogenic dyslipidemia, increased blood pressure, proinflammatory state, and prothrombotic state (*3*).

Although ATP III identified CVD as the primary clinical outcome of the metabolic syndrome, considering that most people with this syndrome have insulin resistance, they are at increased risk for developing type 2 diabetes and when diabetes becomes clinically apparent, the CVD risk rises sharply (*4, 5*). More recently, it became apparent that other conditions such as polycystic ovary syndrome, fatty liver, obstructive sleep apnea, cholesterol gallstones, asthma, and some forms of cancer are strongly associated with the presence of the metabolic syndrome state (*3*). The designated ATP components as metabolic risk factors are briefly described below.

Abdominal obesity is the form of obesity that presents clinically as increased waist circumference and most strongly associated with the metabolic syndrome.

Atherogenic dyslipidemia manifests in routine lipoprotein analysis by raised triglycerides and low concentrations of HDL cholesterol. A more detailed analysis usually reveals other lipoprotein abnormalities, e.g., increased remnant lipoproteins, elevated apolipoprotein B, small LDL particles, and small HDL particles (*3*).

Insulin resistance is one of the main defects accounting for the development of impaired glucose tolerance (IGT), impaired fasting glucose (IFG) and type 2 diabetes and is present in the majority of people with the metabolic syndrome. Both IGT and IFG (*6*) and are considered an intermediate state in the transition from normal glucose tolerance to type 2 diabetes. Subjects with IGT and IFG, although still normoglycemic, manifest the dual defects that are characteristic of type 2 diabetes: reduced insulin sensitivity and impaired β-cell function. As a result, they are at high risk for progression to type 2 diabetes, with an annual conversion rate of 5–10%, depending upon the ethnic group that is studied (*7, 8*).

Insulin resistance correlates univariately with CVD risk (*3*). The relationship between insulin resistance, plasma insulin level, and glucose intolerance is mediated by complex mechanisms including an increase in ambient plasma free-fatty acid (FFA) concentrations (*1*) and subsequent effects on insulin signal transduction increased inflammation, oxidative stress, and subnormal vascular reactivity (9). Because resistance to insulin also results in the relative nonsuppression of adipocyte hormone-sensitive lipase, there is further enhancement of lipolysis, further increase in FFA concentration closing a vicious circle of lipolysis, increased FFA, insulin resistance, and inflammation (9).

Elevated blood pressure strongly associates with obesity and commonly occurs in insulin-resistant persons. Although hypertension is multifactorial and some investigators believe that hypertension is less "metabolic" than other metabolic syndrome components, most consensus panels favor inclusion of elevated blood pressure as one component of the metabolic syndrome (3, 10, 11).

The proinflammatory state, is recognized clinically in general by elevations of C-reactive protein (CRP) and is commonly present in persons with metabolic syndrome. Multiple mechanisms seemingly underlie increased inflammation in metabolic syndrome and will be discussed in more detail later in this chapter.

A *prothrombotic state*, characterized by increased plasma plasminogen-activator inhibitor (PAI)-1 and fibrinogen, also associates with the metabolic syndrome. Fibrinogen, an acute-phase reactant like CRP, rises in response to a high-cytokine state. Thus, prothrombotic and proinflammatory states may be metabolically interconnected (3).

Definition and Diagnostic Criteria of the Metabolic Syndrome

Considering the growing interest in this constellation of closely related CVD risk factors, several expert groups have attempted to produce diagnostic criteria for a timely identification of individuals at high risk of both type 2 diabetes and CVD. Consequently, several definitions and diagnostic criteria were produced by several expert groups and the WHO using more or less various combinations of the risk factors described above which inevitably led to substantial confusion. Prevalence figures for the syndrome have been similar in any given population regardless of which definition is used, but different individuals are identified (12). However it is important to use those criteria, which produce the best prediction of subsequent diabetes and CVD. The first diagnostic criteria were issued by a WHO diabetes group in 1999, which proposed insulin resistance or its surrogates, impaired glucose tolerance or diabetes, as essential components, together with at least two of: raised blood pressure, hypertriglyceridemia and/or low HDL cholesterol, obesity (as measured by waist/hip ratio or body mass index), and microalbuminuria (10).

The European Group for the Study of Insulin Resistance produced a modification of the WHO criteria excluding people with diabetes and requiring hyperinsulinemia to be present and recommending waist circumference as the measure of obesity, with different cutoffs for the other variables (11). The International Diabetes Federation (IDF) felt that different criteria are needed and agreed

Table 5.1
ATP III Clinical Identification of the Metabolic Syndrome

Risk factor	Defining level
Abdominal obesity, given as waist circumference	
Men	>102 cm (>40 in.)
Women	>88 cm (>35 in.)
Triglycerides	≥150 mg/dL
HDL cholesterol	
Men	<40 mg/dL
Women	<50 mg/dL
Blood pressure	≥130/≥85 mmHg
Fasting glucose	≥110 mg/dL[a]

[a]The American Diabetes Association has recently established a cutpoint of 100 mg/dL, above which persons have either prediabetes (impaired fasting glucose) or diabetes (*14*). This new cutpoint should be applicable for identifying the lower boundary to define an elevated glucose as one criterion for the metabolic syndrome (*3*)

that central obesity, as assessed by waist circumference, was the essential component because of the strength of the evidence linking waist circumference with CVD and the other metabolic syndrome components and recommended to use ethnic-specific waist circumference cutoffs in combination with any two other components from specified lipid abnormalities, specified blood pressure cutoffs and blood glucose abnormalities (*10*).

We recommend the revised ATP criteria by the National Heart, Lung, and Blood Institute, in collaboration with the American Heart Association which takes into account several perspectives: (a) major clinical outcomes, (b) metabolic components, (c) pathogenesis, (d) clinical criteria for diagnosis, (e) risk for clinical outcomes, and (f) therapeutic interventions (*3*) shown in Table 5.1.

Interactions Between Metabolic Syndrome, Oxidative Stress, and Inflammation

Oxidative stress and chronic inflammation are important players in the metabolic syndrome state and contribute to subsequent CVD risk and progression to overt type 2 diabetes and chronic complications (*13–15*) (Fig. 5.1). It has also been demonstrated that elevations of inflammation-sensitive plasma proteins precede clinical CVD and are intricately linked with the development of cardiovascular events (*16–18*).

Obesity, one of the key components of the metabolic syndrome, is strongly associated with both increased inflammation and oxidative stress, and was shown that it may lead to subsequent development of abnormal glucose metabolism, dyslipidemia, and hypertension. One reason is that in obesity, the excess adipose tissue releases inflammatory cytokines with a very broad

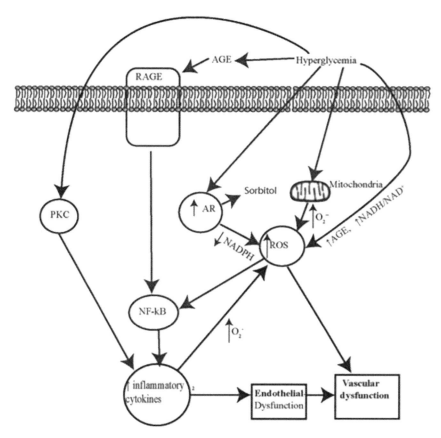

Fig. 5.1 Schematic representation of the cascade of events linking hyperglycemia, increased inflammation, oxidative stress, and vascular dysfunction. *AGE* advanced glycation end-products, *RAGE* receptor for AGE, *AR* aldose reductase, *ROS* reactive oxygen species, *PKC* protein kinase C, *NF-κB* nuclear factor κB, *NADH* nicotinamide adenine dinucleotide, *NADPH* nicotinamide adenine dinucleotide phosphate.

constellation of downstream effects. The traditional view of adipose tissue as a passive energy storage depot is no longer valid after the discovery that adipose tissue secretes a number of bioactive proteins known as adipokines. The proinflammatory adipokines, tumor necrosis factor-α (TNFα) and interleukin-6 (IL-6) have been studied most extensively.

Hotamisligil et al. described that adipocytes constitutively express the proinflammatory cytokine TNFα and that TNFα expression in adipocytes of obese animals (ob/ob mouse, db/db mouse and fa/fa Zucker rat) is markedly increased (19). These data provided also a first evidence of the link between insulin resistance and increased inflammation. Later it was shown that TNFα is constitutively expressed in human adipocytes and that its expression fell after weight loss (20). TNF receptor concentration was found to be elevated in obese patients (21) and a significant correlation was described between the body mass index (BMI) and plasma TNFα concentrations. Further work in the area of obesity has confirmed that obesity is a state of chronic inflammation, as indicated by increased plasma concentrations of CRP (*22*) IL-6 (*23*) or plasminogen-activator inhibitor (*24*).

The association of inflammation with obesity appears to be also modulated by macronutrient and intake as it was described that both a mixed fast-food meal or high glucose intake induced acute cellular and molecular oxidative stress and inflammation lasting for several hours (*25*). Obesity is a major risk factor for metabolic syndrome and type 2 diabetes, and it was therefore proposed that both metabolic syndrome and type 2 diabetes are inflammatory conditions.

There is also growing support for the hypothesis that obesity as an inflammatory condition leads to chronic activation of the innate immune system. Pickup and Crook observed that the "metabolic" dyslipidemia commonly present also in type 2 diabetes (high triglycerides and low HDL cholesterol) is also a feature of experimental and naturally occurring acute-phase reactions and proposed that in individuals with an innately hypersensitive acute-phase response, long-term lifestyle and environmental stressors, such as overnutrition, produce disease (type 2 diabetes) instead of repair (*26*).

Several prospective studies, in diverse human populations, have identified proinflammatory cytokines and acute-phase proteins predict the development of type 2 diabetes (*22, 27–30*). In humans, IL-6 is related to insulin resistance, independent of obesity (*31*). In the Atherosclerosis Risk in Communities study (*28*) and Nurses Health study (*32*). IL-6 at baseline was independently associated with future risk of diabetes. Similar results were reported in the European Prospective Investigation into Cancer and Nutrition-Potsdam study, in which participants with elevated IL-6 and IL-1β had a threefold increase in risk for developing diabetes when compared with the reference group (*33*).

The risk of someone being affected with CVD is elevated even at glucose levels well below the diabetes cut-off (*34–36*). In addition, in a recently reported prospective analysis of the risk of atherosclerosis in a middle-aged population, individuals without diabetes or CVD, but with the metabolic syndrome, were at increased risk for long-term CVD outcomes (*37*).

In addition, autonomic impairment, manifested as abnormal heart rate (HR) variability, has been identified in patients with components of the metabolic syndrome at the time of diagnosis in type 2 diabetes. This suggests that such impairment may be present either after a relatively brief exposure to sustained hyperglycemia or develop in conjunction with obesity, insulin resistance, and/or intermittent episodes of milder glucose elevations (*38, 39*). Some cross-sectional studies in adults without diabetes provided evidence that markers of autonomic function are inversely associated with obesity, insulin resistance, and fasting glucose (*40–43*).

Oxidative stress also plays a central role in the development of diabetes, diabetes complications, and CVD (*44–46*). We have recently demonstrated that systemic oxidative stress is increased and cardiac sympathetic tone and responsiveness is altered early in the course of type 1 diabetes and in concert with impaired perfusion may contribute to the eventual development of myocardial injury (*34*). In addition, in the vascular endothelium, increased oxidative stress and inflammation can promote apoptosis (*47, 48*) and impair the action of vasodilatory agents (*49–51*). There are alterations of NO metabolism in sympathetic ganglia (*46*). Alterations of NO metabolism in sympathetic ganglia and/or vascular endothelium (*52–56*) secondary to oxidative stress (*57*) or subclinical vascular denervation (*58*) could also contribute to the development and progression of sympathetic dysinnervation, since NO has been proposed to function as an inhibitory sympathetic neurotransmitter (*46, 59*). In diabetes, an impaired NO synthase activity (*60*) or ganglionic NO depletion through other mechanisms including the formation of peroxynitrite may further contribute to neurovascular dysfunction.

ROLE OF INFLAMMATION IN METABOLIC SYNDROME AND TYPE 2 DIABETES

Gathering evidence has identified adipose tissue as a dynamic endocrine organ that secretes a number of inflammatory mediators as well as hormones contributing to systemic and vascular inflammation (*61, 62*). Seminal studies have substantiated the involvement of inflammation in the pathogenesis of insulin resistance, obesity and type 2 diabetes (*61, 63–65*). Strong correlations have been shown between inflammatory markers as independent risk factors for disease, but whether inflammatory mediators are simply surrogate markers of an underlying pathological process remains to be elucidated (*66–69*).

The first indirect evidence that diabetes mellitus is associated with inflammation was reported in 1876 by Professor Ebstein who observed that high dose salicylates reduced glycosuria in diabetic patients (*70*). More than one century later, we learned that salicylate prevents the activation of NF-κB, which is a mediator of inflammation and apoptosis (*71, 72*). Several studies in the 1990s suggested a relationship between obesity and inflammation (*19, 26, 64, 73*). These studies showed that type 2 diabetic patients and/or animal models had increased serum levels of acute-phase reactants and that TNFα was increased in adipose tissue from obese rodents. The link between inflammatory cytokines of the innate immune system, such as TNFα, IL-1β, MCP-1, and IL-6, and obesity is now firmly established (*64*). Therefore, metabolic syndrome, obesity and type 2 diabetes are considered to be low-grade inflammatory diseases (*19, 26, 73–76*).

At least three lines of evidence suggest that inflammation plays a key role in the pathogenesis insulin resistance, type 2 diabetes mellitus and metabolic syndrome. Findings from numerous major epidemiologic studies indicate that the presence of different combinations of inflammatory markers, namely C-reactive protein, fibrinogen, IL-6, IL-1β, plasminogen-activator inhibitor-1 (PAI-1), and white blood count, are significant predictors of T2DM. In particular, these studies include the Cardiovascular Health Study (*77*) the Atherosclerosis Risk in Communities study (*68*), the Women's Health Study (*78*), the National Health and Examination Survey (NHANES) (*79*), the US Insulin Resistance and Atherosclerosis Study (*29*), the Scottish men in the West of Scotland Coronary Prevention Study (*30*), the Hoorn Study in the Netherlands (*80*), the Prospective Investigation into Cancer and Nutrition (EPIC)-Postdam Study and the MONICA Ausburg Study both in Germany (*33*), and studies carried out in Pima Indians and in female Mexican populations (*81*).

The second line of evidence relates to the paradigm that inflammation is involved in the pathogenesis of atherosclerosis, a common complication of type 2 diabetes and insulin resistance (*82*). A large number of investigations have convincingly shown that low-grade elevation of circulating markers of inflammation such as CRP, sialic acid, and proinflammatory cytokines are associated with cardiovascular mortality, coronary heart disease, peripheral vascular disease, and stroke (*83*).

The third line of evidence derives from the association of gestational diabetes, a risk factor for type 2 diabetes, and activated innate immunity with increased acute-phase proteins. Elevated CRP levels during the first trimester of pregnancy are more pronounced in women who develop gestational diabetes later in their pregnancy (*64*).

Thus, type 2 diabetes and metabolic syndrome are acute-phase diseases in which increased secretion of cytokines from macrophages, adipose tissue, endothelium, and other cell systems. This increase in circulating cytokines may be genetically programmed (*26, 66, 84–92*). Interleukin-β (IL1-β) may act on pancreatic β cells contributing to impaired insulin secretion. TNFα, may contribute to the development of insulin resistance by inhibiting the tyrosine kinase activity of the insulin receptor (*6*). Importantly, when TNFα action is blocked, insulin sensitivity improves (*19*). The soluble fraction of TNF receptor 2 (sTNFR2) appears to be involved in the pathogenesis of insulin resistance (*74*).

C-Reactive Protein

C-reactive protein is a plasma protein that was initially identified because of its ability to bind to the capsule of pneumococcal bacteria. It belongs to the pentraxin family as it contains five identical globular subunits. C-reactive protein contributes to the activation of the classical pathway of complement through its binding to C1q and it functions as an opsonin. C-reactive protein is an acute-phase reactant that is strongly linked to coronary heart disease (CHD) (*66, 67, 91, 92*). Haffner et al. (*69*) reported that elevated levels of CRP (highest quintile) increased the risk of incident type 2 diabetes 3.4-fold compared to those in quintile 1, even in adjustment for elements of the insulin resistance syndrome. Similar results were noted for fibrinogen.

The Cardiovascular Health Study (CHS) has documented a strong association between high levels of inflammatory markers, such as C-reactive protein (CRP) and fibrinogen, and diabetes, increased waist circumference (a marker of greater visceral or abdominal fat), hypertriglyceridemia and risk of cardiovascular disease (CVD). This risk was conferred independently from traditional CVD risk factors and subclinical disease (*67, 95, 96*). In the CHS a direct relationship between CRP and fibrinogen levels and diabetes has also been found (*67*). The mean CRP level was 2.82 mg/L among nondiabetics, 3.46 mg/L in IGT and 4.97 mg/L in diabetics ($p<0.001$). Fibrinogen levels were also statistically significantly higher among diabetics (333.1 mg/dL) than those with IGT (323.2 mg/dL) or euglycemia.

Additional data from the CHS have further documented that liver enzymes, possibly a marker of hepatic steatosis due to visceral fat flux to the liver, were elevated among diabetics and in nondiabetics who have elevated waist circumference or obesity. As a matter of fact, a direct relationship between elevated liver enzymes and risk of type 2 diabetes has been reported (*97*). A strong association between CRP and blood glucose was demonstrated in the Healthy Women Study (HWS). In particular, in postmenopausal women CRP and plasminogen-activator inhibitor-1 were directly related to waist circumference and other measures of body fat including increased visceral fat (*78*). Prospective data from the HWS reinforce the role of inflammation in the development of diabetes (*98*). In particular, elevated levels of CRP were independently associated with the progression to type 2 diabetes. Positive association persisted after adjustment for body mass index, family history of diabetes, smoking, exercise, use of alcohol, and hormone replacement therapy (*98*).

Furthermore, women on estrogen had higher CRP levels, consistent with a recent report from the Postmenopausal Estrogen/Progestogen Intervention (PEPI) (*99*) and CHS study (*100, 101*) where a positive relationship between waist circumference and estrogen use and higher CRP levels was observed.

We found that in subjects diagnosed as having type 2 diabetes by clinical criteria alone, the presence of GAD65 autoantibodies identifies a pathogenically distinct disease phenotype characterized by the absence of systemic inflammation and its related disorders, the presence of impaired insulin secretion and the high tendency to be treated with insulin therapy (*102*). We found that plasma C-reactive protein and fibrinogen levels were comparable in GAD65 antibody-positive adult diabetic patients to those of control populations (*102, 103*). In this subset of older diabetic patients the primary inflammatory injury seemingly resides in the pancreatic β cells as for type 1 diabetes. We hypothesized that GAD65 antibody-positive diabetics are likely to benefit more from insulin therapy than the obese insulin-resistant, GAD antibody-negative older diabetics, especially early in their disease course. In support of these observations, a recent report indicated that in Latent Autoimmune Diabetes of the Adulthood (LADA) there is no increased frequency of metabolic syndrome in striking contrast with type 2 diabetes (*102*).

PROINFLAMMATORY CYTOKINES

TNFα and IL-1β

Tumor Necrosis Factor α is the primary mediator of the acute inflammatory response to gram-negative bacteria and other pathogens and can cause many of the systemic complications of severe infections. The major cellular source of TNFα is activated mononuclear phagocytes. Antigen-stimulated T cells, NK cells and mast cells can all secrete TNFα. Binding of TNFα to its receptor recruits TRADD (TNF receptor-associated death domain protein), leads to activation NF-κB (Fig. 5.2).

Overproduction of TNFα could be involved in the pathogenesis of type 2 diabetes and insulin resistance (*26*). TNFα may also cause an impairment of insulin secretion in pancreatic islet cells (*105*) and may stimulate IL-6 production leading to β cell destruction (*106*). TNFα signals through two receptors TNFαSR1 and TNFSR2, although the exact role of each has not yet been determined. It has been reported that TNFα interferes with the autophosphorylation of the insulin receptor and inhibits insulin signaling via pathways involving TNFαSR2 (*26*). In one cross-sectional study, levels of both were positively correlated with BMI, fasting glucose, and insulin among elderly men (*107*). In two studies, higher levels of TNFα activity were found among type 2 diabetics compared to nondiabetics (*108*). Correlations with insulin sensitivity were also found in nondiabetic offspring of diabetic parents (*109*).

TNFα is an inflammatory cytokine that appears to be associated with a number of autoimmune disorders (*110*), including type 1 diabetes (*26, 85, 111–113*). This cytokine may be involved in the breakdown of peripheral tolerance to pancreatic islet autoantigens (*114*). To test this hypothesis, the tetracycline-regulated transcriptional control of islet-specific expression of TNFα was applied to analyze the relationship between inflammation and the breaking of peripheral tolerance to islet antigens. Green and Flavell generated a murine model whereby islet-specific expression of TNFα could be repressed/derepressed within 48 h following introduction/removal of tetracycline in drinking water.

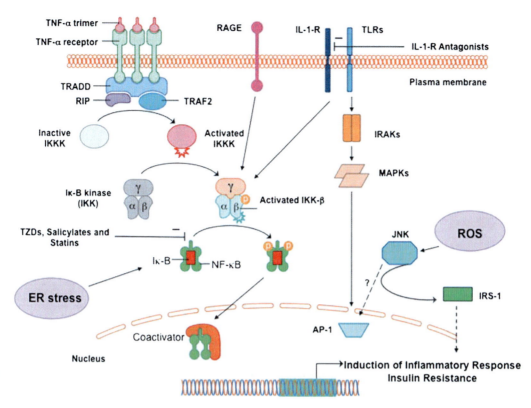

Fig. 5.2 Potential intracellular mechanisms of activation of inflammatory signaling in metabolic syndrome. NF-κB can be activated by a variety of stimuli, including TNFα, IL-1, RAGE, and TLRs. Obesity, high-fat diet and ER stress activate IKKβ/NF-κB and JNK pathways (ROS) in adipocytes, hepatocytes, and macrophages. Mediators activating these pathways include ligands for TNFα, IL-1, Toll, or AGE receptors (TNFR, IL-1R, TLR, or RAGE, respectively). Obesity-induced IKKβ activation leads to NF-κB translocation and the increased expression inflammatory factors that can cause insulin resistance. Obesity-induced JNK activation promotes the phosphorylation of IRS-1 at serine sites that negatively regulate normal signaling through the insulin receptor/IRS-1 axis. Evidence has not been reported for obesity-induced effects on transcription factors such as AP-1 that are regulated by JNK. IKKβ and/or NF-κB are inhibited or repressed by the actions of salicylates, TZDs, and statins. The blockade of the IL-1 pathway with an IL-1 receptor antagonist (Anakinra) in patients with type 2 diabetes, and possibly in metabolic syndrome, resulted in a significant reduction markers of systemic inflammation (*149*).

In this model, the duration of TNFα-mediated inflammatory response seems to play a key role in diabetes progression and therefore in the breakdown of peripheral tolerance to host antigens in animals nongenetically predisposed to develop islet cell autoimmunity. By selectively expressing TNFα for short periods of time, the fate of islet-reactive T cells (activation vs. tolerance) was determined. Initiation of TNFα in neonatal TNFα×RIP-B7-1 mice resulted in diabetes by 6–9 weeks of age, with 100% incidence of disease by 9 weeks of age. Diabetes development was also observed following initiation of TNFα expression in a 6-week-old adult TNFα×RIP-B7-1 mice, with a kinetics similar to that seen in neonates. Interestingly, Green and Flavell also showed that repression of TNFα after initiation of insulitis at 21 days prevented the development of diabetes.

The results of a study carried out by Green and Flavell seem to be in agreement with the findings published earlier by McDevitt and coworkers (*115*), demonstrating that TNFα treated nonobese diabetic (NOD) mice exhibited T cell as well as autoantibody responses to islet autoantigens including GAD65. TNFα may also be involved in the development of insulin resistance by inhibiting the tyrosine kinase activity of the insulin receptor (*26*).

An insulin secretory defect, which resembles that of T1DM, is also seen in transgenic mice expressing elevated serum TNFα levels (*116*). Other observations suggest that TNFα may activate intra-islet resident macrophages, resulting in the release of IL-1β, which generates inducible nitric oxide synthase (iNOS) expression and the overproduction of nitric oxide (NO) in β-cells (*105*) and that alterations in the number and function of CD4$^+$CD25$^+$ T cells may be an additional mechanism by which TNF modulate type 1 diabetes in NOD mice (*117, 118*). The free radical, NO, then downregulates cellular metabolism primarily by interfering with mitochondrial function that leads to β-cell insulin resistance (*105*). In addition, IL-1β may promote an impairment of insulin secretion in pancreatic β cells (*119, 120*). An attractive hypothesis is that β-cell insulin resistance may be a major determinant in creating the insulin secretory defect, which is present in type 2 diabetes (*121*). Thus, metabolic β-cell abnormalities may be the result of elevated serum levels of TNFα in type 2 diabetic patients.

IL-6

IL-6, an important mediator of the acute-phase response, is secreted by adipocytes, myocytes and endothelial cells (*122*). IL-6 may mediate the production of TNFα, but also appears to be a mediator of insulin resistance independent of TNFα (*123*). Data from cross-sectional studies indicate that IL-6 is associated with obesity and TNFα (*124*) and are much higher in diabetic persons with the insulin resistance syndrome (IRS) components than either type 2 diabetes without the IRS features or nondiabetic controls (*26*). Studies performed in vivo, following infusion of human recombinant IL-6 in rats, resulted in the development of hyperglycemia and insulin resistance (*125*). IL-6 seems to have counter regulatory effects on carbohydrate metabolism (*126*).

MCP-1

MCP-1 (also called CCL2) is a chemoattractive protein that recruits immune cells to sites of inflammation. The adipose tissue expression of MCP-1 increases in proportion to adiposity and decreases following treatment with TZDs (*127, 128*) and following bariatric surgery (*129*). Two independent studies convincingly showed that the adipocyte-specific overexpression of MCP-1 in mice was sufficient to increase macrophage recruitment to adipose tissue and cause systemic insulin resistance; notably, MCP-1 expression in adipocytes resulted in hepatic steatosis and insulin resistance in liver and muscle as well as in fat (*130, 131*).

Resistin

Resistin is an proinflammatory cytokine secreted by adipocytes and immune cells whose expression is suppressed by TZDs and upregulated by proinflammatory cytokines and bacterially derived lipopolysaccharide (*62, 132, 133*). Resistin stimulates intracellular signaling through NF-κB activation, which in turn promotes the synthesis of other proinflammatory cytokines, such as TNFα, IL-6, MCP-1, and IL-12, and the surface adhesion molecules intracellular adhesion molecule-1 and vascular-cell adhesion molecule-1 (*133, 134*); various proinflammatory stimuli also induce the expression of resistin, including TNFα, IL-6, IL-1β, and lipopolysaccharide. In addition to its potential roles in insulin resistance, resistin may play a role in the inflammation associated with the pathogenesis of CVD (*135*).

Plasminogen-Activator Inhibitor 1

Plasminogen-activator inhibitor 1 inhibits plasminogen activators, which convert inactive plasminogen into plasmin during fibrinolysis (*26*). PAI-1 is considered to be a cardiovascular risk factor, although PAI-1 concentrations correlate with peripheral insulin resistance in obese type 2 diabetic patients (*64*).

INNATE IMMUNITY IN DIABETES AND OBESITY-RELATED INFLAMMATION

The innate immune system functions as the first line of defense against microbes and infection (*136*). As a general rule, unlike the adaptive immune system, the innate immune system does not generate long-term immunological memory. The innate immune system, once thought to be very nonspecific, illustrates a much greater degree of specificity than previously thought (*136, 137*). This system utilizes multiple cell types including: macrophages, dendritic cells (DCs), NK cells, neutrophils, and epithelial cells, each of which has their own specific function in an innate response, from phagocytosis of infectious pathogens to direct targeted lysis of infected host cells. In order to initiate an innate immune response, the host system first interacts with common surface molecules expressed by an infectious organism. These common microbial surface molecules originally termed Pathogen Associated Molecular Patterns (PAMPs) were predicted to interact with Pattern Recognition Receptors (PRRs) found on the surface of cells. One of the most commonly recognized groups of PRRs are the Toll-like Receptors (TLRs) (*138, 139*). These receptors (TLRs 1, 2, 4, 5, 6, 7, 8, 9, and 11) can promote cell activation via the MyD88 dependent pathway, but some of these TLRs are can also carry out TLR activation in a MyD88 independent manner as well. Though this topic is relatively new, certain TLRs (TLRs 2, 3, 5, and 9) have been categorized as being able to modify and enhance T cell proliferation and cytokine production of TCR-stimulated T cells (*140*).

Cell types involved in obesity such as adipocytes and MΦs are known to express TLR2 and TLR4 (*141*). Studies using TLR4 knock-out or C3H/HeJ mice with a mutant TLR4 receptor and deficient LPS responsiveness have proven extremely useful in understanding the role of TLR4 in obesity-related inflammation (*142*). Importantly, TLR4$^{-/-}$ mice fed a high-fat diet displayed increased feeding efficiency, increased metabolic rates, attenuated increases in serum and adipose tissue concentrations of TNFα, IL-6, and in one case, serum FFA compared to control mice (*141, 143*). In summary, although TLR4 could be implicated with the pathoetiology of inflammatory-related insulin resistance, additional studies are necessary to unravel the role of innate immunity in metabolic syndrome and type 2 diabetes. It would also be important to determine whether or not altered TLR responsiveness (i.e., macrophages from diabetic patients) cause predisposition to many infections, which are commonly seen in patients with type 2 diabetes and metabolic syndrome.

IS THE INFLAMMASOME INVOLVED IN TYPE 2 DIABETES AND METABOLIC SYNDROME?

The Inflammasome is a multiprotein complex consisting of caspase 1 (sometimes caspase 5 or caspase 11), NALP and PYCARD which regulates the cleavage and release of the potent proinflammatory cytokines IL-β, IL-18, and IL-33 (*144*). The inflammasome is involved in the activation of inflammatory processes (*145*) and has been shown to induce cell pyroptosis, a process of programmed cell death distinct from apoptosis (*146*). A recent original observation provides evidence that the innate inflammasome pathway can direct humoral adaptive immune responses (*147*). As a matter of fact, the Nalp3 inflammasome appears to be a crucial factor in the adjuvant effect of aluminum adjuvants. Furthermore, the Nalp3 inflammasome is essential for the development of silicosis (*148*). A better understanding on how stimulation of the inflammasome pathway results in activation of adaptive immune responses has important implications in the design of new and effective adjuvants for treating inflammatory responses in type 2 diabetes and other inflammatory diseases.

The relationship between inflammasome activity and type 2 diabetes provided great potential for insights into the molecular basis for the inflammatory nature of this disease as well as metabolic syndrome (*149*). Indeed, the blockade of IL-1β with an IL-1β receptor antagonist (Anakinra) in patients with type 2 diabetes improved both glycemic homeostasis and β-cell secretory function and resulted in a significant reduction markers of systemic inflammation, namely C-reactive protein and IL-6 (*149*)

Table 5.2
Changes in Inflammatory Mediators After Treatment for Insulin Resistance (Modified from Shoelson et al. (161))

Intervention	Factors changed
Weight loss, diet, and exercise	Decrease in serum CRP, IL-6 after weight lost in postmenopausal women
Bariatric surgery	Decrease in serum CRP, MMP9, VCAM-1, and P-selectin after high-fiber, low-fat diet and exercise Decrease in serum IL-6, PAI-1, E-selectin, P-selectin, TNF-αR2, CRP, CD40L, MCP-1, and adiponectin
Thiazolidinediones	Decrease in serum CRP, PAI-1, MCP-1, resistin after rosiglitazone treatment Decrease in serum TNFα and resistin after pioglitazone treatment
Metformin	Decrease in serum CRP
Sulfonylureas	Decrease in serum IL-6 and E-selectin and increase in adiponectin with gliclazide treatment
IL-1β receptor antagonist	Decrease in serum CRP and IL-6 (*149*)

MMP matrix metalloproteinase; *VCAM-1* vascular-cell adhesion molecule 1. See specific references in refs. (*149, 161*)

(Table 5.2). The rationale of this trial is based on a number of observations providing evidence that in pancreatic β cells high glucose levels determined the release of IL-1β, followed by functional impairment and apoptosis of β cells (*150, 151*). These findings suggested that blocking intra-islet production of proinflammatory cytokines, such as IL-1, could be a potential therapeutic strategy for preserving β-cell mass and function. A similar study is being evaluated by TrialNet to determine whether or not IL-1 blockade decreases inflammatory responses and preserves β-cell function after the clinical of type 1 diabetes.

There is compelling evidence that both hyperinsulinemia and type 2 diabetes are associated with hypertension. Inflammation and oxidative stress have emerged as major factors in hypertension. Polymorphonuclear leukocytes are the main producer of ROS and are involved in the pathogenesis of hypertension in both human and animal models of this disease. Because mutations within the *NALP3* locus were found in patients with essential hypertension, this could explain why insulin resistance and hypertension frequently coexist (*152*).

EFFECTS ON INFLAMMATION BY MOST WIDELY USED DRUGS FOR INSULIN RESISTANCE AND METABOLIC SYNDROME

The anti-inflammatory effects of the hypoglycemic agents thiazolidinediones (TZDs), also known as insulin sensitizers, result from the inhibition of cytokine secretion and macrophage activation. It has been shown that TZD and statins, which alter the secretion of a number of cytokines such as IL-1β and TNFα involved in CRP synthesis, reduce inflammatory markers such as CRP and white blood cell count in type 2 diabetic patients (153, 154) (Table 5.2). The anti-inflammatory effect of aspirin can also be seen in the animal models of diabetes such as the *ob/ob* mouse and the *fa/fa* rat, in which insulin resistance can be reversed by high dose salicylates through an I-κB kinase β-dependent mechanism (155). Thiazolidinediones exert their effects by binding and activating the nuclear hormone receptor PPARγ (153, 156, 157). Thiazolidinediones binding induces the expression of several genes involved in adipocyte differentiation, lipid and glucose uptake, and fatty acid storage (157). The beneficial effects of TZDs as insulin sensitizers are thought to be due primarily to the mobilization of fatty acid storage into the adipose tissue, which decreases circulating FFA and redistributes lipids from other tissues such as muscle and liver into the adipose tissue. Proposed mechanisms for the anti-inflammatory effects of TZDs include PPARγ-independent activation of the glucocorticoid receptor (158), although alternative explanations are possible.

Statins have also been shown to exhibit anti-inflammatory properties (159). These drugs lower circulating cholesterol levels by inhibiting cellular 3-hydroxy-3-methylglutaryl coenzyme A (HMG CoA) reductase, the rate-limiting enzyme in cholesterol biosynthesis. The levels of circulating markers and potential mediators of inflammation are also reduced in subjects treated with statins (159). Because levels of CRP and several proinflammatory cytokines decrease, and these are products of NF-κB genes, it appears that the statins may have modest anti-NF-κB activity. The small decrease in the risk of developing type 2 diabetes that accompanies statin therapy could be related to its anti-inflammatory activity (159, 160). A similar anti-inflammatory mechanism is shared by the potent glucose-lowering drug salicylate (76). Salicylates had been found long ago to lower glucose in patients with diabetes (70) although a potential role for inflammation was not considered until recently (71, 161, 162). The anti-inflammatory effect of salicylates has been attributed to the inhibition of IKK-β and NF-κB (71, 163) and it has been hypothesized that glucose lowering and insulin sensitization might also be due to NF-κB inhibition (163). A recent proof-of-principle study showed that salsalate reduces glycemia and may improve inflammatory cardiovascular risk indexes in overweight individuals. These results support the hypothesis that chronic systemic inflammation may contribute to the pathogenesis of obesity-related hyperglycemia and that targeting inflammation could provide a therapeutic route for diabetes prevention (*162*).

CONCLUDING REMARKS

There is a wide spectrum of inflammatory responses in diabetic syndromes and solid evidence has substantiated that both type 2 diabetes and metabolic syndrome are linked with systemic inflammation, which could be either the cause or simply mark the underlying pathology. Conversely, in autoimmune diabetes inflammatory abnormalities reside mainly in the islets and there appears to be no increased frequency of metabolic syndrome in striking contrast with type 2 diabetes (*102, 104*).

A further understanding of cell inflammatory signaling and genetic functional analyses in metabolic syndrome will provide clues that are indispensable for further progress. A key point is to understand the mechanisms, identify early phenomena, determine the overall effects of modulating the activity of inflammatory mediators, and to use this knowledge to develop targeted interventions.

REFERENCES

1. Reaven GM. Banting lecture. Role of insulin resistance in human disease. Diabetes 1988;37:1595–1607.
2. Third Report of the National Cholesterol Education Program (NCEP) Expert Panel on Detection, Evaluation, and Treatment of High Blood Cholesterol in Adults (Adult Treatment Panel III) final report. Circulation 2002;106:3143–3421.
3. Grundy SM, Brewer HB, Jr, Cleeman JI, Smith SC, Jr, Lenfant C. Definition of metabolic syndrome: Report of the National Heart, Lung, and Blood Institute/American Heart Association conference on scientific issues related to definition. Circulation 2004;109:433–438.
4. Haffner SM, Lehto S, Ronnemaa T, Pyorala K, Laakso M. Mortality from coronary heart disease in subjects with type 2 diabetes and in nondiabetic subjects with and without prior myocardial infarction. N Engl J Med 1998;339:229–234.
5. Stamler J, Vaccaro O, Neaton JD, Wentworth D. Diabetes, other risk factors, and 12-yr cardiovascular mortality for men screened in the Multiple Risk Factor Intervention Trial. Diabetes Care 1993;16:434–444.
6. Diabetes mellitus. Report of a WHO Study Group. World Health Organ Tech Rep Ser 1985;727:1–113.
7. Unwin N, Shaw J, Zimmet P, Alberti KG. Impaired glucose tolerance and impaired fasting glycaemia: the current status on definition and intervention. Diabet Med 2002;19:708–723.
8. Gabir MM, Hanson RL, Dabelea D, Imperatore G, Roumain J, Bennett PH, Knowler WC. Plasma glucose and prediction of microvascular disease and mortality: evaluation of 1997 American Diabetes Association and 1999 World Health Organization criteria for diagnosis of diabetes. Diabetes Care 2000;23:1113–1118.
9. Dandona P, Aljada A. A rational approach to pathogenesis and treatment of type 2 diabetes mellitus, insulin resistance, inflammation, and atherosclerosis. Am J Cardiol 2002;90:27G–33G.

10. Alberti KG, Zimmet P, Shaw J. The metabolic syndrome – a new worldwide definition. Lancet 2005;366:1059–1062.
11. Balkau B, Charles MA, Drivsholm T, Borch-Johnsen K, Wareham N, Yudkin JS, Morris R, Zavaroni I, van Dam R, Feskins E, Gabriel R, Diet M, Nilsson P, Hedblad B. Frequency of the WHO metabolic syndrome in European cohorts, and an alternative definition of an insulin resistance syndrome. Diabetes Metab 2002;28:364–376.
12. Cameron AJ, Shaw JE, Zimmet PZ. The metabolic syndrome: prevalence in worldwide populations. Endocrinol Metab Clin North Am 2004;33:351–375, table of contents.
13. Baynes JW, Thorpe SR. Glycoxidation and lipoxidation in atherogenesis. Free Radic Biol Med 2000;28:1708–1716.
14. Pop-Busui R, Sima A, Stevens M. Diabetic neuropathy and oxidative stress. Diabetes Metab Res Rev 2006;22:257–273.
15. Pennathur S, Heinecke, JW. Mechanisms of oxidative stress in diabetes: implications for the pathogenesis of vascular disease and antioxidant therapy. Front Biosci 2004;9:565–574.
16. Ridker PM, Stampfer MJ, Rifai N. Novel risk factors for systemic atherosclerosis: a comparison of C-reactive protein, fibrinogen, homocysteine, lipoprotein(a), and standard cholesterol screening as predictors of peripheral arterial disease. JAMA 2001; 285:2481–2485.
17. Schonbeck U, Varo N, Libby P, Buring J, Ridker PM. Soluble CD40L and cardiovascular risk in women. Circulation 2001;104:2266–2268.
18. Lobbes,MB, Lutgens E, Heeneman S, Cleutjens KB, Kooi ME, van Engelshoven JM, Daemen MJ, Nelemans PJ. Is there more than C-reactive protein and fibrinogen? The prognostic value of soluble CD40 ligand, interleukin-6 and oxidized low-density lipoprotein with respect to coronary and cerebral vascular disease. Atherosclerosis 2006;187:18–25.
19. Hotamisligil GS, Shargill NS, Spiegelman BM. Adipose expression of tumor necrosis factor-alpha: direct role in obesity-linked insulin resistance. Science 1993;259:87–91.
20. Kern PA, Saghizadeh M, Ong JM, Bosch RJ, Deem R, Simsolo RB. The expression of tumor necrosis factor in human adipose tissue. Regulation by obesity, weight loss, and relationship to lipoprotein lipase. J Clin Invest 1995;95:2111–2119.
21. Mantzoros CS, Moschos S, Avramoulos I, Kaklamani V, Liolios A, Doulgerakis DE, Griveas I, Katsilambros N, Flier JS. Leptin concentrations in relation to body mass index and the tumor necrosis factor-alpha system in humans. J Clin Endocrinol Metab 1997; 82:3408–3413.
22. Yudkin JS, Stehouwer CD, Emeis JJ, Coppack SW. C-reactive protein in healthy subjects: associations with obesity, insulin resistance, and endothelial dysfunction: a potential role for cytokines originating from adipose tissue. Arterioscler Thromb Vasc Biol 1999;19:972–978.
23. Mohamed-Ali V, Goodrick S, Rawesh A, Katz DR, Miles JM, Yudkin JS, Klein S, Coppack SW. Subcutaneous adipose tissue releases interleukin-6, but not tumor necrosis factor-alpha, in vivo. J Clin Endocrinol Metab 1997;82:4196–4200.
24. Lundgren CH, Brown SL, Nordt TK, Sobel BE, Fujii S. Elaboration of type-1 plasminogen activator inhibitor from adipocytes. A potential pathogenetic link between obesity and cardiovascular disease. Circulation 1996;93:106–110.
25. Dandona P, Aljada A, Bandyopadhyay A. Inflammation: the link between insulin resistance, obesity and diabetes. Trends Immunol 2004;25:4–7.
26. Pickup JC, Crook MA. Is type II diabetes mellitus a disease of the innate immune system. Diabetologia 1998;41:1241–1248.
27. Barzilay JI, Abraham L, Heckbert SR, Cushman M, Kuller LH, Resnick HE, Tracy RP. The relation of markers of inflammation to the development of glucose disorders in the elderly: the Cardiovascular Health Study. Diabetes 2001;50:2384–2389.
28. Duncan BB, Schmidt MI, Pankow JS, Ballantyne CM, Couper D, Vigo A, Hoogeveen R, Folsom AR, Heiss G. Low-grade systemic inflammation and the development of type 2 diabetes: the atherosclerosis risk in communities study. Diabetes 2003;52:1799–1805.
29. Festa A, D'Agostino R, Jr, Tracy RP, Haffner SM. Elevated levels of acute-phase proteins and plasminogen activator inhibitor-1 predict the development of type 2 diabetes: the insulin resistance atherosclerosis study. Diabetes 2002;51:1131–1137.
30. Freeman DJ, Norrie J, Caslake MJ, Gaw A, Ford I, Lowe GD, O'Reilly DS, Packard CJ, Sattar N. C-reactive protein is an independent predictor of risk for the development of diabetes in the West of Scotland Coronary Prevention Study. Diabetes 2002;51:1596–1600.
31. Fernandez-Real JM, Vayreda M, Richart C, Gutierrez C, Broch M, Vendrell J, Ricart W. Circulating interleukin 6 levels, blood pressure,

and insulin sensitivity in apparently healthy men and women. J Clin Endocrinol Metab 2001;86:1154–1159.
32. Hu FB, Meigs JB, Li, TY, Rifai N, Manson JE. Inflammatory markers and risk of developing type 2 diabetes in women. Diabetes 2004;53: 693–700.
33. Spranger J, Kroke A, Mohlig M, Hoffmann K, Bergmann MM, Ristow M, Boeing H, Pfeiffer AF. Inflammatory cytokines and the risk to develop type 2 diabetes: results of the prospective population-based European Prospective Investigation into Cancer and Nutrition (EPIC)-Potsdam Study. Diabetes 2003;52:812–817.
34. Pop-Busui R, Kirkwood I, Schmid H, Marinescu V, Schroeder J, Larkin D, Yamada E, Raffel DM, Stevens MJ. Sympathetic dysfunction in type 1 diabetes: association with impaired myocardial blood flow reserve and diastolic dysfunction. J Am Coll Cardiol 2004;44:2368–2374.
35. Gerstein HC, Capes SE. Dysglycemia: a key cardiovascular risk factor. Semin Vasc Med 2002;2:165–174.
36. DECODE Study Group, European Diabetes Epidemiology Group. Is the current definition for diabetes relevant to mortality risk from all causes and cardiovascular and noncardiovascular diseases. Diabetes Care 2003;26:688–696.
37. McNeill AM, Rosamond WD, Girman CJ, Golden SH, Schmidt MI, East HE, Ballantyne CM, Heiss G. The metabolic syndrome and 11-year risk of incident cardiovascular disease in the atherosclerosis risk in communities study. Diabetes Care 2005;28:385–390.
38. Lehtinen JM, Uusitupa M, Siitonen O, Pyorala K. Prevalence of neuropathy in newly diagnosed NIDDM and nondiabetic control subjects. Diabetes 1989;38:1307–1313.
39. Pfeifer MA, Weinberg CR, Cook DL, Reenan A, Halter JB, Ensinck JW, Jr, Porte D. Autonomic neural dysfunction in recently diagnosed diabetic subjects. Diabetes Care 1984;7:447–453.
40. Singh JP, Larson MG, O'Donnell CJ, Wilson PF, Tsuji H, Lloyd-Jones DM, Levy D. Association of hyperglycemia with reduced heart rate variability (The Framingham Heart Study). Am J Cardiol 2000;86:309–312.
41. Liao D, Cai J, Brancati FL, Folsom A, Barnes RW, Tyroler HA, Heiss G. Association of vagal tone with serum insulin, glucose, and diabetes mellitus – The ARIC Study. Diabetes Res Clin Pract 1995;30:211–221.
42. Panzer C, Lauer MS, Brieke A, Blackstone E, Hoogwerf B. Association of fasting plasma glucose with heart rate recovery in healthy adults: a population-based study. Diabetes 2002;51:803–807.
43. Festa A, D'Agostino R, Jr, Hales CN, Mykkanen L, Haffner SM. Heart rate in relation to insulin sensitivity and insulin secretion in nondiabetic subjects. Diabetes Care 2000;23:624–628.
44. Baynes JW, Thorpe SR. Role of oxidative stress in diabetic complications: a new perspective on an old paradigm. Diabetes 1999;48:1–9.
45. Baynes JW. Role of oxidative stress in development of complications of diabetes. Diabetes 1991;40:405–412.
46. Shindo H, Thomas TP, Larkin DD, Karihaloo AK, Inada H, Onaya T, Stevens MJ, Greene DA. Modulation of basal nitric oxide-dependent cyclic-GMP production by ambient glucose, myo-inositol, and protein kinase C in SH-SY5Y human neuroblastoma cells. J Clin Invest 1996;97:736–745.
47. Baumgartner-Parzer SM, Wagner L, Pettermann M, Grillari J, Gessl A, Waldhausl W. High-glucose – triggered apoptosis in cultured endothelial cells. Diabetes 1995;44:1323–1327.
48. Wu QD, Wang JH, Fennessy F, Redmond HP, Bouchier-Hayes D. Taurine prevents high-glucose-induced human vascular endothelial cell apoptosis. Am J Physiol 1999;277:C1229–C1238.
49. Tesfamariam B, Cohen RA. Role of superoxide anion and endothelium in vasoconstrictor action of prostaglandin endoperoxide. Am J Physiol 1992;262:H1915–H1919.
50. Gryglewski RJ, Palmer RM, Moncada S. Superoxide anion is involved in the breakdown of endothelium-derived vascular relaxing factor. Nature 1986;320:454–456.
51. Ward KK, Low PA, Schmelzer JD, Zochodne DW. Prostacyclin and noradrenaline in peripheral nerve of chronic experimental diabetes in rats. Brain 1989;112(Pt 1): 197–208.
52. Vanhoutte PM, Shimokawa H. Endothelium-derived relaxing factor and coronary vasospasm. Circulation 1989;80:1–9.
53. Haefeli WE, Srivastava N, Kongpatanakul S, Blaschke TF, Hoffman BB. Lack of role of endothelium-derived relaxing factor in effects of alpha-adrenergic agonists in cutaneous veins in humans. Am J Physiol 1993;264: H364–H369.
54. Cipolla MJ, Harker CT, Porter JM. Endothelial function and adrenergic reactivity in human type-II diabetic resistance arteries. J Vasc Surg 1996;23:940–949.

55. Tesfamariam B, Cohen RA. Free radicals mediate endothelial cell dysfunction caused by elevated glucose. Am J Physiol 1992;263: H321–H326.
56. Tesfamariam B. Free radicals in diabetic endothelial cell dysfunction. Free Radic Biol Med 1994;16:383–391.
57. Greene DA, Stevens MJ, Obrosova I, Feldman EL. Glucose-induced oxidative stress and programmed cell death in diabetic neuropathy. Eur J Pharmacol 1999;375:217–223.
58. Hogikyan RV, Galecki AT, Halter JB, Supiano MA. Heightened norepinephrine-mediated vasoconstriction in type 2 diabetes. Metabolism 1999;48:1536–1541.
59. Stevens MJ, Dananberg J, Feldman EL, Lattimer SA, Kamijo M, Thomas TP, Shindo H, Sima AA, Greene DA. The linked roles of nitric oxide, aldose reductase and, (Na+,K+)-ATPase in the slowing of nerve conduction in the streptozotocin diabetic rat. J Clin Invest 1994;94:853–859.
60. Nitenberg A. Endothelial dysfunction in patients with diabetes: identification, pathogenesis and treatment. Presse Med 2005;34:1654–1661.
61. Bloomgarden ZT. Adiposity and diabetes. Diabetes Care 2002;25:2342–2349.
62. Lazar MA. How obesity causes diabetes: not a tall tale. Science 2005;307:373–375.
63. Lehrke M, Lazar MA. Inflamed about obesity. Nat Med 2004;10(2):126–127.
64. Pickup JC. Inflammation and activated innate immunity in the pathogenesis of Type 2 diabetes. Diabetes Care 2004;27:813–823.
65. Wellen KE, Hotamisligil GS. Inflammation, stress, and diabetes. J Clin Invest 2005;115:1111–1119.
66. Kuller LH, Tracy RP, Shaten J, Meilahn EN, for the Multiple Risk Factor Intervention Trial Research Group. Relation of C-reactive protein and coronary heart disease in the MRFIT nested case-control study. Am J Epidemiol 1996;144:537–547.
67. Tracy RP, Lemaitre RN, Diane P, Evans RW, Cushman M, Meilahn EN, et al. Relationship of C-reactive proteins to risk of cardiovascular disease in the elderly. Results from the cardiovascular health study and the rural health promotion project. Arterioscler Thromb Vasc Biol 1997;17:1121–1127.
68. Schmidt MI, Duncan BB, Sharret AR, Lindberg G, Savage PJ, Offenbacher S, et al. Markers of inflammation and prediction of diabetes mellitus in adults (Atherosclerosis Risk in Communities study): a cohort study. Lancet 1999;353:1649–1652.
69. Haffner SM, William K, Tracy RP. C-reactive protein: an independent risk factor for type 2 diabetes in the Mexico City diabetes study. Circulation 2000;102: II–871.
70. Ebstein W. Zur therapie des diabetes mellitus, insbesondere über die Anwendung des salicylsauren natron bei demselben. Berliner Klin Wochenschr 1876;24:337–340.
71. Kopp E, Ghosh S. Inhibition of NF-kB by sodium salicylate and aspirin. Science 1994;265:956–959.
72. Schoelson S. Invited comment on W. Ebstein: on the therapy of diabetes mellitus, in particular on the application of sodium salicylate. J Mol Med 2002;80:618–619.
73. Peraldi P, Spiegelman B. TNF-alpha and insulin resistance: summary and future prospects. Mol Cell Biochem 1998;182(1–2):169–175.
74. Fernàndez-Real JM, Broch M, Casamitjana R, Gutirrez C, Vendrell J, Richart C. Plasma levels of the soluble fraction of tumor necrosis factor receptor 2 and insulin resistance. Diabetes 1998;47:1757–1762.
75. Theuma P, Fonseca VA. Inflammation, insulin resistance, and atherosclerosis. Metab Syndr Relat Disord 2004;2:105–113.
76. Shoelson SE, Lee J, Goldfine AB. Inflammation and insulin resistance. J Clin Invest 2006;116(7):1793–1801.
77. Fried LP, Borhani NO, Enright P, Furberg D, Gardin JM, Kronmal RA, et al. The cardiovascular health study: design and rationale. Ann Epidemiol 1991;1:263–276.
78. Barinas-Mitchell E, Cushman M, Meilahn EN, Tracy RP, Kuller LH. Serum levels of C-reactive protein are associated with obesity, weight gain, and hormone replacement therapy in healthy postmenopausal women. Am J Epidemiol 2001;153(11):1094–1101.
79. Harris MI, Flegal KM, Cowie CC, Eberhardt MS, Goldstein DE, Little RR, et al. Prevalence of diabetes, impaired fasting glucose, and impaired glucose tolerance in U.S. adults. The Third National Health and Nutrition Examination Survey, 1988–1994 Diabetes Care 1998;21(4):518–525.
80. Snijder MB, Dekker JM, Visser M, Stehouwer CDA, van Hinsbetrg VWM, Bouter LM, et al. C-reactive protein and diabetes mellitus type 2. Diabetologia 2001;44(Suppl 1): 115A.
81. Han TS, Sattar N, Williams K, Gonzalez-Villapado C, Lean MEJ, Haffner SM. Prospective study of C-reactive protein in relation to the development of diabetes and metabolic syndrome in the Mexico City Diabetes Study. Diabetes Care 2002;25:2016–2021.

82. Willerson JT, Ridker PM. Inflammation as a cardiovascular risk factor. Circulation 2004;109(Suppl II): II-2–II-10.
83. Libby P, Ridker PM, Maseri A. Inflammation and atherosclerosis. Circulation 2002;105: 1135–1143.
84. Fearon DT, Locksley RM. The instructive role of innate immunity in the acquired immune response. Science 1996;272:50–54.
85. Medzhitov R, Janeway CA. Innate immunity: impact on the adaptive immune response. Curr Opin Immunol 1997;9:4–9.
86. Ganda OP, Arkin CF. Hyperfibrinogenemia. An important risk factor for vascular complications in diabetes. Diabetes Care 1992; 15:1245–1250.
87. Kuller LH, Eichner JE, Orchard TJ, Grandits GA, McCallum L, Tracy RP, et al. The relation between serum albumin levels and risk of coronary heart disease in the Multiple Risk Factor Intervention Trial. Am J Epidemiol 1991;134(11):1266–1277.
88. Bruno G, Cavallo-Perin P, Bargero G, Borra M, D'Errico N, Pagano G. Association of fibrinogen with glycemic control and albumin excretion rate in patients with non-insulin-dependent diabetes mellitus. Ann Int Med 1996;125:653–657.
89. Corti MC, Salive ME, Guralnik JM. Serum albumin and physical function as predictors of coronary heart disease mortality and incidence in older persons. J Clin Epidemiol 1996;49(5):519–526.
90. Luoma PV, Näyhä S, Sikkilä K, Hassi J. High serum alpha-tocopherol, albumin, selenium and cholesterol, and low mortality from coronary heart disease in northern Finland. J Int Med 1994;237:49–54.
91. Macy E, Hayes T, Tracy RP. Variability in the measurement of C-reactive protein in healthy subjects: implications for reference interval and epidemiological applications. Clin Chem 1997;43:52–58.
92. Mantovani A, Bussolino F, Intrano M. Cytokine regulation of endothelial cell function: from molecular level to the bedside. Immunol Today 1997;18:231–240.
93. Cushman M, Cornell ES, Howard PR, Bovill EG, Tracy RP. Laboratory methods and quality assurance in the Cardiovascular Health Study. Clin Chem 1995;41:264–270.
94. Ridker PM, Hennekens CH, Buring JE, Rifai N. C-reactive protein and other markers of inflammation in the prediction of cardiovascular disease in women. N Engl J Med 2000;342(12):836–843.
95. Kuller LH, Borhani NO, Furberg CD, Gardin JM, Manolio TA, O'Leary, DH, et al. Prevalence of subclinical atherosclerosis and cardiovascular disease and association with risk factors in the Cardiovascular Health Study. Am J Epidemiol 1994;139: 1164–1179.
96. Kuller LH, Shemanski BM, Psaty BM, Borhani NO, Gardin J, Haan MN, et al. Subclinical disease as an independent risk factor for cardiovascular disease. Circulation 1995;92:720–726.
97. Perry IJ, Wannamethee SG, Shaper AG. Prospective study of serum g-glutamyltransferase and risk of NIDDM. Diabetes Care 1998;21(2):732–737.
98. Pradhan AD, Manson JE, Rifai N, Buring JE, Ridker PM. C-reactive protein, interleukin 6, and risk of developing type 2 diabetes mellitus. JAMA 2001;286(3):327–334.
99. Fineberg SE. Glycaemic control and hormone replacement therapy: implications of the Postmenopausal Estrogen/Progestogen Intervention (PEPI) study. Drugs Aging 2000;17(6):453–461.
100. Cushman M, Psaty BM, Kuller LH, Dobs AS, Tracy RP. Hormone replacement therapy, inflammation, and homeostasis in elderly women. Arterioscler Thromb Vasc Biol 1999;19:893–899.
101. Cushman M, Arnold AM, Psaty BM, Manolio TA, Kuller LH, Burke GL, et al. C-reactive protein and the 10-year incidence of coronary heart disease in older men and women: the cardiovascular health study. Circulation 2005;112:25–31.
102. Pietropaolo M, Barinas-Mitchell E, Kuller LH. The heterogeneity of diabetes: unraveling a dispute: is systemic inflammation related to islet autoimmunity. Diabetes 2007;56(5):1189–1197.
103. Zinman B, Kahn SE, Haffner SM, O'Neill MC, Heise MA, Freed MI. Phenotypic characteristics of GAD antibody-positive recently diagnosed patients with type 2 diabetes in North America and Europe. Diabetes 2004;53(12):3193–3200.
104. Hawa MI, Thivolet C, Mauricio D, Alemanno I, Cipponeri E, Collier D, Hunter S, Buzzetti R, de Leiva A, Pozzilli P, Leslie RD; Action LADA Group. Metabolic syndrome and autoimmune diabetes: action LADA 3. Diabetes Care 2009;32(1):160–164.
105. Kwon G, Xu G, Marshall CA, McDaniel ML. Tumor necrosis factor a-induced pancreatic b-cell insulin resistance is mediated by nitric oxide and prevented by 15-deoxy-D^{12,14}-prostaglandin J$_2$ and aminoguanidine. J Biol Chem 1999;274(26):18702–18708.

106. Pakala SV, Chivetta M, Kelly CB, Katz JD. In autoimmune diabetes the transition from benign to pernicious insulitis requires an islet cell response to tumor necrosis factor alpha. J Exp Med 1999;189:1053–1062.
107. Saghizadeh M, Ong GM, Garvey WT, Henry RR, Kern PA. The expression of TNF-alpha by human muscle: relationship to insulin resistance. J Clin Invest 2001;97:1111–1116.
108. Winkler G, Salamon F, Salamon D, Speer G, Simon K, Cseh K. Elevated serum tumor necrosis factor-alpha levels contribute to the insulin resistance in type 2 (non-insulin-dependent) diabetes and in obesity. Diabetologia 1998;41:860–861.
109. Kellerer M, Rett K, Renn W, Groop L, Haring HU. Circulating TNF-alpha and leptin levels in offspring of NIDDM patients do not correlate to individual insulin sensitivity. Horm Metab Res 1996;28:737–743.
110. Ehl S, Hombach J, Aichele P, Odermatt B, Hengartner H, Zinkernagel RM, et al. Viral and bacterial infections interfere with peripheral tolerance induction and activate CD8+ T cells to cause immunopathology. J Exp Med 1998;5:763–774.
111. Berliner J, Navab M, Fogelman A, Frank J, Demer L, Edwards P, et al. Atherosclerosis: basic mechanisms. Oxidation, inflammation, and genetics. Circulation 1995;91:2488–2496.
112. Locksley RM, Killeen N, Lenardo MJ. The TNF and TNF receptor superfamilies: integrating mammalian biology. Cell 2001; 104:487–501.
113. Meade T, Brozovic M, Chakrabarti R, Haines A, Imerson J, Mellows S, et al. Haemostatic function and ischaemic heart disease: principal results of the Northwick Park Heart Study. Lancet 1986;ii(533):537.
114. Green EA, Flavell RA. The temporal importance of TNFa expression in the development of diabetes. Immunity 2000;12:459–469.
115. Yang X-D, Tisch R, Singer SM, Cao ZA, Liblau R, Schreiber RD, et al. Effect of tumor necrosis factor a on insulin-dependent diabetes mellitus in NOD mice. I. The early development of autoimmunity and the diabetogenic process. J Exp Med 1994;180:995–1004.
116. Augustine KA, Rossi RM, Van G, Housman J, Stark K, Danilenko D, et al. Noninsulin-dependent diabetes mellitus occurs in mice ectopically expressing the human Axl tyrosine kinase receptor. J Cell Physiol 1999;181(433):447.
117. Wu AJ, Hua H, Munson SH, McDevitt HO. Tumor necrosis factor-alpha regulation of CD4+CD25+ T cell levels in NOD mice. Proc Natl Acad Sci USA 2002;99(19): 12287–12292.
118. Stassi G, De Maria R, Trucco G, Rudert W, Testi R, Galluzzo A, et al. Nitric oxide primes pancreatic beta cell destruction for Fas-mediated destruction in IDDM. J Exp Med 1997;186(8):1193–1200.
119. Mandrup-Poulsen T, Egeberg J, Nerup J, Bendtzen K, Nielsen JH, Dinarello C. Interleukin-1 effects on isolated islets: kinetics and specificity of ultrastructural changes. Acta Endocrinol Suppl 1986;275:29A.
120. Arnush M, Heitmeier MR, Scarim AL, Marino MH, Manning PT, Corbett J. A. IL-1 produced and released endogenously within human islets inhibits b cell function. J Clin Invest 1998;102:516–526.
121. Kulkarni RN, Winnay JN, Postic C, Magnuson MA, Kahn CR. Tissue-specific knockout of the insulin receptor in pancreatic b cells creates an insulin secretory defect similar to that in Type 2 diabetes. Cell 1999;96:329–339.
122. Papanicolaou DA, Wilder RL, Manolagas SC, Chrousos GP. The pathophysiologic roles of interleukin-6 in human disease. Ann Int Med 1998;128:127–137.
123. Mohamed-Ali V, Goodrick S, Rowesh A. Subcutaneous adipose tissue releases interleukin-6, but not tumor necrosis factor-alpha, in vivo. J Clin Endocrinol Metab 1997; 82:4196–4200.
124. Yudkin J, Yajnik C, Mohamed-Ali V, Bulmer K. High levels of circulating proinflammatory cytokines and leptin in urban, but not rural, Indians: a potential explanation for increased risk of diabetes and coronary heart disease. Diabetes Care 1999;22:363–364.
125. Sandler S, Bentzen K, Eizirik DL, Welsh M. Interleukin-6 affects insulin secretion and glucose metabolism of rat pancreatic islets in vitro. Endocrinology 1990;126:1288–1294.
126. Kanemaki T, Kitade H, Kaibori M. Interleukin 1 beta and interleukin 6, but not tumor necrosis factor alpha, inhibit insulin-stimulated glycogen synthesis in rat hepatocytes. Hepatology 1998;27:1296–1303.
127. Weisberg SP, Hunter D, Huber R, Lemieux J, Slaymaker S, Vaddi, K, et al. CCR2 modulates inflammatory and metabolic effects of high-fat feeding. J Clin Invest 2006;116(1):115–124.
128. Tsou CL, Peters W, Si Y, Slaymaker S, Aslanian AM, Weisberg SP, et al. (2007) Critical roles for CCR2 and MCP-3 in monocyte mobilization from bone marrow and recruitment to inflammatory sites. J Clin Invest 2007;117(4):902–909.

129. Schernthaner GH, Kopp HP, Krzyzanowska K, Kriwanek S, Koppensteiner R, Schernthaner G. Soluble CD40L in patients with morbid obesity: significant reduction after bariatric surgery. Eur J Clin Invest 2006;36(6):395–401.
130. Kanda H, Tateya S, Tamori Y, Kotani K, Hiasa K, Kitazawa R, et al. MCP-1 contributes to macrophage infiltration into adipose tissue, insulin resistance, and hepatic steatosis in obesity. J Clin Invest 2006;116(6):1494–1505.
131. Kamei N, Tobe K, Suzuki R, Ohsugi M, Watanabe T, Kubota N, et al. Overexpression of monocyte chemoattractant protein-1 in adipose tissues causes macrophage recruitment and insulin resistance. J Biol Chem 2006;281(36):26602–26614.
132. Steppan CM, Bailey ST, Bhat S, Brown EJ, Banerjee RR, Wright CM, et al. The hormone resistin links obesity to diabetes. Nature 2001;409(6818):307–312.
133. Kaser S, Kaser A, Sandhofer A, Ebenbichler CF, Tilg H, Patsch JR. Resistin messenger-RNA expression is increased by proinflammatory cytokines in vitro. Biochem Biophys Res Commun 2003;309(2):286–290.
134. Verma S, Li SH, Wang CH, Fedak PW, Li RK, Weisel RD, et al. Resistin promotes endothelial cell activation: further evidence of adipokine-endothelial interaction. Circulation 2003;108(6):736–740.
135. Reilly MP, Lehrke M, Wolfe ML, Rohatgi A, Lazar MA, Rader DJ. Resistin is an inflammatory marker of atherosclerosis in humans. Circulation 2005;111(7):932–939.
136. Janeway CA, Jr, Medzhitov R. Innate immune recognition. Annu Rev Immunol 2002;20:197–216.
137. Wen L, Wong FS. How can the innate immune system influence autoimmunity in type 1 diabetes and other autoimmune disorders. Crit Rev Immunol 2005;25(3):225–250.
138. Takeda K, Kaisho T, Akira S. Toll-like receptors. Annu Rev Immunol 2003;21:335–376.
139. Akira S, Uematsu S, Takeuchi O. Pathogen recognition and innate immunity. Cell 2006;124(4):783–801.
140. Kabelitz D. Expression and function of Toll-like receptors in T lymphocytes. Curr Opin Immunol 2007;19(1):39–45.
141. Shi H, Kokoeva MV, Inouye K, Tzameli I, Yin H, Flier JS. TLR4 links innate immunity and fatty acid-induced insulin resistance. J Clin Invest 2006;116(11):3015–3025.
142. Suganami T, Tanimoto-Koyama K, Nishida J, Itoh M, Yuan X, Mizuarai S, et al. Role of the Toll-like receptor 4/NF-kappaB pathway in saturated fatty acid-induced inflammatory changes in the interaction between adipocytes and macrophages. Arterioscler Thromb Vasc Biol 2007;27(1):84–91.
143. Tsukumo DM, Carvalho-Filho MA, Carvalheira JB, Prada PO, Hirabara SM, Schenka AA, et al. Loss-of-function mutation in Toll-like receptor 4 prevents diet-induced obesity and insulin resistance. Diabetes 2007;56(8):1986–1998.
144. Martinon F, Burns K, Tschopp J. The inflammasome: a molecular platform triggering activation of inflammatory caspases and processing of proIL-beta. Mol Cell 2002;10(2):417–426.
145. Mariathasan S, Newton K, Monack DM, Vucic D, French DM, Lee WP, et al. (2004) Differential activation of the inflammasome by caspase-1 adaptors ASC and Ipaf. Nature 2004;430(6996):213–218.
146. Fink SL, Cookson BT. Apoptosis, pyroptosis, and necrosis: mechanistic description of dead and dying eukaryotic cells. Infect Immun 2005;73(4):1907–1916.
147. Eisenbarth SC, Colegio OR, O'Connor W, Sutterwala FS, Flavell RA. Crucial role for the Nalp3 inflammasome in the immunostimulatory properties of aluminium adjuvants. Nature 2008;453(7198):1122–1126.
148. Cassel SL, Eisenbarth SC, Iyer SS, Sadler JJ, Colegio OR, Tephly LA, et al. The Nalp3 inflammasome is essential for the development of silicosis. Proc Natl Acad Sci USA 2008;105(26):9035–9040.
149. Larsen CM, Faulenbach M, Vaag A, Volund A, Ehses JA, Seifert, B, et al. Interleukin-1-receptor antagonist in type 2 diabetes mellitus. N Engl J Med 2007;356(15):1517–1526.
150. Maedler K, Sergeev P, Ris F, Oberholzer J, Joller-Jemelka HI, Spinas GA, et al. Glucose-induced beta cell production of IL-1beta contributes to glucotoxicity in human pancreatic islets. J Clin Invest 2002;110(6):851–860.
151. Welsh N, Cnop M, Kharroubi I, Bugliani M, Lupi R, Marchetti P, et al. Is there a role for locally produced interleukin-1 in the deleterious effects of high glucose or the type 2 diabetes milieu to human pancreatic islets. Diabetes 2005;54(11):3238–3244.
152. Omi T, Kumada M, Kamesaki T, Okuda H, Munkhtulga L, Yanagisawa Y, et al. An intronic variable number of tandem repeat polymorphisms of the cold-induced autoinflammatory syndrome 1 (CIAS1) gene modifies gene expression and is associated with essential hypertension. Eur J Hum Genet 2006;14(12):1295–1305.

153. Jiang C, Ting AT, Seed B. PPAR-gamma agonists inhibit production of monocyte inflammatory cytokines. Nature 1998;391(6662):82–86.
154. Murphy GJ, Holder JC. PPAR-g agonists: therapeutic role in diabetes, inflammation and cancer. Trends Pharmacol Sci 2000;21:469–474.
155. Yuan M, Konstanopoulos N, Lee J, Hansen L, Li Z-W, Karin M, et al. Reversal of obesity- and diet-induced insulin resistance with salicylates or targeted disruption of Ikk-β. Science 2001;293:1673–1677.
156. Mohanty P, Aljada A, Ghanim H, Hofmeyer D, Tripathy D, Syed T, et al. Evidence for a potent antiinflammatory effect of rosiglitazone. J Clin Endocrinol Metab 2004;89(6):2728–2735.
157. Yki-Jarvinen H. Thiazolidinediones. N Engl J Med 2004;351(11):1106–1118.
158. Ialenti A, Grassia G, Di Meglio P, Maffia P, Di Rosa M, Ianaro, A. Mechanism of the anti-inflammatory effect of thiazolidinediones: relationship with the glucocorticoid pathway. Mol Pharmacol 2005;67(5):1620–1628.
159. Weitz-Schmidt G. Statins as anti-inflammatory agents. Trends Pharmacol Sci 2002;23(10):482–486.
160. Kimura T, Mogi C, Tomura H, Kuwabara A, Im DS, Sato K, et al. Induction of scavenger receptor class B type I is critical for simvastatin enhancement of high-density lipoprotein-induced anti-inflammatory actions in endothelial cells. J Immunol 2008;181(10):7332–7340.
161. Shoelson SE, Herrero L, Naaz A. Obesity, inflammation, and insulin resistance. Gastroenterology 2007;132(6):2169–2180.
162. Fleischman A, Shoelson SE, Bernier R, Goldfine AB. Salsalate improves glycemia and inflammatory parameters in obese young adults. Diabetes Care 2008;31(2):289–294.
163. Yin MJ, Yamamoto Y, Gaynor RB. The anti-inflammatory agents aspirin and salicylate inhibit the activity of I(kappa)B kinase-beta. Nature 1998;396(6706):77–80.

Part II

Syndromes

Chapter 6

The Mouse Model of Autoimmune Polyglandular Syndrome Type 1

James Gardner and Mark Anderson

Summary

Autoimmune polyglandular syndrome type 1 (APS-1) is a monogenic autoimmune disease caused by mutations in the autoimmune regulator (*AIRE*) gene. Here we describe the mouse models of APS-1 generated by targeted mutation of the mouse *Aire* gene, and how these models recapitulate the autoimmunity seen in APS-1. Further, we discuss how the study of these mouse systems has shed light on the pathogenesis of the disease and some of the basic mechanisms of self-tolerance in the immune system. Aire promotes self-antigen expression within the thymus, and failure to express such antigens in the thymus leads to autoimmunity. We discuss how the AIRE protein may function at a molecular and cellular level to accomplish this remarkable feat. We then address the identification of organ-specific antigens and the characterization of specific cell populations involved in this disease model, and how these discoveries in the mouse may lead to improved therapies for APS-1 and other autoimmune diseases. Finally, we present a number of current and prospective topics in autoimmunity and self-tolerance that have emerged from the study of these mouse models.

Key Words: Autoimmune regulator, FoxP3, Thymic deletion, Thymic epithelial cells, Self-antigens

THE *Aire*-KNOCKOUT MOUSE AS A MODEL OF HUMAN APS-1

APS-1 in Humans: A Monogenic Autoimmune Disease Resulting from Mutations in the AIRE Gene

Autoimmune polyglandular syndrome type 1 (APS-1) is an autoimmune disease characterized principally by immune-mediated destruction of the endocrine organs. Clinically, the diagnosis is made by meeting two of the following three criteria – hypoparathyroidism, adrenal insufficiency, and mucocutaneous candidiasis. In addition, most APS-1 patients exhibit a diverse range of other autoimmune symptoms including type I diabetes, gonadal atrophy, hypothyroidism, autoimmune hepatitis, and autoimmune pneumonitis, among others (*1, 2*). The disease generally manifests during childhood, but the diverse symptoms may emerge throughout a patient's life. Though the precise manifestations vary from individual to individual, and even between siblings (*1*), the overall clinical picture is one of a profound failure in the immune system's ability to properly distinguish self- from non-self-tissues, and a consequently devastating attack on primarily the endocrine organs.

While the manifestations of this disease are diverse, the genetics are uniquely simple. APS-1 is an autosomal recessive disease caused by mutations in a single gene, the autoimmune regulator (AIRE). Though rare, with an estimated total of 500 cases worldwide, APS-1 has uniquely elevated frequency among genetically isolated groups including Sardinians (1/14,400), Iranian Jews (1/9,000), and Finns (1/25,000) (*3*). Linkage analysis of families with the disorder led to the identification of AIRE (*4, 5*), with almost all affected APS-1 patients containing either homozygous or compound heterozygous mutations of the gene. To date over 40 such mutations have been identified, the majority of which are either premature stop codons or large exon deletions (*6*).

The *AIRE* gene itself encodes a ~57-kDa protein of 545 amino acids comprised of multiple domains common to transcriptional regulators and nuclear proteins (Fig. 6.1). Located on chromosome 21 in humans and chromosome 10 in mice, *Aire* is a single-copy gene whose orthologues have been identified in all gnathostome (jawed vertebrate) classes except the cartilaginous fish, and whose sequence and structure is broadly conserved

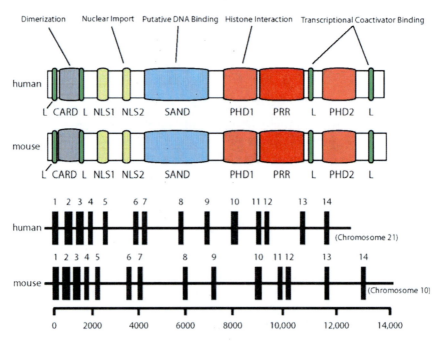

Fig. 6.1 The mouse and human AIRE protein and gene.

between these classes (*7*). Suggestively, this places the emergence of the *Aire* gene approximately 500 million years ago, roughly coincident with the emergence of the adaptive immune system (*8*). This relationship between Aire and the adaptive immune system is likely to be central to its role in preventing autoimmunity.

The murine *Aire* gene, in particular, is highly homologous to the human gene, sharing all major protein domains, all exons, and having 71% nucleotide and 73% amino-acid sequence homology (Fig. 6.1) (*9, 10*). As such, and because the mouse is such a well-characterized system for the study of the immunology, it has proven an attractive candidate for modeling human APS-1, and for studying the mechanisms of Aire biology and immune self-tolerance in general.

The Mouse Model of APS-1 Broadly Recapitulates the Autoimmunity Observed in Human APS-1

Due to the significant interest in the mechanisms underlying APS-1 upon the identification of the *AIRE* gene and its murine homologue Aire, a number of independent groups generated Aire-knockout mice. In all cases, these mice exhibited significant autoimmunity including multiorgan lymphocytic infiltration, autoreactive antibodies in serum, and tissue destruction, though the precise phenotypes differed somewhat depending on the strain and the influence of genetic background.

The first Aire-knockout mouse was generated by insertion of a termination codon in exon 6, replicating a common mutation observed in APS-1 patients (*11*). This knockout, though generated in a relatively autoimmune-resistant Sv/129/C57BL/6 mixed background, still exhibited both multiorgan lymphocytic infiltration and the presence of autoreactive antibodies in serum, as well as infertility among both males and females. Specific endocrine organs including the ovaries and liver showed distinct lymphocytic infiltrates, and consistent with human APS-1, adrenal glands were absent in a significant portion of the Aire-knockout mice suggesting their complete destruction. Further, Aire-knockout mouse serum demonstrated antibody reactivity against the liver, testis, pancreas, and adrenal glands. A second Aire-knockout mouse, also in the Sv/129/C57BL/6 mixed background, was generated by targeted deletion of exon 2 of the murine *Aire* gene which resulted in a frameshift early termination (*12*). These mice demonstrated lymphocytic infiltrates of the salivary gland, ovary, retina, thyroid, liver, and stomach, and serum autoantibodies were also detected against the salivary gland, ovary, retina, thyroid, pancreas, and stomach (Fig. 6.2). Further, this study showed a distinct correlation between organ-specific autoantibodies and lymphocytic infiltrates of that organ. Finally a third group generated a unique Aire knockout by targeted deletion of a region spanning from exon 5 to exon 12, removing the sequences coding for the SAND domain as well as both PHD domains (*13*). This third knockout showed a similar phenotype of

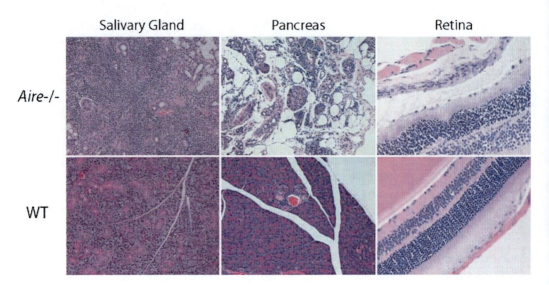

Fig. 6.2 Histology of *Aire*-knockout tissues shows multiorgan lymphocytic infiltrate and tissue destruction (images courtesy of J. DeVoss).

infertility and autoimmune lymphocytic infiltrates of the salivary and lacrimal glands, as well as some infiltration of the pancreas and stomach.

Overall, these overlapping models suggest a consistent picture of the Aire-knockout mouse as predisposed to autoimmunity that generally resembles the diverse but organ-specific autoimmunity seen in APS-1 patients. As in APS-1 patients, Aire-knockout mice begin with relatively mild disease that spreads in both the number of targeted organs and the severity of tissue damage. Further, the disease seen in Aire-knockout mice is both disseminated and organ-specific – while numerous and diverse organs can be targeted, specific organs are affected while others are spared, and the organs targeted differ from individual to individual or strain to strain.

The influence of genetic modifier loci on the disease phenotype of Aire-knockout mice was further demonstrated when the Aire mutation was backcrossed into diverse genetic backgrounds (*14*). In autoimmune-prone strains like the non-obese diabetic (NOD) mouse, for example, lymphocytic infiltration affects a diverse set of organs including the retina, cornea, stomach, salivary gland, lung, liver, prostate, ovary, pancreas, and thyroid gland, while only a small subset of these organs (retina, salivary gland, lung, and prostate) are infiltrated in the autoimmune-resistant C57BL/6 strain (Fig. 6.3). Further, Aire-knockout NOD mice experience wasting and die by 15 weeks of age, while Aire-knockout C57BL/6 mice do not waste and have survival curves similar to wildtype. Thus, the presence or absence of other genetic

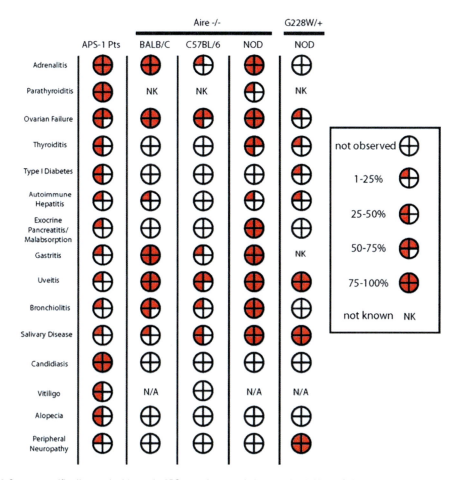

Fig. 6.3 Organ-specific disease incidence in APS-1 patients and characterized *Aire*-deficient mouse strains (*1, 2, 14, 44, 75, 76*; M. Su, J. DeVoss, M. Cheng, T. Shum, personal communication).

modifiers affects both the spectrum of organs targeted and the severity of tissue damage.

In this sense, the Aire-knockout mouse broadly reflects the heterogeneity of disease manifestations in human APS-1, where genetic modifiers and environmental factors likely influence the spectrum of affected organs (though it should be noted that the exacerbation or elimination of innate immune stimuli appears to have little to no discernable effect on the spectrum of disease in Aire-knockout mice) (*15*). However, some of the targeted organs clearly seem to differ between humans and mice; for example, the endocrine pancreas is targeted in many APS-1 patients but spared in mice, while the retina is targeted in mice but rare in humans. Indeed even among those organs that are shared between man and mouse, the precise antigens recognized may in fact differ between the species (*16*). Some disease manifestations of APS-1 in humans are never observed in mice, for example mucocutaneous candidiasis, though this may be partly explained by the fact that Candida is a commensal organism in humans but not in mice (17, 18). Regardless of these differences, however, the mouse model of APS-1 provides a broad recapitulation of the autoimmunity seen in the human disease, and therefore presents an invaluable tool to learn about both the pathogenesis of this disease as well as more fundamental mechanisms of immune self-tolerance.

THE MECHANISM OF Aire-DEFICIENCY UNRAVELED IN MICE

Aire's Expression in the Thymus Provides Clues to Its Function

While the phenotypic characterization of Aire-knockout mice demonstrated a broad recapitulation of the autoimmunity seen in APS-1, this still did not provide immediate answers to the fundamental pathogenesis of the disease. Indeed, while the described Aire-knockout mouse models all reported autoimmune sequellae, they also reported few or no detectable changes in the immune system itself. The number of thymocytes and lymphocytes, the ratios of CD4+ and CD8+ T cells and B cells, the activation and death of thymocytes, the responsiveness of T cells to in vitro stimulation, and the number and function of regulatory T cells are all grossly normal in Aire-knockout mice (11–13).

One clue to Aire's function, however, lay in its highly tissue-restricted expression pattern. While early attempts to characterize this expression were somewhat discordant, all concurred that Aire was most highly expressed in the thymus (9, 19, 20). As the organ in which T cells develop and are selected, the thymus plays an important role in shaping a T-cell repertoire. Because the adaptive immune system generates individual receptors for each T-cell precursor essentially at random through V(D)J recombination, many T-cell precursors are born with either a completely non-functional receptor or with a receptor that recognizes self. One of the principal functions of the thymus, therefore, is to provide permissive signals for those developing T cells that express a functional T-cell receptor (positive selection), while eliminating those that recognize self-antigen (negative selection), or diverting such self-reactive T cells to a regulatory lineage (21, 22).

The thymus therefore shoulders a heavy burden in trying to prevent the development of self-reactive effector T cells – it must eliminate not just T cells that recognize ubiquitous self-antigens expressed in all cells, but also those T cells that might recognize tissue-specific antigens (TSAs) like insulin or thyroglobulin, which are normally expressed only in very restricted and specialized tissues like the beta cells of the pancreas or the principal cells of the thyroid. Without some mechanism to account for this, T cells specific for such antigens might escape thymic negative selection simply because the self-antigen was sequestered in the target organ. Numerous complementary systems could, and do, exist to prevent the development and activation of such tissue-specific autoreactive T cells, including the migration of antigen-presenting cells from the periphery back to the thymus (23), the peripheral development of regulatory T cells (24), and the inactivation or anergy of those naïve T cells that undergo inappropriate activation upon exposure to self-antigen (reviewed in 25). However the immune system has also found an additional elegant solution to this problem.

Thymic Epithelial Cells Are Unique Sources of TSA Expression

In order to produce a T-cell repertoire which is tolerant of all the body's diverse tissues, the thymus has developed a specialized cell population which expresses a vast array of otherwise tissue-specific self-antigens from the entire body. These cells, called medullary thymic epithelial cells (mTECs), produce a broad sample of the body's otherwise tissue-specific self-antigens like insulin and thyroglobulin, and thus recreate within the thymus a microcosm of the entire body's proteome against which to screen developing T cells.

The unique epithelial cells of the thymus have long been known to play an indispensable role in the positive and negative selection of T-cell precursors. Unlike most epithelium, thymic epithelial cells (TECs) do not form a continuous barrier or define a topological space; rather, they are interdigitated among the developing T-cell precursors throughout the entire parenchyma of the thymus. Broadly speaking, cortical thymic epithelial cells (cTECs) play an important role in the positive selection of T-cell precursors, while mTECs play a role in the negative selection of those T cells that recognize self-antigen (reviewed in 8). While ectopic expression of individual TSAs like insulin in the thymus was first described more than a decade ago (26, 27), until recently the scope of such TSA expression, its physiologic significance, and the cell populations responsible were unknown. Thus, the discovery that mTECs were in fact the principal cell population responsible for this thymic TSA expression, and that mTECs expressed thousands of such TSAs (28), suggested that these cells might play an important role not only in tolerizing the immune system against ubiquitous antigens but also against many tissue-restricted ones as well. However, this theory, while compelling, lacked evidence of physiologic relevance as no examples of autoimmunity caused by defects in thymic TSA expression were known.

Aire Regulates Expression of TSAs in mTECs

The contemporaneous discoveries that APS-1 was caused by mutations in the AIRE gene, that mTECs were the source of TSA expression in the thymus, and that AIRE was highly expressed in mTECs led investigators to hypothesize that perhaps the autoimmunity observed in APS-1 patients and Aire-knockout mice resulted from a failure of TSAs expression in the thymus (*12, 28*). Indeed, using microarrays and quantitative PCR to compare TSA expression in mTECs from Aire-wildtype and Aire-knockout mice it was shown that Aire is required for mTECs to produce this diverse set of TSAs, and in the absence of Aire this reduction in expression of "peripheral self" in the thymus leads to autoimmunity in these mice (*12*). Thus in Aire-knockout mice, mTECs are unable to promiscuously transcribe TSAs like insulin, thyroglobulin, and interphotoreceptor retinoid-binding protein, and therefore T cells reactive against these antigens can escape thymic negative selection without ever seeing these antigens (Fig. 6.4). Further, loss of Aire in the thymic epithelium is sufficient to cause this autoimmunity, as transplantation of Aire-deficient thymic stroma into Nude mice (which lack a thymus due to mutation of the FoxN1 gene) causes these mice to develop autoimmunity that resembles the complete Aire-knockout mouse (*12*).

To confirm that loss of thymic TSA expression in Aire-knockout mice leads directly to autoimmunity, additional studies have been done using Aire-dependent TSA promoters to drive expression of exogenous neo-antigens in the thymus and study negative selection of T-cell receptor transgenic T cells specific for those antigens in the presence and absence of Aire. For example, investigators used the insulin promoter to drive expression of hen egg lysozyme (HEL) in both the pancreas and the thymus, and then examined the thymic negative selection of HEL-specific T cells

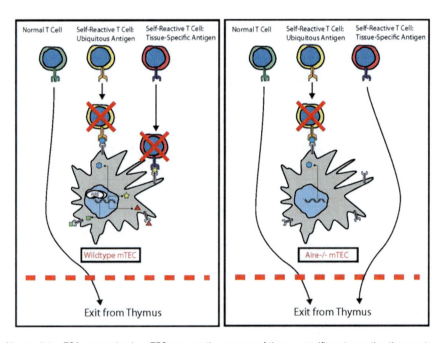

Fig. 6.4 *Aire* regulates TSA expression in mTECs, preventing escape of tissue-specific autoreactive thymocytes.

in Aire-wildtype and Aire-knockout mice (*29, 30*). Because mTECs normally transcribe insulin at low levels in an Aire-dependent manner, these transgenic mice produce insulin promoter-driven HEL within the thymus, and when HEL-specific T-cell precursors are introduced, they are negatively selected and die before leaving the thymus. However, in the absence of Aire, mTECs no longer produce this insulin-driven HEL, and thus HEL-specific T cells do not undergo negative selection in the Aire-knockout thymus. Instead, these cells now mature normally and exit the thymus, encountering HEL protein in the pancreatic islets and causing autoimmune diabetes. Such transgenic approaches provide direct mechanistic insight into the breakdown of tolerance that occurs in the absence of Aire, offering clear evidence that the autoimmunity seen in Aire-knockout mice is a result of failures in thymic TSA expression.

It is important to note that while promiscuous expression of TSAs in the thymus represents a large sample of the body's transcriptome, and Aire regulates a significant percentage of these TSAs, it is also clear that both these sets are incomplete – that some TSAs, like islet-specific glucose-6-phosphatase-related protein (IGRP), a major autoantigen in type I diabetes, are not expressed at all in mTECs (*31*), while others like C-reactive protein (CRP) from the liver, are clearly expressed in mTECs but in an Aire-independent fashion (*12*). Indeed, mature mTECs themselves appear to promiscuously express at least 3,000 TSA genes, of which Aire regulates perhaps 250–1,000, in addition to other, non-TSA genes (*12, 32, 33*). Thus Aire appears to regulate the thymic expression of a subset of the TSAs expressed in mTECs, and these TSAs themselves represent a subset of the body's total transcriptome. This incredibly diverse but incomplete representation of self in the thymus suggests, not surprisingly, that other complementary mechanisms must also be in place to help reinforce self-tolerance.

Such transcriptional de-regulation is itself a remarkable feat, as it requires uncoupling the normally tissue-restricted expression program of specific genes, allowing them all to be simultaneously expressed in this one remarkable cell population. Precisely how Aire functions to accomplish this is still not completely understood, though the molecular mechanism of AIRE's action has been the subject of significant research.

The Molecular Mechanism of AIRE Function

Long before Aire was implicated as a regulator of TSAs gene transcription in mTECs, the homology of its predicted domains to other known proteins (Fig. 6.1) led investigators to speculate that it might act as a transcriptional regulator (*4, 5*). Like other transcriptional regulators, AIRE contains a nuclear localization sequence that is necessary (*34*) and sufficient (*35*) to target it to the nucleus; a caspase recruitment domain (CARD) involved in homodimerization (*36*); four LXXLL nuclear receptor boxes that mediate interaction with transcriptional coactivators (*37*); a SAND (Sp100, AIRE, NucP41/P75, and DEAF1) domain whose other family members have DNA-binding ability (*38*); and two zinc-finger containing plant homeodomains (PHD1 and 2) that may be involved in histone binding (*39, 40*).

The subcellular localization of AIRE also provides clues that suggest it might act to regulate transcription. Immunofluorescent staining shows that AIRE in mTECs localizes to the nucleus, specifically into punctate nuclear bodies (*41, 42*) that may associate with the nuclear matrix (*43*). More specifically, AIRE appears to localize within or adjacent to nuclear speckles, which are often sites of splicing, polyadenylation, capping, and other RNA processing, as well as sites of RNA polymerase II stabilization and elongation (*44*). Indeed, AIRE has been suggested to play a role in transcriptional elongation through recruitment of P-TEFb, a positive elongation factor (*45*). Further, in in vitro assays AIRE has been shown to interact with the transcriptional coactivator CBP, and to have direct and cooperative transcriptional transactivation capabilities (*46, 47*) as well as direct DNA-binding activity (*39, 48*). However, the relevance of these in vitro findings to AIRE's function in vivo is still uncertain, and its role in directly binding to *cis*-acting regulatory sequences of target genes remains unclear. Further, genomic analyses of the thousands of Aire-regulated gene promoters have failed to identify any common sequence elements that might define a consensus binding site for AIRE.

Because AIRE exerts such large-scale effects on transcription of diverse genes across the genome, it has also been suggested that it may exert its effects epigenetically, perhaps by interacting with and modifying chromatin. Indeed, a number of groups have observed that Aire-regulated genes cluster into groups within a chromosome (*33, 49*). However, the clustering of Aire-regulated genes is not a simple case of broad transcriptional derepression. For example, in the casein gene cluster (normally expressed in mammary epithelium of lactating females but also in Aire-expressing mTECs), individual Aire-repressed genes sit between groups of Aire-induced genes, while other genes within the same cluster are unaffected by the presence or absence of Aire (*33*). This suggests that while AIRE may mediate large-scale epigenetic changes such as chromatin remodeling, this alone is not sufficient to explain its transcriptional regulatory effects.

The most illustrative recent data regarding the molecular basis of AIRE's function relates to interactions between the PHD1 domain of AIRE and unmethylated histones. The importance of the PHD1 domain to AIRE's function is underscored by the fact that it is highly conserved between species (*7*), and is also the site of a number of deleterious point mutations in human

APS-1 patients (*50*). Furthermore, other PHD domains have been found in chromatin-associated proteins and these domains appear to bind histones in a manner that is sensitive to the methylation status of specific lysine residues on the histone (*51, 52*). Indeed, reports have now shown that the PHD1 domain of mouse and human AIRE bind directly to histone H3 and that methylation of this histone on lysine 4 inhibits interactions with AIRE and AIRE's ability to bind chromatin-associated DNA (*40, 53*). Importantly, these groups have shown that transfected AIRE directly binds to and upregulates expression of a number of TSA genes in vitro, that this effect is dependent on the histone-binding residues of its PHD1 domain, and that those genes upregulated by AIRE also show a higher ratio of unmethylated to methylated histone H3. Strong evidence therefore exists that AIRE is acting directly or indirectly as a transcriptional regulator, and is likely interacting with chromatin in order to do so.

There is also growing evidence that AIRE regulates transcription in a stochastic manner, turning on certain genes in some mTECs and other genes in others. Only mature mTECs make Aire, these cells are largely postmitotic (*54*), and these mature mTECs collectively express by far the greatest number of TSAs of the thymic cell populations (*33*). However, there is substantial animal-to-animal variability in transcription of AIRE-regulated genes in the thymus between mice of the same background, and even significant variability between the two thymic lobes of individual animals (*55*). Furthermore, single-cell sorting of Aire-expressing mTECs has shown similar variability between individual cells, suggesting each mature mTEC may only produce a small number of these TSAs (*56, 57*). Within an AIRE-regulated locus like the casein gene cluster, for example, one mTEC will express one casein gene and not others, while another mTEC will express different casein genes or none at all. Single-cell sorting also reveals that the TSAs expressed in each mTEC do not appear to follow any tissue-specific regulatory pattern – a cell that expresses some lactation genes like the caseins will simultaneously express genes from other tissues, like insulin. This stochastic mechanism even applies at the individual gene level; whereas autosomal genes in differentiated tissues are normally expressed biallelically, in single mTECs there is often expression of only one allele (*57*). Together, these data suggest that while AIRE acts to globally stimulate transcription of a wide range of genes in mTECs, in any one cell it appears to activate only a small and random subset of these genes. Much work therefore remains to resolve the molecular mechanisms of AIRE's function, and to understand how a single protein exerts such broad-ranging but pleiotropic transcriptional effects. In contrast, much more is now known about the cellular mechanisms of disease.

Cellular Mechanisms of Disease in Aire-Deficient Mice

While early studies of Aire-knockout mice implicated TSA expression in the thymic stroma as playing a causative role in disease pathogenesis, the cellular mechanisms of the resulting disease were not immediately clear. One question that arose was whether the disease resulted from a failure to delete autoreactive effector T cells that destroyed self-tissue, or a failure to produce autoreactive regulatory T cells that protected self-tissue. Indeed, the thymic development of regulatory T cells is indispensable in maintaining self-tolerance (22), and the expression of a self-antigen within the thymus does lead to the development of regulatory T cells specific for that antigen (58, 59).

Aire-deficient mice, however, appear to have no gross defects in regulatory T cells, as the number and percent of FoxP3+ Tregs are unchanged in Aire-knockout animals from multiple strains (12, 13). Further, the ability of Tregs to suppress proliferation of effector T cells in a dose-dependent manner, a classic hallmark of Treg function, is equivalent in Aire-wildtype and Aire-knockout mice, as is the ability to rescue immunodeficient recipients from Treg-depleted adoptive transfer mediated autoimmunity (13, 60). Because the tolerance mediated by regulatory T cells is a dominant form of tolerance which can be transferred (as opposed to deletion of effector T cells which is recessive, and cannot), experiments have also been done to combine equal numbers of Aire-wildtype and Aire-knockout thymi or splenocytes and determine whether the presence of Aire-wildtype Tregs can therefore complement the tolerance defect observed in Aire-knockout animals. In all such cases, the presence of Aire-wildtype thymic stroma or Aire-wildtype splenocytes does not prevent the autoimmunity caused by the Aire-knockout counterpart, suggesting that the autoimmunity in the Aire-knockout could not be rescued by replacing the regulatory T-cell compartment (60). Finally, crossing the Aire knockout onto the Scurfy knockout strain, which lacks FoxP3 and therefore functional regulatory T cells, accelerates disease over either individual knockout alone (61), suggesting that the defects are complementary and not redundant. Thus, while an altered regulatory T-cell repertoire may still play some role in the pathogenesis of autoimmunity in Aire-knockout mice, it appears secondary to a defect in negative selection of autoreactive effector T cells.

The effector cells themselves that mediate disease in Aire-knockout mice have also been characterized. Since the initial description of the Aire-knockout mouse it has been known that the transfer of bulk lymphocytes from an Aire-deficient mouse into an immunodeficient recipient causes autoimmunity in the recipient, and therefore that lymphocytes themselves are sufficient to mediate disease (12). Histological examination of affected organs in Aire-knockout mice also shows a clear lymphocytic infiltrate, with a preponderance of CD4+ T cells but also some CD8+

T cells and B cells (62, 63), with the relative ratios depending on the tissue targeted and the severity of the lesion. Further, the pathogenesis of disease has been shown to require T cells, as Aire-knockout mice that lack T cells do not develop autoimmunity (63). Among T cell subsets, CD4+ T cells appear to play the most important role, as depletion of CD4+ T cells, but not CD8+ T cells, before transfer of Aire-deficient bulk lymphocytes, prevents autoimmunity. The CD4+ T cells isolated from the infiltrated tissues of Aire-knockout mice show a distinct skewing toward a Th1-like phenotype, and produce high levels of INF-γ and TNF-α but low levels of Th2 or Th17 cytokines like IL-4, IL-10, and IL-17 (63). In support of the relevance of Th1-skewing in the pathogenesis of Aire-deficiency, Aire-knockout mice lacking the Stat4 gene, which is necessary for Th1-like polarization, exhibit significantly reduced autoimmunity, while those lacking the Stat6 gene, which is necessary for Th2-like polarization, exhibit in some cases worse disease.

The role of CD4+ T cells in the pathogenesis of autoimmunity in Aire-knockout mice is further supported by the fact that treatment with a depleting anti-CD4 antibody dramatically reduces the tissue infiltration and organ destruction across a range of organs from the eye to the liver, lung, pancreas, and salivary glands (63). As in other models of autoimmune disease (64), treatment with a depleting anti-CD4 antibody appears to largely prevent the severe manifestations of disease in Aire-knockout mice, and may be of future therapeutic interest in the treatment of APS-1. The role of B cells in the model is currently less clear (63, 65). Sera transfers are unable to promote autoimmunity, suggesting a limited role for autoantibodies. However, B-cell depletion with Rituximab appears to ameliorate disease in the mouse model (65). Taken together, these results suggest that B cells may serve as a contributor through their APC function, but more detailed study is needed.

Defining the Antigen-Specific Response in Aire-Knockout Mice: Identification of Disease-Relevant Autoantigens

While the role of B cells and antibodies in the pathogenesis of disease in the Aire-knockout mouse appears to be limited, these autoantibodies can be used as tools to identify disease-relevant autoantigens. One such example from the Aire-knockout mouse is the identification of the retinal antigen interphotoreceptor retinoid-binding protein (IRBP), whose Aire-dependent thymic expression is both necessary and sufficient to prevent retinal autoimmunity in mice (62). Using serum from Aire-deficient mice as a tool, the investigators found a ~150-kD protein that was the target of consistent antibody reactivity in Aire-knockout mice, and identified this protein as IRBP. To test whether IRBP expression in the thymus was required to prevent uveitis, thymic tissue from IRBP-knockout mice (which still retain functional Aire) was then transplanted into athymic recipient mice, and surprisingly it was found that these mice did in fact develop retinal autoimmunity. Thus, IRBP presents both a promising model antigen to study central tolerance and a potentially exciting therapeutic target for antigen-specific therapy of autoimmune uveitis.

Additional organ-specific antigens have also been identified in Aire-knockout mice using similar techniques. A stomach antigen, Mucin 6, was shown to be the target of autoantibodies in Aire-knockout serum and to be Aire-regulated in the thymic stroma (*66*). Other organ-specific autoantigens identified include an exocrine pancreatic protein, protein disulfide isomerase, PDIp (*67*), and as well as a salivary antigen, α-fodrin (*13*), though these last two are not Aire-regulated in the thymus, and their causative role in the pathogenesis of organ-specific autoimmunity is therefore less clear. It is perhaps surprising, given the vast array of self-antigens regulated by Aire in the thymus, that only a restricted number of organs are targeted in Aire-knockout mice and in APS-1 patients, and within those organs only specific antigens are recognized. The reason for this telescoping, oligoclonal immune response to self is not entirely clear, but may reflect the limited autoreactive T-cell repertoire in the model.

Finally, it is important to note that there may be some differences in autoantibody reactivity profiles between APS-1 patients and Aire-knockout mouse strains (*16*). Indeed, some of the proteins recognized by APS-1 patient serum may be different than those targeted in Aire-knockout mice; this would, in fact, not be surprising given the significant divergence in MHC molecules observed between the two species. However some overlap clearly exists, as evidenced by the recent identification of the NALP5 protein as an important parathyroid antigen in APS-1, and the parallel reactivity to NALP5 seen in Aire-knockout mouse serum (*68*; T. Shum, M. Cheng, O. Kampe, M. Anderson, unpublished results).

Unique Autosomal Dominant AIRE Allele Modeled in Mouse

Recently, a novel inheritance pattern of AIRE mutations was described in an Italian family that suggested an autosomal dominant form of transmission. This disease manifested a unique phenotype including predominant thyroiditis as well as some of the conventional hallmarks of APS-1, but all affected family members were reported to be heterozygotes with one functional AIRE allele (*69*). The other allele carried a missense mutation causing substitution of a tryptophan for a glycine at amino acid 228, within the putatively DNA-binding SAND domain of AIRE. This mutation was subsequently knocked into the Aire locus to generate a mouse model of this APS-1-like disease (*44*). As in humans, G228W heterozygous mice developed spontaneous autoimmunity targeting a diverse range of organs including the lacrimal and salivary glands, as well as background-dependent infiltration of the retina, exocrine pancreas, thyroid gland, and sciatic nerve (Fig. 6.3).

In addition to confirming the unique genetics of this mutation, two interesting observations have arisen out of the generation of this mouse. First, this study suggests a link between AIRE's subnuclear localization and its function, because the introduction of the G228W allele causes AIRE, which is normally distributed in nuclear dots adjacent to nuclear speckles, to form large, ubiquitin-containing aggregates within the nucleus that resemble nuclear inclusion bodies. Second, this G228W system provides unique insight into the levels of thymic TSA expression that are required to maintain self-tolerance. For each Aire-regulated TSA gene examined, the presence of the heterozygous G228W mutation reduced but did not abolish expression of that gene in mTECs, whereas complete Aire-knockout mice showed undetectable or nearly undetectable expression. For example, the retinal antigen IRBP, which is both necessary and sufficient to prevent autoimmunity against the target organ, was still expressed in mTECs of the G228W mouse but at lower levels. In the complete absence of thymic IRBP, all examined strains develop uveitis, but in the G228W mouse, this lower level of IRBP expression led to uveitis in only certain, autoimmune-prone backgrounds like the NOD mouse (*44*). This finding illustrates that not only do the presence or absence of thymic TSAs matter, but the levels of expression may be critically important as well. This is indirectly supported in human autoimmunity, where it has been found that type I diabetes is associated with decreased levels of intrathymic insulin expression (*70, 71*).

Extrathymic Aire Expression and Peripheral Self-Tolerance

In addition to its established role in thymic tolerance, there is longstanding evidence that Aire is also expressed outside the thymus, particularly in the spleen and lymph nodes, also known as the secondary lymphoid organs (*12, 19*). The identity and function of these cells, however, has been uncertain, with some reports of Aire expression in dendritic cells, some of Aire expressed in lymphocytes, and some in tissues entirely outside the lymphatic system (*19, 42, 72*). Recent evidence, however, has suggested that the same promiscuous TSA expression used by the thymus to prevent autoimmunity may also occur in the secondary lymphoid organs (*31, 73, 74*). These studies have shown that tissue-specific promoters can drive expression of transgenes in the lymphoid stroma, and that this self-antigen expression is sufficient to mediate deletion of naïve T cells specific for that antigen. Furthermore, one such extrathymic Aire-expressing stromal population was recently defined, and Aire in these cells was found to regulate the expression of a large number of TSAs (*31*). Interestingly, however, the Aire-regulated genes in these extrathymic stromal cells were almost completely distinct from the set of Aire-regulated genes in the thymus, suggesting these cells may serve as a "backup" or "safety net" to prevent the escape of autoreactive T cell clones that evade thymic negative selection. However, the physiologic relevance of these cells, their usefulness as therapeutic targets, and the role of Aire in the periphery remain to be discovered.

CONCLUSIONS

The adaptive immune system provides a powerful tool to combat the incredible diversity and rapid evolution of prokaryotic pathogens like bacteria and viruses. The price of generating this diversity, however, is the greatly increased risk of autoimmunity presented by self-reactive T- and B-cell clones of one's own making. Indeed, the vast preponderance of T-cell precursors born in the bone marrow do not survive the process thymic positive and negative selection (8), suggesting the thymus acts as an indispensable gatekeeper in preventing the maturation of faulty and autoreactive T-cell clones.

The discovery of the AIRE gene as the site of causative mutations in APS-1, while recent, has heralded a wealth of insight into the fundamental mechanisms of thymic immune tolerance. Mouse models of Aire-deficiency, in particular, have provided a unique perspective into the function of Aire and the immunologic significance of promiscuous gene expression within the thymus. Further, the Aire-knockout mouse offers a powerful tool to identify pathogenic tissue-specific autoantigens that may be important both for our understanding of the basic mechanisms of APS-1, and more generally for the diagnosis and the treatment of a broad range of autoimmune diseases. Finally, Aire-knockout mouse models are now serving as tools to develop more effective treatment regimens for APS-1 itself. Numerous exciting questions remain, including the precise molecular mechanism of Aire's regulation of TSA transcription, the organ-specific autoantigens involved, the relationship between the diversity of genes regulated by Aire in the thymus and the relative oligoclonality of immune reactivity in target organs, and the role of Aire, of any, outside the thymus.

REFERENCES

1. Perheentupa J. Autoimmune polyendocrinopathy-candidiasis-ectodermal dystrophy. J Clin Endocrinol Metab 2006;91:2843–2850.
2. Perheentupa J. APS-I/APECED: the clinical disease and therapy. Endocrinol Metab Clin North Am 2002;31:295–320, vi.
3. Peterson P, Peltonen L. Autoimmune polyendocrinopathy syndrome type 1 (APS1) and AIRE gene: new views on molecular basis of autoimmunity. J Autoimmun 2005;25(Suppl):49–55.
4. Nagamine K, Peterson P, Scott HS, et al. Positional cloning of the APECED gene. Nat Genet 1997;17:393–398.
5. The Finnish-German APECED Consortium. An autoimmune disease, APECED, caused by mutations in a novel gene featuring two PHD-type zinc-finger domains. Nat Genet 1997;17:399–403.
6. Heino M, Peterson P, Kudoh J, et al. APECED mutations in the autoimmune regulator

(AIRE) gene. Hum Mutat 2001;18: 205–211.
7. Saltis M, Criscitiello MF, Ohta Y, et al. Evolutionarily conserved and divergent regions of the autoimmune regulator (Aire) gene: a comparative analysis. Immunogenetics 2008;60:105–114.
8. Kyewski B, Klein L. A central role for central tolerance. Annu Rev Immunol 2006;24:571–606.
9. Blechschmidt K, Schweiger M, Wertz K, et al. The mouse Aire gene: comparative genomic sequencing, gene organization, and expression. Genome Res 1999;9:158–166.
10. Mittaz L, Rossier C, Heino M, et al. Isolation and characterization of the mouse Aire gene. Biochem Biophys Res Commun 1999;255: 483–490.
11. Ramsey C, Winqvist O, Puhakka L, et al. Aire deficient mice develop multiple features of APECED phenotype and show altered immune response. Hum Mol Genet 2002;11:397–409.
12. Anderson MS, Venanzi ES, Klein L, et al. Projection of an immunological self shadow within the thymus by the Aire protein. Science 2002;298:1395–1401.
13. Kuroda N, Mitani T, Takeda N, et al. Development of autoimmunity against transcriptionally unrepressed target antigen in the thymus of Aire-deficient mice. J Immunol 2005;174:1862–1870.
14. Jiang W, Anderson MS, Bronson R, Mathis D, Benoist C. Modifier loci condition autoimmunity provoked by Aire deficiency. J Exp Med 2005;202:805–815.
15. Gray DH, Gavanescu I, Benoist C, Mathis D. Danger-free autoimmune disease in Aire-deficient mice. Proc Natl Acad Sci USA 2007;104:18193–18198.
16. Pontynen N, Miettinen A, Arstila TP, et al. Aire deficient mice do not develop the same profile of tissue-specific autoantibodies as APECED patients. J Autoimmun 2006;27: 96–104.
17. Lacasse M, Fortier C, Trudel L, Collet AJ, Deslauriers N. Experimental oral candidosis in the mouse: microbiologic and histologic aspects. J Oral Pathol Med 1990;19: 136–141.
18. Phillips AW, Balish E. Growth and invasiveness of Candida albicans in the germ-free and conventional mouse after oral challenge. Appl Microbiol 1966;14:737–741.
19. Heino M, Peterson P, Sillanpaa N, et al. RNA and protein expression of the murine autoimmune regulator gene (Aire) in normal, RelB-deficient and in NOD mouse. Eur J Immunol 2000;30:1884–1893.
20. Zuklys S, Balciunaite G, Agarwal A, Fasler-Kan E, Palmer E, Hollander GA. Normal thymic architecture and negative selection are associated with Aire expression, the gene defective in the autoimmune-polyendocrinopathy-candidiasis-ectodermal dystrophy (APECED). J Immunol 2000;165:1976–1983.
21. Kim JM, Rasmussen JP, Rudensky AY. Regulatory T cells prevent catastrophic autoimmunity throughout the lifespan of mice. Nat Immunol 2007;8:191–197.
22. Sakaguchi S, Yamaguchi T, Nomura T, Ono M. Regulatory T cells and immune tolerance. Cell 2008;133:775–787.
23. Bonasio R, Scimone ML, Schaerli P, Grabie N, Lichtman AH, von Andrian UH. Clonal deletion of thymocytes by circulating dendritic cells homing to the thymus. Nat Immunol 2006;7:1092–1100.
24. Apostolou I, von Boehmer H. In vivo instruction of suppressor commitment in naive T cells. J Exp Med 2004;199:1401–1408.
25. Schwartz RH. T cell anergy. Annu Rev Immunol 2003;21:305–334.
26. Jolicoeur C, Hanahan D, Smith KM. T-cell tolerance toward a transgenic beta-cell antigen and transcription of endogenous pancreatic genes in thymus. Proc Natl Acad Sci USA 1994;91:6707–6711.
27. Smith KM, Olson DC, Hirose R, Hanahan D. Pancreatic gene expression in rare cells of thymic medulla: evidence for functional contribution to T cell tolerance. Int Immunol 1997;9:1355–1365.
28. Derbinski J, Schulte A, Kyewski B, Klein L. Promiscuous gene expression in medullary thymic epithelial cells mirrors the peripheral self. Nat Immunol 2001;2:1032–1039.
29. Liston A, Gray DH, Lesage S, et al. Gene dosage – limiting role of Aire in thymic expression, clonal deletion, and organ-specific autoimmunity. J Exp Med 2004;200:1015–1026.
30. Liston A, Lesage S, Wilson J, Peltonen L, Goodnow CC. Aire regulates negative selection of organ-specific T cells. Nat Immunol 2003;4:350–354.
31. Gardner JM, Devoss JJ, Friedman RS, et al. Deletional tolerance mediated by extrathymic Aire-expressing cells. Science 2008;321:843–847.
32. Kyewski B, Derbinski J. Self-representation in the thymus: an extended view. Nat Rev Immunol 2004;4:688–698.
33. Derbinski J, Gabler J, Brors B, et al. Promiscuous gene expression in thymic

epithelial cells is regulated at multiple levels. J Exp Med 2005;202:33–45.
34. Ilmarinen T, Melen K, Kangas H, Julkunen I, Ulmanen I, Eskelin P. The monopartite nuclear localization signal of autoimmune regulator mediates its nuclear import and interaction with multiple importin alpha molecules. FEBS J 2006;273:315–324.
35. Pitkanen J, Vahamurto P, Krohn K, Peterson P. Subcellular localization of the autoimmune regulator protein. Characterization of nuclear targeting and transcriptional activation domain. J Biol Chem 2001;276: 19597–19602.
36. Meloni A, Fiorillo E, Corda D, Perniola R, Cao A, Rosatelli MC. Two novel mutations of the AIRE protein affecting its homodimerization properties. Hum Mutat 2005;25:319.
37. Savkur RS, Burris TP. The coactivator LXXLL nuclear receptor recognition motif. J Pept Res 2004;63:207–212.
38. Bottomley MJ, Collard MW, Huggenvik JI, Liu Z, Gibson TJ, Sattler M. The SAND domain structure defines a novel DNA-binding fold in transcriptional regulation. Nat Struct Biol 2001;8:626–633.
39. Purohit S, Kumar PG, Laloraya M, She JX. Mapping DNA-binding domains of the autoimmune regulator protein. Biochem Biophys Res Commun 2005;327:939–944.
40. Org T, Chignola F, Hetenyi C, et al. The autoimmune regulator PHD finger binds to non-methylated histone H3K4 to activate gene expression. EMBO Rep 2008;9: 370–376.
41. Heino M, Peterson P, Kudoh J, et al. Autoimmune regulator is expressed in the cells regulating immune tolerance in thymus medulla. Biochem Biophys Res Commun 1999;257:821–825.
42. Bjorses P, Pelto-Huikko M, Kaukonen J, Aaltonen J, Peltonen L, Ulmanen I. Localization of the APECED protein in distinct nuclear structures. Hum Mol Genet 1999;8:259–266.
43. Tao Y, Kupfer R, Stewart BJ, et al. AIRE recruits multiple transcriptional components to specific genomic regions through tethering to nuclear matrix. Mol Immunol 2006;43:335–345.
44. Su MA, Giang K, Zumer K, et al. Mechanisms of an autoimmunity syndrome in mice caused by a dominant mutation in Aire. J Clin Invest 2008;118:1712–1726.
45. Oven I, Brdickova N, Kohoutek J, Vaupotic T, Narat M, Peterlin BM. AIRE recruits P-TEFb for transcriptional elongation of target genes in medullary thymic epithelial cells. Mol Cell Biol 2007;27:8815–8823.
46. Pitkanen J, Doucas V, Sternsdorf T, et al. The autoimmune regulator protein has transcriptional transactivating properties and interacts with the common coactivator CREB-binding protein. J Biol Chem 2000;275:16802–16809.
47. Pitkanen J, Rebane A, Rowell J, et al. Cooperative activation of transcription by autoimmune regulator AIRE and CBP. Biochem Biophys Res Commun 2005;333:944–953.
48. Kumar PG, Laloraya M, Wang CY, et al. The autoimmune regulator (AIRE) is a DNA-binding protein. J Biol Chem 2001;276:41357–41364.
49. Johnnidis JB, Venanzi ES, Taxman DJ, Ting JP, Benoist CO, Mathis DJ. Chromosomal clustering of genes controlled by the Aire transcription factor. Proc Natl Acad Sci USA 2005;102:7233–7238.
50. Halonen M, Kangas H, Ruppell T, et al. APECED-causing mutations in AIRE reveal the functional domains of the protein. Hum Mutat 2004;23:245–257.
51. Li H, Ilin S, Wang W, et al. Molecular basis for site-specific read-out of histone H3K4me3 by the BPTF PHD finger of NURF. Nature 2006;442:91–95.
52. Pena PV, Davrazou F, Shi X, et al. Molecular mechanism of histone H3K4me3 recognition by plant homeodomain of ING2. Nature 2006;442:100–103.
53. Koh AS, Kuo AJ, Park SY, et al. Aire employs a histone-binding module to mediate immunological tolerance, linking chromatin regulation with organ-specific autoimmunity. Proc Natl Acad Sci USA 2008;105:15878–15883.
54. Gray D, Abramson J, Benoist C, Mathis D. Proliferative arrest and rapid turnover of thymic epithelial cells expressing Aire. J Exp Med 2007;204:2521–2528.
55. Venanzi ES, Melamed R, Mathis D, Benoist C. The variable immunological self: genetic variation and nongenetic noise in Aire-regulated transcription. Proc Natl Acad Sci USA 2008;105:15860–15865.
56. Derbinski J, Pinto S, Rosch S, Hexel K, Kyewski B. Promiscuous gene expression patterns in single medullary thymic epithelial cells argue for a stochastic mechanism. Proc Natl Acad Sci USA 2008;105:657–662.
57. Villasenor J, Besse W, Benoist C, Mathis D. Ectopic expression of peripheral-tissue antigens in the thymic epithelium: probabilistic, monoallelic, misinitiated. Proc Natl Acad Sci USA 2008;105:15854–15859.
58. Jordan MS, Boesteanu A, Reed AJ, et al. Thymic selection of CD4+CD25+ regulatory

T cells induced by an agonist self-peptide. Nat Immunol 2001;2:301–306.
59. Aschenbrenner K, D'Cruz LM, Vollmann EH, et al. Selection of Foxp3+ regulatory T cells specific for self antigen expressed and presented by Aire+ medullary thymic epithelial cells. Nat Immunol 2007;8:351–358.
60. Anderson MS, Venanzi ES, Chen Z, Berzins SP, Benoist C, Mathis D. The cellular mechanism of Aire control of T cell tolerance. Immunity 2005;23:227–239.
61. Chen Z, Benoist C, Mathis D. How defects in central tolerance impinge on a deficiency in regulatory T cells. Proc Natl Acad Sci USA 2005;102:14735–14740.
62. DeVoss J, Hou Y, Johannes K, et al. Spontaneous autoimmunity prevented by thymic expression of a single self-antigen. J Exp Med 2006;203:2727–2735.
63. Devoss JJ, Shum AK, Johannes KP, et al. Effector mechanisms of the autoimmune syndrome in the murine model of autoimmune polyglandular syndrome type 1. J Immunol 2008;181:4072–4079.
64. Makhlouf L, Grey ST, Dong V, et al. Depleting anti-CD4 monoclonal antibody cures new-onset diabetes, prevents recurrent autoimmune diabetes, and delays allograft rejection in nonobese diabetic mice. Transplantation 2004;77:990–997.
65. Gavanescu I, Benoist C, Mathis D. B cells are required for Aire-deficient mice to develop multi-organ autoinflammation: A therapeutic approach for APECED patients. Proc Natl Acad Sci USA 2008;105:13009–13014.
66. Gavanescu I, Kessler B, Ploegh H, Benoist C, Mathis D. Loss of Aire-dependent thymic expression of a peripheral tissue antigen renders it a target of autoimmunity. Proc Natl Acad Sci USA 2007;104:4583–4587.
67. Niki S, Oshikawa K, Mouri Y, et al. Alteration of intra-pancreatic target-organ specificity by abrogation of Aire in NOD mice. J Clin Invest 2006;116:1292–1301.
68. Alimohammadi M, Bjorklund P, Hallgren A, et al. Autoimmune polyendocrine syndrome type 1 and NALP5, a parathyroid autoantigen. N Engl J Med 2008;358:1018–1028.
69. Cetani F, Barbesino G, Borsari S, et al. A novel mutation of the autoimmune regulator gene in an Italian kindred with autoimmune polyendocrinopathy-candidiasis-ectodermal dystrophy, acting in a dominant fashion and strongly cosegregating with hypothyroid autoimmune thyroiditis. J Clin Endocrinol Metab 2001;86:4747–4752.
70. Pugliese A, Zeller M, Fernandez A, Jr., et al. The insulin gene is transcribed in the human thymus and transcription levels correlated with allelic variation at the INS VNTR-IDDM2 susceptibility locus for type 1 diabetes. Nat Genet 1997;15:293–297.
71. Vafiadis P, Bennett ST, Todd JA, et al. Insulin expression in human thymus is modulated by INS VNTR alleles at the IDDM2 locus. Nat Genet 1997;15:289–292.
72. Zheng X, Yin L, Liu Y, Zheng P. Expression of tissue-specific autoantigens in the hematopoietic cells leads to activation-induced cell death of autoreactive T cells in the secondary lymphoid organs. Eur J Immunol 2004;34:3126–3134.
73. Lee JW, Epardaud M, Sun J, et al. Peripheral antigen display by lymph node stroma promotes T cell tolerance to intestinal self. Nat Immunol 2007;8:181–190.
74. Nichols LA, Chen Y, Colella TA, Bennett CL, Clausen BE, Engelhard VH. Deletional self-tolerance to a melanocyte/melanoma antigen derived from tyrosinase is mediated by a radio-resistant cell in peripheral and mesenteric lymph nodes. J Immunol 2007;179:993–1003.
75. DeVoss JJ, Anderson MS. Lessons on immune tolerance from the monogenic disease APS1. Curr Opin Genet Dev 2007;17:193–200.
76. De Luca F, Valenzise M, Alaggio R, et al. Sicilian family with autoimmune polyendocrinopathy-candidiasis-ectodermal dystrophy (APECED) and lethal lung disease in one of the affected brothers. Eur J Pediatr 2008;167:1283–1288.

Chapter 7

Autoimmune Polyendocrine Syndrome Type I: Man

Eystein S. Husebye and Olle Kämpe

Summary

Autoimmune polyendocrine syndrome type I (APS-I) is a monogenic disease with the three main components: chronic mucocutaneous candidiasis, hypoparathyroidism, and adrenal insufficiency. In addition, a number of other endocrine, gastrointestinal, and ectodermal tissues are targeted. There is a huge variability in clinical phenotype, but in typical cases main components appear in childhood and adolescence. The main diagnostic criterion is still the presence of two of the three main components, but diagnosis can be aided by the mutational analysis of the autoimmune regulator (*AIRE*) gene and assay of specific autoantibodies, particularly against interferon omega and alpha. Many patients are diagnosed late or not at all, and the management is not optimal. An overview of the main clinical aspects, diagnostic approaches, and treatment will hopefully contribute to improved care for APS-I patients.

Key Words: Autoimmune, Polyglandular, Autoantibodies, Autoimmune regulator, Candidiasis, Hypoparathyroidism, Addison's disease

INTRODUCTION

Autoimmune polyendocrine syndrome type I (APS-I) (OMIM 240300) is one of a few monogenic autosomal recessive diseases characterized by polyglandular autoimmunity. The diagnosis is made clinically when two of the three main components chronic mucocutaneous candidiasis, hypoparathyroidism, and primary adrenal insufficiency (Addison's disease) are present (*1–3*), except in first-degree relatives in whom the presence of any of the main components is sufficient. In addition, a host of minor components may present in patients mainly in endocrine glands, the gastrointestinal tract, and in the ectoderm (Table 7.1), explaining the alternative name autoimmune polyendocrinopathy-candidiasis-ectodermal dystrophy (APECED). APS-I is rare; in Norway, the prevalence is reported to be 1:90,000 (*4*), but higher frequencies are found in

Table 7.1
Diagnosis of Autoimmune Polyendocrine Syndrome Type I

Definite APS-I	Main components	Definition/remark
1. Two of the three main manifestations	Hypoparathyroidism	Low calcium and PTH, high phosphate
	Addison's disease	High ACTH and renin; low cortisol and aldosterone
	Mucocutaneous candidiasis	Chronic mucocutaneous candidiasis
2. One main component and affected sibling	Any of the three main components	
3. Mutation in the autoimmune regulator gene (AIRE)		Any component
Suspected APS-I	Component	Definition/remark
1. Interferon omega or alpha antibodies	Any component	
2. One major component		For Addison's disease, debut before age 30
3. Affected sibling	Any minor component	
4. Minor component typical of APS-I	Keratitis	Eye examination
	Enamel dysplasia	Orthopantogram and dental examination
	Autoimmune hepatitis	Autoimmune hepatitis on biopsy, increased alanine amino transferase (ALAT)
	Intestinal malabsorption	
Polyglandular autoimmunity	Two or more manifestations	Except type 1 diabetes, autoimmune thyroid disease, and celiac disease

Finland (1:25,000) (*1*), on Sardinia (1:14,000) (*5*), and among Iranian Jews (*6*).

Identification and characterization of a number of autoantibodies against tissue-specific autoantigens have improved our ability to diagnose APS-I (*7*). The autoantigens are typically intracellular enzymes with a restricted tissue expression. A typical autoantigen is tryptophan hydroxylase (TPH), which is expressed in serotonin-producing cells in the intestinal mucosa (*8*). Autoantibodies against TPH are found in about 50% of patients and are correlated to intestinal malabsorption (*8*). In addition, patients generate high-titer antibodies against type I interferons, notably interferon ω and α$_2$, which turns out to be the most sensitive and specific disease marker (*9, 10*). Although autoantibodies are highly suggestive of APS-I, the identification of mutations in the disease-causing gene, autoimmune regulator (AIRE) (*11, 12*), is the ultimate proof and can be found in over 95% of the cases. More than 60 different mutations have now been reported including several large deletions, one encompassing the whole gene (*13*). The Finnish major mutation and the 13 bp deletion in exon 8 are the most common worldwide.

Even if APS-I is diagnosed early, its treatment and follow-up is challenging even in the best of hands. Treatment is complicated by the use of multiple and interacting drugs, and the risk of developing new debilitating and life-threatening complications throughout life. This overview of the main clinical aspects, diagnostic approaches, and treatment will hopefully contribute to improved care for these patients.

ENDOCRINE MANIFESTATIONS

Hypoparathyroidism

Hypoparathyroidism is the most common and often earliest endocrine component found in about 90% of Scandinavian patients (*3, 4*). Hypoparathyroidism can present as severe hypocalcemia with tetany and seizures of grand mal type; but can also give only slight symptoms for a long time, i.e., paresthesias and muscle cramps during infections and dehydration. Renal failure is excluded, and the combination of hypocalcemia, hyperphosphatemia, and often hypomagnesemia is typical. Parathyroid hormone (PTH) may be normal or low. As non-iatrogenic hypoparathyroidism is extremely rare, APS-I should be considered in every patient with hypoparathyroidism. The immunological target in the parathyroid cells was recently identified as NALP5 (nacht leucine-rich repeat protein 5) (*7*), a protein with an unknown function. NALP5 is also expressed, albeit at a much lower level, in ovaries. Interestingly, the presence of autoantibodies against NALP5 does not only correlate with hypoparathyroidism, but also with ovarian failure.

Hypoparathyroidism is treated with vitamin D, calcium, and magnesium supplementation. Either long-acting ergocalciferol or the more potent short-acting calcidiol or calcitrol preparations are used. The short-acting drugs are to be preferred, since long-acting analogs give a higher risk of hypercalcemia and permanent damage of kidney function. However, they may be of value in patients with large and frequent fluctuations in calcium values. Calcium supplementation at 200–1,000 mg daily divided in

3–4 doses, preferably as the citrate salt, is recommended, and gives the opportunity to rapidly lower the calcium when needed. Many patients also lack magnesium, and magnesium supplementation of 50–200 mg per day should be given. Treatment should be aimed at calcium concentrations in lower end of the normal range or slightly below provided that disturbing hypocalcemic symptoms are avoided. The main problem is that vitamin D increases calcium excretion in the urine with the risk of renal stones, nephrocalcinosis. Urinary calcium should therefore be followed, and ultrasound of kidneys should be performed at regular intervals to screen for calcifications. A high water intake is recommended to lower urinary calcium concentrations. Patients should be educated about the symptoms of both hypo- and hypercalcemia, and mature and knowledgeable patients should be given the opportunity to check their calcium levels and to adjust medication at their own discretion. Febrile illness, diarrhea, and an increase in cortisol medication may all lower the calcium levels. Vitamin D intoxication may require forced diuresis and steroid treatment of hypercalcemia. Recently, twice daily administration of synthetic PTH has been shown to give reasonably stable calcium levels and normalized urinary calcium (*14*).

Adrenal Insufficiency

Adrenal failure commonly becomes evident after hypoparathyroidism, commonly in adolescent and early adult years. It is reported in 80% of Finnish and other European patients (*2, 4*), but more infrequent among Iranian Jews (*6*). The typical symptoms and signs are fatigue, salt craving, hypotension, weight loss, increased pigmentation of the skin and mucous membranes, hyponatremia, and hypokalemia. Once suspected, adrenal failure can be confirmed by finding low morning cortisol and high adrenocorticotropic hormone (ACTH) values. Moreover, plasma renin activity is high and aldosterone levels are low. It is rarely necessary to do a short ACTH-stimulation test. Sometimes a dissociation of hypocortisolism and hypoaldosteronism is seen (*3*). Most patients display autoantibodies against 21-hydroxylase (*15*).

Adrenal failure is treated with hydrocortisone or cortisone acetate and fludrocortisone in near physiological doses. The recommended doses for adults are 20 mg hydrocortisone (or 25 mg cortisone acetate); for children 10–15 mg/m^2 hydrocortisone and 0.1 mg fludrocortisone once daily. We recommend a thrice daily regimen with the first dose of hydrocortisone taken as early as possible in the morning, the next dose at lunchtime, and the last dose in the late afternoon or early evening. A weight-adjusted regimen can also be used (*16*). A very important point is to instruct the patients to increase the glucocorticoid dose in acute stress situation, e.g., infections, major surgery, and myocardial infarction. Patients can be given syringes with 100 mg hydrocortisone for emergency use, and should always carry a steroid card.

Gonadal Insufficiency

They are extremely vulnerable to adrenal crisis when they get travelers' diarrhea as they lose water and sodium, and the ability to absorb medication is reduced.

Ovarian insufficiency is an early and common manifestations found in 40–60% in the Finnish and Italian series (*2, 3*). It manifests itself as primary amenorrhea with delayed or arrested pubertal development or as early menopause before 30 years of age. Low estrogen and high gonadotropin are the typical biochemical findings. Testicular insufficiency is also seen, albeit more seldom and at a later age (*3*). A clear correlation to antibodies against side-chain cleavage enzyme is found (*15*). Moreover, gonadal failure is also correlated to NALP5, also expressed in the ovaries (*7*). Patients with primary amenorrhea or pubertal arrest should be given estrogen to initiate puberty, followed by cyclical estrogen and gestagen replacement therapy. Women who wish to have a child should not delay their plans.

Type 1 Diabetes

Type 1 diabetes occurs in APS-I, but the frequency varies between different populations. It is found in 12% of the Finnish (*1*) and 8% of the Norwegian patients (*4*), but is much rarer in the Italian (2%) (*2*) and American (4%) series (*17*). This can explained in part by the high prevalence of type 1 diabetes in Scandinavia. The presence of autoantibodies against IA-2 tyrosine phosphatase-like protein (IA-2) and insulin, but not glutamic acid decarboxylase (GAD), is predictive for the development of diabetes (15).

Thyroid Disease

Autoimmune thyroid disease is rarely seen in young APS-I patients, but the prevalence increases with age and is reported to be 30% among individuals aged 50 or more in the Finnish series (*3*). Those with high titers of thyroid peroxidase, autoantibodies need to be monitored for hypothyroidism. A high frequency of autoimmune thyroid disease was reported in an Italian kindred with a dominant negative AIRE mutation (*18*). Intriguingly, a mouse model harboring the same mutation also displays a high frequency of thyroiditis (*19*). Hypothyroidism is treated with L-thyroxine replacement.

MUCOCUTANEOUS CANDIDIASIS

Chronic Mucocutaneous Candidiasis

Chronic candida infections are usually the first main component to become evident (*1*), typically in childhood and as early as the first year of life. The candida infection is typically seen on the skin and mucous membranes, and varies in severity from mild angular chelitis to candida infections affecting most of the mucous membranes, nails, esophagus, and sometimes the intestines and the skin (*20*). In the mouth, lesions can be hypertrophic with thick white coatings on the tongue and mucus membranes or they can be atrophic. Candidiasis in the esophagus causes chest pain and odynophagia, and in rare cases stricture (*1, 2*). Nails are commonly affected, and post-pubertal females commonly experience vulvo-vaginitis. Systemic candida infection is only seen in APS-I patients on immunosuppressive treatment.

A vigilant treatment approach is warranted because chronic oral candida lesions are linked to the development of oral and esophageal squamous carcinoma, especially in smokers (*21*). Good mouth hygiene is mandatory. Candida of the mouth can be treated with topical polyene solutions such as nystatin and amphotericin B, while skin candidiasis responds to azole treatment. However, drug resistance can become a problem, especially if azole preparations are used prophylactically over extended periods (*22*).

GASTRO-INTESTINAL MANIFESTATIONS

Autoimmune hepatitis is a serious complication which affects children and can have a fatal outcome. It is rarely seen after the age of 15. Even slightly elevated alanine amino transferase (ALAT) levels indicate a need for a close follow-up. Increasing and very high ALAT levels should prompt liver biopsy to secure the diagnosis, since the course of the disease may be rapid and fatal (*1, 3*). Autoantibodies against a number of cytochrome P450 (CYP) enzymes have been found in patients with APS-I, notably CYP1A1, CYP1A2, CYP2A6, and CYP2B6. Only anti-CYP1A2 correlates to the presence of autoimmune hepatitis in APS-I with high sensitivity, but low specificity (*23, 24*). Autoantibodies against TPH and aromatic L-amino acid decarboxylase are not only associated with autoimmune hepatitis, but also with other components of APS-I, i.e., malabsorption and vitiligo, respectively (*15*). Autoimmune hepatitis is initially treated with high-dose glucocorticoid therapy. When ALAT values decrease to 2–3 times the upper reference limit, azathioprine is added and the steroid treatment is reduced. Careful evaluation for side-effects of steroid treatment is important, especially in children since it affects their growth.

Intestinal malabsorption is common. Symptoms include chronic or recurrent diarrhea and steatorrhea, as well as periods with constipation. Histology may reveal lymphocytic infiltration, with and without lymphangiectasia or normal villous architecture (*25–27*). Intestinal malabsorption is correlated to TPH antibodies (*8*), and in duodenal biopsies the serotonin-producing enterochromaffin cells are lacking (*8, 25*). The absence of local serotonin provides an explanation for altered motility in the bowel. In case of loose stools or overt diarrhea, calcium levels should be checked because hypocalcemia can give diarrhea. Pancreatic insufficiency evidenced by decreased secretin-stimulated lipase can also contribute to malabsorption (*25*). The workup of patients with gastrointestinal symptoms should include duodenoscopy, and test of exocrine pancreatic function and stool cultures for candida. Malabsorption can seriously affect the absorption of drugs, and the patient needs to be followed closely. Immunosuppressive treatment with cyclosporin A has been shown to improve the pancreatic function in one case (*25*).

About 15% of patients are affected with autoimmune gastritis and pernicious anemia (*2, 3, 17*). Appearance of autoantibodies to parietal cells and/or intrinsic factor should prompt the investigation of vitamin B12 status, and if necessary gastroduodenoscopy, to look for autoimmune gastritis. B12 deficiency is treated by the conventional replacement therapy either parentally or orally.

ECTODERMAL MANIFESTATIONS

Eye Manifestations

Keratitis, cataract, iridocyclitis, retinal detachment, optic atrophy, and reduced tear production have been reported (*28, 29*). Keratitis is seen in about 25% of patients and is an early and feared complication that may lead to blindness. In a survey of 69 Finnish patients, the oldest age at the presentation of keratitis was 11 years (*28*). Initial symptoms include intense photophobia, blepharospasm, and reduced lacrimation. The etiology is unknown, but may be caused by autoimmunity. Topical treatment with steroids and cyclosporin A may improve keratitis (*25*). Corneal transplantation can help, but the transplanted tissue may become affected (*30*). Limbal stem cell treatment has proven effective (*31*).

Skin Manifestations

Alopecia is observed in 30–40% of patients; severity varies from local hair loss on the scalp to complete loss of scalp or body hair (*2, 3*). Vitiligo is seen in 8–15% of patients (*2*). The extent and distribution is variable. Affected areas should be shielded from excessive sun exposure. Transient episodes of maculopapular, morbilliform, or urticarial rashes, together with fever, have been noted in children (*3*).

Enamel Dysplasia

Enamel dysplasia is commonly seen in up to 70% of patients (*1*). It is only observed in permanent teeth and of variable extent; from grooves or rows of pits of variable width and depth can be seen often running horizontally across the teeth to a near total lack of crown (*32*). The teeth are especially vulnerable to the harmful effects of sweets and abrasive toothpastes, and hypoparathyroidism can contribute to enamel damage. Prompt repair of damaged teeth is highly recommended.

Other and Rare Manifestations

Hypoplasia or aplasia of the spleen is not an uncommon finding (*3*), but the frequency is not known. We must assume that APS-I patients are susceptible to bacterial infections, especially with capsule-bearing microbes such as pneumococcus pneumoniae. Presence of Howell–Jolly bodies in a peripheral blood smear should prompt imaging of the spleen. As splenic hypotrophy can develop silently, we recommend vaccination for all patients against pneumococci. Autoimmune hemolytic anemia (*2, 3*), hypoplastic anemia (*3*), and autoimmune thrombocytopenia (*33*) have been reported in a few patients. Hypokalemia and hypertension indicate high-sensitivity fludrocortisone, over consumption of salted licorice (*3*). Yet others have tubulointerstitial nephritis, which can lead to terminal renal failure (*33*). Autoimmune hypophysitis is reported, but uncommon (*2, 3, 25*). Immunoreactivity against tudor domain containing protein 6 indicates autoimmunity (*34*). Bronchiolitis obliterance has recently been reported as a rare and sometimes fatal complication (*35*). Intriguingly, Aire knockout mice on the non-obese diabetic (NOD) background also develop severe autoimmune destruction of lung tissue (*36*). Reversible metaphyseal dysplasia with growth retardation (*37*) and severe progressive myopathy (*38*) are rare manifestations, probably linked to *AIRE* mutations.

Diagnosis

Improved diagnostic criteria are required to identify patients who present with only one major component or one of the minor components. Autoantibodies against interferon ω or interferon α_2 occur in almost all patients, but is not entirely specific as these autoantibodies occur in other disorders such as myasthenia gravis and thymomas (*9*). If a patient does not fulfill the clinical criteria (Table 7.1), but APS-I is suspected due to the occurrence of any of its components, we propose that autoantibodies against interferon omega or alpha be measured (*39*). A list of clinically relevant antibody assays is given in Table 7.2.

Natural Course and Follow-Up

The course of the disease varies substantially, both in terms of debut age and the number of manifestations exemplified by data from the Norwegian series (Table 7.3) (*4*). The average patient has four manifestations (*1, 40*), and the disease has an increased mortality (*41*). Typically, reports of siblings who have died unexpectedly turn out to be undiagnosed APS-I patients (*4*). APS-I-related causes of death are squamous carcinoma of the oral and esophageal mucosa, fulminant autoimmune hepatitis, renal failure, bronchiolitis, and acute adrenal failure (*3, 21, 41*).

Table 7.2
Clinically Relevant Autoantibodies

Antibody specificity	Characteristic
Interferon omega and alpha	Virtually diagnostic in patients with one of the main components; strongly suggestive of APS-I in patients with a minor component
21-Hydroxylase	Correlated to adrenal insufficiency, also common in isolated autoimmune Addison's disease and APS-II
Side-chain cleavage enzyme	Correlated to ovarian insufficiency; both APS-I and APS-II
Nacht leucine-rich repeat protein 5 (NALP5) antibodies	Correlated to hypoparathyroidism and ovarian insufficiency
Tryptophan hydroxylase antibodies	Correlated to intestinal malabsorption and autoimmune hepatitis
Aromatic L-amino acid decarboxylase	Correlated to autoimmune hepatitis and vitiligo

Specialists should follow patients at a large medical center with experience in treating all aspects of the disease. Patients should be seen at least twice yearly and often more frequently. Endocrinopathies must be treated with replacement therapy, while keratitis, autoimmune hepatitis, and pancreatic insufficiency may improve on immunosuppressive therapy (25, 33). New manifestations can develop throughout life which must be reflected in the follow-up program. Physicians should be alerted to the possible need of psychological counseling (20).

Future Prospects

After the seminal papers identifying *AIRE* as the disease-causing gene was published in 1997, APS-I has been under intense scrutiny as a model disease of autoimmunity. Using mouse models, it has been shown that the expression of tissue-specific proteins in thymic medullary epithelial cells is regulated by Aire (42), leading to negative selection of autoreative T cells (43). Moreover, Aire may also play a role in peripheral tolerance by utilizing a similar mechanism of modulated antigen presentations in peripheral lymphoid organs (44). Future research should focus on new treatment modalities, particularly immunomodulatory therapy that can halt and/or even reverse the autoimmune manifestations.

Table 7.3
Clinical Details, Autoantibodies, and *AIRE* Mutations in the Coding Region in 36 Norwegian Patients with APS-I – Follow-Up After 5–10 Years

Family no	Pat. no	Sex	Age	Age of debut[a]	Autoantibodies[b]	Manifestations[c]	Aire mutations
I	1	M	11	3	AADC+	HP(3), C(3), Al, K	c.967-979del13/c.769C>T
I	2	M	14	2	21OH+	HP(5), C(2)	c.967-979del13/c.769C>T
II	3	F	16	0	SCC+, (21OH-), 17OH	A(5), HP(5), C(0), E	c.769C>T/ c.1242_1243insA
II	4	F	20	9	21OH, 17OH	A(9)	c.769C>T/ c.1242_1243insA
II	5	F	25	14	21OH, SCC, 17OH	A(14), C(14), V, N, G	c.769C>T/ c.1242_1243insA
III	6	M	16	4	21OH, TH	A(4), HP(4), C(4), E, M	c.967-979del13/c.967-979del13
IV	7	M	19	4	21OH, SCC, 17OH	A(11), HP(4), C(9), E	c.967-979del13/c.967-979del13
IV	8	M	26	9	21OH, AADC, GAD	A(12), HP(9), C, E	c.967-979del13/c.967-979del13
IV	9	F	30	4	21OH, AADC, GAD, TPH	HP(4), C, AT,V, E	c.967-979del13/c.967-979del13
V	10	M	22	9	21OH, AADC, TPH, TH	HP(9), C(14), N, E	c.1163_1164insA/c.967-979del13
VI	11	M	30	0	21OH, AADC	A(10), HP(10), C(0), Al, H, M	c.967-979del13/ c.1244_1245insC
VII	12	F	39	13	21OH, SCC, 17OH	A(14), HP(13), G, Al, C, AT	c.1244_1245insC/ c.1244_1245insC
VIII	13	M	35[d]	4	21OH, SCC, AADC, TH	A(4), HP(4), C(26), Al, E, SC	c.967-979del13/c.967-979del13
IX	14	M	44	20	SCC, AADC, GAD, TPH	A(20), HP(27), C(30)	c.967-979del13/c.967-979del13
IX	15	F	10[d]	9	n.d.	A(9), HP?	n.d.
X	16	F	44	7	21OH	A(22), C(7), V, Al, M, E	Not found
XI	17	F	48	10	21OH, SCC	A(13), HP(10), C(10), G	c.967-979del13/c.967-979del13
XII	18	F	49	1	21OH, SCC, AADC+, GAD, TPH, 17OH	A(17), HP(15), C(1), G	c.967-979del13/c.967-979del13

(continued)

Table 7.3 (continued)

Family no	Pat. no	Sex	Age	Age of debut[a]	Autoantibodies[b]	Manifestations[c]	Aire mutations
XIII	19	F	55	13	21OH, GAD	A(13), HP(13), C(13), G, AT, Al, E, D	c.769C>T/c.1336T>G
XIV	20	M	58	9	21OH, SCC, AADC, **GAD+**	A(16), HP(9), V, Al, C	c.769C>T/c.769C>T
XIV	21	F	6[d]	Not known	n.d.	n.d.	n.d.
XIV	22	M	12[d]	Not known	n.d.	n.d.	n.d.
XV	23	M	61	5	21OH	A(17), HP(20), C(5), K, V, Al	c.967-979del13/c.967-979del13
XVI	24	F	30	1	AADC, GAD, TPH	HP(1), C(5), G, N, Al, E	c.769C>T/c.769C>T
XVII	25	F	46	9	Not found	HP(9), G(17), Al, N, E, C	c.22C>T/c.290T>C
XVIII	26	M	36	12	(**21OH-**), SCC, (**GAD-**)	A(12)	c.967-979del13/c.967-979del13
XIX	27	M	55	Not known	21OH, SCC	A, HP, Al	c.22C>T/c.402delC
XX	28	F	32	21	21OH, TPH	A, C	c.879+1G>A/c.879+1G>A
XX	29	M	47	43	AADC, GAD, TPH	HP(43), D(32), V(14)	c.879+1G>A/c.879+1G>A
XXI	30	M	49[d]	13	21OH, SCC, AADC, TPH	A(13), HP, C, Al	c.967-979del13/c.1249dupC
XXII	31	M	42	14	AADC, GAD, TPH	HP(14), C(22), D, K, N, V, Al	c.769C>T/c.1249dupC
XXIII	32	M	39[d]	14	n.d.	A, C	c.967-979del13/c.769C>T
XXIV	33	M	48	Not known	Not found	C, HP	c.967-979del13/c.967-979del13
XXIV	34	F	3[d]	3	n.d.	HP	n.d.[e]
XXIV	35	M	17[d]	5	n.d.	A, HP, C, Al, E	n.d.[e]
XXIV	36	F	34[d]	8	n.d.	HP, AT, E	n.d.[e]

Reproduced from Ref 4, *Copyright 2007, The Endocrine Society*
21OH 21-hydroxylase, *SCC* side-chain cleavage enzyme, *AADC* aromatic L-amino acid decarboxylase, *GAD* glutamic acid decarboxylase, *TPH* tryptophan hydroxylase, *17OH* 17α-hydroxylase, *TH* tyrosine hydroxylase, *A* adrenal insufficiency, *HP* hypoparathyroidism, *C* mucocutaneous candidiasis, *G* primary gonadal insufficiency, *V* vitiligo, *Al* alopecia,

(continued)

Table 7.3 (continued)

AT autoimmune thyroid disease, *M* malabsorption, *N* nail pitting, *E* dental enamel hypoplasia, *K* keratopathy, *H* autoimmune hepatitis, *SC* oral squamous cell carcinoma, *D* diabetes type 1, *n.d.* not done
[a]The age of debut denotes the age at which the first APS-I main component appear
[b]The year of diagnosis for the manifestations is written within brackets
[c]Autoantigen *written in bold with a plus sign* signifies that reactivity against a given antigen has appeared, whereas autoantigen *written in bold within brackets with a minus sign* denotes that reactivity against a given autoantigen was lost, compared with earlier analyses
[d]Deceased (at age *x*)
[e]Mother is heterozygous for c.967-979del13

ACKNOWLEDGMENTS

The work was supported by The European Union FP 6 research project EurAPS, The Swedish Research Council, The Norwegian Research Council, and The Western Regional Health Authorities, Norway.

Conflict of interest: None declared.

REFERENCES

1. Ahonen P, Myllarniemi S, Sipila I, Perheentupa J. Clinical variation of autoimmune polyendocrinopathy-candidiasis-ectodermal dystrophy (APECED) in a series of 68 patients. N Engl J Med 1990;322(26):1829–1836.
2. Betterle C, Greggio NA, Volpato M. Clinical review 93: Autoimmune polyglandular syndrome type 1. J Clin Endocrinol Metab 1998;83(4):1049–1055.
3. Perheentupa J: Autoimmune polyendocrinopathy-candidiasis-ectodermal dystrophy. J Clin Endocrinol Metab 2006;91(8):2843–2850.
4. Wolff AS, Erichsen MM, Meager A, et al. Autoimmune polyendocrine syndrome type 1 in Norway: phenotypic variation, autoantibodies, and novel mutations in the autoimmune regulator gene. J Clin Endocrinol Metab 2007;92(2):595–603.
5. Rosatelli MC, Meloni A, Devoto M, et al. A common mutation in Sardinian autoimmune polyendocrinopathy-candidiasis-ectodermal dystrophy patients. Hum Genet 1998;103(4):428–434.
6. Zlotogora J, Shapiro MS. Polyglandular autoimmune syndrome type I among Iranian Jews. J Med Genet 1992;29(11):824–826.
7. Alimohammadi M, Bjorklund P, Hallgren A, et al. Autoimmune polyendocrine syndrome type 1 and NALP5, a parathyroid autoantigen. N Engl J Med 2008;358(10):1018–1028.
8. Ekwall O, Hedstrand H, Grimelius L, et al. Identification of tryptophan hydroxylase as an intestinal autoantigen. Lancet 1998;352(9124):279–283.
9. Meager A, Visvalingam K, Peterson P, et al. Anti-interferon autoantibodies in autoimmune polyendocrinopathy syndrome type 1. PLoS Med 2006;3(7):e289.
10. Meloni A, Furcas M, Cetani F, et al. Autoantibodies against type I interferons as an additional diagnostic criterion for autoimmune polyendocrine syndrome type I. J Clin Endocrinol Metab 2008;93(11):4389–4397.
11. Finnish-German APECED Consortium. Autoimmune polyendocrinopathy-Candidiasis-Ectodermal Dystrophy. An autoimmune disease, APECED, caused by mutations in a novel gene featuring two PHD-type zinc-finger domains. Nat Genet 1997;17(4):399–403.
12. Nagamine K, Peterson P, Scott HS, et al. Positional cloning of the APECED gene. Nat Genet 1997;17(4):393–398.
13. Trebusak Podkrajsek K, Milenkovic T, Odink R, et al. Detection of a complete AIRE gene deletion and two additional novel mutations

in a cohort of patients with atypical phenotypic variants of APS-1. Eur J Endocrinol 2008;159(5):633–639.
14. Winer KK, Sinaii N, Peterson D, Sainz B, Jr., Cutler GB, Jr. Effects of once versus twice-daily parathyroid hormone 1-34 therapy in children with hypoparathyroidism. J Clin Endocrinol Metab 2008;93(9):3389–3395.
15. Söderbergh A, Myhre AG, Ekwall O, et al. Prevalence and clinical associations of 10 defined autoantibodies in autoimmune polyendocrine syndrome type I. J Clin Endocrinol. Metab 2004;89(2):557–562.
16. Mah PM, Jenkins RC, Rostami-Hodjegan A, et al. Weight-related dosing, timing and monitoring hydrocortisone replacement therapy in patients with adrenal insufficiency. Clin Endocrinol (Oxf) 2004;61(3):367–375.
17. Neufeld M, Maclaren NK, Blizzard RM. Two types of autoimmune Addison's disease associated with different polyglandular autoimmune (PGA) syndromes. Medicine (Baltimore) 1981;60(5):355–362.
18. Cetani F, Barbesino G, Borsari S, et al. A novel mutation of the autoimmune regulator gene in an Italian kindred with autoimmune polyendocrinopathy-candidiasis-ectodermal dystrophy, acting in a dominant fashion and strongly cosegregating with hypothyroid autoimmune thyroiditis. J Clin Endocrinol Metab 2001;86(10):4747–4752.
19. Su MA, Giang K, Zumer K, et al. Mechanisms of an autoimmunity syndrome in mice caused by a dominant mutation in Aire. J Clin Invest 2008;118(5):1712–1726.
20. Perheentupa J. APS-I/APECED: the clinical disease and therapy. Endocrinol Metab Clin North Am 2002;31(2):295–320, vi.
21. Rautemaa R, Hietanen J, Niissalo S, Pirinen S, Perheentupa J. Oral and oesophageal squamous cell carcinoma – a complication or component of autoimmune polyendocrinopathy-candidiasis-ectodermal dystrophy (APECED, APS-I). Oral Oncol 2007;43(6):607–613.
22. Rautemaa R, Richardson M, Pfaller M, Perheentupa J, Saxen H. Reduction of fluconazole susceptibility of Candida albicans in APECED patients due to long-term use of ketoconazole and miconazole. Scand J Infect Dis 2008;23:1–4.
23. Gebre-Medhin G, Husebye ES, Gustafsson J, et al. Cytochrome P450IA2 and aromatic L-amino acid decarboxylase are hepatic autoantigens in autoimmune polyendocrine syndrome type I. FEBS Lett 1997;412(3): 439–445.
24. Obermayer-Straub P, Perheentupa J, Braun S, et al. Hepatic autoantigens in patients with autoimmune polyendocrinopathy-candidiasis-ectodermal dystrophy. Gastroenterology 2001;121(3):668–677.
25. Ward L, Paquette J, Seidman E, et al. Severe autoimmune polyendocrinopathy-candidiasis-ectodermal dystrophy in an adolescent girl with a novel AIRE mutation: response to immunosuppressive therapy. J Clin Endocrinol Metab 1999;84(3):844–852.
26. Bereket A, Lowenheim M, Blethen SL, Kane P, Wilson TA. Intestinal lymphangiectasia in a patient with autoimmune polyglandular disease type I and steatorrhea. J Clin Endocrinol Metab 1995;80(3):933–935.
27. Makharia GK, Tandon N, Stephen Nde J, Gupta SD, Tandon RK: Primary intestinal lymphangiectasia as a component of autoimmune polyglandular syndrome type I: a report of 2 cases. Indian J Gastroenterol 2007;26(6): 293–295.
28. Merenmies L, Tarkkanen A. Chronic bilateral keratitis in autoimmune polyendocrinopathy-candidiadis-ectodermal dystrophy (APECED). A long-term follow-up and visual prognosis. Acta Ophthalmol Scand 2000;78(5): 532–535.
29. Chang B, Brosnahan D, McCreery K, Dominguez M, Costigan C. Ocular complications of autoimmune polyendocrinopathy syndrome type 1. J AAPOS 2006;10(6):515–520.
30. Tarkkanen A, Merenmies L. Corneal pathology and outcome of keratoplasty in autoimmune polyendocrinopathy-candidiasis-ectodermal dystrophy (APECED). Acta Ophthalmol Scand 2001;79(2):204–207.
31. Shah M, Holland E, Chan CC. Resolution of autoimmune polyglandular syndrome-associated keratopathy with keratolimbal stem cell transplantation: case report and historical literature review. Cornea 2007;26(5):632–635.
32. Perniola R, Tamborrino G, Marsigliante S, De Rinaldis C. Assessment of enamel hypoplasia in autoimmune polyendocrinopathy-candidiasis-ectodermal dystrophy (APECED). J Oral Pathol Med 1998;27(6):278–282.
33. Ulinski T, Perrin L, Morris M, et al. Autoimmune polyendocrinopathy-candidiasis-ectodermal dystrophy syndrome with renal failure: impact of posttransplant immunosuppression on disease activity. J Clin Endocrinol Metab 2006;91(1):192–195.
34. Bensing S, Fetissov SO, Mulder J, et al. Pituitary autoantibodies in autoimmune polyendocrine syndrome type 1. Proc Natl Acad Sci U S A 2007;104(3):949–954.
35. De Luca F, Valenzise M, Alaggio R, et al. Sicilian family with autoimmune polyendocrinopathy-candidiasis-ectodermal dystrophy

(APECED) and lethal lung disease in one of the affected brothers. Eur J Pediatr 2008;167(11):1283–1288.
36. Jiang W, Anderson MS, Bronson R, Mathis D, Benoist C. Modifier loci condition autoimmunity provoked by Aire deficiency. J Exp Med 2005;202(6):805–815.
37. Harris M, Kecha O, Deal C, et al. Reversible metaphyseal dysplasia, a novel bone phenotype, in two unrelated children with autoimmunepolyendocrinopathy-candidiasis-ectodermal dystrophy: clinical and molecular studies. J Clin Endocrinol Metab 2003;88(10):4576–4585.
38. Evans RA, Carter JN, Shenston B, et al. Candidiasis-endocrinopathy syndrome with progressive myopathy. Q J Med 1989;70(262):139–144.
39. Oftedal BE, Wolff AS, Bratland E, et al. Radioimmunoassay for autoantibodies against interferon omega; its use in the diagnosis of autoimmune polyendocrine syndrome type I. Clin Immunol 2008;129(1):163–169.
40. Myhre AG, Halonen M, Eskelin P, et al. Autoimmune polyendocrine syndrome type 1 (APS I) in Norway. Clin Endocrinol (Oxf) 2001;54(2):211–217.
41. Bensing S, Brandt L, Tabaroj F, et al. Increased death risk and altered cancer incidence pattern in patients with isolated or combined autoimmune primary adrenocortical insufficiency. Clin Endocrinol (Oxf) 2008;69(5):697–704.
42. Anderson MS, Venanzi ES, Klein L, et al. Projection of an immunological self shadow within the thymus by the aire protein. Science 2002;298(5597):1395–1401.
43. Liston A, Lesage S, Wilson J, Peltonen L, Goodnow CC. Aire regulates negative selection of organ-specific T cells. Nat Immunol 2003;4(4):350–354.
44. Gardner JM, Devoss JJ, Friedman RS, et al. Deletional tolerance mediated by extrathymic Aire-expressing cells. Science 2008;321(5890):843–847.

Chapter 8

IPEX Syndrome: Clinical Profile, Biological Features, and Current Treatment

Rosa Bacchetta, Laura Passerini, and Maria Grazia Roncarolo

Summary

Children carrying mutations in the forkhead box p3 (*FOXP3*) gene are affected by the syndrome known as Immune dysregulation, polyendocrinopathy, enteropathy, X-linked (IPEX). Early onset severe enteropathy, Type-1 diabetes (T1D) and eczema with elevated IgE serum levels are the hallmarks of the disease. Mortality is generally high within the first year of life, although some patients can partially respond to conventional immunosuppression showing clinical improvement. Progress in understanding the pathogenesis of IPEX have been made possible by the recognition that FOXP3 is the driving force for the function of naturally occurring regulatory T cells, a T-cell subset specialized in controlling immune responses. However, many open questions concerning the disease mechanisms, the indications for genetic screening and appropriate treatment of IPEX syndrome remain unanswered. In addition, several patients presenting IPEX-like symptoms do not carry mutations in the *FOXP3* gene.

In the present chapter, we will (1) summarize the latest findings on the biologic function of FOXP3 and its role in immune regulation, (2) highlight the most relevant signs for a correct diagnosis of IPEX syndrome, and (3) provide indications for the development of more targeted therapeutic strategies for the treatment of this devastating pediatric autoimmune disease.

Key Words: Regulatory T cells, FOXP3, CD25, Hyper-IgE, Neonatal diabetes, Enteritis, X-linked, Immunosuppression, HSCT

INTRODUCTION

The syndrome of Immune dysregulation, polyendocrinopathy, enteropathy, X-linked (IPEX) is due to mutations of the gene encoding for the transcription factor forkhead box p3 (FOXP3) and is characterized by multiorgan autoimmunity (*1–3*). The disease is rare, but since the defective gene and its relevance in immunological tolerance have been increasingly acknowledged, more and more patients have been identified. The precise incidence of the disease is unknown, but retrospective data from clinical cases of early autoimmune enteritis or neonatal diabetes of unknown origin, suggest that the occurrence of the disease may be underestimated. The frequency of IPEX does not seem to correlate with a particular geographic distribution. To date less than 50 different mutations have been reported worldwide (4), including missense, splice site mutations, and deletions. It is currently unknown whether the observed variability of the clinical manifestations can be attributed to different mutations (5). Since the gene is located on the X-chromosome, only males are affected, whereas the mother carriers are healthy. Prenatal diagnosis is available for women with positive family history of the disease.

CLINICAL MANIFESTATIONS AND LABORATORY FINDINGS

Based on the cases reported in past and recent literature, the onset of IPEX syndrome occurs in males usually within the first year and mostly in the first month of life (1, 2, 4, 5). Severe enteropathy is always present, manifests with refractory secretory diarrhea and it is typically associated with detection of anti-enterocyte antibodies in the serum and villous atrophy with mucosal lymphocyte infiltration at histology. Enteritis manifests during breast-feeding and, therefore, is independent from cow milk or gluten introduction in the diet. The onset of this symptom can precede or follow Type-1 diabetes (T1D), which is present in the majority of the patients, even in newborns. Elevated serum IgE and dermatitis, usually eczema, are also present. Other autoimmune symptoms, such as thyroiditis with either hyper- or, most frequently, hypo-thyroidism, Coombs positive haemolytic anemia, thrombocytopenia and neutropenia, can be variably present, often with detectable autoantibodies against the respective target tissues. Less commonly, renal disease with interstitial nephritis, can occur as primarily associated to the syndrome and not only secondary to treatments. Early onset, with severe acute enteritis and/or T1D, commonly (but not exclusively) occurs in patients carrying mutations within the forkhead (FKH) domain or null mutations (5). However, the site of the mutation is not always predictive of the disease severity and course and, regardless of the mutation site, IPEX can be rapidly fatal, especially early after onset. In addition, patients show different outcomes, despite the presence of similar mutations. In particular, some patients overcome the first severe phase of the disease and respond to immunosuppressive therapy (5).

Among the clinical symptoms, severe infections or pneumonia have been reported, although these symptoms were less frequent than the more prominent signs described above. A clear causative link between pathogens and the onset of autoimmunity has not been demonstrated in IPEX and often infections can be the consequence of multiple immunosuppressive therapy.

Although rarely, milder forms can be observed, presenting with less severe diarrhea, sometimes intermittent, and symptoms such as arthritis, lymphoadenopathy, alopecia and liver insufficiency. In several patients with typical or milder forms of IPEX, *FOXP3* mutations are not detected. These patients are generally defined as IPEX-like and they also comprise female subjects. The IPEX-like autoimmune manifestations have been correlated to mutations in the *FOXP3* promoter region (*6*) or to mutations in the gene encoding *CD25* (*7, 8*), the alpha-chain of the IL-2 receptor, whose expression is closely related to that of FOXP3 (*9*). This latter observation suggests that mutations in other genes relevant for the regulation of FOXP3 expression or function, can determine pathogenic tissue modifications similar to those found in IPEX syndrome.

Patients in the acute phase of the disease, prior to immunosuppressive therapy, can have a white blood cell count normal or increased. Despite immune dysregulation, there are no clear alterations in the main lymphocyte subsets. $CD4^+$ and $CD8^+$ T- and B-lymphocyte percentages are within the normal ranges (*10*). In addition, lymphocytes display normal in vitro proliferative responses to mitogens. Similarly, normal serum levels of IgG, IgA, and IgM are detected, unless there is intestinal protein loss due to enteropathy. On the contrary, markedly elevated IgE levels and increased eosinophil counts are observed in all patients, already in the early stages of the disease. Autoantibodies are often present and their presence usually correlates with signs of pathology in the target organs. For example, early presence of detectable serum autoantibodies against insulin, pancreatic islet cells, or anti-glutamate decarboxylase, correlates with occurence of neonatal T1D.

Although the clinical presentation of IPEX syndrome, with the typical triad of symptoms, should be easily distinguishable from other pathologies, in infants with enteropathy the most common causes of persistent diarrhea should be excluded, including infections, food-sensitive enteritis, transport system disorders, anatomical or motility abnormalities, and metabolic diseases (*11*). In the presence of T1D as the only symptom, neonatal T1D of different origin should be ruled out (*12*). The clinical severity of protracted diarrhea, possibly with septic complications, should also lead to exclude a primary immunodeficiency, such as severe combined immunodeficiency (*13*). In addition, the association with elevated serum IgE, eosinophilia, and eczema may question the differential diagnosis with Wiskott–Aldrich syndrome, Omenn's syndrome or Hyper-IgE syndrome, whereas celiac disease can usually be excluded because of the early time of onset of IPEX enteropathy, prior to gluten exposure. Parathyroid or adrenal glands are rarely involved in IPEX, whereas they are the main target organs in autoimmune polyglandular syndromes. Most of the relevant features of IPEX that can help in the differential diagnosis are summarized in Table 8.1.

Table 8.1
Main signs and symptoms for the differential diagnosis of genetic autoimmune syndromes and primary immunodeficiencies with immune dysregulation

Symptoms/signs	IPEX	IPEX-like	APECED	Omenn's	WAS	HIES
Time of onset	Neonatal/1 year	1 year/infant	Childhood	Neonatal/1 year	1 year/infant	Neonatal/1 year
Enteropathy	Always present	Frequent	Rare	Frequent	Possible	Rare
Endocrinopathy	Frequent T1D Possible thyroiditis	Frequent T1D Possible thyroiditis	Frequent parathyroid/adrenal deficiency Possible T1D and/or thyroiditis	Absent	Absent	Absent
Skin lesions	Frequent eczema	Possible eczema	Possible candidiasis	Erythroderma	Frequent eczema	Always eczema
Infections	Rare/secondary	Rare/increased viral	Rare	Severe	Frequent	Skin/lung *Staphylococcus aureus*
Anemia	Possible	Possible	Rare	Frequent	Possible	Absent
Trombocytopenia	Possible	Possible	Rare	Possible	Always present	Absent
Neutropenia	Possible	Possible	Possible	Rare	Rare	Rare
Lymphocyte number	Normal/increased	Normal/increased	Normal	Normal/low T cells Low/absent B cells	Normal/low	Normal/increased
Serum IgG-IgA-IgM	Normal	Normal	Normal	Low	IgG normal/high IgA and IgM low	Normal/low
Serum IgE	Elevated	Elevated	Normal	Elevated	Elevated	Elevated
Eosinophil number	Elevated	Elevated	Normal	Elevated	Elevated	Elevated
Autoantibodies	Commonly present	Commonly present	Always present	Absent	Possibly present	Absent

Inheritance	X-linked	Autosomal recessive/ unknown	Autosomal recessive	Autosomal recessive	X-linked	Autosomal dominant/ unknown
Gene mutation	FOXP3	IL-2RA or unknown	AIRE	RAG1/RAG2 (90%) DCLREIC/LigaseIV RMRP/IL7RA/ADA	WASP	STAT3, Tyk-2 or unknown

IPEX Immune dysregulation, polyendocrinopathy, enteropathy, X-linked syndrome, *APECED* Autoimmune polyendocrinopathy candidiasis ectodermal dysplasia, *WAS* Wiskott–Aldrich syndrome, *HIES* Hyper-IgE syndrome, *T1D* Type-1 diabetes, *Ig* Immunoglobulin

FOXP3 STRUCTURE AND FUNCTION

FOXP3 is a member of the FKH family of transcription factors containing, in addition to a proline-rich amino-terminal and a central zinc finger domains, a leucine zipper domain, important for protein–protein interactions, and a carboxyl-terminal FKH domain, required for nuclear localization and DNA-binding activity (14). Most of the missense mutations reported in IPEX patients are located in these specific functional domains. In human subjects, two isoforms, FOXP3FL encoding the full-length protein and FOXP3Δ(DELTA)2 lacking exon 2, are co-expressed (15, 16). The differential function of the two isoforms is not yet fully understood (15, 17), although recent reports indicate interaction of the FOXP3Δ(DELTA)2 form with RORα(alpha), transcription factor expressed in IL-17-producing cells (16).

In both humans and mice FOXP3 is preferentially expressed by CD4+CD25+ naturally occurring (n) regulatory T (Treg) cells, a specific subset of CD4+ T cells that plays a crucial role in preventing responses to self-antigens (Ags) and in regulating effector immune responses to foreign Ags, by a variety of possible mechanisms (18–21). FoxP3 mutation in mice causes the development of a severe autoimmune pathology due to complete lack of functional CD4+CD25+ Treg cells (22–24). Based on these observations, FOXP3 has been indicated as the master gene regulator for nTreg cell development and function.

FOXP3 was originally thought to be a transcriptional repressor that suppressed cytokine production in T cells by direct binding to DNA in proximity to nuclear factor of activated T cell (NFAT)-binding sites (25). FOXP3 indeed forms heterodimers with NFAT, and the two proteins act in concert to regulate gene transcription (26). By gene expression array or chromatin immunoprecipitation (ChIP) array (27–30) it has been demonstrated that FOXP3 can also act as a transactivator. Therefore, transcription of target genes such as IL-2 and IL7R is directly suppressed by FOXP3, whereas other targets, such as CTLA4, IL2RA, and TNFRSF18 (GITR), are activated by FOXP3.

The assumption that FOXP3 is the master regulator for nTreg cells has been recently challenged by the hypothesis that FOXP3 drives regulatory program together with other genes (31). Indeed, recent work indicates that the early stages of nTreg development do not require FOXP3, which is indeed necessary to maintain Treg cells in the periphery by modulating expression of cell surface and signalling molecules (28).

FOXP3 is preferentially expressed by Treg cells, but it is now well accepted that FOXP3 can also be expressed transiently at low levels in human activated effector T (Teff) cells (32–35). A specific role for FOXP3 in non-Treg cells has not yet been identified. It has been reported that transient FOXP3 expression cannot convert Teff cells into Treg cells (*9, 33, 36–38*), but only stable and high FOXP3 expression can generate suppressor T cells (*39*). Therefore, simple expression of FOXP3 is not sufficient for the stable development of Treg cells. Importantly, nTreg cells are subject to epigenetic modifications involving demethylation of CpG motifs. Indeed, a specific region of the *FOXP3* gene is constitutively demethylated exclusively in Treg cells, thus allowing to distinguish Treg from other T cells transiently expressing FOXP3 (*37, 40–42*).

REGULATORY T CELLS IN IPEX

In human subjects, relatively pure populations of FOXP3⁺ Treg cells can be obtained by sorting the brightest 1–2% of CD25⁺ cells (*43*). A clear correlation between autoimmunity, mutation of *foxp3*, and CD4⁺CD25⁺ Treg cell dysfunction, has been demonstrated in the mouse (*24, 44*). Natural *foxp3*-mouse mutants, called scurfy mice, are considered the murine counterpart of IPEX. Adoptive transfer of Treg cells can correct the autoimmune phenotype and rescue affected mice from lethality (*23, 45*). Therefore, the lack of Treg cells caused by *foxp3* mutations has been considered the key pathogenic event sustaining lack of tolerance and development of autoimmunity in scurfy mice.

Differently from scurfy mice, CD4⁺CD25⁺ FOXP3⁺ T cells can be present in normal percentage in the peripheral blood of IPEX patients, since the majority of the mutations so far identified does not abrogate FOXP3 expression (*5, 46, 47*). Indeed, despite the presence of a mutation, FOXP3 can be expressed, but, importantly, FOXP3 expression does not correlate with the severity of the disease (*5*). In some patients, CD4⁺CD25⁺FOXP3⁺ T cells are detectable in peripheral blood (Fig. 8.1) and also in the intestinal mucosa, during the acute stage of the disease (*5*). FOXP3 in peripheral blood mononuclear cells (PBMC) can be undetectable if the mutation abrogates protein expression (Fig. 8.1) or in patients under immunosuppression (*5*). The inconsistent correlation between FOXP3 expression and disease severity makes the genetic analysis for *FOXP3* mutations essential for infants presenting with a combination of autoimmune enteropathy and/or neonatal diabetes with elevated IgE levels with or without eczema.

In IPEX patients the degree of functional Treg impairment, as measured by their suppressive activity, varies among different patients, being more severe in patients with null mutations (*46*). Interestingly, the impaired function of *FOXP3*-mutated Treg cells could be reversed by in vitro activation and expansion in long-term cultures, in the presence of exogenous IL-2 (*46*). It may therefore be possible that in some patients, residual protein

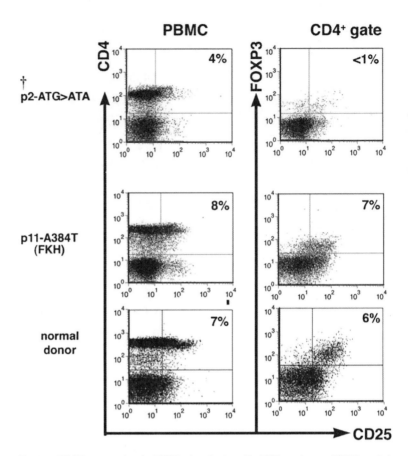

Fig. 8.1 FOXP3 expression in PBMC of patients with IPEX syndrome. FOXP3 protein expression was detected by flow cytometry in PBMC of two IPEX patients carrying different *FOXP3* mutations. A representative age-matched normal donor (ND) is also shown. Numbers in the plots indicate the percentage of positive cells in the relative quadrant. Analysis of CD4 and CD25 expression was performed in the lymphocyte gate; analysis of CD25 and FOXP3 expression was performed in the CD4+ T cell gate. The site of the mutation is reported for each patient. *Dagger*: patient posttransplant, with donor chimerism below 10% in the CD4+ T-cell compartment, at the time of determination.

activity exists and, under favorable circumstances (i.e., different immunosuppressive drugs or antigenic stimulation), could still lead to partial function with modulation of the disease course. To date there are no easily feasible tests allowing the determination of residual FOXP3 function. Therefore, when a *FOXP3* mutation is detected in patients, the functional impairment remains difficult to evaluate.

It is well known that in human subjects, in addition to nTreg cells, "adaptive" Treg cells, the IL-10-producing Type 1 regulatory T (Tr1) cells, can be induced in the periphery upon T-cell encounter with the antigen. Evidence from studies on humans and murine models, show that both Treg cell subsets have the capacity to suppress the development of autoimmunity, allergy, graft rejection, and responses to commensal flora (*19, 20, 48*).

We previously demonstrated that CD4⁺CD25⁺ T cells are not required for the normal differentiation of Tr1 cells (*49*) and we recently observed that Tr1 cells can also develop in IPEX patients even when FOXP3 expression is completely abrogated (Passerini L., unpublished data). It can therefore be hypothesized that once the IPEX patient has recovered from the acute onset, FOXP3 independent pathways of active immune regulation can contribute to disease control, providing that their development is not hampered by the use of immunosuppression.

As mentioned, in humans, as well as in mice, *FOXP3* mutations are responsible for the dysfunction of nTreg cells contributing to the autoimmune pathogenesis of the disease. In addition, in contrast to what is reported for mice, in IPEX patients in vitro production of Th1 cytokines, especially IL-2 and IFN-γ (gamma), by Teff cells activated via the TCR is also defective (*46, 50, 51*). This supports the idea that FOXP3 has a complex role in immune regulation not confined to that of thymic differentiation of nTreg cells. Whether expression of a mutated FOXP3 by Teff cells contributes to the pathology remains to be clarified. Recently, a new subset of IL-17-producing T helper (Th17) cells has been identified (*52, 53*). Th17 cells have been involved in the pathogenesis of autoimmune manifestations, such as rheumatoid arthritis (*54–56*) and multiple sclerosis (*57, 58*). A direct involvement of Th17 cells in the pathogenesis of IPEX has not yet been demonstrated, but based on growing evidence indicating an active role for FOXP3 in the inhibition of Th17 development (*59–61*), it could be hypothesized that upon antigen exposure *FOXP3*-mutated T cells could preferentially differentiate into Th17 cells, which contribute to the pathogenesis of the disease.

THERAPIES FOR IPEX: CURRENT LIMITATIONS AND FUTURE PERSPECTIVES

Despite multiple side effects, in IPEX patients pharmacological immunosuppression is required to control symptoms at the onset, together with supportive and replacement therapies. Parenteral nutrition is often required, although it is not sufficient to reverse the severe failure to thrive. Corticosteroids are used as first choice immunosuppressive drugs, but they are usually not sufficient if administered alone. Among different corticosteroids, methylprednisolone is most commonly used, although betamethasone has been described as more efficacious (*62*).

Calcineurin inhibitors, in particular cyclosporine and tacrolimus, or azathioprine are most commonly associated with corticosteroids. Outcomes are inconsistent, without permanent control of the clinical manifestations, especially early onset diarrhea, for most of the patients (*2, 63, 64*). Patients surviving under immunosuppression have usually experienced multiple treatments in combination or sequence, with consequent difficulty to identify single drug's best efficacy. However, some patients better responding to therapy in the early acute phase of the disease, require less immunosuppression to control the symptoms over time (5).

Importantly, rapamycin or mycophenolate mofetil (MMF) has been effectively used in place of calcineurin-dependent agents for early onset IPEX patients and also for patients with IPEX symptoms but no detectable *FOXP3* mutations (5, 65, 66). The clinical efficacy of rapamycin correlates with the knowledge that rapamycin suppresses Teff cell function and selectively induces or expands Treg cells (67–69). Indeed, there is suggestive evidence that administration of rapamycin and MMF facilitates the induction of active tolerance mediated by Treg cells (67). Therefore, early treatment of IPEX patients with non-calcineurin inhibitor drugs deserves further attention. Furthermore, it should be clarified whether these agents are effective only in IPEX patients with residual Treg cell function. Better definition of immunosuppressive therapies aimed at "boosting" Treg cell function in patients with dysregulated immune responses would represent an important improvement over current therapies that typically rely on general immune suppression.

At present, the only effective cure for IPEX is hematopoietic stem cell transplantation (HSCT) (3, 5, 6, 70–73), although there are no well-defined conditioning protocols. Both HLA-identical and matched unrelated HSCT have been successful, with the longest follow-up of approximately 6 years (5). HSCT should be always considered for patients carrying mutations that abrogate FOXP3 expression or that are located in critically functional domain of the protein and most likely alter Treg function. The procedure should possibly be performed early, before severe autoimmunity develops, since extensively compromised patients have high risk of mortality due to conditioning. Results from IPEX transplanted patients indicate that full donor chimerism is not required to overcome the autoimmune pathology, suggesting that a small number of functional Treg cells may be sufficient to control the disease (5, 6, 74).

Although, longer follow-up studies are necessary for absolute conclusions, the efficacy of mixed chimerism after HSCT would suggest that transfer of functional Treg cells could control the pathology. Based on these observations, cellular therapy could represent a promising approach, since it would allow maintenance of long-term immune modulation, while avoiding general immunosuppression and systemic toxicity. In the last 5 years, much effort has been expended to understand which Treg population is suitable for cellular therapy approaches in different pathologies, how to effectively isolate them and/or expand them ex vivo, and in which pathology their usage would be most appropriate (75).

Currently, answers for all these issues are progressively generated and IPEX patients would certainly be elective candidates for these innovative therapies. One possible future cell therapy approach could involve in vivo transfer of autologous T cells after in vitro *FOXP3* gene transfer, which would allow conversion of pathogenic T cells into potent suppressor cells specific for self-Ags (*39, 67*).

CONCLUSIONS

Severe autoimmune enteropathy and T1D, often associated with increased IgE in serum and eosinophilia, are the most prominent early manifestations in male patients affected with IPEX syndrome. Genetic analysis of FOXP3 should be performed to ensure an accurate diagnosis, since FOXP3 expression is not consistently abrogated. Prompt treatment should be administered to control the severity of the autoimmune symptoms and search for an available HSC donor should be considered early postdiagnosis.

Although IPEX is a primary immunodeficiency, because of the impairment of a T-cell subset committed to immune regulation, it shares several different features with autoimmune diseases of different origins. Thus, IPEX represents a unique disease model that bridges immunodeficiency to autoimmunity and further studies on this disease will bring insights into the mechanisms responsible for immune dysregulation in autoimmune pathologies other than IPEX syndrome.

ACKNOWLEDGMENTS

This work was supported by the Italian Telethon Foundation, Rome (Grants GGP07241 and TELEA3).

REFERENCES

1. Powell BR, Buist NR, Stenzel P. An X-linked syndrome of diarrhea, polyendocrinopathy, and fatal infection in infancy. J Pediatr 1982;100(5):731–737.
2. Wildin RS, Smyk-Pearson S, Filipovich AH. Clinical and molecular features of the immunodysregulation, polyendocrinopathy, enteropathy, X linked (IPEX) syndrome. J Med Genet 2002;39(8):537–545.
3. Ochs HD, Ziegler SF, Torgerson TR. FOXP3 acts as a rheostat of the immune response. Immunol Rev 2005;203:156–164.
4. Torgerson TR, Ochs HD. Immune dysregulation, polyendocrinopathy, enteropathy, X-linked: forkhead box protein 3 mutations and lack of regulatory T cells. J Allergy Clin Immunol 2007;120(4):744–750; quiz 751–742.
5. Gambineri E, Perroni L, Passerini L, et al. Clinical and molecular profile of a new series of patients with immune dysregulation, polyendocrinopathy, enteropathy, X-linked syndrome: inconsistent correlation between forkhead box protein 3 expression and disease severity. J Allergy Clin Immunol 2008;122(6):1105–1112.

6. Mazzolari E, Forino C, Fontana M, et al. A new case of IPEX receiving bone marrow transplantation. Bone Marrow Transplant 2005;35:1033–1034.
7. Sharfe N, Shahar M, Roifman CM. An interleukin-2 receptor gamma chain mutation with normal thymus morphology. J Clin Invest 1997;100(12):3036–3043.
8. Caudy AA, Reddy ST, Chatila T, Atkinson JP, Verbsky JW. CD25 deficiency causes an immune dysregulation, polyendocrinopathy, enteropathy, X-linked-like syndrome and defective IL-10 expression from CD4 lymphocytes. J Allergy Clin Immunol 2007;119(2):482–487.
9. Passerini L, Allan SE, Battaglia M, et al. STAT5-signaling cytokines regulate the expression of FOXP3 in CD4+CD25+ regulatory T cells and CD4+CD25- effector T cells. Int Immunol 2008;20(3):421–431.
10. Bakke AC, Purtzer MZ, Wildin RS. Prospective immunological profiling in a case of immune dysregulation, polyendocrinopathy, enteropathy, X-linked syndrome (IPEX). Clin Exp Immunol 2004;137(2):373–378.
11. Murch S. Advances in the understanding and management of autoimmune enteropathy. Curr Paediatr 2006;16:305–316.
12. Marquis E, Robert JJ, Bouvattier C, Bellanne-Chantelot C, Junien C, Diatloff-Zito C. Major difference in aetiology and phenotypic abnormalities between transient and permanent neonatal diabetes. J Med Genet 2002;39(5):370–374.
13. Geha RS, Notarangelo LD, Casanova JL, et al. Primary immunodeficiency diseases: an update from the International Union of Immunological Societies Primary Immunodeficiency Diseases Classification Committee. J Allergy Clin Immunol 2007;120(4):776–794.
14. Ziegler SF. FOXP3: of mice and men. Annu Rev Immunol 2006;24:209–226.
15. Allan SE, Passerini L, Bacchetta R, et al. The role of two FOXP3 isoforms in the generation of human CD4+ T regulatory cells. J Clin Invest 2005;115:3275–3284.
16. Du J, Huang C, Zhou B, Ziegler SF. Isoform-specific inhibition of ROR alpha-mediated transcriptional activation by human FOXP3. J Immunol 2008; 180(7):4785–4792.
17. Aarts-Riemens T, Emmelot ME, Verdonck LF, Mutis T. Forced overexpression of either of the two common human Foxp3 isoforms can induce regulatory T cells from CD4(+) CD25(-) cells. Eur J Immunol 2008;38(5):1381–1390.
18. Levings MK, Allan S, d'Hennezel E, Piccirillo CA. Functional dynamics of naturally occurring regulatory T cells in health and autoimmunity. Adv Immunol 2006;92:119–155.
19. Sakaguchi S, Ono M, Setoguchi R, et al. Foxp3+ CD25+ CD4+ natural regulatory T cells in dominant self-tolerance and autoimmune disease. Immunol Rev 2006;212:8–27.
20. Shevach EM. From vanilla to 28 flavors: multiple varieties of T regulatory cells. Immunity 2006;25(2):195–201.
21. Vignali D. How many mechanisms do regulatory T cells need? Eur J Immunol 2008;38(4):908–911.
22. Hori S, Nomura T, Sakaguchi S. Control of regulatory T cell development by the transcription factor Foxp3. Science 2003;299(5609):1057–1061.
23. Fontenot JD, Gavin MA, Rudensky AY. Foxp3 programs the development and function of CD4+CD25+ regulatory T cells. Nat Immunol 2003;4(4):330–336.
24. Khattri R, Cox T, Yasayko SA, Ramsdell F. An essential role for Scurfin in CD4+CD25+ T regulatory cells. Nat Immunol 2003;4(4):337–342.
25. Schubert LA, Jeffery E, Zhang Y, Ramsdell F, Ziegler SF. Scurfin (FOXP3) acts as a repressor of transcription and regulates T cell activation. J Biol Chem 2001;276(40):37672–37679.
26. Wu Y, Borde M, Heissmeyer V, et al. FOXP3 controls regulatory T cell function through cooperation with NFAT. Cell 2006;126(2):375–387.
27. Zheng Y, Josefowicz SZ, Kas A, Chu TT, Gavin MA, Rudensky AY. Genome-wide analysis of Foxp3 target genes in developing and mature regulatory T cells. Nature 2007;445(7130):936–940.
28. Gavin MA, Rasmussen JP, Fontenot JD, et al. Foxp3-dependent programme of regulatory T-cell differentiation. Nature 2007;445(7129): 771–775.
29. Williams LM, Rudensky AY. Maintenance of the Foxp3-dependent developmental program in mature regulatory T cells requires continued expression of Foxp3. Nat Immunol 2007;8(3):277–284.
30. Marson A, Kretschmer K, Frampton GM, et al. Foxp3 occupancy and regulation of key target genes during T-cell stimulation. Nature 2007;445(7130):931–935.
31. Hill JA, Feuerer M, Tash K, et al. Foxp3 transcription-factor-dependent and -independent regulation of the regulatory T cell transcriptional signature. Immunity 2007;27(5): 786–800.

32. Allan SE, Crome SQ, Crellin NK, et al. Activation-induced FOXP3 in human T effector cells does not suppress proliferation or cytokine production. Int Immunol 2007;19(4):345–354.
33. Wang J, Ioan-Facsinay A, van der Voort EI, Huizinga TW, Toes RE. Transient expression of FOXP3 in human activated nonregulatory CD4+ T cells. Eur J Immunol 2007;37(1): 129–138.
34. Pillai V, Ortega SB, Wang CK, Karandikar NJ. Transient regulatory T-cells: a state attained by all activated human T-cells. Clin Immunol 2007;123(1):18–29.
35. Gavin MA, Torgerson TR, Houston E, et al. Single-cell analysis of normal and FOXP3-mutant human T cells: FOXP3 expression without regulatory T cell development. Proc Natl Acad Sci USA 2006;103(17):6659–6664.
36. Roncarolo MG, Gregori S. Is FOXP3 a bona fide marker for human regulatory T cells? Eur J Immunol 2008;38(4):925–927.
37. Polansky JK, Kretschmer K, Freyer J, et al. DNA methylation controls Foxp3 gene expression. Eur J Immunol 2008;38(6):1654–1663.
38. Tran DQ, Ramsey H, Shevach EM. Induction of FOXP3 expression in naive human CD4+FOXP3 T cells by T-cell receptor stimulation is transforming growth factor-beta dependent but does not confer a regulatory phenotype. Blood 2007;110(8):2983–2990.
39. Allan SE, Alstad AN, Merindol N, et al. Generation of potent and stable human CD4+ T regulatory cells by activation-independent expression of FOXP3. Mol Ther 2008;16(1):194–202.
40. Floess S, Freyer J, Siewert C, et al. Epigenetic control of the foxp3 locus in regulatory T cells. PLoS Biol 2007;5(2):e38.
41. Nagar M, Vernitsky H, Cohen Y, et al. Epigenetic inheritance of DNA methylation limits activation-induced expression of FOXP3 in conventional human CD25-CD4+ T cells. Int Immunol 2008;20(8):1041–1055.
42. Baron U, Floess S, Wieczorek G, et al. DNA demethylation in the human FOXP3 locus discriminates regulatory T cells from activated FOXP3(+) conventional T cells. Eur J Immunol 2007;37(9):2378–2389.
43. Baecher-Allan C, Brown JA, Freeman GJ, Hafler DA. CD4+CD25 high regulatory cells in human peripheral blood. J Immunol 2001;167(3):1245–1253.
44. Brunkow ME, Jeffery EW, Hjerrild KA, et al. Disruption of a new forkhead/winged-helix protein, scurfin, results in the fatal lymphoproliferative disorder of the scurfy mouse. Nat Genet 2001;27(1):68–73.
45. Smyk-Pearson SK, Bakke AC, Held PK, Wildin RS. Rescue of the autoimmune scurfy mouse by partial bone marrow transplantation or by injection with T-enriched splenocytes. Clin Exp Immunol 2003;133(2): 193–199.
46. Bacchetta R, Passerini L, Gambineri E, et al. Defective regulatory and effector T cell functions in patients with FOXP3 mutations. J Clin Invest 2006;116(6):1713–1722.
47. Lopes JE, Torgerson TR, Schubert LA, et al. Analysis of FOXP3 reveals multiple domains required for its function as a transcriptional repressor. J Immunol 2006;177(5):3133–3142.
48. Roncarolo MG, Gregori S, Battaglia M, Bacchetta R, Fleischhauer K, Levings MK. Interleukin-10-secreting type 1 regulatory T cells in rodents and humans. Immunol Rev 2006;212:28–50.
49. Levings MK, Gregori S, Tresoldi E, Cazzaniga S, Bonini C, Roncarolo MG. Differentiation of Tr1 cells by immature dendritic cells requires IL-10 but not CD25+CD4+ Tr cells. Blood 2005;105(3):1162–1169.
50. Chatila TA, Blaeser F, Ho N, et al. JM2, encoding a fork head-related protein, is mutated in X-linked autoimmunity-allergic disregulation syndrome. J Clin Invest 2000;106(12):R75–R81.
51. Nieves DS, Phipps RP, Pollock SJ, et al. Dermatologic and immunologic findings in the immune dysregulation, polyendocrinopathy, enteropathy, X-linked syndrome. Arch Dermatol 2004;140(4):466–472.
52. Park H, Li Z, Yang XO, et al. A distinct lineage of CD4 T cells regulates tissue inflammation by producing interleukin 17. Nat Immunol 2005;6(11):1133–1141.
53. Harrington LE, Hatton RD, Mangan PR, et al. Interleukin 17-producing CD4+ effector T cells develop via a lineage distinct from the T helper type 1 and 2 lineages. Nat Immunol 2005;6(11):1123–1132.
54. Fossiez F, Djossou O, Chomarat P, et al. T cell interleukin-17 induces stromal cells to produce proinflammatory and hematopoietic cytokines. J Exp Med 1996;183(6): 2593–2603.
55. Kotake S, Udagawa N, Takahashi N, et al. IL-17 in synovial fluids from patients with rheumatoid arthritis is a potent stimulator of osteoclastogenesis. J Clin Invest 1999;103(9): 1345–1352.
56. Kim KW, Cho ML, Lee SH, et al. Human rheumatoid synovial fibroblasts promote

osteoclastogenic activity by activating RANKL via TLR-2 and TLR-4 activation. Immunol Lett 2007;110(1):54–64.
57. Kebir H, Kreymborg K, Ifergan I, et al. Human TH17 lymphocytes promote blood-brain barrier disruption and central nervous system inflammation. Nat Med 2007;13(10): 1173–1175.
58. Tzartos JS, Friese MA, Craner MJ, et al. Interleukin-17 production in central nervous system-infiltrating T cells and glial cells is associated with active disease in multiple sclerosis. Am J Pathol 2008; 172(1):146–155.
59. Ichiyama K, Yoshida H, Wakabayashi Y, et al. Foxp3 inhibits RORgammat-mediated IL-17A mRNA transcription through direct interaction with RORgammat. J Biol Chem 2008;283(25):17003–17008.
60. Zhou L, Lopes JE, Chong MM, et al. TGF-beta-induced Foxp3 inhibits T(H)17 cell differentiation by antagonizing RORgammat function. Nature 2008;453(7192):236–240.
61. Zhang F, Meng G, Strober W. Interactions among the transcription factors Runx1, RORgammat and Foxp3 regulate the differentiation of interleukin 17-producing T cells. Nat Immunol 2008;9(11):1297–1306.
62. Taddio A, Faleschini E, Valencic E, et al. Medium-term survival without haematopoietic stem cell transplantation in a case of IPEX: insights into nutritional and immunosuppressive therapy. Eur J Pediatr 2007;166(11): 1195–1197.
63. Bennett CL, Christie J, Ramsdell F, et al. The immune dysregulation, polyendocrinopathy, enteropathy, X-linked syndrome (IPEX) is caused by mutations of FOXP3. Nat Genet 2001;27(1):20–21.
64. Owen CJ, Jennings CE, Imrie H, et al. Mutational analysis of the FOXP3 gene and evidence for genetic heterogeneity in the immunodysregulation, polyendocrinopathy, enteropathy syndrome. J Clin Endocrinol Metab 2003;88(12):6034–6039.
65. Yong PL, Russo P, Sullivan KE. Use of sirolimus in IPEX and IPEX-like children. J Clin Immunol 2008;28(5):581–587.
66. Bindl L, Torgerson T, Perroni L, et al. Successful use of the new immune-suppressor sirolimus in IPEX (immune dysregulation, polyendocrinopathy, enteropathy, X-linked syndrome). J Pediatr 2005;147(2):256–259.
67. Allan SE, Broady R, Gregori S, et al. CD4+ T-regulatory cells: toward therapy for human diseases. Immunol Rev 2008;223:391–421.
68. Battaglia M, Stabilini A, Roncarolo MG. Rapamycin selectively expands CD4+CD25+FOXP3+ regulatory T cells. Blood 2005;105(12):4743–4748.
69. Battaglia M, Stabilini A, Migliavacca B, Horejs-Hoeck J, Kaupper T, Roncarolo MG. Rapamycin promotes expansion of functional CD4+CD25+FOXP3+ regulatory T cells of both healthy subjects and type 1 diabetic patients. J Immunol 2006;177(12):8338–8347.
70. Baud O, Goulet O, Canioni D, et al. Treatment of the immune dysregulation, polyendocrinopathy, enteropathy, X-linked syndrome (IPEX) by allogeneic bone marrow transplantation. N Engl J Med 2001;344(23):1758–1762.
71. Zhan H, Sinclair J, Adams S, et al. Immune reconstitution and recovery of FOXP3 (forkhead box P3)-expressing T cells after transplantation for IPEX (immune dysregulation, polyendocrinopathy, enteropathy, X-linked) syndrome. Pediatrics 2008;121(4):e998–e1002.
72. Lucas KG, Ungar D, Comito M, Bayerl M, Groh B. Submyeloablative cord blood transplantation corrects clinical defects seen in IPEX syndrome. Bone Marrow Transplant 2007;39(1):55–56.
73. Rao A, Kamani N, Filipovich A, et al. Successful bone marrow transplantation for IPEX syndrome after reduced-intensity conditioning. Blood 2007;109(1):383–385.
74. Serdel MG, Fntsch G, Lion T, et al. Selective engragtment of donor CD4+CD2Shigh FoxP3-Positive T cells in IPEX syndrome after nonmyeloablative hematopoletic stem cell transplantation. Blood 2009;113(22): 5689–5691.
75. Roncarolo MG, Battaglia M. Regulatory T-cell immunotherapy for tolerance to self antigens and alloantigens in humans. Nat Rev Immunol 2007;7(8):585–598.

Chapter 9

Autoimmune Polyendocrine Syndrome Type 2: Pathophysiology, Natural History, and Clinical Manifestations

Jennifer M. Barker

Summary

Autoimmune Polyendocrine Syndrome Type 2 (APS-2) is the association of multiple organ-specific autoimmune diseases including but not limited to type 1 diabetes, Addison's disease, and autoimmune thyroid disease. Additional autoimmune diseases are associated with APS-2, in particular celiac disease. The diseases share a common pathophysiology characterized by T-cell mediated destruction of the target organ. The component diseases of APS-2 have overlapping genetic risk factors. The natural history is characterized by a long preclinical phase, identifiable by the presence of organ-specific autoantibodies and normal gland function. Over time, destruction of the gland progresses and clinical disease develops. Treatment addresses the underlying hormonal abnormalities. Subjects with one autoimmune disease are at risk for the development of additional autoimmune diseases and therefore careful clinical and laboratory screening is required for follow-up.

Key Words: Autoimmune polyendocrine syndrome type 2, Type 1 diabetes, Autoimmune thyroid disease, Addison's disease, Celiac disease

Autoimmune Polyendocrine Syndrome Type 2 (APS-2) is the association of multiple organ-specific autoimmune diseases in one patient. Schmidt first recognized the association of Addison's disease and chronic lymphocytic thyroiditis in 1926 and the combination of these two diseases has been termed Schmidt's syndrome (*1*). Over the years, associations with other autoimmune diseases including type 1 diabetes have been identified. Additionally, organ-specific autoimmune diseases outside the endocrine system (e.g., celiac disease) have been associated with type 1 diabetes, autoimmune thyroid disease, and Addison's disease. Table 9.1 shows the prevalence of autoimmune diseases by disease state.

For the purpose of this chapter, we will define APS-2 as the combination of two or more organ-specific autoimmune diseases and not APS-1 (*2*), which has a distinct genetic cause and phenotype.

Table 9.1
Overlap of Components of the Autoimmune Polyendocrine System

Prevalence	Autoimmune thyroid disease	Type 1 diabetes	Celiac disease	Addison's disease
General population	5%	0.2–0.3%	1%	0.005%
Autoimmune thyroid disease	–	20%	10–15%	20%
Type 1 diabetes	4%	–	7% with multiple antibodies	10–15%
Celiac disease	5–10%	5–10%	–	5%
Addison's disease	?	0.5%	0.25%	–

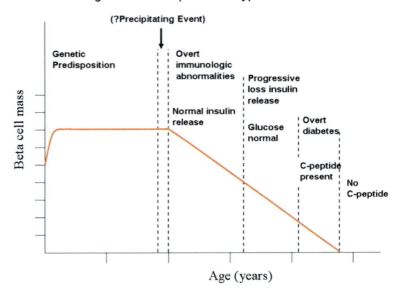

Fig. 9.1 Stages in the development of type 1A diabetes.

Other authors have subdivided this definition of APS-2 into APS-2 (Addison's disease plus autoimmune thyroid disease or type 1 diabetes), APS-3 (autoimmune thyroid disease plus another autoimmune disease – not Addison's diseases or type 1 diabetes), and APS-4 (any combination of two other organ-specific autoimmune diseases not APS-1, 2, or 3) (3).

A paradigm for disease development has been proposed by several authors including Drs. Eisenbarth (4) and Betterle (5). This model serves as a framework for understanding the pathophysiology of these autoimmune diseases (Fig. 9.1). In this model, in a subset of subjects at increased risk for autoimmunity, an autoimmune attack is triggered (potentially via an environmental exposure). Over a period of time that may extend for years, the autoimmune attack proceeds and the organ is destroyed. The disease does not manifest itself clinically until the remaining tissue is inadequate to provide a normal function. At this point, the silent disease becomes clinically evident. We will use this model to discuss the pathophysiology of the disease components of APS-2, focusing on genetic risk, environmental triggers, markers of the autoimmune disease, and gland failure and briefly touch on diagnosis and treatment. We will focus on the most common components of APS-2: Addison's disease, type 1 diabetes, and autoimmune thyroid disease and will also discuss celiac disease.

PATHO-PHYSIOLOGY

The fundamental defect in the development of autoimmunity is the breakdown of immunologic tolerance (6). Immunologic tolerance is the process by which the immune system recognizes an immune response as against self and deletes or modifies this response. Tolerance occurs centrally (within the thymus). T-lymphocytes that recognize self-antigens presented by peripheral antigen presenting cells are deleted. If self-reactive T-lymphocytes escape deletion in the thymus, they are subject to regulation in the form of anergy or the development of regulatory T-cells in peripheral immunologic tissues such as the spleen and lymph nodes. Tolerance is a complex and on-going process, vulnerable to errors at several different time points.

Overlapping Genetic Risk (Table 9.2)

APS-2 is a polygenic disorder. Many of the genes associated with APS-2 and its component disorders are active in the immune system and play important roles in the development of immunologic tolerance. The genes that are involved can increase the risk for autoimmunity in general or increase the risk for a specific autoimmune disease. For example, the human leukocyte antigen (HLA) DR3 has been associated with type 1 diabetes (7), celiac disease (8), and autoimmune thyroid disease (9). In contrast, polymorphisms of the variable tandem number repeat (VNTR) of the insulin gene are associated with type 1 diabetes, not with other autoimmune diseases (10).

Proteins encoded by HLA loci play a vital role in the acquired immune system (6). They bind polypeptides in their groove and are on the cell surface for interaction with T-lymphocytes through the T-cell receptor (TCR). Class I HLA molecules interact with TCR of CD8 T-cells, and Class II HLA molecules interact with the TCR of CD4 T-cells. The specific polypeptides to which the HLA

Table 9.2
Disease Components of Autoimmune Polyendocrine Syndrome Type 2: Genetic Associations, Autoantibodies, Diagnostic Criteria, and Prevalence in Type 1 Diabetes

Disease	Genetic Associations	Autoantibodies	Diagnostic criteria	Prevalence in T1D
Type 1 diabetes	HLA DR/DQ Insulin VNTR PTPN22	ICA Insulin GAD65 IA2 ZnT8	*Fasting glucose* ≥ 126 mg/dL *Random glucose* ≥ 200 mg/dL *2-h glucose on oral glucose tolerance test* ≥ 200 mg/dL	N/A
Autoimmune thyroid disease	HLA DR/DQ CTLA-4	Thyroid peroxidase Thyroglobulin Thyroid stimulating Ig	*TSH* – elevated or suppressed *T4 or T3* – low or elevated	30% with antibodies Up to 20–30% with disease
Addison's disease	HLA DR/DQ PTPN22	21-Hydroxylase	*ACTH* – elevated *PRA* – elevated *Cortisol* – <18–20 mg/dL 30–60 min post cortrosyn stimulation test	1.5% antibodies <0.5% with disease
Celiac disease	HLA DR/DQ	Anti-endomysial antibody Tissue transglutaminase	Biopsy with characteristic changes	10% with antibodies 4–9% with disease

molecule can bind are influenced by the amino acid structure of both the HLA molecule and the protein from which the polypeptide is derived. Different HLA molecules confer risk to different autoimmune diseases, possibly by their ability to bind differing molecules. Thus, an HLA molecule that is high risk for one autoimmune disease may be low risk for another (e.g., DQB1 0602, which is low risk for type 1 diabetes but high risk for multiple sclerosis).

The DR and DQ loci of the class II HLA are important for risk for the component disorders of APS-2. The highest risk genotype for type 1 diabetes is DR3-DQA 0501 DQB 0201/DR4-DQA 0301 DQB 0302 (DR3-DQ2/DR4-DQ8). Approximately 1/20 subjects in the general population with this genotype develop type 1 diabetes by the age of 15 years (*11*), an increase over the general population risk of 1 in 300 subjects by 18 years (*12*). The strength of this association is influenced by the presence of a family history of type 1 diabetes. Siblings with the high-risk diabetes genotype (DR3-DQ2/DR4-DQ8) have a higher risk for type 1 diabetes, compared to offsprings of patients with type 1 diabetes with this high-risk genotype. This relationship has been further explored in prospective studies following children for the development of type 1 diabetes. Children who are siblings with a subject who has type 1 diabetes and are identical by descent for this high-risk HLA genotype (i.e., have inherited the same chromosomes of DR3-DQ2/DR4-DQ8 as their sibling with diabetes) have a risk for the development of diabetes-related autoimmunity of 80% and diabetes of 55% by the age of 15 years (13). These data suggest that there are additional linked-genetic factors within the HLA influencing the risk for type 1 diabetes. Celiac disease and autoimmune thyroid disease share the HLA risk for type 1 diabetes. A full 98% of subjects with celiac disease have at least one of the high-risk HLA DR haplotypes (14). In children with type 1 diabetes homozygous for DR3-DQ2, the risk for celiac disease related autoantibodies is 1/3 (15). Autoimmune thyroid disease has been associated with the DR3 haplotype.

Genes outside the HLA region associated with autoimmune disease have odds ratios much less than that observed for DR and DQ, on the order of 1.1–1.5. However, some genes have shown a consistent relationship with autoimmune diseases. A single nucleotide polymorphism in the gene PTPN22 has been associated with multiple autoimmune diseases, including type 1 diabetes (16), autoimmune thyroid disease (17), Addison's disease (18), and celiac disease (19). PTPN22 encodes a protein called the lymphoid tyrosine phosphatase (LYP) and this particular SNP results in an amino acid change at position 620 of arginine to tryptophan. LYP is an important molecule in the signaling cascade of the T-cell receptor, and the polymorphism associated with autoimmunity is associated with an alteration of the signaling cascade of the T-cell receptor. Recently, genome-wide association scans in which patients with type 1 diabetes and autoimmune thyroid disease were considered as affected identified linkage with a region of the genome on 2q. Further positional candidate analysis strongly suggested that CTLA-4 was responsible for this linkage. The linkage was not found when patients with only type 1 diabetes or only autoimmune thyroid disease were considered affected (20). Thus, we may be able to identify genes that are associated with the risk for multiple autoimmune diseases.

Disease-specific genes such as the insulin VNTR and polymorphisms within the thyroglobulin gene are associated with type 1 diabetes (10) and autoimmune thyroid disease (21), respectively. Polymorphisms within the VNTR affect the level of insulin produced in the thymus such that polymorphisms associated with type 1 diabetes have lower levels of insulin in the thymus (22). This may then play a role in central tolerance.

Environmental Factors

Celiac disease is the one organ-specific autoimmune disease in which the environmental cause is known. In a genetically susceptible individual, the ingestion of gluten can, but does not always, result in the development of an autoimmune response in the small intestine (*9*). Complete removal of gluten from the diet results in the resolution of symptoms of celiac disease and healing of the pathologic changes on small intestinal biopsy. Celiac disease therefore serves as a model for autoimmune diseases, such as type 1 diabetes, in which an environmental trigger is not known..

The incidence of type 1 diabetes has increased in multiple geographic locations over the past four to five decades (*23*). This increase in incidence of type 1 diabetes has been argued to be too rapid to be accounted for by genetic changes alone. Therefore, environmental factors have been evaluated as a potential cause of the increase in incidence of type 1 diabetes and are being studied in prospective cohort studies of young children at risk for type 1 diabetes (e.g., DAISY (*24*), TEDDY (*25*), DIPP (*26*), and BABY DIAB (*27*)). These studies have evaluated factors from infant diet to immunizations and viral infections.

No clear environmental trigger of type 1 diabetes has been identified, but there are intriguing hints emerging from these studies. Early suspicion for the influence of cow's milk formula playing a role in the development of type 1 diabetes has not been confirmed by all studies (*28*). Two independent studies have found that the timing of cereal introduction is associated with the development of diabetes-related autoimmunity (*29, 30*). The timing of cereal introduction has also been linked to celiac disease (*31*) and wheat allergy (*32*), providing evidence for environmental overlap in susceptible individuals. Case-control studies have associated lower levels of vitamin D and omega-3 fatty acids with the increase in incidence of type 1 diabetes (*33*). Preliminary data from prospective cohort studies have suggested a link between dietary levels of omega-3 fatty acids and diabetes-related autoimmunity (*34*). Intriguing reports of epidemics of type 1 diabetes and enteroviruses occurring simultaneously suggest that viral infections may play an important role in triggering diabetes-related autoimmunity, although no specific virus has been identified. The environment also plays a role in the development of autoimmune thyroid disease. Iodine has been associated, but not in every study, with triggering hyperthyroidism in subjects with thyroid-related autoimmunity in iodine insufficient areas (*35*). Given the rarity of Addison's disease, environmental associations have not been systematically studied.

Markers of the Autoimmune Process (Table 9.2)

The autoimmune process can be detected years prior to the development of signs or symptoms of the disease. Markers of the autoimmune process include organ-specific autoantibodies and T-cell assays. While the autoimmune process is largely T-cell mediated, autoantibodies (products of B-cells) have been used for decades to follow subjects at risk for these autoimmune diseases.

Islet cell autoantibodies (ICA) were first detected over 30 years ago and were identified by reacting sera of patients with type 1 diabetes with sections of pancreas (*36*). There are now four specific autoantibodies that are associated with type 1 diabetes: those to insulin (IAA), GAD65, IA2, and the recently described ZnT8 (*37*). Characteristics of the autoantibodies including number (*38*), level (*39*), affinity for antigen (*40*), and IgG subtype (*41*) have all been associated with differing diabetes risk. These autoantibodies have been used in studies to identify subjects at risk for type 1 diabetes for prevention trials (e.g., DPT-1 and TrialNet) and as an outcome for cohort studies attempting to define the natural history of the prediabetic period.

Antibodies against thyroid peroxidase (TPO) and thyroglobulin (TG) have also been identified and are useful in predictive models of autoimmune thyroid disease (*42*). Graves' disease is unique in that the autoantibody against the thyroid hormone receptor, thyroid stimulating immunoglobulin (TSI) is the cause of the hyperthyroidism and is therefore pathogenic. People with type 1 diabetes are at high risk for both thyroid autoimmunity and hypothyroidism (*43*). Patients with celiac disease are also at risk for thyroid disease, with up to 25% showing evidence for thyroid autoimmunity (*44*).

Antibodies against tissue transglutaminase (TTG) are associated with celiac disease. TTG antibodies can be identified in as many as 1/100 people, and people with type 1 diabetes have a risk for TTG antibodies of approximately 10% (*45*). Evidence for celiac disease is present in 8% of children with autoimmune thyroid disease (*46*).

Addison's disease is associated with 21-hydroxylase autoantibodies (*47*). While Addison's disease is very rare in the general population, 1.5% of people with type 1 diabetes have antibodies against 21-hydroxylase (*43*).

Because the autoimmune process is largely mediated by T-cells, T-cell assays are under development. The identification of a T-cell assay that is robust and accurately predicts the development of type 1 diabetes or other autoimmune diseases will be invaluable in the ability to understand the pathogenesis of these autoimmune diseases and ultimately may aid in the prediction of disease (*48*).

Markers of Gland Failure

Autoantibodies associated with type 1 diabetes, autoimmune thyroid disease, and Addison's disease may be present before any metabolic abnormalities are detected. The majority of the destruction of the gland by the autoimmune process is clinically silent. However, as the destruction progresses subtle metabolic abnormalities may be detected.

The β-cell is nestled within the pancreatic islet, and measuring the β-cell mass in humans is to date very difficult. Imaging methods are currently being explored to quantitate the β-cell mass in humans. Therefore, methods of estimating the β-cell mass in humans currently rely on provocative testing, including oral and intravenous glucose tolerance testing (OGTT and IVGTT, respectively). In the IVGTT, subjects receive a bolus of glucose, and levels of insulin are followed. In a subject without diabetes, insulin is released in two phases known as the first and second phase of insulin release. Follow-up of subjects with diabetes-related autoimmunity shows a decline in the first-phase insulin response (FPIR) (*49*). This decline can precede the diagnosis of diabetes by many years but is a strong risk factor for the development of type 1 diabetes in at risk subjects. On OGTT, subjects usually proceed through a series of abnormalities starting with impaired glucose tolerance (levels greater than or equal to 140 mg/dL 2 h after a glucose load), progressing to impaired fasting glucose, levels consistent with diabetes and fasting hyperglycemia (*50, 51*). Levels of hemoglobin A1c increase in the period prior to the diagnosis of diabetes (*52*). Up to the point of fasting hyperglycemia, subjects are usually asymptomatic or mildly symptomatic of the disease.

Measurement of thyroid gland function relies on assessing levels of thyroid hormone (measured as free T4, total T4, and/or T3) and thyroid stimulating hormone (TSH). Subjects often pass through a phase of compensated hypothyroidism with TSH above normal and normal thyroid hormone levels prior to developing frank hypothyroidism. In large-scale epidemiologic studies of the risk for frank hypothyroidism, increases in TSH above 10 mIU/L are associated with a greatly increased risk for frank hypothyroidism (*42*). TPO and TG antibodies may be present for many years prior to the development of hypothyroidism (*42, 53*).

Metabolic abnormalities leading to Addison's disease also progress through a fairly typical pattern. Abnormalities of aldosterone synthesis often develop first, and the first detectable metabolic abnormality is often an increase in the plasma renin activity (PRA). Abnormalities of glucocorticoid function are then first manifested by the presence of an increase in ACTH. As glandular failure progresses, electrolyte abnormalities such as hyponatremia, hyperkalemia, and hypoglycemia develop, and the person is at risk for an adrenal crisis (*54*).

Clinical Disease (Table 9.2)

The clinical presentation of type 1 diabetes, Addison's disease, and autoimmune thyroid disease can be fulminant and lifethreatening. Type 1 diabetes typically presents with symptoms of hyperglycemia and if unrecognized can culminate in diabetic ketoacidosis (DKA). Symptoms of Addison's disease may be present for years prior to the diagnosis. Unrecognized Addison's disease can lead to an Addisonian crisis characterized by electrolyte abnormalities, hypotension, hypoglycemia, and increased skin pigmentation. Autoimmune thyroid disease may present with thyroid storm or myxedema coma. More frequently, symptoms of thyroid disease are elicited, and the diagnosis is confirmed on laboratory screening. In all conditions, the diagnosis depends on the clinician having a high index of clinical suspicion. Significant morbidity and even mortality can be prevented by an astute clinician recognizing the symptoms and screening for the disease.

DIAGNOSIS AND TREATMENT

Diabetes is diagnosed when blood glucose levels are 126 mg/dL or greater fasting or 200 mg/dL randomly or after an oral glucose challenge. In the absence of symptoms of diabetes, the measurement must be repeated (55). In the presence of symptoms, a single blood glucose value is needed to confirm the diagnosis. Some have argued for the use of hemoglobin A1c for the diagnosis of type 2 diabetes; its use for diagnosis of type 1 diabetes has not been thoroughly evaluated. Autoimmune thyroid disease is diagnosed with abnormalities of thyroid function testing. Addison's disease can be diagnosed with random levels of cortisol, ACTH, PRA, and electrolytes, especially in the setting of an Addisonian crisis. If the diagnosis is unclear, stimulation testing with cosyntropin may be necessary, and Addison's disease is diagnosed with elevated ACTH levels and failure to stimulate cortisol above 18–20 μg/dL 30–60 min after provocation with cosyntropin 250 mcg IV. Small intestinal biopsy is required for the diagnosis of celiac disease. Characteristic changes include blunting of the intestinal villi with intraepithelial lymphocytes. Changes are graded on a Marsh score from 0 (normal) to 5. Diagnosis of celiac disease is confirmed with a Marsh score greater than 2 and positive TTG antibodies with resolution of small intestinal biopsy changes with implementation of a gluten free diet. It is important to think about a second autoimmune disease in a person diagnosed with a first. Adrenal crises can be precipitated by initiating treatment for hypothyroidism.

The principle of treatment for type 1 diabetes, autoimmune hypothyroidism, and Addison's disease is the replacement of the missing hormone. However, hormonal replacement is at best an approximation of physiology. Treatment with insulin requires blood glucose monitoring and close attention to diet. Technological advances such as the use of continuous subcutaneous insulin infusions and glucose sensor technology will likely revolutionize diabetes management and may open the door for near normal glycemic control. Treatment of Addison's disease requires oral replacement with florinef (usually once daily) and cortef (usually two to three times daily) with increases in cortef doses with significant physiological stress such as febrile illness and surgical stress. Hypothyroidism is treated with levothyroine and at times triiodothyroxine. Levels of TSH and thyroid hormone are used to assess the efficacy of treatment. Celiac disease is treated by removing gluten from the diet.

CONCLUSION

APS-2 is characterized by the presence of multiple autoimmune diseases including type 1 diabetes, Addison's disease, and autoimmune thyroid disease. These diseases share a common pathophysiology, characterized by T-cell-mediated autoimmune attack of the target gland. The coexistence of these diseases may be in part due to shared genetic and environmental risk factors. The diseases tend to have a long preclinical period and are diagnosed when the majority of the gland is destroyed. At this point, subjects present clinically. The diseases are treated by replacing the missing hormone. Patients with one autoimmune disease are at risk for developing additional autoimmune diseases and therefore benefit from careful history, physical, and laboratory screening to identify these diseases.

ACKNOWLEDGMENTS

Dr. Barker is supported by the Juvenile Diabetes Research Foundation (JDRF) grant number 11-2005-15.

REFERENCES

1. Schmidt MB. Eine biglandulare Erkrankung (Nebennieren und Schilddruse) bei Morbus Addisonii. Verh Dtsch Ges Pathol 1926;21:212–221.
2. Eisenbarth GS, Gottlieb PA. Autoimmune polyendocrine syndromes. N Engl J Med 2004;350:2068–2079.
3. Betterle C, Zanchetta R. Update on autoimmune polyendocrine syndromes (APS). Acta Biomed 2003;74:9–33.
4. Eisenbarth GS. Type I diabetes mellitus. A chronic autoimmune disease. N Engl J Med 1986;314:1360–1368.
5. Betterle C, Dal Pra C, Mantero F, Zanchetta R. Autoimmune adrenal insufficiency and autoimmune polyendocrine syndromes: autoantibodies, autoantigens, and their applicability in diagnosis and disease prediction. Endocr Rev 2002;23:327–364.
6. Eisenbarth SC, Eisenbarth GS. Primer: immunology/autoimmunity. Adv Exp Med Biol 2004;552:1–15.
7. Noble JA, Valdes AM, Cook M, Klitz W, Thomson G, Erlich HA. The role of HLA class II genes in insulin-dependent diabetes mellitus: Molecular analysis of 180 Caucasian, multiplex families. Am J Hum Genet 1996;59:1134–1148.
8. Ban Y, Davies TF, Greenberg DA, Concepcion ES, Tomer Y. The influence of human

leucocyte antigen (HLA) genes on autoimmune thyroid disease (AITD): results of studies in HLA-DR3 positive AITD families. Clin Endocrinol (Oxf) 2002;57:81-88.
9. Hoffenberg EJ, Mackenzie T, Barriga KJ, Eisenbarth GS, Bao F, Haas JE, Erlich H, Bugawan TT, Sokol RJ, Taki I, Norris JM, Rewers M. A prospective study of the incidence of childhood celiac disease. J Pediatr 2003;143:308–314.
10. Tait KF, Collins JE, Heward JM, Eaves I, Snook H, Franklyn JA, Barnett AH, Todd JA, Maranian M, Compston A, Sawcer S, Gough SCL. Evidence for a Type 1 diabetes-specific mechanism for the insulin gene-associated IDDM2 locus rather than a general influence on autoimmunity. Diabet Med 2004;21:267–270.
11. Lambert AP, Gillespie KM, Thomson G, Cordell HJ, Todd JA, Gale EA, Bingley PJ. Absolute risk of childhood-onset type 1 diabetes defined by human leukocyte antigen class II genotype: a population-based study in the United Kingdom. J Clin Endocrinol Metab 2004;89:4037–4043.
12. Liese AD, D'Agostino RB, Jr, Hamman RF, Kilgo PD, Lawrence JM, Liu LL, Loots B, Linder B, Marcovina S, Rodriguez B, Standiford D, Williams DE. The burden of diabetes mellitus among US youth: prevalence estimates from the SEARCH for Diabetes in Youth Study. Pediatrics 2006;118:1510–1518.
13. Aly TA, Ide A, Jahromi MM, Barker JM, Fernando MS, Babu SR, Yu L, Miao D, Erlich HA, Fain PR, Barriga KJ, Norris JM, Rewers MJ. Eisenbarth, GS. Extreme genetic risk for type 1A diabetes. Proc Natl Acad Sci USA 2006;103:14074–14079.
14. Bao F, Yu L, Babu S, Wang T, Hoffenberg EJ, Rewers M, Eisenbarth GS. One third of HLA DQ2 homozygous patients with type 1 diabetes express celiac disease associated transglutaminase autoantibodies. J Autoimmun 1999;13:143–148.
15. Hanneman MJ, Sprangers MA, De Mik EL, Ernest van Heurn LW, De Langen ZJ, Looyaard N, Madern GC, Rieu PN, van der Zee DC, van Silfhout M, Aronson DC. Quality of life in patients with anorectal malformation or Hirschsprung's disease: development of a disease-specific questionnaire. Dis Colon Rectum 2001;44:1650–1660.
16. Bottini N, Musumeci L, Alonso A, Rahmouni S, Nika K, Rostamkhani M, MacMurray J, Meloni GF, Lucarelli P, Pellecchia M, Eisenbarth GS, Comings D, Mustelin T. A functional variant of lymphoid tyrosine phosphatase is associated with type I diabetes. Nat Genet 2004;36:337–338.
17. Skorka A, Bednarczuk T, Bar-Andziak E, Nauman J, Ploski R. Lymphoid tyrosine phosphatase (PTPN22/LYP) variant and Graves' disease in a Polish population: association and gene dose-dependent correlation with age of onset. Clin Endocrinol (Oxf) 2005;62: 679–682.
18. Kubo T, Hatton RD, Oliver J, Liu XF, Elson CO, Weaver CT. Regulatory T cell suppression and anergy are differentially regulated by proinflammatory cytokines produced by TLR-activated dendritic cells. J Immunol 2004;173: 7249–7258.
19. Santin I, Castellanos-Rubio A, Aransay AM, Castano L, Vitoria JC, Bilbao JR. The functional R620W variant of the PTPN22 gene is associated with celiac disease. Tissue Antigens 2008;71(3):247–249.
20. Villano MJ, Huber AK, Greenberg DA, Golden BK, Concepcion E, Tomer Y. Autoimmune thyroiditis and diabetes: dissecting the joint genetic susceptibility in a large cohort of multiplex families. J Clin Endocrinol Metab 2009;94(4):1458–1466.
21. Ban Y, Tomer Y. Susceptibility genes in thyroid autoimmunity. Clin Dev Immunol 2005;12:47–58.
22. Pugliese A, Zeller M, Fernandez A, Zalcberg LJ, Bartlett RJ, Ricordi C, Pietropaolo M, Eisenbarth GS, Bennett ST, Patel DD. The insulin gene is transcribed in the human thymus and transcription levels correlate with allelic variation at the INS VNTR-IDDM2 susceptibility locus for type I diabetes. Nat Genet 1997;15:293–297.
23. Rewers M, Zimmet P. The rising tide of childhood type 1 diabetes – what is the elusive environmental trigger? Lancet 2004;364: 1645–1647.
24. Rewers M, Norris JM, Eisenbarth GS, Erlich HA, Beaty B, Klingensmith G, Hoffman M, Yu L, Bugawan TL, Blair A, Hamman RF, Groshek M, Mc Duffie RS, Jr. Beta-cell autoantibodies in infants and toddlers without IDDM relatives: diabetes autoimmunity study in the young (DAISY) J Autoimmun 1996;9:405–410.
25. TEDDY Study Group. The Environmental Determinants of Diabetes in the Young (TEDDY) study: study design. Pediatr Diabetes 2007;8:286–298.
26. Nejentsev S, Sjoroos M, Soukka T, Knip M, Simell O, Lovgren T, Ilonen J. Population-based genetic screening for the estimation of Type 1 diabetes mellitus risk in Finland: selective genotyping of markers in the HLA-DQB1, HLA-DQA1 and HLA-DRB1 loci. Diabet Med 1999;16:985–992.

27. Ziegler AG, Hummel M, Schenker M, Bonifacio E. Autoantibody appearance and risk for development of childhood diabetes in offspring of parents with type 1 diabetes. The 2-year analysis of the German BABYDIAB study. Diabetes 1999;48:460–468.
28. Norris JM, Beaty B, Klingensmith G, Yu L, Hoffman M, Chase HP, Erlich HA, Hamman RF, Eisenbarth GS, Rewers M. Lack of association between early exposure to cow's milk protein and b-cell autoimmunity: Diabetes Autoimmunity Study in the Young (DAISY). JAMA 1996;276:609–614.
29. Norris JM, Barriga K, Klingensmith G, Hoffman M, Eisenbarth GS, Erlich HA, Rewers M. Timing of initial cereal exposure in infancy and risk of islet autoimmunity. JAMA 2003;290:1713–1720.
30. Ziegler AG, Schmid S, Huber D, Hummel M, Bonifacio E. Early infant feeding and risk of developing type 1 diabetes-associated autoantibodies. JAMA 2003;290:1721–1728.
31. Norris JM, Barriga K, Hoffenberg EJ, Taki I, Miao D, Haas JE, Emery LM, Sokol RJ, Erlich HA, Eisenbarth GS, Rewers M. Risk of celiac disease autoimmunity and timing of gluten introduction in the diet of infants at increased risk of disease. JAMA 2005;293:2343–2351.
32. Poole JA, Barriga K, Leung DY, Hoffman M, Eisenbarth GS, Rewers M, Norris JM. Timing of initial exposure to cereal grains and the risk of wheat allergy. Pediatrics 2006;117:2175–2182.
33. Stene LC, Joner G. Use of cod liver oil during the first year of life is associated with lower risk of childhood-onset type 1 diabetes: a large, population-based, case-control study. Am J Clin Nutr 2003;78:1128–1134.
34. Norris JM, Yin X, Lamb MM, Barriga K, Seifert J, Hoffman M, Orton HD, Baron AE, Clare-Salzler M, Chase HP, Szabo NJ, Erlich H, Eisenbarth GS, Rewers M. Omega-3 polyunsaturated fatty acid intake and islet autoimmunity in children at increased risk for type 1 diabetes. JAMA 2007;298:1420–1428.
35. Roti E, Uberti ED. Iodine excess and hyperthyroidism. Thyroid 2001;11:493–500.
36. Bottazzo GF, Florin-Christensen A, Doniach D. Islet-cell antibodies in diabetes mellitus with autoimmune polyendocrine deficiencies. Lancet 1974;2:1279–1283.
37. Wenzlau JM, Juhl K, Yu L, Moua O, Sarkar SA, Gottlieb P, Rewers M, Eisenbarth GS, Jensen J, Davidson HW, Hutton JC. The cation efflux transporter ZnT8 (Slc30A8) is a major autoantigen in human type 1 diabetes. Proc Natl Acad Sci USA 2007;104:17040–17045.
38. Verge CF, Gianani R, Kawasaki E, Yu L, Pietropaolo M, Jackson RA, Chase HP, Eisenbarth GS. Prediction of type I diabetes in first-degree relatives using a combination of insulin, GAD, and ICA512bdc/IA-2 autoantibodies. Diabetes 1996;45:926–933.
39. Barker JM, Barriga K, Yu L, Miao D, Erlich H, Norris JN, Eisenbarth GS, Rewers M. Prediction of autoantibody positivity and progression to type 1 diabetes: Diabetes Autoimmunity Study in the Young (DAISY). J Clin Endocrinol Metab 2004;89:3896–3902.
40. Achenbach P, Koczwara K, Knopff A, Naserke H, Ziegler AG, Bonifacio E. Mature high-affinity immune responses to (pro)insulin anticipate the autoimmune cascade that leads to type 1 diabetes. J Clin Invest 2004;114:589–597.
41. Achenbach P, Warncke K, Reiter J, Naserke HE, Williams AJ, Bingley PJ, Bonifacio E, Ziegler AG. Stratification of type 1 diabetes risk on the basis of islet autoantibody characteristics. Diabetes 2004;53:384–392.
42. Vanderpump MP, Tunbridge WM, French JM, Appleton D, Bates D, Clark F, Grimley EJ, Hasan DM, Rodgers H, Tunbridge F. The incidence of thyroid disorders in the community: a twenty-year follow-up of the Whickham Survey. Clin Endocrinol (Oxf) 1995;43:55–68.
43. Barker JM, Yu J, Yu L, Wang J, Miao D, Bao F, Hoffenberg E, Nelson JC, Gottlieb PA, Rewers M, Eisenbarth GS. Autoantibody "sub-specificity" in type 1 diabetes: Risk for organ specific autoimmunity clusters in distinct groups. Diabetes Care 2005;28:850–855.
44. Ansaldi N, Palmas T, Corrias A, Barbato M, D'Altiglia MR, Campanozzi A, Baldassarre M, Rea F, Pluvio R, Bonamico M, Lazzari R, Corrao G. Autoimmune thyroid disease and celiac disease in children. J Pediatr Gastroenterol Nutr 2003;37:63–66.
45. Farrell RJ, Kelly CP. Celiac sprue. N Engl J Med 2002;346:180–188.
46. Larizza D, Calcaterra V, De Giacomo C, De Silvestri A, Asti M, Badulli C, Autelli M, Coslovich E, Martinetti M. Celiac disease in children with autoimmune thyroid disease. J Pediatr 2001;139:738–740.
47. Falorni A, Laureti S, Nikoshkov A, Picchio ML, Hallengren B, Vandewalles CL, Gorus FK, Tortoioli C, Luthman H, Brunetti P, Santeusanio F. 21-hydroxylase autoantibodies in adult patients with endocrine autoimmune diseases are highly specific for Addison's disease. Clin Exp Immunol 1997;107:341–346.

48. Di Lorenzo TP, Peakman M, Roep BO. Translational mini-review series on type 1 diabetes: systematic analysis of T cell epitopes in autoimmune diabetes. Clin Exp Immunol 2007;148:1–16.
49. Bingley PJ, Colman P, Eisenbarth GS, Jackson RA, McCulloch DK, Riley WJ, Gale EAM. Standardization of IVGTT to predict IDDM. Diabetes Care 1992;15:1313–1316.
50. Barker JM, McFann K, Harrison LC, Fourlanos S, Krischer J, Cuthbertson D, Chase HP, Eisenbarth GS. Pre-type 1 diabetes dysmetabolism: maximal sensitivity achieved with both oral and intravenous glucose tolerance testing. J Pediatr 2007;150:31–36.
51. Greenbaum CJ, Cuthbertson D, Krischer JP. Type I diabetes manifested solely by 2-h oral glucose tolerance test criteria. Diabetes 2001;50:470–476.
52. Stene LC, Barriga K, Hoffman M, Kean J, Klingensmith G, Norris JM, Erlich HA, Eisenbarth GS, Rewers M. Normal but increasing hemoglobin A1c levels predict progression from islet autoimmunity to overt type 1 diabetes: Diabetes Autoimmunity Study in the Young (DAISY). Pediatr Diabetes 2006;7:247–253.
53. Umpierrez GE, Latif KA, Murphy MB, Lambeth HC, Stentz F, Bush A, Kitabchi AE. Thyroid dysfunction in patients with type 1 diabetes: a longitudinal study. Diabetes Care 2003;26:1181–1185.
54. Betterle C, Scalici C, Presotto F, Pedini B, Moro L, Rigon F, Mantero F. The natural history of adrenal function in autoimmune patients with adrenal autoantibodies. J Endocrinol 1988;117:467–475.
55. American Diabetes Association. Diagnosis and classification of diabetes mellitus. Diabetes Care 2004;27 Suppl 1:S5–S10.

Chapter 10

Drug-Induced Endocrine Autoimmunity

Paolo Pozzilli, Rocky Strollo, and Nicola Napoli

Summary

Drug-induced autoimmune syndromes have been recognized for a long time and their frequency and complexity have increased in recent years. Many of these conditions are associated with autoantibodies that have been classically defined as limited to idiopathic disease states. Several medications are known to induce endocrine autoimmunity in genetically predisposed individuals, but the mechanisms to which they owe this effect are different.

Several molecules used for different clinical conditions have a physiological role in immune response (e.g., IFNα and IL-2) or are capable of modifying (blocking or stimulating) one or more phases of immune response. Given its particular immune-modeling properties, IFNα is the most common therapeutic agent that induces endocrine autoimmunity, but, according to recent developments, other molecules may alter immune response and generate endocrine autoimmunity and disease. They can act at several steps in the immune response: by disturbing the phase of antigen presentation (sulfhydryl compounds), costimulation (anti-CTLA4 antibody, IL-2), T-cell activation (IL-2), or Th1/Th2 balance generation (Campath-1H). They may trigger autoimmunity and autoimmune diseases in subjects with specific vulnerability (usually genetically determined) in one of the stages of immune response (Table 10.1).

Therefore, the recent development of new molecules that may modulate immune response to treat immune-mediated disease or cancer makes it imperative for endocrinologists and physicians to know about this risk. In this chapter, we review the role of drugs that are capable of inducing endocrine autoimmunity. Thus, we will attempt to give an updated and simple interpretation of current knowledge on the subject and focus on the most common conditions in clinical practice and the use of new medications.

Key Words: Diabetes, Animal model diabetes, Genetics diabetes, Lymphopenia, T cells, Regulatory T cells, Biobreeding diabetes resistant rat

Table 10.1
Drugs Associated with Induction of Endocrine Autoimmunity

Drug	Mechanism	Endocrine dysfunction
IFNα	Stimulation of ADCC	Graves' disease
	Activation of Th1 cells	Hashimoto's thyroiditis, diabetes mellitus
IL-2	Activation of T cells	Hashimoto's thyroiditis
Ipilimumab	Blockage of CTLA4, an inhibitor of T cell proliferation and function	Hypophysitis
GM-CSF	Activation of mature leukocytes	Thyroid dysfunction
Campath-1H	Decrease in Th1/Th2 ratio	Graves' disease
Amiodarone	Thyroid damage, iodine excess	Uncertain: Hashimoto's thyroiditis
HAART	Changes in CD4+ cells	Graves' disease
Sulfhydryl compounds	Changes in conformation of proteins of immune response	Insulin autoimmune syndrome

Modified from Prummel MF, Strieder T, Wiersinga W. The environment and autoimmune thyroid diseases. *Eur J Endocrinol.* 2004;150:605–18

INTERFERON ALPHA

The interferons are a group of proteins that are characterized by antiviral activity, growth regulatory properties, and a wide variety of immunomodulatory activities. At the moment, several interferon-induced proteins have been identified and used as therapeutic agents (1). So far, interferon alpha (IFNα) has been associated most often with induction of endocrine autoimmunity (Table 10.1).

Once IFNα binds its transmembrane receptors (containing cytoplasmic domains), it activates important signaling pathways, such as JAK-STAT, Crk, IRS, and MAP kinase (2, 3).

The most common disease treated with IFNα is the hepatitis C virus (HCV) infection, which today affects millions of people worldwide. Limitations to a more widespread use of IFNα are related to a high incidence of side effects related to this treatment. In fact, although it has been shown in randomized trials that approximately 50% of patients with chronic hepatitis C were successfully treated with virologic response [in association with Ribavirin (Riba)] (4, 5), flu-like symptoms, endocrine dysfunctions, hematologic abnormalities, and neuropsychiatry symptoms caused both dose reductions in up to 40% of cases and treatment discontinuation in up to 14% (6). In the next paragraph, we will discuss the effects of IFNα on endocrine dysfunctions.

THYROID DYSFUNCTION

The association between IFNα and thyroiditis, called interferon-induced thyroiditis (IIT), is one of the most common and well-described side effects of IFNα therapy. The association was diagnosed for the first time more than 20 years ago in patients treated with IFNα for carcinoid tumors and breast cancer (7, 8). IIT has been the object of several studies since then. Studies have shown that the majority of patients with IIT develop thyroid peroxidase (TPO) antibodies (87%), indicating the autoimmune nature of this event. During treatment, thyroid autoantibodies tend to increase and subjects with circulating TPO autoantibodies have an increased risk of developing thyroid dysfunction, a condition that can interfere with an adequate IFNα therapeutic response (9–12). Moreover, physicians may be misled, considering that fatigue, weight gain, and depression might be attributable to IFNα therapy and not to a low thyroid function (6), thus increasing the risk of late diagnosis and further complications. According to most studies, hypothyroidism can be transient and subside after discontinuation of IFNα.

The subtypes of induced disease are autoimmune IIT and nonautoimmune IIT. Autoimmune IIT includes autoimmune hypothyroidism (Hashimoto's thyroiditis) and Graves' disease (GD). Nonautoimmune IIT includes destructive thyroiditis and nonautoimmune hypothyroidism. These abnormalities can occur at any time during IFNα therapy, from as early as 4 weeks to as late as 23 months after initiation (7), with a median date of onset of 17 weeks after the start of IFNα treatment.

AUTOIMMUNE IFNα-INDUCED THYROIDITIS

The most common autoimmune IIT disease occurs in patients who are treated for HCV infection. However, IFNα therapy has also been known to cause autoimmune thyroid disease in malignancies such as breast cancer, carcinoid, and hematological disorders (7, 8, 13–15).

AUTOIMMUNE HYPOTHYROIDISM

The most common form of thyroid autoimmunity is characterized by asymptomatic thyroiditis with the presence of thyroid antibodies (TPO-Ab and thyroglobulin antibodies) (16). The presence of TAbs is usually a preclinical phase of autoimmune thyroid disease (*17*), and the risk of thyroid disease is significantly higher in patients with preexisting positive antithyroid antibodies. However, 9% of IFNα-treated patients who were negative for TAbs without clinical disease developed TAbs during treatment. Therefore, circulating TAbs positivity can be a de novo condition during IFNα or it can be significantly increased in individuals who are already positive prior to IFNα therapy, resulting in an exacerbation of a preexisting thyroid autoimmunity (*18–20*).

The percentage of patients who develop de novo TAbs secondary to IFNα varies according to studies and ranges from 1.9 to 40% (*21*). Most patients who develop de novo TAbs during IFNα therapy remain positive even years after the treatment is discontinued. Long-term TAbs positivity was shown in a clinical study in which 72% of patients, followed as long as up to 8 years after the end of IFNα treatment, were still TAbs positive (*22*). In fact, authors found that ten of 36 (28%) patients with TPO antibodies became antibody negative 6 years after discontinuation, while 26 patients remained antibody positive. Subclinical hypothyroidism was diagnosed in seven of the latter. The IFNα-induced TAbs positivity is more common in women (14.8% vs. 1%) and directly related to age (*18*). However, over 60% of patients who had or developed TAbs during treatment developed thyroid disease. Similarly, in a review of the literature by Koh et al. (*23*), it was reported that 56% of the patients had permanent hypothyroidism. The high rate of thyroid autoimmunity was independent of the kind of interferon used, leukocyte-derived or recombinant. Another study treating carcinoid with leukocyte-derived interferon obtained similar results, with 14.3% of the patients developing autoimmune IIT and 16.3% developing positive TAbs on IFNα.

GRAVES' DISEASE

GD is a less common complication in patients treated with IFNα (*10*). In a retrospective analysis of 321 patients treated with IFNα for hepatitis B virus (HBV) and HCV infections, ten patients had GD with suppressed TSH and symptomatic thyrotoxicosis. Considering this subgroup of patients, thyroid scintigraphy showed a diffusely increased uptake and thyroid-stimulating antibody positivity in six of them. More importantly, even after the discontinuation of IFNα therapy, thyrotoxicosis did not resolve in all patients (*24*) and required definitive treatment. Similar results were found in another large multicenter study in which 1.3% of patients on IFNα developed permanent GD (*25*). Graves' ophthalmopathies have rarely been reported. However, the lack of remission of thyrotoxicosis after IFNα therapy discontinuation

Predisposition

highlights the severity of thyroid damage and how this condition should be considered by physicians (*9*).

The pattern of thyroid disease observed during IFNα treatment is similar to that observed during the "endogenous" immunostimulation in the postpartum period. As stated above, circulating levels of TAbs tend to increase during IFNα treatment and predispose these patients to the development of thyroid dysfunction. Thyroid function may normalize in some patients after the withdrawal of therapy.

Several factors have been suggested that predispose an individual to the development of IIT, including the patient's underlying condition, the dose and duration of IFNα treatment, and genetic factors. In patients treated with IFNα because of HCV infection, some authors have indicated that the virus itself was a direct cause (*26–29*), but a dose-dependent effect of IFNα and duration of treatment also seem to play a main role (*23*). Other risk factors are related to prior TAb positivity, female gender, stress, iodine intake, and pregnancy (*10, 23, 30–34*).

Interestingly, in vitro studies have shown that IFNα upregulates major histocompatibility complex (MHC) class I and II expression on xenografted thyroid tissues from Graves' patients only when local infiltrating lymphocytes are in the graft. This suggests that IFNα may be capable of aggravating an immune response only in predisposed subjects with some degree of preexisting thyroiditis.

GENETIC FACTORS

Hypothesizing that IFNα may be involved in triggering IIT in genetically susceptible individuals, several studies have investigated a genetic predisposition in the development of IIT in patients treated with IFNα (*20, 21, 23*), including studies carried out on twins. The rationale of these studies was based on evidence revealing that women are more predisposed to developing this complication than men. Combining data from several studies, it has been calculated that the risk is 4.4 times higher in females than in males. This evidence has opened several suppositions about a potential chromosome X-related gene. It should be also mentioned that estrogen may play a role in this regard, making the scenario more complex (*35*). Even ethnicity has been the object of studies, and it has been found that the Asian race is an independent predictor of IIT (*36*).

However, most of the studies have focused on genes involved in immune regulation, such as HLA-DR (*37, 38*), CTLA4 (*2, 39–41*), and PTPN22 (*42, 43*) and thyroid-specific genes, including thyroglobulin. Currently, the most consistent data support a higher risk of IIT in patients bearing the HLA-A2 and DRB1*11 alleles (9). Preliminary evidence shows a possible association between polymorphisms in the CTLA4 and CD40 genes with IIT (44).

NONGENETIC FACTORS

While genetic factors are important in IIT, nongenetic factors may also play an important role, and viral infections have been considered triggering factors (45, 46). Some of the nongenetic factors that have been found to contribute to the development of IIT include the HCV genotype, the therapeutic regimen, and the presence of TAbs prior to the initiation of IFNα therapy.

Viral genotype: Even if IIT has been diagnosed in patients receiving IFNα for a variety of diseases (47), most cases have been described in HCV positive patients, suggesting that HCV may play an independent role. The potential role of the virus is also sustained by some studies that found a higher susceptibility to IIT in patients infected with HCV than those with HBV (24, 30, 48, 49). However, no certain conclusions can be drawn since HCV patients require longer regimens of IFNα.

Given the homology between some HCV quasispecies sequences and thyroglobulin sequences and that HCV is classified into six major genotypes over 70 subtypes (50), several investigators have looked at a possible association between viral genotype and the susceptibility of patients in developing IIT (51, 52). However, clinical studies linking the hepatitis viruses to the development of IIT are lacking (18), and no correlation between HCV genotypes and the development of TAbs or IIT has been found. Current data support the notion that viral genotype does not influence a predisposition to thyroid autoimmunity in patients infected with HCV during IFNα therapy (53, 66).

Ribavirin (Riba): The independent correlation between Riba and IIT has been tested in a clinical study on the base of the effect of this compound on the immune system. In fact, it has been found that it may induce a T helper (Th) 1 polarization of Th cells by augmenting interleukin 2 (IL-2), IFNγ, and tumor necrosis factor-alpha (TNFα) production and suppressing IL-4, IL-5, and IL-10 production (54–57). However, when 72 patients who were treated with IFNα and Riba were compared to 75 on IFNα alone, no significant difference was found between the two groups in terms of thyroid autoimmunity (23.6% vs. 22.7%) (58).

Presence of baseline TAbs: The presence of baseline TAbs is considered an independent risk factor in the development of IIT in patients treated with IFNα. In fact, it has been estimated that 84% of patients with IIT were TAbs prior to the treatment and the data from pooled studies show a higher risk of IIT in TAb positive patients, compared to those who were negative at baseline (46.1% vs. 5.4%) (23). In addition, the presence of TPO-Ab before treatment was a statistically significant risk factor in the development of thyroid disease in patients treated with IFNα (10). Similarly, Watanabe et al. showed that the incidence of thyroid disease in patients with pretreatment TPO-Ab was much higher compared to patients with negative TPO-Ab levels (60% vs. 3.3%) (20). According to Roti et al., positive TPO-Abs before the IFNα treatment had a predictive value of 67% for the development of IIT (10). Therefore, the authors recommended a TAb screening before initiating IFNα treatment, as well strict thyroid monitoring in patients who were TPO-Ab positive.

Pathogenesis

IFNα-induced thyroiditis is a complex mechanism that involves both direct and immune-mediated effects. However, this condition still remains unclear for many reasons.

Through the activation of the JAK–STAT pathway (51), IFNα activates several genes coding for cytokines and adhesion molecules (60). The immune-mediated mechanism should be considered in light of the many immune effects exerted by IFNα. IFNα can also enhance MHC class I antigens in thyroid cells, activating cytotoxic T cells, lymphocytes, natural killer cells, neutrophils, and monocytes. IFN also plays an important role on cell activity, it being an important cofactor in the development of Th1 immune reaction, inducing thyroid autoimmune inflammatory response, and consequently, tissue damage. It has also been reported that thyroid damage may be mediated by the release of IFNγ and IL-2, and tumor necrosis factor-beta (TNFβ) through the activation of Th1. IFNα can induce the activation of other cytokines, such as IL-6, which has been shown to have specific binding sites in the thyroid tissue, thus decreasing TSH-mediated iodine uptake, and thyroid hormone release in vitro (61, 62).

Direct Effects of IFNα

Evidence of thyroid damage without release of thyroid antibodies have raised the doubt that IFNα may directly have a toxic effect on thyroid tissue. In vitro data indicate, however, that IFNα inhibits levels of TG and TPO in thyroid cell lines inducing thyroid cell death (63, 64).

Table 10.2 summarizes the potential mechanisms for the development of IIT.

Table 10.2
Potential Mechanisms for the Development of IIT

Immune-mediated effects of IFNα
Enhanced expression of class I MHC antigens on thyrocytes
Activation of cytotoxic T cells
Enhanced expression of cellular adhesion molecules (ICAM, B7.1)
Increased activity of lymphocytes, macrophages, NK cells, neutrophils, monocytes
Increased activity of IL-6
Modulation of immunoglobulin production
Inhibition of T regulatory cells
Th1 polarization
Direct effects of IFNα on the thyroid
Inhibition of TSH-induced gene expression of Tg, TPO, and NIS
Decreased iodine organification
Decreased thyroxine (T4) release

From Mandac JC, et al. The clinical and physiological spectrum of interferon-alpha induced thyroiditis: Toward a new classification. *Hepatology*. 2006;43(4):661–72

NONAUTO-IMMUNE INTERFERON-INDUCED THYROIDITIS

IFNα may play an independent role in thyroid dysfunction and this would explain the reason why nonautoimmune thyroiditis affects up to 50% of patients with IIT (*48*). This form of IIT is characterized by a destructive thyroiditis, which is a self-limited inflammatory disorder of the gland. This condition is characterized by an initial thyrotoxicosis followed by hypothyroidism that usually evolves to resolution after a few weeks (*65*). Very rarely, patients (less than 5%) develop permanent hypothyroidism and require a lifelong replacement with thyroid hormones (*66*). Many cases of these forms of thyroiditis are not symptomatic, and therefore, they may occur more frequently than reported. However, in some cases, patients may undergo atrial fibrillation. In this case, thyroid ablation is necessary before an IFNα rechallenge. The diagnosis is based on negative TSH-receptor antibodies (TRAb) and low thyroid iodine uptake. Even after recovering from this complication, and in patients who have a normal thyroid functioning, thyroid hormones should be monitored to avoid further recidivisms (*67*). The clinical course of the disease is often reversible but it becomes permanent, mostly when the TAbs are developed.

Diabetes Mellitus

While the role of IFNα in inducing thyroid disease has been widely studied, the onset of type 1 diabetes (T1D) has been reported several times, yet no consistent data are available on explaining a direct causative effect. The role that IFNα exerts in T1D is unclear, given the complex properties of IFNα on immune modulation and individual variability, for example, the rate of basal activation of the immune system and the presence of viral infections. Several studies indicate that IFNα plays a primary role in the pathogenesis of autoimmune diabetes, triggering the autoimmune process or modifying the natural history of diabetes.

The first case of T1D developed during IFNα therapy was published in 1992 (*2, 68*) and before initiating the treatment this patient was positive for glutamic acid decarboxylase (GAD) antibodies and insulin autoantibodies (IAAs). In most cases, T1D developed in those patients who are already anti-GAD positive prior to starting the treatment (*69, 70*). Thus, several authors agree that IFNα can cause T1D in patients who are genetically and immunologically predisposed. In one series of 70 patients with hepatitis C receiving IFNα, only one developed T1D (5 months after the beginning of treatment) and that patient was anti-GAD positive before treatment. However, according to other studies, IFNα may also prevent autoimmune diabetes (*71*). Hence, further studies are needed to clarify the role of IFNα in autoimmune diabetes.

In the following paragraphs, we will review the epidemiology and role of IFNα treatment in the induction of autoimmune diabetes and the natural history of diabetes in treated patients.

EPIDEMIOLOGY

A large, Italian, retrospective study, conducted on 11,241 patients with chronic HCV infection treated with IFNα, reported ten new diagnoses (0.08%) of diabetes after at least 16 weeks of treatment (*72*). In another retrospective study on 667 Japanese treated patients, only five (0.7%) developed diabetes (*70*). Although the reported incidences are significantly higher than those in the normal population of Italy and Japan (*72, 73*), authors have not provided data on antibodies, limiting the interest of these findings.

In these studies, the distinction between autoimmune and nonautoimmune diabetes mellitus could not be made because (a) beta-cell autoimmunity was not investigated and (b) the aims of these studies were to evaluate the incidence and prognosis of various IFNα-related side effects, not only diabetes.

These data were recently confirmed in a prospective study on the development of diabetes in chronic HCV patients treated with Peg-IFNα/Riba. In this study, Schreuder et al. studied 207 patients treated for chronic hepatitis. The population was stratified under the type of therapy given, 189 received standard therapy (Peg-IFNα-2b or Peg-IFNα-2a and Riba) and 100 received triple therapy with amantadine. Nine of the 189 patients (4.8%) developed diabetes, five patients (1.6%) developed autoantibodies [anti-GAD65, tyrosine phosphatase autoantibodies (IA-2), or islet cell autoantibodies (ICA)], and two of the nine patients who developed diabetes tested positive for T1D-associated autoantibodies (anti-GAD65 or ICA) before IFNα (74).

PATHOGENESIS

The role of IFNα in diabetogenesis is still controversial, and experimental models have not given unequivocal responses. Besides its immunomodulatory properties, it has been found that IFNα increases insulin resistance and induces hyperglycemia (75–80). Transgenic mice overexpressing IFNα develop a form of T1D that can be prevented using neutralizing antibodies. In these models, IFNα induces inflammation and autoreactive T cells preceding the development of diabetes. On the contrary, it has been shown in other animal studies that IFNα seems to prevent glucose intolerance and even cure the disease in nonobese diabetic (NOD) mice (81, 82).

In 1987, Foulis et al. studied pancreases that were removed from deceased newly diagnosed T1D. In most cases, the beta cells were positive for immunoreactive IFNα, a finding related to hyperexpression of MHC antigens (83). Huang et al., using a reverse transcriptase–polymerase chain reaction protocol to examine the expression of TNFα, IL-1β, IL-2, IL-4, and IL-6 in the islets of patients with T1D, concluded that only IFNα was significantly increased in diabetic patients (84).

In human studies, pancreatic islet cells of patients affected with T1D have an enhanced expression of IFNα. However, in most cases, patients who develop T1D bear HLA haplotypes associated with increased susceptibility to T1D (DR3, DQ2, DR4, and DQ8).

In fact, Fabris et al. (69) found that all of the 13 HCV patients who developed T1D during IFNα therapy had an HLA haplotype associated with increased susceptibility. In the prospective study by Schreuder et al. (74), four of the nine patients diagnosed with T1D had HLA haplotypes increasing the risk of T1D and three patients also tested positive for one or more autoantibodies. Given that Riba is not associated with the development of diabetes, it seems that IFNα plays an independent role. Taken together, these results suggest that HCV positive patients may be predisposed to T1D during IFNα therapy if they have certain high-risk HLA haplotypes. Considering the limited data available, more studies are needed to further investigate the role of IFNα on pathogenesis of T1D in these patients. Figure 10.1 summarizes the role that IFN exerts on pathogenesis of T1D.

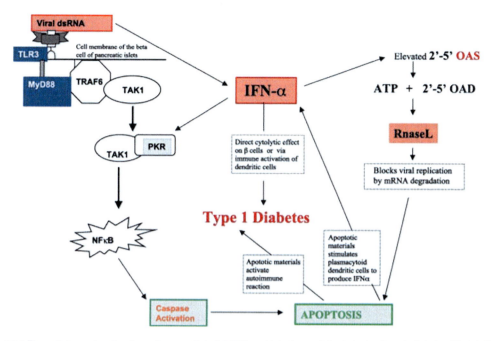

Fig. 10.1 The cellular and molecular pathways of viral dsRNA and interferon alpha inducing type 1 diabetes. Viral dsRNA activates the toll-like receptor-3 (TLR3) and via various differentiating factors activates the nuclear factor NFκB to induce apoptosis. Viral dsRNA also activates the production of IFNα in various cells, which is directly cytotoxic to beta cells of the pancreas. IFNα also induces apoptosis by activating the oligoadenylate synthase (OAS)–RNAase L pathway and the protein kinase R (PKR) pathway. Apoptotic materials induce more IFNα and activate the immune system. *TAK-1*, transforming growth factor β activated protein kinase 1; *TLR-3*, toll-like receptor 3; *MyD88*, myeloid differentiation factor; *PKR*, protein kinase R; *OAS*, oligoadenylate synthase; *TRAF-6*, tumor necrosis factor receptor-associated factor 6; *NFκB*, nuclear factor κB. From Devendra D, Eisenbarth GS. Interferon alpha – a potential link in the pathogenesis of viral-induced type 1 diabetes and autoimmunity. *Clin Immunol.* 2004;111(3):225–33. Review.

THE NATURAL HISTORY OF T1D DURING IFNα TREATMENT

Several clinical cases of T1D during or soon after IFNα therapy have been reported (*69, 85–108*). The majority of these reports are in regard to patients on IFNα for chronic hepatitis C, while a few reports on patients treated for chronic hepatitis B or with an adjuvant therapy for cancer are also available. Most of these cases relate to patients treated with IFNα in monotherapy or combination with Riba. The total dose of interferon ranged from 65 to 1,350 MU, with a duration of treatment that lasted from 10 days to 4 years. An important aspect that should be considered is that approximately 50% of the patients tested were already positive for at least one marker of pancreatic autoimmunity and 77% of those who developed diabetes had at least one marker of pancreatic autoimmunity (in particular, anti-GAD and ICA). The majority (89%) of subjects studied presented a predisposing genetic background (assessed by HLA genotype). The clinical presentation of the disease followed the typical symptoms, such as polyuria, polydipsia, weight loss, and in some cases, ketoacidosis and hyperosmolar coma. In most cases, permanent insulin treatment was required, although in some cases, the condition may have been reversible, implying that the interruption of IFNα treatment may at least partially reverse the autoimmune attack in some cases. More importantly, some patients who initially tested negative for pancreatic autoimmunity seroconverted during therapy. A fulminant onset after 8.5 months of IFNα has been described by Bosi et al. in a subject genetically predisposed with autoantibodies appearing at high titer when the disease was clinically manifest.

Besides these clinical cases, the effect of IFNα therapy on pancreatic autoimmunity has been evaluated in several studies and almost always in patients with chronic hepatitis C infection (*19, 108–115*). However, results may not be consistent, given the different types of IFN, dosages and durations used. Betterle et al. studied the prevalence of clinical and latent autoimmune diseases in 70 Italian patients with HCV chronic infection, for 6 months before and after treatment with IFNα, using ICA, glucagon-cell antibodies (GCA), and anti-GAD as markers of pancreatic autoimmunity. None of the patients studied had evidence of clinical disease before treatment, although one (1.4%) patient was positive for ICA, two (2.8%) were positive for GCA, two (2.8%) for anti-GAD, without a significant difference compared to healthy control subjects. Only one patient, whose ICA/GAD titers increased during the IFNα therapy, developed T1D, 5 months after the beginning of treatment. In another study that analyzed pancreatic islet autoantibodies from 62 patients treated for 6 months with IFNα, Wesche et al. found GAD65 positivity in five patients and IA2 in one patient. In a long-term study, Di Cesare et al. found in 60 HCV patients that IAA appeared in eight of 60 (13.3%) and four of 30 (13.3%) patients, after 6 and 12 months of therapy, respectively. As stated above, in a large prospective study by Schreuder et al., only two of the nine patients who developed diabetes were positive for T1D-associated autoantibodies (anti-GAD65 or ICA) before IFNα therapy was started (*74*).

These results indicate that IFNα therapy may enhance pancreatic autoimmunity, and some of those antibody positive may develop T1D.

In summary, (a) a small portion of patients with chronic HCV hepatitis is positive for one or more markers of pancreatic autoimmunity, (b) these patients are at relative risk of developing diabetes if treated with IFNα, (c) a small number of patients can develop de novo pancreatic autoimmunity and fall in the group of patients at risk of developing diabetes, (d) certain HLA haplotypes may predispose patients to the development of T1D during Peg-IFNα/Riba therapy in chronic HCV patients, (e) a timely suspension of IFNα therapy is rarely accompanied by a regression of clinical diabetes, (f) no correlation has been documented between the response to anti-viral therapy and the development of diabetes mellitus, (g) routine assessment of blood glucose levels in all outpatient visits before, during, and in the first month after Peg-IFNα/Riba treatment may be useful to detect diabetes without delay, and (h) both the positive and the negative predictive values of beta-cell autoantibodies seem too low to identify patients at high risk or to effectively rule out the possibility of developing IFNα-associated T1D.

Adrenal Dysfunction

Little data are available on this condition. A 4.8% prevalence of anti-21-hydroxylase antibodies in hepatitis C patients receiving interferon therapy has been reported, but without clinical symptoms of adrenal dysfunction. On the other hand, some case reports have increased knowledge on the natural history of Addison's disease during IFNα therapy. However, adrenal dysfunction symptoms may be difficult to distinguish from the common side effects of IFNα, so that this complication should be considered in patients with persistent symptoms after IFNα therapy and especially in those who have a history of autoimmune diseases (*116, 117*).

Pituitary Dysfunction

To date, IFN-induced hypopituitarism is considered a rare condition and few reports are available. In the first report of IFN-induced hypopituitarism (*118*), a patient with the hepatitis C infection, who was treated with IFNα2b for 3 months, reported the symptoms of generalized fatigue, edema, and amenorrhea after 2 weeks of treatment, with laboratory evidence of secondary hypothyroidism and hypoadrenalism. No signs of anatomical damage were evidenced in the MRI scan and the hypopituitarism resolved after stopping treatment. In another patient, reported by Concha (*119*), pituitary impairment was permanent even 1 year after having stopped IFNα therapy, and replacement therapy was necessary. The pathogenesis of this condition is unclear, through the involvement of the immune system is likely.

INTERLEUKIN 2

IL-2 has antitumor activity and it has been used in the treatment of HIV, metastatic malignant melanoma, and renal cell carcinoma (*120*). The mechanism of action includes T-cell proliferation, B-cell growth, and natural killer cell and monocyte activation (*121*). IL-2 is, however, involved in autoimmunity, and labeled IL-2 is used to visualize sites of autoimmune inflammation in patients with Hashimoto's thyroiditis or diabetes. An immune-mediated thyroid disease may occur in patients with cancer, who are treated with interleukin either alone or in conjunction with lymphokine-activated killer cells or IFNα. Thyroid dysfunction is frequently reversible occurring in as many as 16% of patients (*122*). Short-term IL-2 administration through the direct central stimulation of the pituitary may induce an increase in serum T4, T3, and TSH levels. Interestingly, this form of thyroiditis has been associated with a higher rate of long-term survival in patients with metastatic renal cell carcinoma (*123*). In fact, in this study, TAbs antibodies positivity, which was detected in 18% of the patients studied had a 5-year survival rate of 54% compared to 15% who were negative for these antibodies. The authors proposed that a cross-reaction autoimmune response between thyroid and renal cells may be involved.

IPILIMUMAB (ANTI-CTLA4 ANTIBODY)

Cytotoxic T-lymphocyte-associated protein 4 (CTLA4, CD152) is an inducible receptor expressed by T cells which ligates CD80 and CD86 on antigen-presenting cells that, when activated, inhibit T-cell proliferation and function. In animal models, it has been shown that CTLA4 blockade induces antitumor immunity, leading to the development of CTLA4 blocking antibodies, which are used in cancer immunotherapy (*124*).

Patients treated with IV ipilimumab every 3 weeks developed autoimmune disorders, like enteritis (21%) and hypophysitis, which occurred in 5% of patients. In this study of over 163 patients (113 with metastatic melanoma and 50 with metastatic renal cancer), hypophysitis was found in 5% of the patients with melanoma and 4% of those with renal cancer. This condition occurred on average after four doses of ipilimumab and only in male subjects. Clinical presentation was based on panhypopituitarism symptoms, such as fatigue, headache, and loss of memory. The pituitary gland was enlarged in seven cases with an increase over 100% than normal. However, immune-mediated adverse events were associated with tumor regression, although the mechanism of this phenomenon is still unknown. The association between autoimmunity and tumor regression may reflect the presence of a genetic pattern that may explain differences in immune reactivity. In fact, polymorphisms in the *CTLA4* gene have been associated with autoimmune endocrine diseases, such as T1D, GD, and autoimmune hypothyroidism (*125*).

GRANULOCYTE-MACROPHAGE COLONY-STIMULATING FACTOR

Granulocyte-macrophage colony-stimulating factor (GM-CSF) plays a major role in the proliferation and differentiation of progenitor cells and neutrophils in bone marrow but also exerts multiple effects, including the activation of mature leukocyte and immune cell functions (*126*). The effect on mature leukocytes may explain the induction of thyroid autoimmunity, which has been reported in a few studies, showing rare and transient thyroid dysfunction (*127*). In a report on 25 cancer patients with previously normal thyroid function receiving GM-CSF, two patients developed reversible hypothyroidism or biphasic thyroiditis, respectively (*128*). Both patients had TPO antibodies before treatment and required thyroxin therapy for 2 months. The author proposed that the stimulation of antigen-presenting cells by GM-CSF may cause this phenomenon.

CAMPATH-1H (ALEMTUZUMAB)

Campath-1H is a humanized anti-CD52 monoclonal antibody and suppresses Th1 lymphocytes, shifting the Th1/Th2 balance toward antibody production and enhancing an immune response against the TSH receptor (*129*). In a study conducted on 29 patients with multiple sclerosis treated with this compound, nine developed GD after 6–31 months of treatment. The clinical features were typically related to suppressed TSH, high FT4, positivity for TRAb, and a diffused pattern of thyroidal uptake with TC99 (*130*). In patients treated with Campath-1H, the study revealed profound lymphopenia with a CD4 and CD8 count that was 30–40% lower than before the treatment. Interestingly, GD has never been reported in patients who were not affected with MS, suggesting that these patients are uniquely susceptible to this complication. However, in 2006, the first case of GD in a patient who underwent a kidney transplant and then treated with Campath-1H was reported. It is not clear if the apparent association between the treatment and the GD is secondary to a specific effect of the medication or to generalized lymphocyte depletion.

AMIODARONE

Thyroid dysfunction is a frequent side effect of amiodarone, and this condition is more frequent in women who are positive for TAbs. The high iodine content has been considered the most important cause of amiodarone-thyroid impairment. Nevertheless, in recent years, it has been suggested that amiodarone may induce thyroid disease, triggering an autoimmune process. Accordingly, Weetman proposed that amiodarone may modulate preexisting thyroid autoantibody titers, suggesting that this may cause autoantigen release. However, according to other authors, it seems that amiodarone does not induce thyroid autoimmunity and even the occurrence of TPO antibodies during the treatment is uncertain (*131–133*).

ANTIRETROVIRAL THERAPY

Highly active antiretroviral therapy (HAART) has been found to be associated with GD, occurring 16–19 months after initiation of a combined treatment with indanavir, stavudine, lamivudine, and ritonavir. The prevalence of this condition is small, and autoimmunity is likely the consequence of the HAART-induced changes in CD4 T cells with an incomplete or unbalanced immune restoration. In patients on HAART, CD4 naive and memory T cells contribute to immune restoration. In addition to retrafficking, the increase in peripheral CD4 T cells may result from peripheral expansion, thymus input, occurrence of revertant memory T cells, or all of these mechanisms. In a case series reported by Gilquin et al., the delayed occurrence of autoimmune hyperthyroidism may indicate an escape of autoreactive T cells and an immune regulatory process dependent upon incomplete immune reconstitution, despite sustained viral suppression and increased CD4 T cell count (*134*).

SULFHYDRYL COMPOUNDS AND INSULIN AUTOIMMUNE SYNDROME

Insulin autoimmune syndrome (IAS) has been mostly described in Japan and it is clinically characterized by fasting hypoglycemia, high concentration of total serum immunoreactive insulin, and serum positivity to antibodies to native human insulin (*135, 136*). IAS is strongly associated to susceptible HLA loci as HLA-DR4, and all patients present an haplotype DR B1*0406, DQ A1*0301, and DQ B1*0302 (vs. 14% of controls). The DR B1*0406 allele plays an important role on presenting insulin peptides to T cells and its high frequency in the Japanese population may explain the risk of the disease in this population (*137, 138*).

This condition is one of the most frequent causes of hypoglycemia in the Japanese population and is often linked to other autoimmune disorders (e.g., GD and rheumatoid arthritis). Medications containing sulfhydryl groups have been associated with Hirata's syndrome, such as methimazole, pyritinol for rheumatoid arthritis (*139*), imipenem (beta-lactam antibiotic) (*140*), and penicilline G (beta-lactam antibiotic) (*141*). Table 10.3 summarizes sulfhydryl compounds associated with the induction of IAS. Sulfhydryl groups have a reductive effect and are associated with the induction of autoimmunity, probably for their strong reducing capacity, which may modify the conformation of proteins involved in the immune response. Because Hirata's syndrome is rare and develops particularly in Japanese individuals (subjects with genetic background), it is thought that these

Table 10.3
Drugs Exposure Ahead of Development of IAS and Associated Diseases from 1970 to September 2007 in Japan

Drugs	Diseases	n
Methimazole[a]	Graves' disease	63
Alfa-mercaptopropionyl glycine (tiopronin)[a]	Chronic liver function/cataract/dermatitis/rheumatoid arthritis	45
Glutathione[a]	Urticaria	8
Gold thioglucose[a]	Bronchial asthma	1
Captopril[a]	Hypertension	1
Penicillamine[a]	Rheumatoid arthritis	1
Acegratone	Urinary balder carcinoma	1
Steroid	Polymyositis	1
Interferon alfa	Renal cell carcinoma	1
Loxoprofen sodium	Rheumatoid polymyositis/lumbar pain	2
Alfa lipoic acid[a]	Dieting/anti-aging supplement	17
Miscellaneous		48

From Uchigata Y, Hirata Y, Iwamoto Y. Drug-induced insulin autoimmune syndrome. *Diabetes Res Clin Pract.* 2009;83(1):e19–20
[a]Contains sulfhydryl compounds itself or after decomposition

medications may induce insulin autoimmunity in genetically predisposed subjects (HLA genotype). In the last 5 years, several cases of IAS induced by alpha lipoic acid (ALA) have been described. ALA is a coenzyme of an enzyme subunit (E2) of enzymes that catalyze oxidative decarboxylation of pyruvic acid and alpha-ketoglutaric acid in mitochondria. ALA possesses two sulfur atoms and it has strong antioxidative effects, which are 400 times higher than vitamin C or vitamin E (*142*). For this reason, besides the natural intake from food, it has been used as part of supplements in the American and Japanese market. In some cases, it is also used as a treatment for diabetic neuropathy, subacute necrotizing encephalopathy, hearing impairment, and Reye's syndrome (*143*). ALA is an example of IAS induced by sulfhydryl compounds. Although this medication may induce this syndrome, the high frequency in some subjects, like the Japanese, indicates the importance of genetic background and, more specifically, particular HLA haplotypes.

REFERENCES

1. Baron S, Tyring SK, Fleischmann WR, Jr, Coppenhaver DH, Niesel DW, Klimpel GR, et al. The interferons. Mechanisms of action and clinical applications. JAMA 1991;266(10):1375–1383.
2. Parmar S, Platanias LC. Interferons: mechanisms of action and clinical applications. Curr Opin Oncol 2003;15(6):431–439.
3. Jonasch E, Haluska FG. Interferon in oncological practice: review of interferon biology, clinical applications, and toxicities. Oncologist 2001;6(1):34–55.
4. Manns MP, McHutchison JG, Gordon SC, Rustgi VK, Shiffman M, Reindollar R, et al. Peginterferon alfa-2b plus ribavirin compared with interferon alfa-2b plus ribavirin for initial treatment of chronic hepatitis C: a randomised trial. Lancet 2001;358(9286):958–965.
5. Fried MW, Shiffman ML, Reddy KR, Smith C, Marinos G, Goncales FL, Jr, et al. Peginterferon alfa-2a plus ribavirin for chronic hepatitis C virus infection. N Engl J Med 2002;347(13):975–982.
6. Russo MW, Fried MW. Side effects of therapy for chronic hepatitis C. Gastroenterology 2003;124(6):1711–1719.
7. Burman P, Totterman TH, Oberg K, Karlsson FA. Thyroid autoimmunity in patients on long term therapy with leukocyte-derived interferon. J Clin Endocrinol Metab 1986;63(5):1086–1090.
8. Fentiman IS, Thomas BS, Balkwill FR, Rubens RD, Hayward JL. Primary hypothyroidism associated with interferon therapy of breast cancer. Lancet 1985;1(8438):1166.
9. Kryczka W, Brojer E, Kowalska A, Zarebska-Michaluk D. Thyroid gland dysfunctions during antiviral therapy of chronic hepatitis C. Med Sci Monit 2001;7(Suppl 1):221–225.
10. Roti E, Minelli R, Giuberti T, Marchelli S, Schianchi C, Gardini E, et al. Multiple changes in thyroid function in patients with chronic active HCV hepatitis treated with recombinant interferon-alpha. Am J Med 1996;101(5):482–487.
11. Mazziotti G, Sorvillo F, Stornaiuolo G, Rotondi M, Morisco F, Ruberto M, et al. Temporal relationship between the appearance of thyroid autoantibodies and development of destructive thyroiditis in patients undergoing treatment with two different type-1 interferons for HCV-related chronic hepatitis: a prospective study. J Endocrinol Invest 2002;25(7):624–630.
12. Villanueva RB, Brau N. Graves' ophthalmopathy associated with interferon-alpha treatment for hepatitis C. Thyroid 2002;12(8):737–738.
13. Ronnblom LE, Alm GV, Oberg KE. Autoimmunity after alpha-interferon therapy for malignant carcinoid tumors. Ann Intern Med 1991;115:178–183.
14. Silvestri F, Virgolini L, Mazzolini A, et al. Development of autoimmune thyroid diseases during long-term treatment of hematological malignancies with alpha-interferons. Haematologica 1994;79:367–370.
15. Vallisa D, Cavanna L, Berte R, Merli F, Ghisoni F, Buscarini L. Autoimmune thyroid dysfunctions in hematologic malignancies treated with alpha-interferon. Acta Haematol 1995;93:31–35.
16. Hollowell JG, Staehling NW, Flanders WD, Hannon WH, Gunter EW, Spencer CA, et al. Serum TSH, T(4), and thyroid antibodies in the United States population (1988 to 1994): National Health and Nutrition Examination Survey (NHANES III). J Clin Endocrinol Metab 2002;87(2):489–499.
17. Vanderpump MPJ, Tunbridge WMG, French JM, Appleton D, Bates D, Clark F, et al. The incidence of thyroid disorders in the community: a twenty-year follow-up of the Whickham survey. Clin Endocrinol (Oxf) 1995;43:55–68.
18. Marazuela M, Garcia-Buey L, Gonzalez-Fernandez B, Garcia-Monzon C, Arranz A, Borque MJ, et al. Thyroid autoimmune disorders in patients with chronic hepatitis C before and during interferon-alpha therapy. Clin Endocrinol (Oxf) 1996;44(6):635–642.
19. Imagawa A, Itoh N, Hanafusa T, Oda Y, Waguri M, Miyagawa J, et al. Autoimmune endocrine disease induced by recombinant interferon-alpha therapy for chronic active type C hepatitis. J Clin Endocrinol Metab 1995;80(3):922–926.
20. Watanabe U, Hashimoto E, Hisamitsu T, Obata H, Hayashi N. The risk factor for development of thyroid disease during interferon-alpha therapy for chronic hepatitis C. Am J Gastroenterol 1994;89(3):399–403.
21. Carella C, Amato G, Biondi B, Rotondi M, Morisco F, Tuccillo C, et al. Longitudinal study of antibodies against thyroid in patients undergoing interferon-alpha therapy for HCV chronic hepatitis. Horm Res 1995;44(3):110–114.
22. Carella C, Mazziotti G, Morisco F, Manganella G, Rotondi M, Tuccillo C, et al. Long-term outcome of interferon-alpha-induced thyroid autoimmunity and prognostic influence of

thyroid autoantibody pattern at the end of treatment. J Clin Endocrinol Metab 2001;86(5):1925–1929.
23. Koh LK, Greenspan FS, Yeo PP. Interferon-alpha induced thyroid dysfunction: three clinical presentations and a review of the literature. Thyroid 1997;7(6):891–896.
24. Wong V, Fu AX, George J, Cheung NW. Thyrotoxicosis induced by alpha-interferon therapy in chronic viral hepatitis. Clin Endocrinol (Oxf) 2002;56(6):793–798.
25. Lisker-Melman M, Di Bisceglie AM, Usala SJ, Weintraub B, Murray LM, Hoofnagle JH. Development of thyroid disease during therapy of chronic viral hepatitis with interferon alfa. Gastroenterology 1992;102(6):2155–2160.
26. Tran A, Quaranta JF, Benzaken S, et al. High prevalence of thyroid autoantibodies in a prospective series of patients with chronic hepatitis C before interferon therapy. Hepatology 1993;18:253–257.
27. Pateron D, Hartmann DJ, Duclos-Vallee JC, Jouanolle H, Beaugrand M. Latent autoimmune thyroid disease in patients with chronic HCV hepatitis. J Hepatol 1993;17:417–419.
28. Prummel MF, Laurberg P. Interferon-a and autoimmune thyroid disease. Thyroid 2003;13:547–551.
29. Ganne-Carrie N, Medini A, Coderc E, et al. Latent autoimmune thyroiditis in untreated patients with HCV chronic hepatitis: a case-control study. J Autoimmun 2000;14:189–193.
30. Preziati D, La Rosa L, Covini G, et al. Autoimmunity and thyroid function in patients with chronic active hepatitis treated with recombinant interferon alpha-2a. Eur J Endocrinol 1995;132:587–593.
31. Kakizaki S, Takagi H, Ichikawa T, et al. Histological change after interferon therapy in chronic hepatitis C in view of iron deposition in the liver. Biol Trace Elem Res 2000;73:151–162.
32. Dumoulin FL, Leifeld L, Sauerbruch T, Spengler U. Autoimmunity induced by interferon-alpha therapy for chronic viral hepatitis. Biomed Pharmacother 1999;53:242–254.
33. Fernandez-Soto L, Gonzalez A, Escobar-Jimenez F, et al. Increased risk of autoimmune thyroid disease in hepatitis C vs. hepatitis B before, during, and after discontinuing interferon therapy. Arch Intern Med 1998;158:1445–1448.
34. N. Custro, G. Montalto, V. Scafidi, et al. Prospective study on thyroid autoimmunity and dysfunction related to chronic hepatitis C and interferon therapy. J Endocrinol Invest 1997;20:374–380.
35. Ansar AS, Penhale WJ, Talal N. Sex hormones, immune responses, and autoimmune diseases. Mechanisms of sex hormone action. Am J Pathol 1985;121:531–551.
36. Dalgard O, Bjoro K, Hellum K, Myrvang B, Bjoro T, Haug E, et al. Thyroid dysfunction during treatment of chronic hepatitis C with interferon alpha: no association with either interferon dosage or efficacy of therapy. J Intern Med 2002;251:400–406.
37. Stenszky V, Kozma L, Balazs C, Rochkitz S, Bear JC, Farid NR. The genetics of Graves' disease: HLA and disease susceptibility. J Clin Endocrinol Metab 1985;61:735–740.
38. Ban Y, Davies TF, Greenberg DA, Concepcion ES, Osman R, Oashi T, et al. Arginine at position 74 of the HLA-DRb1 chain is associated with Graves' disease. Genes Immun 2004;5:203–208.
39. Yanagawa T, Hidaka Y, Guimaraes V, Soliman M, DeGroot LJ. CTLA-4 gene polymorphism associated with Graves' disease in a caucasian population. J Clin Endocrinol Metab 1995;80:41–45.
40. Vaidya B, Imrie H, Perros P, Young ET, Kelly WF, Carr D, et al. The cytotoxic T lymphocyte antigen-4 is a major Graves' disease locus. Hum Mol Genet 1999;8:1195–1199.
41. Tomer Y, Greenberg DA, Barbesino G, Concepcion ES, Davies TF. CTLA-4 and not CD28 is a susceptibility gene for thyroid autoantibody production. J Clin Endocrinol Metab 2001;86:1687–1693.
42. Smyth D, Cooper JD, Collins JE, Heward JM, Franklyn JA, Howson JM, et al. Replication of an association between the lymphoid tyrosine phosphatase locus (LYP/PTPN22) with type 1 diabetes, and evidence for its role as a general autoimmunity locus. Diabetes 2004;53:3020–3023.
43. Velaga MR, Wilson V, Jennings CE, Owen CJ, Herington S, Donaldson PT, et al. The codon 620 tryptophan allele of the lymphoid tyrosine phosphatase (LYP) gene is a major determinant of Graves' disease. J Clin Endocrinol Metab 2004;89(11):5862–5865.
44. Jacobson EM, Chaudhry S, Mandac JC, Concepcion E, Tomer Y. Immune-regulatory gene involvement in the etiology of interferon induced thyroiditis (IIT). Thyroid 2006;16:926.
45. Tomer Y, Davies TF. Searching for the autoimmune thyroid disease susceptibility genes: From gene mapping to gene function. Endocr Rev 2003;24:694–717.

46. Tomer Y, Davies TF. Infection, thyroid disease and autoimmunity. Endocr Rev 1993;14:107–120.
47. Oppenheim Y, Ban Y, Tomer Y. Interferon induced Autoimmune Thyroid Disease (AITD): a model for human autoimmunity. Autoimmun Rev 2004;3:388–393.
48. Monzani F, Caraccio N, Dardano A, Ferrannini E. Thyroid autoimmunity and dysfunction associated with type I interferon therapy. Clin Exp Med 2004;3:199–210.
49. Antonelli A, Ferri C, Pampana A, Fallahi P, Nesti C, Pasquini M, et al. Thyroid disorders in chronic hepatitis C. Am J Med 2004;117:10–13.
50. Hsieh MC, Yu ML, Chuang WL, Shin SJ, Dai CY, Chen SC, et al. Virologic factors related to interferon-alpha-induced thyroid dysfunction in patients with chronic hepatitis C. Eur J Endocrinol 2000;142:431–437.
51. Codes L, de Freitas LA, Santos-Jesus R, Vivitski L, Silva LK, Trepo C, et al. Comparative study of hepatitis C virus genotypes 1 and 3 in Salvador, Bahia Brazil. Braz J Infect Dis 2003;7:409–417.
52. Huang MJ, Tsai SL, Huang BY, Sheen IS, Yeh CT, Liaw YF. Prevalence and significance of thyroid autoantibodies in patients with chronic hepatitis C virus infection: a prospective controlled study. Clin Endocrinol (Oxf) 1999;50:503–509.
53. Zusinaite E, Metskula K, Salupere R. Autoantibodies and hepatitis C virus genotypes in chronic hepatitis C patients in Estonia. World J Gastroenterol 2005;11:488–491.
54. Picardi A, Gentilucci UV, Zardi EM, D'Avola D, Amoroso A, Afeltra A. The role of ribavirin in the combination therapy of hepatitis C virus infection. Curr Pharm Des 2004;10:2081–2092.
55. Shiina M, Kobayashi K, Satoh H, Niitsuma H, Ueno Y, Shimosegawa T. Ribavirin upregulates interleukin-12 receptor and induces T cell differentiation towards type 1 in chronic hepatitis C. J Gastroenterol Hepatol 2004;19:558–564.
56. Tam RC, Pai B, Bard J, Lim C, Averett DR, Phan UT, et al. Ribavirin polarizes human T cell responses towards a Type 1 cytokine profile. J Hepatol 1999;30:376–382.
57. Tam RC, Lim C, Bard J, Pai B. Contact hypersensitivity responses following ribavirin treatment in vivo are influenced by type 1 cytokine polarization, regulation of IL-10 expression, and costimulatory signaling. J Immunol 1999;163:3709–3717.
58. Carella C, Mazziotti G, Morisco F, Rotondi M, Cioffi M, Tuccillo C, et al. The addition of ribavirin to interferon-alpha therapy in patients with hepatitis C virus-related chronic hepatitis does not modify the thyroid autoantibody pattern but increases the risk of developing hypothyroidism. Eur J Endocrinol 2002;146:743–749.
59. Nguyen KB, Watford WT, Salomon R, Hofmann SR, Pien GC, Morinobu A, et al. Critical role for STAT4 activation by type 1 interferons in the interferon-gamma response to viral infection. Science 2002;297(5589):2063–2066.
60. You X, Teng W, Shan Z. Expression of ICAM-1, B7. 1 and TPO on human thyrocytes induced by IFN-alpha. Chin Med J (Engl) 1999;112(1):61–66.
61. Corssmit EP, de Metz J, Sauerwein HP, Romijn JA. Biologic responses to IFN-alpha administration in humans. J Interferon Cytokine Res 2000;20(12):1039–1047.
62. Sato K, Satoh T, Shizume K, Ozawa M, Han DC, Imamura H, et al. Inhibition of 125I organification and thyroid hormone release by interleukin-1, tumor necrosis factor-alpha, and interferon-gamma in human thyrocytes in suspension culture. J Clin Endocrinol Metab 1990;70(6):1735–1743.
63. Caraccio N, Giannini R, Cuccato S, Faviana P, Berti P, Galleri D, et al. Type I interferons modulate the expression of thyroid peroxidase, sodium/iodide symporter, and thyroglobulin genes in primary human thyrocyte cultures. J Clin Endocrinol Metab 2005;90(2):1156–1162.
64. Akeno N, Tomer Y. Dissecting the mechanisms of interferon induced thyroiditis (IIT): Direct effects of interferon alpha on thyroid epithelial cells. The 89th Meeting of the Endocrine Society; Toronto, Canada, 2007.
65. Volpe R. Etiology, pathogenesis, and clinical aspects of thyroiditis. Pathol Annu 1978;13:399–413.
66. Weetman AP, Smallridge RC, Nutman TB, Burman KD. Persistent thyroid autoimmunity after subacute thyroiditis. J Clin Lab Immunol 1987;23:1–6.
67. Parana R, Cruz M, Lyra L, Cruz T. Subacute thyroiditis during treatment with combination therapy (interferon plus ribavirin) for hepatitis C virus. J Viral Hepat 2000;7(5):393–395.
68. Fabris P, Betterle C, Floreani A, et al. Development of type 1 diabetes mellitus during interferon alpha therapy for chronic HCV hepatitis. Lancet 1992;340:548.
69. Okanoue T, Sakamoto S, Itoh Y, et al. Side effects of high-dose interferon therapy for chronic hepatitis C. J Hepatol 1996;25:283–91.

70. Garancini P, Gallus G, Calori G, Formigaro F, Micossi P. Incidence and prevalence of diabetes mellitus in Italy from routine data: a methodological assessment. Eur J Epidemiol 1991;7:55–63.
71. Wong FS, Wen L. IFN-alpha can both protect against and promote the development of type 1 diabetes. Ann N Y Acad Sci 2008;1150:187–189.
72. Fattovich G, Giustina G, Favarato S, Ruol A, Investigators of the Italian Association for the Study of the Liver. A survey of adverse events in 11241 patients with chronic viral hepatitis. J Hepatol 1996;24:34–87.
73. Atkinson MA, Maclaren K. The pathogenesis of insulin-dependent diabetes mellitus. New Engl J Med 1994;331:1428–1436.
74. Schreuder TC, Gelderblom HC, Weegink CJ, Hamann D, Reesink HW, Devries JH, Hoekstra JB, Jansen PL. High incidence of type 1 diabetes mellitus during or shortly after treatment with pegylated interferon alpha for chronic hepatitis C virus infection. Liver Int 2008;28(1):39–46.
75. Koivisto VA, Peklonen R, Cantel K. Effect of interferon on glucose tolerance and insulin sensitivity. Diabetes 1989;38:641–647.
76. Frankart L, Jejeune D, Donckier J. Diabetes mellitus and interferon therapy. Diabet Med 1997;14:405.
77. Hayakawa M, Gando S, Morimoto Y, Kemmottsu O. Development of severe diabetic keto-acidosis with shock after changing interferon-β into interferon-α for chronic hepatitis C. Intensive Care Med 2000;26:1008.
78. Konrad T, Zeuzem S, Vicini P, et al. Evaluation of factors controlling glucose tolerance in patients with HCV infection before and after 4 months therapy with interferon-α. Eur J Clin Invest 2000;30:111–121.
79. Nemesanszky E, Pusztay M, Cspregi A. Effect of interferon treatment on the glucose metabolism of patients with chronic hepatitis C. Eur J Intern Med 2000;11:151–155.
80. Imano E, Kanda T, Ishigami Y, et al. Interferon induces insulin resistance in patients with chronic hepatitis C. J Hepatol 1998;28:189–193.
81. Sobel DO, Ahvazi B. Alpha-interferon inhibits the development of diabetes in NOD mice. Diabetes 1998;47:1867–1972.
82. Brod SA, Malone M, Darcan S, Papolla M, Nelson L. Ingested interferon alpha suppresses type 1 diabetes in non-obese diabetic mice. Diabetologia 1998;41:1227–1232.
83. Foulis AK, Farquharson MA, Meager A. Immunoreactive α-interferon on insulin-secreting β-cells in type I diabetes mellitus. Lancet.1987;2:1423–1427.
84. Huang X, Yuan J, Goddard A, et al. Interferon-α expression in the pancreases of patients with type I diabetes. Diabetes 1995;44:658–664.
85. Gross U, Seifert E. Insulinpflichitiger diebets mellitus unter alpha-interferon therapie bein chronish aktiver hepatitis. Z Gastroenterol 1993;31:609–611.
86. Guerci AP, Guerci B, Lovy-Marshall C, et al. Onset of insulin-dependent diabetes mellitus after interferon alpha therapy for hairy cell leukemia. Lancet 1994;343:1167–1168.
87. Waguri M, Hanafusa T, Itoh N, et al. Occurrence of IDDM during interferon therapy for chronic viral hepatitis. Diabetes Res Clin Pract 1994;23:33–36.
88. Gori A, Caredda F, Franzetti F, Ridolfo A, Ruscon F, Moroni M. Reversible diabetes in patients with AIDS-related Kaposi's sarcoma treated with interferon-α 2a. Lancet 1994;345:1438–1439.
89. Giuntoli P, Mariani S, Avoli D, Giammarco V. Diabete mellito insulino-dipendente indotto da interferon-alfa. Minerva Endocrinol 1995;20:243–245.
90. Murakami M, Iriuchijima T, Mori M. Diabetes mellitus and interferon-alpha therapy. Ann Intern Med 1995;123:318.
91. Okada K, Kikuoka H, Kokawa M, et al. A case of insulin-dependent diabetes mellitus (IDDM) following interferon alpha therapy for type C chronic hepatitis. J Jpn Diab Soc 1995;38:625–630.
92. Yanagisawa K, Anemiya S, Morita Y, et al. A case of insulin-dependent diabetes mellitus developing during interferon therapy for chronic hepatitis type C. J Jpn Diab Soc 1995;38:283–288.
93. Whitehead RP, Hauschild A, Christophers E, Figlin R. Diabetes mellitus in cancer patients treated with combination interleukin 2 and α-interferon. Cancer Biother 1995;1: 45–50.
94. Mathieu E, Fain O, Sitbom M, Thomas M. Diabète auto-immun après traitement par interféron alpha. Presse Med 1995;24:238.
95. Chedin P, Cahen-Varsaux J, Boyer N. Non-insulin-dependent diabetes mellitus developing during interferon-alpha therapy for chronic hepatitis C. Ann Int Med 1996;125:521.
96. Shiba T, Morino Y, Tagawa K, Fujino H, Unuma T. Onset of diabetes with high titer anti-GAD antibody after IFN therapy for chronic hepatitis. Diabetes Res Clin Pract 1995;30:237–241.
97. Rostaing L, Oksman F, Izopet J, et al. Serological markers of autoimmunity in renal transplant patients before and after alpha

interferon treatment for chronic viral hepatitis. Am J Nephrol 1996;16:478–483.
98. Fabris P, Betterle C, Greggio NA, et al. Insulin-dependent diabetes mellitus during alpha-interferon therapy for chronic viral hepatitis. J Hepatol 1998;28:514–517.
99. Tohda G, Oida K, Higashi S, et al. Interferon-α and development of type 1 diabetes. Diabetes Care 1998;21:1774.
100. Seifarth C, Benningere J, Bohm BO, Wiest-Ladenburger U, Hahn EJ. Augmentation of the immune response to islet cell antigens development of diabetes mellitus caused by interferon-alpha in chronic hepatitis C. Z Gastroenterol 1999;37:235–239.
101. Kado S, Miyamoto J, Komatsu N, et al. Type 1 diabetes mellitus induced by treatment with interferon. Intern Med 2000;39:146–149.
102. Eibl N, Gschwantler M, Ferenci P, Eibl M, Weiss W, Schernthaner G. Development of insulin-dependent diabetes mellitus in a patient with chronic hepatitis C during therapy with interferon-α. Eur J Gastroenterol Hepatol 2001;13:295–298.
103. Uto H, Matsuoka H, Murata M, et al. A case of chronic hepatitis C developing insulin-dependent diabetes mellitus associated with various autoantibodies during interferon therapy. Diabetes Res Clin Pract 2000;49:101–106.
104. Bosi E, Minelli R, Bazzigaluppi E, Salvi M. Fulminant autoimmune type 1 diabetes during interferon-α therapy: a case of Th1-mediated disease? Diabet Med 2001;18:329–332.
105. Bhatti A, McGarrity TJ, Gabbay R. Diabetic ketoacidosis induced by alpha interferon and ribavirin in a patient with hepatitis C. Am J Gastroenterol 2001;96:604–605.
106. Figge E, Reiser M, Schmiegel W, Nauck MA. Manifestation eines Typ-1-Diabetes bei einem patienten mit hepatitis C während einer therapie mit interferon-a and ribavirin. Diabetes Stoffwechsel 2001;10:133–138.
107. Recasens M, Aguilera E, Ampurandanés S, et al. Abrupt onset of diabetes during interferon-alpha therapy in patients with chronic hepatitis C. Diabet Med 2001;18:764–767.
108. Mofredj A, Howaizi M, Grasset D, et al. Diabetes mellitus during interferon therapy for chronic viral hepatitis. Dig Dis Sci 2002;47:1648–1654.
109. Fattovich G, Betterle C, Brollo L, et al. Autoantibodies during alpha-IFN therapy for chronic hepatitis B. J Med Virol 1991;34:321–325.

110. Di Cesare E, Previti M, Russo F, et al. Interferon-α therapy may induce insulin autoantibodies development in patients with chronic viral hepatitis. Dig Dis Sci 1996;41:1672–1677.
111. Imagawa A, Itoh H, Hanafusa T, et al. Antibodies to glutamic acid decarboxylase induced by interferon-alpha therapy for chronic viral hepatitis. Diabetologia 1996;39:126.
112. Floreani A, Chiaramonte M, Greggio NA, et al. Organ-specific autoimmunity and genetic predisposition in interferon-treated HCV-related chronic hepatitis patients. Ital J Gastroenterol 1998;30:71–76.
113. Betterle C, Fabris P, Zanchetta R, et al. Autoimmunity against pancreatic islets and other tissues before and after interferon-α therapy in patients with hepatitis C virus chronic infection. Diabetes Care 2000;23:117–181.
114. Wesche B, Jaechel E, Trautwein C, et al. Induction of autoantibodies to adrenal cortex and pancreatic islet cells by interferon alpha therapy for chronic hepatitis C. Gut 2001;48:378–383.
115. Wasmuth HB, Stolte C, Geier A, Gartung C, Matern S. Induction of multiple autoantibodies to islet cell antigens during treatment with interferon alpha for chronic hepatitis C. Gut 2001;49:596–597.
116. Oshimoto K, Shimizu H, Sato N, Mori M. A case of Addison's disease which became worse during interferon therapy: [insulin secretion under hyposmolarity]. Nippon Naibunpi Gakkai Zasshi 1994;70:511–516.
117. Knost JA, Sherwin S, Abrams P, Oldham RK. Increased steroid dependence after recombinant leucocyte interferon therapy. Lancet 1981; ii:1287–1288.
118. Sakane N, Yoshida T, Yoshioka K, Umekawa T, Kondo M, Shimatsu A. Reversible hypopituitarism after interferon alfa therapy. Lancet 1995;345:1305.
119. Concha LB. Interferon-induced hypopituitarism. Am J Med 2003;114(2):161–163.
120. Rosenberg SA, Lotze MT, Muul LM, et al. A progress report on the treatment of 157 patients with advanced cancer using lymphokine-activated killer cells and interleukin-2 or high-dose interleukin-2 alone. N Engl J Med 1987;316:889–897.
121. Roitt I, Brostoff J, Male D. Cell cooperation in antibody response. In: Roitt I, Brostoff J, Male D, eds. Immunology. 5th ed. London, UK: Mosby, 1998:139–153.
122. Weijl NI, Van der Harst D, Brand A, et al. Hypothyroidism during immunotherapy with interleukin-2 is associated with antithyroid

antibodies and response to treatment. J Clin Oncol 1993;11:1376–1383.
123. Franzke D, Peest M, Probst K, et al. Autoimmunity resulting from cytokine treatment predicts long-term survival in patients with metastatic renal cell cancer. J Clin Oncol 1999;17:529–533.
124. Chambers CA, Kuhns MS, Egen JG, et al. CTLA-4-mediated inhibition in regulation of T cell responses: mechanisms and manipulation in tumor immunotherapy. Annu Rev Immunol 2001;19:565–594.
125. Yang JC, Hughes M, Kammula U, Royal R, Sherry RM, Topalian SL, Suri KB, Levy C, Allen T, Mavroukakis S, Lowy I, White DE, Rosenberg SA. Ipilimumab (anti-CTLA4 antibody) causes regression of metastatic renal cell cancer associated with enteritis and hypophysitis. J Immunother 2007;30(8):825–830.
126. Vial T, Descotes J. Immune-mediated side-effects of cytokines in humans. Toxicology 1995;105:31–57.
127. Hansen PB, Johnsen HE, Hippe E. Autoimmune hypothyroidism and granulocyte-macrophage colony-stimulating factor. Eur J Haematol 1993;50(3):183–184.
128. Hoekman K, von Blomberg-van der Flier BM, Wagstaff J, Drexhage HA, Pinedo HM. Reversible thyroid dysfunction during treatment with GM-CSF. Lancet 1991;338(8766):541–542.
129. Jones JL, Coles AJ. Campath-1H treatment of multiple sclerosis. Neurodegener Dis 2008;5(1):27–31.
130. Kirk AD, Hale DA, Swanson SJ, Mannon RB. Autoimmune thyroid disease after renal transplantation using depletional induction with alemtuzumab. Am J Transplant 2006;6(5 Pt 1):1084–1085.
131. Monteiro E, Galvão-teles A, Santos ML, Mourão L, Correia MJ, Lopo Tuna J, Ribeiro C. Antithyroid antibodies as an early marker for thyroid disease induced by amiodarone. Br Med J (Clin Res Ed) 1986;292(6515):227–228.
132. Trip MD, Düren DR, Wiersinga WM. Two cases of amiodarone-induced thyrotoxicosis successfully treated with a short course of antithyroid drugs while amiodarone was continued. Br Heart J 1994;72(3):266–268.
133. Weetman AP, Bhandal SK, Burrin JM, Robinson K, McKenna W. Amiodarone and thyroid autoimmunity in the United Kingdom. BMJ 1988;297(6640):33.
134. Gilquin J, Viard JP, Jubault V, Sert C, Kazatchkine MD. Delayed occurrence of Graves' disease after immune restoration with HAART. Highly active antiretroviral therapy. Lancet 1998;352(9144):1907–1908.
135. Hirata Y, Ishizu H, Ouchi N, et al. Insulin autoimmunity in a case of spontaneous hypo-glycemia. J Jpn Diabetes Soc 1970;13:312–320.
136. Uchigata Y, Hirata Y. Insulin autoimmune syndrome (IAS, Hirata disease). Ann Med Interne (Paris) 1999;150:245–253.
137. Uchigata Y, Kuwata S, Tokunaga K, et al. Strong association of insulin autoimmune syndrome with HLA-DR4. Lancet 1992;339:393–394.
138. Uchigata Y, Kuwata S, Tsushima T, Tokuhinaga K, Miyamoto M, Tshuchikawa K, et al. Patients with Graves' disease who developed insulin autoimmune syndrome (Hirata Disease) possess HLA-Bw62/CW4/DR4 carrying DRB1*0406. J Clin Endocrinol Metab 1993;77:246–254.
139. Archambeaud-Mouveroux F, Canivet B, Fressinaud C, de Buhan B, Treves R, Laubie B. [Autoimmune hypoglycemia: the fault of pyritinol?] Presse Med 1988;17(34):1733–1736.
140. Lidar M, Rachmani R, Half E, Ravid M. Insulin autoimmune syndrome after therapy with imipenem. Diabetes Care 1999;22(3):524–525.
141. Cavaco B, Uchigata Y, Porto T, Amparo-Santos M, Sobrinho L, Leite V. Hypoglycaemia due to insulin autoimmune syndrome: report of two cases with characterisation of HLA alleles and insulin autoantibodies. Eur J Endocrinol 2001;145(3):311–316.
142. The Merck Index. 11th ed. Merck & Co., Inc. p703, 780, 789790, 942, 1122, 1123 and 1490.
143. Furukawa N, Miyamura N, Nishida K, Motoshima H, Takeda K, Araki E, Possible relevance of alpha lipoic acid contained in a health supplement in a care of insulin autoimmune syndrome. Diabetes Res Clin Prac 2007;75:366–367.

Part III

Specific Diseases

Chapter 11

The BB Rat

Ulla Nøhr Dalberg, Claus Haase, Lars Hornum, and Helle Markholst

Key Words: Diabetes, Animal model diabetes, Genetics diabetes, Lymphopenia, T cells, Regulatory T cells, Biobreeding diabetes-resistant rat

INTRODUCTION

Diabetes-prone BioBreeding (BBDP) rats develop a spontaneous diabetic syndrome resembling human type 1 diabetes (T1D). Foremost, BBDP rats lose the majority of their beta cells during a rapid and aggressive inflammation of the islets during the last 2 weeks prior to overt hyperglycemia (*1*). Once hyperglycemia occurs, the rats become highly polyuric – they may lose well over 20 g (10–15% of body weight) overnight despite an excessive drinking behavior – and they proceed within 24–48 h to become ketotic. They die in ketoacidosis unless rescued by exogenous insulin therapy within the first 2 days of hyperglycemia (*2, 3*) – i.e. this clearly separates their diabetic phenotype from that of NOD mice that can easily survive for longer time after the onset of clinical diabetes. Indeed, within the first week, all insulin release and immunoreactivity in the pancreas is entirely lost – i.e. the phenotype of hypoinsulinemia is complete in BBDP rats (*4–7*).

Some substrains of BBDP rats also exhibit other autoimmune phenomena like anti-parietal cell autoantibodies, inflammation of salivary glands, and thyroiditis – i.e. based on their specific genetic background, they may have primarily a diabetic phenotype or exhibit multiple endocrinopathologies of autoimmune nature (*8–10*).

In colonies of BBDP rats where the microbial environment is strictly controlled and remains the same for generations, it is normal to observe consistent and high percentage (>90%) of diabetes during early adolescence and just after puberty, i.e. between 60 and 120 days of age (*11*). Diabetes is genetically linked to the major histocompatibility locus, RT1 (*12*), and this locus has – in accordance with the nomenclature in man and mouse – been named Iddm1. The locus has been refined to the MHC class II region by congenic breeding (*13*). The importance of MHC class II for diabetes development was confirmed by the prevention of disease with an anti-RT1D antibody (*14*).

DESCRIPTION OF THE INSULITIS IN BBDP RATS

Histological examination of pancreata from diabetic BB rats is characterized by two principal findings: the mononuclear infiltration of the islets of Langerhans (termed insulitis) and the absence or ongoing destruction of insulin-positive beta cells. The inflammatory reaction is focused on the islets, and the end-result is islets that are devoid of beta cells but still contain alpha cells, delta cells, and PP cells. Insulitis usually precedes clinical diabetes by up to 16 days (*1*), and the antigen-presenting cells (APCs), macrophages, and dendritic cells (DCs) are thought to be the first cells to arrive in the islets, as discussed below (*15–17*). APCs are immediately followed by NK cells which are the pre-dominant cell type during pre-diabetes, and by CD4+ and CD8+ T cells and finally by B cells (*18*). Interestingly, activated T cells only account for the minority of T cells; however, intra-islet lymphocytes have been shown to be much more cytotoxic than splenic effector cells, indicating an enrichment of cytotoxic leukocytes in the islets (*19*). Generally, the sequence of events described above is similar to what is seen in the NOD mouse (*20–23*) – albeit the process is far more prolonged in time in NOD mice. In humans, the knowledge about infiltrating cells is more limited, but CD4+ and CD8+ T cells, macrophages, and B cells have all been identified in pancreatic sections from patients with recent-onset type 1 diabetes (*24–27*). Thus, taken together, the beta cell-specific inflammatory response pattern in the BB rat correlates well with the NOD mouse model of type 1 diabetes, and both models are thought to model the histopathology seen during the destruction of human beta cells in type 1 diabetes.

BETA CELLS IN THE DEVELOPMENT OF DIABETES IN THE BBDP RAT

The target of spontaneous autoimmunity in BBDP rats, the beta cells, appears to be altered even before the insulitis process is clearly detectable. Reddy et al. found that the first-phase insulin in response to iv glucose was blunted already from the time of weaning (*28*), and Markholst et al. detected a reduced glucose-induced insulin release during pancreatic perfusions already at the age of 30–45 days, i.e. well before the detectable insulitis (*1, 29*). The latter was independently confirmed (*30*). Indeed, the local pancreatic exposure to insulin – normally much higher than the systemic exposure, due to first-pass removal of insulin in the liver, – appears to be reduced at an early age in BBDPs as well (*31*) inasmuch as pancreatic amylase production (dependent on insulin) is reduced. Similar to human T1D, BBDP rats maintain some responsiveness to arginine-induced insulin release when glucose-induced release is gone; however, this is short-lived as the beta cells disappear entirely (*32*).

ANTIGEN-PRESENTING CELLS IN THE DEVELOPMENT OF DIABETES IN THE BBDP RAT

Antigen-presenting cells are involved early in the disease process in the BBDP rat. Normal islets – in man, mice, and rats – contain a limited number of both macrophages and DCs, which are thought to play an important role in tissue homeostasis and in the induction of peripheral tolerance to islet-associated antigens, respectively (*33–37*). However, early insulitis in the BBDP rat is characterized by an increased presence of macrophages and DCs, which has been found to precede infiltration by T and B cells (*15–17, 38*).

It is not entirely clear whether DCs arrive before macrophages or vice versa and this has been controversial mostly due to the overlap of surface markers between the two cell types. Histological evaluation using a putative DC-specific marker suggests that DCs do in fact precede macrophages in the initiation of insulitis (*39*). In any case, the increased number of macrophages and DCs is also observed in other animal models of type 1 diabetes, including the NOD mouse (*21, 23*). Functionally, the presence of APCs in the islets is required for disease development, as in vivo depletion of these cells abrogates the development of insulitis (*18, 38, 40*), and it is highly likely that both DCs and macrophages will contribute to the onset of insulitis.

The reason(s) for the gradual increase in the number of APCs in the islets with the age of BBDPs has not been clearly identified. A single study showing that islets transplanted from adult BB rats to acutely diabetic animals are rejected, whereas islets transplanted from neonatal BB rats are not, suggests that a contributing factor to the disease process may indeed be change in the presentation of islet-associated antigens (*41*). One explanation could be that accumulating APCs contribute to the changes in the islet microenvironment, e.g. by the production of pro-inflammatory mediators, which may render beta cells more susceptible to autoimmune destruction because of increased antigen presentation and specific sensitivity of rat beta cells to pro-inflammatory mediators such as TNF-alpha and IL-1-beta (*42, 43*).

In line with this, it has been shown that macrophages from the BBDP rats have an increased activity of the arginine-citrulline cycle, which leads to an increased production of nitric oxide (NO), a free-radical molecule toxic for beta cells (*44, 45*). This phenotype of BBDP macrophages is secondary to their inherited T-cell lymphopenia (see next section), since correction of lymphopenia results in normalization of the NO response (*46*). Regarding DCs, BBDP-derived DCs are hyper-responsive to macrophage-derived factors such as IL-1 and GM-CSF when compared with WF-derived DCs, resulting in increased APC function of BBDP-derived DCs. Moreover, this phenotype is dependent on the BBDP genetic background since BBDPxWF F1 DCs have an intermediate phenotype (*47*). Interestingly, the increased responsiveness to macrophage-derived factors is combined with a more immature phenotype of BBDP-derived DCs when measured by a decreased expression of MHC-II, a decreased ability to form clusters with T cells and an impairment in the ability to activate CD4$^+$RT6$^+$ T cells – a subset of cells thought to contain regulatory T cells. Still, it has not been formally demonstrated that BBDP-derived DCs are deficient in their ability to induce natural or adaptive T_{regs} (*48, 49*). Nevertheless, it has been demonstrated that DCs have a decreased ability to produce IL-10 in response to microbial stimuli and that this phenotype is linked to a locus on rat chromosome 4 outside the *Lyp*-region (see elsewhere) (*50, 51*). As IL-10 is an important immunomodulatory cytokine, this may also contribute to disease development, e.g. by defective downmodulation of an induced immune-response.

Taken together, these studies clearly demonstrate that the differences in the phenotype of both macrophages and DCs in the BBDP rat, and the combination of (*1*) increased production of pro-inflammatory mediators, (*2*) hyper-responsiveness of DCs to macrophage-derived cytokines, and (*3*) a potential decreased ability to induce regulatory T cells and IL-10, are likely to contribute to the development of diabetes. Moreover, upon initiation of insulitis by macrophages and DCs, an increased production of NO may lead to increased beta-cell stress. This combined with an increased response by DCs to IL-1 and GM-CSF and a decreased ability to produce IL-10 may tip the balance in favor of a pro-inflammatory microenvironment in the islets. Finally, as DCs from BBDP rats may be impaired in supporting the function and activity of regulatory T cells, autoreactive T cells may prevail, thereby strengthening the auto-reactive response.

T CELLS IN THE DEVELOPMENT OF DIABETES IN THE BBDP RAT

Diabetes development in the BBDP rat is T-cell dependent since depletion of T cells by thymectomy or anti-T-cell serum or impairment of T-cell function by Cyclosporine A inhibits their spontaneous diabetes (*52–54*). A substantial number of T cells are detected in the pancreatic islets during insulitis, and Th1 cytokines such as IFN-γ and IL-12 are upregulated (*10, 55, 56*). Paradoxically, the BBDP rat has a very low number of T cells. In the BBDP rat, 11–13% of total splenic mononuclear cells are CD4⁺ T cells and 3–4% are CD8⁺ T cells, whereas Wistar-Furth and diabetes-resistant BB (BBDR) rats contain 33–35% CD4⁺ and 11–17% CD8⁺ T cells (*57*). Chromosome 4 is linked to T-cell lymphopenia (*58*), and only rats that are homozygous for the BBDP allele of the *lyp* region develop diabetes spontaneously (*11*). The *lyp* region contains several genes but the only identified difference in this region when compared to the BBDR rat is a frameshift mutation in *Gimap5* that results in a severely truncated protein (*59, 60*).

The cause of T-cell lymphopenia is supposed to be both a reduced thymic output and a shortened lifespan of the recent thymic emigrants (RTEs) (*61*). The latter is shown in vitro where an increased percentage of thymocytes and T cells from the BBDP rat undergo apoptosis (*62–64*), and overexpression of *Gimap5* with the BBDP mutation results in increased cell death (*65*). Similar observations were made in vivo because significantly more apoptotic RTEs are detected in the liver (*62*). However, the RTEs can be rescued from apoptosis by antigen activation both in vivo and in vitro (*63, 64*). The BBDP rats have both effector and memory T cells further demonstrating that not all RTEs undergo apoptosis. At first, the combination of a severely reduced number of T cells and the development of a T-cell-dependent disease appear contradictory, but in the following we will try to elucidate this paradox.

A lymphopenic environment induces homeostatic proliferation of naïve T cells (*66*). Naïve T cells undergoing many cell divisions in the course of lymphopenia-induced proliferation develop memory/effector cell characteristics. The cells can become independent of CD28 costimulation and thereby develop resistance to tolerance induction (*67*). Moreover, the lymphopenia-induced proliferation has the potential to skew the TCR repertoire toward greater self-reactivity (*67*) which could explain why adolescent BBDP rat-derived T cells express only a limited number of TCRvb genes when compared with similar T cells from control rats (*68*). In short, homeostatic expansion induces changes in the T-cell repertoire which may promote autoreactivity. Nevertheless, it has been shown that homeostatic expansion is less in autoimmune-prone animals that harbor some memory cells and regulatory T cells (*69*). As the BBDP rat contains none or few regulatory T cells albeit some memory cells, we expect a certain contribution of homeostatic proliferation to the diabetes process in the BBDP; however, this is not thoroughly investigated. Thus, the expansion of T cells in a lymphopenic animal can cause autoimmunity, but the importance of this in the BBDP rat is not entirely clear.

The phenotype of T cells from rats with the *lyp* region (rats$^{lyp/lyp}$) is altered compared to wt rats. Both BBDP and F344$^{lyp/lyp}$ T cells spontaneously become semi-activated in vivo which is characterized by a downregulation of L-selectin (CD62L) and a semi-blast morphology (*70*). The semi-activated state of the T cells is not due to homeostatic expansion in the lymphopenic animals; when T cells from the lymphopenic rats develop in a normal environment they still adopt the semi-activated state (*71*), i.e. it is a T-cell intrinsic feature inherent of the BBDP genome. When BBDP T cells are activated through the TCR, they express the activation markers OX40 and CD25 and enter S-phase of the cell cycle (*70, 72*), whereas T cells from wt rats require costimulation along with the TCR stimulation. Thus, in the BBDP rat, the interaction of naïve T cells with self-peptide-MHC bearing cells might lead to the activation of T cells, whereas in wt rats this interaction would induce tolerance due to lack of costimulation. It is unknown why T cells from the BBDP rat have an increased response to TCR signaling. Interestingly, PTPN22 mutations confirmed to be linked to human T1D as well as RA and SLE, and other autoimmune diseases are also associated with altered TCR signaling responses (*38, 73, 74*). It could thus be highly interesting to study possible allelic variants of this gene in BBDPs versus other rat strains. In connection to this issue of TCR-signal threshold, Moore et al. suggest that a reduced level of the cell cycle inhibitor p27^{Kip1} in RTEs from BBDP and F344$^{lyp/lyp}$ rats could contribute since signaling through CD28 normally results in downregulation of p27^{Kip1} (*75, 76*). Recent data have shown that p27^{Kip1} is also involved in the induction of anergy and tolerance. Anergic CD4$^+$ T cells have an increased level of p27^{Kip1}, and murine T cells lacking functional p27^{Kip1} are resistant to tolerance induction by blockade of costimulatory signals in vivo (*77, 78*). Altogether, these results may explain the presence of an autoreactive potential in T cells from BBDP and defective tolerance induction via superantigen has been indeed shown (*79*). In contrast to the independence of costimulation observed in in vitro studies, an in vivo study showed that inhibition of some types of costimulation prevented or delayed diabetes in the BBDP rat (*80*). On the contrary, inhibition of other types of costimulation accelerated diabetes (*80*), thus underscoring the complexity of activation of the T cells. In summary, the T cells in the BBDP rat have a reduced dependence on costimulation, which may decrease the threshold for activation and impair induction of tolerance; however, they still require some costimulation to mediate their diabetogenic effect in vivo.

Induction of tolerance to self-antigens occurs both in the thymus by interactions between developing T cells and MHC expressing APCs (leading to deletion of autoreactive T cells) and in the periphery by immature DCs and natural regulatory T cells which induce T-cell anergy, deletion or differentiation into adaptive regulatory T cells. Both of these processes are impaired in the BBDP rat and both contribute to the development of diabetes. Both BBDP and BBDR rats contain regions in the thymic cortex which lack MHC class II expression and it is very likely that this affects the selection of thymocytes (*81, 82*). Moreover, both BBDP and BBDR rats contain thymocyte populations which are predisposed to autoreactivity (*83*). Also, BBDP thymic macrophages display reduced stimulatory capacity (*84*). The major importance of the changed thymic selection in the BBDP rat is emphasized by the fact that transplantation of fetal thymic tissue from diabetes-resistant rats into BBDP rats reduced the incidence of insulitis and prevented the development of diabetes (*85*). Whether thymocyte subsets are changed due to the changed selection is not fully known because different results have been published. A reduction in mature CD8 SP thymocytes has been found (*86, 87*), but in two other studies no differences in thymocyte subsets were detected (*81, 88*). In conclusion, thymic selection is changed in the BBDP rat, and this contributes to the development of autoreactive T cells.

Regulatory T cells can be identified by the expression of transcription factor Foxp3 and a high surface level of CD25. In the BBDP rat, the percentage of CD4$^+$CD25$^+$ cells is increased but a closer scrutiny of these cells reveals reduced FoxP3 expression and reduced suppressive capacity in vitro compared with wt CD4$^+$CD25$^+$ cells, indicating that they are activated T cells and not regulatory T cells (*89, 90*). Indeed, BBDP rats have for many years been viewed as having increased levels of activated T cells (*91*), and they exhibit blast morphology, OX34 expression, and increased MHC II surface levels (our own unpublished data). We and others have shown that the lack of regulatory T cells indeed contribute to the development of diabetes because transfer of regulatory T cells can prevent the development of diabetes in the BBDP rat (*89, 90, 92*). Furthermore, diabetes can be induced in the BBDR rat by depletion of the RT6$^+$ cells, which includes the regulatory T cells (*93*). Thus, regulatory T cells are important for the prevention of diabetes in the BBDR rat. Both the lack of FoxP3$^+$ regulatory T cells and the defective thymic APCs in the BBDP rat are linked to the lyp-locus (*84, 89*).

As described above, the BBDP rat has very few CD8$^+$ T cells; however, these cells are necessary for the development of diabetes as adoptive transfer-induced diabetes development is dependent on CD8⁺ T cells (*94*), and depletion of CD8⁺ cells from BBDP rats inhibits the development of disease (*53, 95*). Interestingly, CD8⁺ cells are only important for the initiation of disease because depletion of CD8⁺ cells after 8 weeks of age does not affect disease progression (*95*). Although massive lymphocytic insulitis is not detected in BBDP rats less than 8 weeks of age, some activated autoreactive CD8⁺ T cells may have already infiltrated and damaged some of the islets at a young age. Thus, the most important role of CD8⁺ T cells in diabetes development is most likely in the initial steps of disease.

In summary, the T-cell compartment in the BBDP rat has many alterations that skew them toward autoreactivity. The T cells are more apoptosis-prone which creates T-cell lymphopenia, and the lymphopenic environment induces homeostatic proliferation, which in turn may increase the autoreactive potential of the remaining T cells. Furthermore, the combination of a decrease in the requirement for costimulation and the lack of regulatory T cells may contribute to an increased autoreacitve potential. Finally, the thymic selection is altered in an autoimmune-prone direction. In addition, important factors influencing diabetes expression in BBDP rats are diet, viral infections, and the MHC class II alleles (described in Crisá et al. (*55*)).

T-cell lymphopenia is not an absolute prerequisite for diabetes development in the BB rat. Even the non-lymphopenic BBDR rat can develop diabetes if an adequate immunostimulatory signal is given. One such signal is infection with the ssDNA parvovirus RV (formerly Kilham's rat virus; KRV) (*96*). The diabetogenic effect was shown not to be dependent on direct infection or virus-dependent lysis of beta cells, but rather to be an effect of immune-stimulation resulting in IL-6 and IL-12p40 (but not TNF-alpha) upregulation via toll-like receptor (TLR) 9 (*97*), although down-regulation of T_{reg} number and immune deviation (upregulation of the Th1:Th2 ratio) may also be of importance (*98, 99*). By treating with the TLR3 agonist poly(I:C) (mimicking dsRNA) on top of an RV infection, diabetes incidence was increased from 30 to 100% (*100*) with simultaneous upregulation of IFN-γ, IP-10, and IL-12p40 (but not IL-12p70 – perhaps indicating IL-23 expression). Poly(I:C) treatment alone is sufficient to induce diabetes in the BBDR rat (*101*), and Wistar-Furth (WF) rats carrying at least one (permissive) BB-rat allele of the diabetes susceptibility gene *Iddm4* (*102*). *Iddm4* is also a susceptibility gene for RV-induced diabetes (*103*), and recently a nonsense mutation in the T-cell receptor beta variable gene *TCRVB4* (positioned in the Iddm4 genomic region) was identified in the non-permissive WF rat (*104*). This positional candidate gene could be necessary for the development of autoreactive T cells with high specificity for a beta cell-specific antigen.

OTHER LEUKOCYTES IN THE DEVELOPMENT OF DIABETES IN THE BBDP RAT

BBDP rats harbor many B cells (*105*) and are able to mount B cell responses to viral infections (*106–109*). Nevertheless, the entire Ig –subclass repertoire develop more slowly in BBDP (*110*), possibly due to insufficient help of T cells to Ig-subclass switching. Although autoantibodies to islet cell antigens were reported in the BB rat before the inbreeding program (*111*), these autoantibodies are no longer detectable in the inbred BB strains, including anti-insulin antibodies (IAA) (*112, 113*). The function of B cells as APCs has not been studied in any detail in BBDP.

As mentioned earlier, NK cells are very abundant in the inflammatory infiltrate of the islets of BBDP rats, both before and after the onset of diabetes (*19*). However, although their presence in the islets during the autoimmune attack on the beta cells would suggest an important role in the destructive process, the precise role and importance of NK cells in BBDP rat diabetes is unclear. Indeed, the cytotoxicity of BBDP rat splenocytes toward islet cells is greatly increased when compared with other rat strains such as the WF (*114*), and NK cells isolated from diabetic or diabetes-prone BB rats are cytotoxic to beta cell lines and islet cells in vitro (*115*). The increased NK cytotoxicity correlates with the ability of BB sublines to develop diabetes as both the DR and W substrain of BB rats have lower NK cell activity than the DP substrain (*115, 116*). Still, due to the lack of specific NK cell markers in the rat, it has not been possible to directly examine the functional role of NK cytotoxicity in diabetes development. Depleting antibodies against OX8 and anti-asialo-GM1 have been shown to inhibit diabetes development, but these antibodies are not specific for NK cells but also recognize other immune cells including macrophages and T cells, the depletion of which – as discussed above – will also inhibit diabetes development (*53, 117*). A more recent study where NK cells were targeted using a monoclonal antibody toward NKR-P1 demonstrated no effect on spontaneous or poly(I:C)-induced diabetes development, despite a clear (but not complete) effect on NK cell number and activity (*118*). Thus, until depletion of NK cells in the BB rat can be obtained by using a monoclonal antibody, which specifically depletes NK cells in an efficient manner, the importance of NK cells in diabetes development in the BB rat remains controversial.

CONCLUSION

In this selective rather than comprehensive review, we hope to have illustrated the complexity of the multiple factors interacting toward the development of diabetes in BBDP rat – despite them being inbred and exhibiting a consistent, rather synchronized "single" path toward diabetes. Interestingly, intervention studies in BBDP rats are less likely to be positive when compared with similar studies in NOD mice. That is, the highly aggressive nature and the short time interval from the initiation of appreciable loss of beta cells until total loss of beta cells appear to heighten the therapeutic bar. This underscores to us how important it is to elucidate multiple animal models and whenever possible to compare to human data to distinguish important drivers of disease development. Apparently, discreet aberrancies at the level of beta cells, APCs, and T cells, soluble factors and possibly also NK cells play together toward total beta-cell loss with remaining life-long intolerance to beta cells in BBDP rats.

REFERENCES

1. Logothetopoulos J, Valiquette N, Madura E, Cvet D. The onset and progression of pancreatic insulitis in the overt, spontaneously diabetic, young adult BB rat studied by pancreatic biopsy. Diabetes. 1984; 33(1):33–36.
2. Mordes JP, Desemone J, Rossini AA. The BB rat. Diabetes Metab Rev. 1987; 3(3):725–750.
3. Markholst H, Eastman S, Wilson D, Fisher L, Lernmark A. Decreased weight gain in BB rats before the clinical onset of insulin-dependent diabetes. Diabetes Res Clin Pract. 1993; 21(1):31–38.
4. Tannenbaum GS, Colle E, Wanamaker L, Gurd W, Goldman H, Seemayer TA. Dynamic time-course studies of the spontaneously diabetic BB Wistar rat. II. Insulin-, glucagon-, and somatostatin-reactive cells in the pancreas. Endocrinology. 1981; 109(6):1880–1887.
5. Seemayer TA, Tannenbaum GS, Goldman H, Colle E. Dynamic time course studies of the spontaneously diabetic BB Wistar rat. III. Light-microscopic and ultrastructural observations of pancreatic islets of Langerhans. Am J Pathol. 1982; 106(2):237–249.
6. Svenningsen A, Dyrberg T, Markholst H, Binder C, Lernmark A. Insulin release and pancreatic insulin is reduced in young prediabetic BB rats. Acta Endocrinol (Copenh). 1986; 112(3):367–371.
7. Löhr M, Markholst H, Dyrberg T, Klöppel G, Oberholzer M, Lernmark A. Insulitis and diabetes are preceded by a decrease in beta cell volume in diabetes-prone BB rats. Pancreas. 1989; 4(1):95–100.
8. Colle E, Guttmann RD, Seemayer TA. Association of spontaneous thyroiditis with the major histocompatibility complex of the rat. Endocrinology. 1985; 116(4):1243–1247.
9. Awata T, Guberski DL, Like AA. Genetics of the BB rat: association of autoimmune disorders (diabetes, insulitis, and thyroiditis) with lymphopenia and major histocompatibility complex class II. Endocrinology. 1995; 136(12):5731–5735.
10. Zipris D. Evidence that Th1 lymphocytes predominate in islet inflammation and thyroiditis in the BioBreeding (BB) rat. J Autoimmun. 1996; 9(3):315–319.
11. Markholst H, Eastman S, Wilson D, Andreasen BE, Lernmark A. Diabetes segregates as a single locus in crosses between inbred BB rats prone or resistant to diabetes. J Exp Med. 1991; 174(1):297–300.
12. Colle E, Guttmann RD, Seemayer TA, Michel F. Spontaneous diabetes mellitus syndrome in the rat. IV. Immunogenetic interactions of MHC and non-MHC components of the syndrome. Metabolism. 1983; 32(7 Suppl 1):54–61.
13. Colle E, Ono SJ, Fuks A, Guttmann RD, Seemayer TA. Association of susceptibility to spontaneous diabetes in rat with genes of major histocompatibility complex. Diabetes. 1988; 37(10):1438–1443.
14. Boitard C, Michie S, Serrurier P, Butcher GW, Larkins AP, McDevitt HO. In vivo prevention of thyroid and pancreatic autoimmunity in the BB rat by antibody to class II major histocompatibility complex gene products. Proc Natl Acad Sci USA. 1985; 82(19):6627–6631.
15. Lee KU, Kim MK, Amano K, et al. Preferential infiltration of macrophages during early

stages of insulitis in diabetes-prone BB rats. Diabetes. 1988; 37(8):1053–1058.
16. Voorbij HA, Jeucken PH, Kabel PJ, De HM, Drexhage HA. Dendritic cells and scavenger macrophages in pancreatic islets of prediabetic BB rats. Diabetes. 1989; 38(12):1623–1629.
17. Walker R, Bone AJ, Cooke A, Baird JD. Distinct macrophage subpopulations in pancreas of prediabetic BB-E rats. Possible role for macrophages in pathogenesis of IDDM. Diabetes. 1988; 37(9):1301–1304.
18. Hanenberg H, Kolb-Bachofen V, Kantwerk-Funke G, Kolb H. Macrophage infiltration precedes and is a prerequisite for lymphocytic insulitis in pancreatic islets of pre-diabetic BB rats. Diabetologia. 1989; 32(2):126–134.
19. Hosszufalusi N, Chan E, Teruya M, Takei S, Granger G, Charles MA. Quantitative phenotypic and functional analyses of islet immune cells before and after diabetes onset in the BB rat. Diabetologia. 1993; 36(11):1146–1154.
20. Jarpe AJ, Hickman MR, Anderson JT, Winter WE, Peck AB. Flow cytometric enumeration of mononuclear cell populations infiltrating the islets of Langerhans in prediabetic NOD mice: development of a model of autoimmune insulitis for type I diabetes. Reg Immunol. 1990; 3(6):305–317.
21. Jansen A, Homo-Delarche F, Hooijkaas H, Leenen PJ, Dardenne M, Drexhage HA. Immunohistochemical characterization of monocytes-macrophages and dendritic cells involved in the initiation of the insulitis and beta-cell destruction in NOD mice. Diabetes. 1994; 43(5):667–675.
22. Debussche X, Lormeau B, Boitard C, Toublanc M, Assan R. Course of pancreatic beta cell destruction in prediabetic NOD mice: a histomorphometric evaluation. Diabetes Metab. 1994; 20(3):282–290.
23. Dahlen E, Dawe K, Ohlsson L, Hedlund G. Dendritic cells and macrophages are the first and major producers of TNF-alpha in pancreatic islets in the nonobese diabetic mouse. J Immunol. 1998; 160(7):3585–3593.
24. Foulis AK, Liddle CN, Farquharson MA, Richmond JA, Weir RS. The histopathology of the pancreas in type 1 (insulin-dependent) diabetes mellitus: a 25-year review of deaths in patients under 20 years of age in the United Kingdom. Diabetologia. 1986; 29(5):267–274.
25. Foulis AK, McGill M, Farquharson MA. Insulitis in type 1 (insulin-dependent) diabetes mellitus in man–macrophages, lymphocytes, and interferon-gamma containing cells. J Pathol. 1991; 165(2):97–103.
26. Santamaria P, Nakhleh RE, Sutherland DE, Barbosa JJ. Characterization of T lymphocytes infiltrating human pancreas allograft affected by isletitis and recurrent diabetes. Diabetes. 1992; 41(1):53–61.
27. Itoh N, Hanafusa T, Miyazaki A, et al. Mononuclear cell infiltration and its relation to the expression of major histocompatibility complex antigens and adhesion molecules in pancreas biopsy specimens from newly diagnosed insulin-dependent diabetes mellitus patients. J Clin Invest. 1993; 92(5):2313–2322.
28. Reddy S, Bibby NJ, Fisher SL, Elliott RB. Longitudinal study of first phase insulin release in the BB rat. Diabetologia. 1986; 29(11):802–807.
29. Markholst H, Lernmark A. Reduced pancreatic insulin is associated with retarded growth of the pancreas in young prediabetic BB rats. Pancreas. 1988; 3(2):140–144.
30. Kanazawa M, Ikeda J, Sato J, et al. Alteration of insulin and glucagon secretion from the perfused BB rat pancreas before and after the onset of diabetes. Diabetes Res Clin Pract. 1988; 5(3):201–204.
31. Markholst H, Laursen HV. Decreased levels of serum alpha-isoamylase prior to diabetes onset in BB rats. Pancreas. 1990; 5(2):144–150.
32. Komiya I, Unger RH. Absence of glucopenic inhibition of the insulin response to arginine at the onset of diabetes in BB/W rats. Diabetologia. 1988; 31(4):225–227.
33. Faustman DL, Steinman RM, Gebel HM, Hauptfeld V, Davie JM, Lacy PE. Prevention of rejection of murine islet allografts by pretreatment with anti-dendritic cell antibody. Proc Natl Acad Sci USA. 1984; 81(12):3864–3868.
34. Nocera A, Leprini A, Fontana I. HLA-DR-bearing cells in the human pancreas. Transplant Proc. 1985; 17(Suppl 2):144–145.
35. Pipeleers DG, In't Veld PA, Pipeleers-Marichal MA, Gepts W, van de Winkel M. Presence of pancreatic hormones in islet cells with MHC-class II antigen expression. Diabetes. 1987; 36(7):872–876.
36. In't Veld PA, Pipeleers DG. In situ analysis of pancreatic islets in rats developing diabetes. Appearance of nonendocrine cells with surface MHC class II antigens and cytoplasmic insulin immunoreactivity. J Clin Invest. 1988; 82(3):1123–1128.
37. Charre S, Rosmalen JG, Pelegri C, et al. Abnormalities in dendritic cell and macrophage accumulation in the pancreas of

nonobese diabetic (NOD) mice during the early neonatal period. Histol Histopathol. 2002; 17(2):393–401.
38. Lee KU, Pak CY, Amano K, Yoon JW. Prevention of lymphocytic thyroiditis and insulitis in diabetes-prone BB rats by the depletion of macrophages. Diabetologia. 1988; 31(6):400–402.
39. Ziegler AG, Erhard J, Lampeter EF, Nagelkerken LM, Standl E. Involvement of dendritic cells in early insulitis of BB rats. J Autoimmun. 1992; 5(5):571–579.
40. Oschilewski U, Kiesel U, Kolb H. Administration of silica prevents diabetes in BB-rats. Diabetes. 1985; 34(2):197–199.
41. Ihm SH, Lee KU, Yoon JW. Studies on autoimmunity for initiation of beta-cell destruction. VII. Evidence for antigenic changes on beta-cells leading to autoimmune destruction of beta-cells in BB rats. Diabetes. 1991; 40(2):269–274.
42. Nerup J, Mandrup-Poulsen T, Helqvist S, et al. On the pathogenesis of IDDM. Diabetologia. 1994; 37(Suppl 2):S82–89.
43. Kay TWH, Thomas HE, Harrison LC, Allison J. The beta cell in autoimmune diabetes: Many mechanisms and pathways of loss. Trends Endocrinol Metab. 2000; 11(1):11–15.
44. Wu G, Flynn NE. The activation of the arginine-citrulline cycle in macrophages from the spontaneously diabetic BB rat. Biochem J. 1993; 294(1):113–118.
45. Lee KU. Nitric oxide produced by macrophages mediates suppression of ConA-induced proliferative responses of splenic leukocytes in the diabetes-prone BB rat. Diabetes. 1994; 43(10):1218–1220.
46. Lau A, Ramanathan S, Poussier P. Excessive production of nitric oxide by macrophages from DP-BB rats is secondary to the T-lymphopenic state of these animals. Diabetes. 1998; 47(2):197–205.
47. Tafuri A, Bowers WE, Handler ES, et al. High stimulatory activity of dendritic cells from diabetes-prone biobreeding/Worcester rats exposed to macrophage-derived factors. J Clin Invest. 1993; 91(5):2040–2048.
48. Delemarre FG, Simons PJ, de Heer HJ, Drexhage HA. Signs of immaturity of splenic dendritic cells from the autoimmune prone biobreeding rat: consequences for the in vitro expansion of regulator and effector T cells. J Immunol. 1999; 162(3):1795–1801.
49. Delemarre FGA, Hoogeveen PG, de Haan-Meulman M, Simons PJ, Drexhage HA. Homotypic cluster formation of dendritic cells, a close correlate of their state of maturation. Defects in the biobreeding diabetes-prone rat. J Leukoc Biol. 2001; 69(3):373–380.
50. Sommandas V, Rutledge EA, Van YB, Fuller J, Lernmark A, Drexhage HA. Aberrancies in the differentiation and maturation of dendritic cells from bone-marrow precursors are linked to various genes on chromosome 4 and other chromosomes of the BB-DP rat. J Autoimmun. 2005; 25(1):1–12.
51. Sommandas V, Rutledge EA, Van YB, Fuller J, Lernmark A, Drexhage HA. Defects in differentiation of bone-marrow derived dendritic cells of the BB rat are partly associated with IDDM2 (the lyp gene) and partly associated with other genes in the BB rat background. J Autoimmun. 2005; 25(1):46–56.
52. Like AA, Kislauskis E, Williams RR, Rossini AA. Neonatal thymectomy prevents spontaneous diabetes mellitus in the BB/W rat. Science. 1982; 216(4546):644–646.
53. Like AA, Biron CA, Weringer EJ, Byman K, Sroczynski E, Guberski DL. Prevention of diabetes in BioBreeding/Worcester rats with monoclonal antibodies that recognize T lymphocytes or natural killer cells. J Exp Med. 1986; 164(4):1145–1159.
54. Rabinovitch A, Sumoski WL. Theophylline protects against diabetes in BB rats and potentiates cyclosporine protection. Diabetologia. 1990; 33(8):506–508.
55. Crisá L, Mordes JP, Rossini AA. Autoimmune diabetes mellitus in the BB rat. Diabetes Metab Rev. 1992; 8(1):4–37.
56. Zipris D, Greiner DL, Malkani S, Whalen B, Mordes JP, Rossini AA. Cytokine gene expression in islets and thyroids of BB rats. IFN-gamma and IL-12p40 mRNA increase with age in both diabetic and insulin-treated nondiabetic BB rats. J Immunol. 1996; 156(3):1315–1321.
57. Hosszufalusi N, Chan E, Granger G, Charles MA. Quantitative analyses comparing all major spleen cell phenotypes in BB and normal rats: autoimmune imbalance and double negative T cells associated with resistant, prone and diabetic animals. J Autoimmun. 1992; 5(3):305–318.
58. Jacob HJ, Pettersson A, Wilson D, Mao Y, Lernmark A, Lander ES. Genetic dissection of autoimmune type I diabetes in the BB rat. Nat Genet. 1992; 2(1):56–60.
59. Hornum L, Rømer J, Markholst H. The diabetes-prone BB rat carries a frameshift mutation in Ian4, a positional candidate of Iddm1. Diabetes. 2002; 51(6):1972–1979.

60. MacMurray AJ, Moralejo DH, Kwitek AE, et al. Lymphopenia in the BB rat model of type 1 diabetes is due to a mutation in a novel immune-associated nucleotide (Ian)-related gene. Genome Res. 2002; 12(7):1029–1039.
61. Zadeh HH, Greiner DL, Wu DY, Tausche F, Goldschneider I. Abnormalities in the export and fate of recent thymic emigrants in diabetes-prone BB/W rats. Autoimmunity. 1996; 24(1):35–46.
62. Iwakoshi NN, Goldschneider I, Tausche F, Mordes JP, Rossini AA, Greiner DL. High frequency apoptosis of recent thymic emigrants in the liver of lymphopenic diabetes-prone BioBreeding rats. J Immunol. 1998; 160(12):5838–5850.
63. Ramanathan S, Norwich K, Poussier P. Antigen activation rescues recent thymic emigrants from programmed cell death in the BB rat. J Immunol. 1998; 160(12):5757–5764.
64. Hernández-Hoyos G, Joseph S, Miller NG, Butcher GW. The lymphopenia mutation of the BB rat causes inappropriate apoptosis of mature thymocytes. Eur J Immunol. 1999; 29(6):1832–1841.
65. Dalberg U, Markholst H, Hornum L. Both Gimap5 and the diabetogenic BBDP allele of Gimap5 induce apoptosis in T cells. Int Immunol. 2007; 19(4):447–453.
66. Bell EB, Sparshott SM, Drayson MT, Ford WL. The stable and permanent expansion of functional T lymphocytes in athymic nude rats after a single injection of mature T cells. J Immunol. 1987; 139(5):1379–1384.
67. Khoruts A, Fraser JM. A causal link between lymphopenia and autoimmunity. Immunol Lett. 2005; 98(1):23–31.
68. Gold DP, Bellgrau D. Identification of a limited T-cell receptor beta chain variable region repertoire associated with diabetes in the BB rat. Proc Natl Acad Sci USA. 1991; 88(21):9888–9891.
69. Bourgeois C, Stockinger B. CD25+CD4+ regulatory T cells and memory T cells prevent lymphopenia-induced proliferation of naive T cells in transient states of lymphopenia. J Immunol. 2006; 177(7):4558–4566.
70. Lang JA, Kominski D, Bellgrau D, Scheinman RI. Partial activation precedes apoptotic death in T cells harboring an IAN gene mutation. Eur J Immunol. 2004; 34(9):2396–2406.
71. Kupfer R, Lang J, Williams-Skipp C, Nelson M, Bellgrau D, Scheinman RI. Loss of a gimap/ian gene leads to activation of NF-kappaB through a MAPK-dependent pathway. Mol Immunol. 2007; 44(4):479–487.
72. Moore JK, Bellgrau D. Promiscuous activation and cell cycle entry in T cells from autoimmune animals. Transplant Proc. 1999; 31(3):1606–1610.
73. Bottini N, Musumeci L, Alonso A, et al. A functional variant of lymphoid tyrosine phosphatase is associated with type I diabetes. Nat Genet. 2004; 36(4):337–338.
74. Kyogoku C, Langefeld CD, Ortmann WA et al. Genetic association of the R620W polymorphism of protein tyrosine phosphatase PTPN22 with human SLE. Am J Hum Genet. 2004; 75(3):504–507.
75. Moore JK, Scheinman RI, Bellgrau D. The identification of a novel T cell activation state controlled by a diabetogenic gene. J Immunol. 2001; 166(1):241–248.
76. Appleman LJ, Berezovskaya A, Grass I, Boussiotis VA. CD28 costimulation mediates T cell expansion via IL-2-independent and IL-2-dependent regulation of cell cycle progression. J Immunol. 2000; 164(1):144–151.
77. Kubsch S, Graulich E, Knop J, Steinbrink K. Suppressor activity of anergic T cells induced by IL-10-treated human dendritic cells: association with IL-2- and CTLA-4-dependent G1 arrest of the cell cycle regulated by p27Kip1. Eur J Immunol. 2003; 33(7):1988–1997.
78. Li L, Iwamoto Y, Berezovskaya A, Boussiotis VA. A pathway regulated by cell cycle inhibitor p27Kip1 and checkpoint inhibitor Smad3 is involved in the induction of T cell tolerance. Nat Immunol. 2006; 7(11):1157–1165.
79. Sellins KS, Gold DP, Bellgrau D. Resistance to tolerance induction in the diabetes-prone biobreeding rat as one manifestation of abnormal responses to superantigens. Diabetologia. 1996; 39(1):28–36.
80. Beaudette-Zlatanova BC, Whalen B, Zipris D, et al. Costimulation and autoimmune diabetes in BB rats. Am J Transplant. 2006; 6(5 Pt 1):894–902.
81. Rozing J, Coolen C, Tielen FJ, et al. Defects in the thymic epithelial stroma of diabetes prone BB rats. Thymus. 1989; 14(1–3):125–135.
82. Doukas J, Mordes JP, Swymer C et al. Thymic epithelial defects and predisposition to autoimmune disease in BB rats. Am J Pathol. 1994; 145(6):1517–1525.
83. Whalen BJ, Rossini AA, Mordes JP, Greiner DL. DR-BB rat thymus contains thymocyte populations predisposed to autoreactivity. Diabetes. 1995; 44(8):963–967.
84. Sommandas V, Rutledge EA, Van YB, Fuller J, Lernmark A, Drexhage HA. Low-density cells isolated from the rat thymus resemble

branched cortical macrophages and have a reduced capability of rescuing double-positive thymocytes from apoptosis in the BB-DP rat. J Leukoc Biol. 2007; 82(4):869–876.
85. Georgiou HM, Bellgrau D. Thymus transplantation and disease prevention in the diabetes-prone Bio-Breeding rat. J Immunol. 1989; 142(10):3400–3405.
86. Plamondon C, Kottis V, Brideau C, Metroz-Dayer MD, Poussier P. Abnormal thymocyte maturation in spontaneously diabetic BB rats involves the deletion of CD4⁻8⁺ cells. J Immunol 1990; 144(3):923–928.
87. Groen H, Klatter FA, Brons NH, Mesander G, Nieuwenhuis P, Kampinga J. Abnormal thymocyte subset distribution and differential reduction of CD4⁺ and CD8⁺ T cell subsets during peripheral maturation in diabetes-prone BioBreeding rats. J Immunol. 1996; 156(3):1269–1275.
88. Jung CG, Kamiyama T, Agui T. Elevated apoptosis of peripheral T lymphocytes in diabetic BB rats. Immunology. 1999; 98(4):590–594.
89. Poussier P, Ning T, Murphy T, Dabrowski D, Ramanathan S. Impaired post-thymic development of regulatory CD4⁺25⁺ T cells contributes to diabetes pathogenesis in BB rats. J Immunol. 2005; 174(7):4081–4089.
90. Hillebrands JL, Whalen B, Visser JT et al. A regulatory CD4⁺ T cell subset in the BB rat model of autoimmune diabetes expresses neither CD25 nor Foxp3. J Immunol. 2006; 177(11):7820–7832.
91. Francfort JW, Barker CF, Kimura H, Silvers WK, Frohman M, Naji A. Increased incidence of Ia antigen-bearing T lymphocytes in the spontaneously diabetic BB rat. J Immunol. 1985; 134(3):1577–1582.
92. Lundsgaard D, Holm TL, Hornum L, Markholst H. In vivo control of diabetogenic T-cells by regulatory CD4⁺CD25⁺ T-cells expressing Foxp3. Diabetes. 2005; 54(4):1040–1047.
93. Greiner DL, Mordes JP, Handler ES, Angelillo M, Nakamura N, Rossini AA. Depletion of RT6.1⁺ T lymphocytes induces diabetes in resistant biobreeding/Worcester (BB/W) rats. J Exp Med. 1987; 166(2):461–475.
94. Whalen BJ, Greiner DL, Mordes JP, Rossini AA. Adoptive transfer of autoimmune diabetes mellitus to athymic rats: synergy of CD4⁺ and CD8⁺ T cells and prevention by RT6⁺ T cells. J Autoimmun. 1994; 7(6):819–831.
95. Groen H, Klatter F, Pater J, Nieuwenhuis P, Rozing J. Temporary, but essential requirement of CD8⁺ T cells early in the pathogenesis of diabetes in BB rats as revealed by thymectomy and CD8 depletion. Clin Dev Immunol. 2003; 10(2–4):141–151.
96. Guberski DL, Thomas VA, Shek WR, et al. Induction of type I diabetes by Kilham's rat virus in diabetes-resistant BB/Wor rats. Science. 1991; 254(5034):1010–1013.
97. Zipris D, Lien E, Nair A, et al. TLR9-signaling pathways are involved in Kilham rat virus-induced autoimmune diabetes in the biobreeding diabetes-resistant rat. J Immunol. 2007; 178(2):693–701.
98. Chung YH, Jun HS, Son M, et al. Cellular and molecular mechanism for Kilham rat virus-induced autoimmune diabetes in DR-BB rats. J Immunol. 2000; 165(5):2866–2876.
99. Zipris D, Hillebrands JL, Welsh RM, et al. Infections that induce autoimmune diabetes in BBDR rats modulate CD4⁺CD25⁺ T cell populations. J Immunol. 2003; 170(7):3592–3602.
100. Zipris D, Lien E, Xie JX, Greiner DL, Mordes JP, Rossini AA. TLR activation synergizes with Kilham rat virus infection to induce diabetes in BBDR rats. J Immunol. 2005; 174(1):131–142.
101. Sobel DO, Newsome J, Ewel CH, et al. Poly I:C induces development of diabetes mellitus in BB rat. Diabetes. 1992; 41(4):515–520.
102. Hornum L, Lundsgaard D, Markholst H. PolyI:C induction of diabetes is controlled by Iddm4 in rats with a full regulatory T cell pool. Ann N Y Acad Sci. 2007; 1110:65–72.
103. Blankenhorn EP, Rodemich L, Martin-Fernandez C, Leif J, Greiner DL, Mordes JP. The rat diabetes susceptibility locus Iddm4 and at least one additional gene are required for autoimmune diabetes induced by viral infection. Diabetes. 2005; 54(4):1233–1237.
104. Blankenhorn EP, Descipio C, Rodemich L, et al. Refinement of the Iddm4 diabetes susceptibility locus reveals TCRVbeta4 as a candidate gene. Ann N Y Acad Sci. 2007; 1103:128–131.
105. Elder ME, Maclaren NK. Identification of profound peripheral T lymphocyte immunodeficiencies in the spontaneously diabetic BB rat. J Immunol. 1983; 130(4):1723–1731.
106. Dyrberg T, Schwimmbeck P, Oldstone M. The incidence of diabetes in BB rats is decreased following acute LCMV infection. Adv Exp Med Biol. 1988; 246: 397–402.
107. Dyrberg T, Schwimmbeck PL, Oldstone MB. Inhibition of diabetes in BB rats by virus infection. J Clin Invest. 1988; 81(3): 928–931.
108. Oldstone MB, Tishon A, Schwimmbeck PL, Shyp S, Lewicki H, Dyrberg T. Cytotoxic T lymphocytes do not control lymphocytic

choriomeningitis virus infection of BB diabetes-prone rats. J Gen Virol. 1990; 71(Pt 4): 785–791.
109. Schwimmbeck PL, Dyrberg T, Oldstone MB. Abrogation of diabetes in BB rats by acute virus infection. Association of viral-lymphocyte interactions. J Immunol. 1988; 140(10):3394–3400.
110. Tullin S, Farris P, Petersen JS, Hornum L, Jackerott M, Markholst H. A pronounced thymic B cell deficiency in the spontaneously diabetic BB rat. J Immunol. 1997; 158(11):5554–5559.
111. Dyrberg T, Poussier P, Nakhooda F, Marliss EB, Lernmark A. Islet cell surface and lymphocyte antibodies often precede the spontaneous diabetes in the BB rat. Diabetologia. 1984; 26(2):159–165.
112. Markholst H, Klaff LJ, Klöppel G, Lernmark A, Mordes JP, Palmer J. Lack of systematically found insulin autoantibodies in spontaneously diabetic BB rats. Diabetes. 1990; 39(6):720–727.
113. DeSilva MG, Jun HS, Yoon JW, Notkins AL, Lan MS. Autoantibodies to IA-2 not detected in NOD mice or BB rats. Diabetologia. 1996; 39(10):1237–1238.
114. Kitagawa Y, Greiner DL, Reynolds CW et al. Islet cells but not thyrocytes are susceptible to lysis by NK cells. J Autoimmun. 1991; 4(5):703–716.
115. MacKay P, Jacobson J, Rabinovitch A. Spontaneous diabetes mellitus in the Bio-Breeding/Worcester rat. Evidence in vitro for natural killer cell lysis of islet cells. J Clin Invest. 1986; 77(3):916–924.
116. Woda BA, Biron CA. Natural killer cell number and function in the spontaneously diabetic BB/W rat. J Immunol 1986; 137(6):1860–1866.
117. Jacobson JD, Markmann JF, Brayman KL, Barker CF, Naji A. Prevention of recurrent autoimmune diabetes in BB rats by anti-asialo-GM1 antibody. Diabetes. 1988; 37(6):838–841.
118. Sobel DO, Azumi N, Creswell K, et al. The role of NK cell activity in the pathogenesis of poly I: C accelerated and spontaneous diabetes in the diabetes prone BB rat. J Autoimmun. 1995; 8(6):843–857.

Chapter 12

Immunopathogenesis of the NOD Mouse

Li Zhang and George S. Eisenbarth

Key Words: Diabetes mouse model, Major histocompatibility complex, Insulin autoantibodies, Insulin autoimmunity, T-cell receptors, T cells, Genetics

INTRODUCTION

The NOD mouse model of type 1A (immune-mediated) diabetes and genetic derivatives of this strain are probably the most extensively studied autoimmune animal models (1–4). NOD mice spontaneously develop insulitis. This is followed in the great majority of female mice by sufficient beta-cell destruction to result in overt diabetes and approximately 50% of male mice develop diabetes. Insulitis develops between 4 and 8 weeks and over a prolonged period of time increasing numbers of mice develop severe hyperglycemia. In addition, the mice develop sialitis and other autoimmune disorders, such as thyroiditis, retinitis, and autoimmune neuropathy, depending upon the genetic backgrounds (5–7). Multiple derivatives of the NOD model (congenic strains of mice with specific mutations and transgenes) are available from repositories at the Jackson Laboratories and Taconic and from individual investigators. There is no doubt that type 1A diabetes is the result of T cell-mediated destruction of beta cells with genetic mutations and therapies that eliminate (e.g., Rag and SCID mutations) T cells preventing disease and ability to transfer the disease with autoreactive T cells.

Insights derived from the model have provided important preclinical data for a series of trials in man that have led to successful interventions delaying but not yet permanently preventing immune-mediated islet beta-cell destruction (*8*). A criticism of the NOD model is that many interventions prevent diabetes, some of which have not shown efficacy in clinical trials (e.g., nicotinamide, BCG) (*9*).

GENETICS

Genetic determinants of diabetes of the NOD mouse have their relevant expression in bone marrow-derived cells and not in islet or stromal cells. Transplantation of bone marrow cells from NOD mice induces diabetes in control strains of mice, and bone marrow from control strains transplanted into NOD mice prevents diabetes (*10*).

As in man, the dominant genetic determinant of islet autoimmunity and diabetes is genes within the major histocompatibility complex on chromosome 17, in particular class II MHC alleles (*11–13*). Both the NODs, unique sequence of I-A (homologous to DQ of man) and lack of expression of I-E (a lack shared with many standard mouse strains), are essential for the development of diabetes. The sequence of NOD I-A^{g7} differs from many strains by having a serine rather than aspartic acid at position 57 of the I-A beta chain and a proline at position 56 (*13, 14*). Altering of either of these positions decreases the development of diabetes. The crystal structure of I-A^{g7} with a bound peptide is available allowing the modeling of the binding of autoantigenic peptides to I-A^{g7} (*15*).

There are alternative hypotheses as to why I-A^{g7} is associated with islet autoimmunity. One hypothesis is that I-A^{g7} is a poor binder of peptides and potentially unstable (*16, 17*). Such instability or defective binding might limit the deletion of autoimmune T cells within the thymus. Alternatively, the hypothesis we prefer is that I-A^{g7} is critical for the selection of anti-islet T cells within the thymus and/or the presentation of specific autoantigenic peptide(s) in the periphery and thus enhances the development of diabetes (*18–21*). Congenic NOD mice with different I-A molecules such as I-A^{k} do not develop diabetes but have alternative autoimmune disorders, suggesting that class II alleles determine the specific organ targeted rather than general susceptibility to autoimmunity (*22, 23*).

The MHC region by itself is not sufficient for the development of diabetes. For example, a congenic strain having I-A^{g7} on a C57 genetic background does not develop diabetes (*24*). Polymorphisms of multiple genes are important for disease. The NOR mouse that shares approximately 80% of the genome of NOD mice including I-A^{g7} develops insulitis and insulin autoantibodies but does not develop diabetes (*25*). Even within the

MHC, there is evidence of additional loci contributing to diabetes in addition to class II MHC alleles (*26–28*). Though a large number of loci contribute to diabetes risk in crosses of NOD mice with multiple standard strains relatively, few genes within the defined loci have been conclusively demonstrated to underlie susceptibility. This may relate to the observation that multiple subloci contributing to diabetes risk are present within defined loci. Genes with the evidence of pathogenic polymorphisms include a variant of beta-2 microglobulin (*29*), the IDD3 NOD locus associated with decreased IL-2 expression, and a synonymous single-nucleotide polymorphism of cytotoxic T lymphocyte-associated antigen-4 (CTLA4) exon 2 of CTLA4 (iddm 5.1) (*30*).

The gene encoding CTLA4 has been suggested as a candidate gene for conferring susceptibility to type 1A diabetes. CTLA4 is encoded as a 223 amino acid precursor protein. As in the mouse, the human *CTLA4* and *CD28* genes are closely linked. CTLA4 has an important function (*31*). It is considered the most likely candidate gene for murine iddm 5.1 on chromosome 1 through mapping studies (*32*). It is hypothesized that the NOD variant of CTLA4 contributes to diabetes by increasing the ligand-independent isoform of CTLA4 that deliveries a negative signal to T cells. NOD CTLA4-Ig transgenic mice have a more rapid onset of diabetes and higher incidence (100%) than control mice (*33*). Treatment with CTLA4-Ig in NOD mice at 2–3 weeks of age prevents the development of IDDM. T cells from CTLA4$^{-/-}$ deficient mice show a similar resistance to gamma irradiation-induced apoptosis as observed in NOD mice (*34*).

A large number of genes of man are also associated with type 1A diabetes, while only a subset of these have been implicated in diabetes of the NOD mouse (*35*). A polymorphism of a variable-nucleotide tandem repeat (VNTR) of the insulin gene is quantitatively the most important locus of man after the MHC. The insulin locus of different mouse strains in simple crosses does not influence the development of diabetes (*36*). In contrast to humans with one insulin gene, mice have two insulin genes. Knockouts of either the insulin 1 or insulin 2 gene have a dramatic effect upon the development of diabetes of NOD mice (*21, 37*). A knockout of the insulin 1 gene prevents almost all progression to diabetes whereas a knockout of the insulin 2 gene accelerates the development of diabetes (*21*). Though both insulin genes are expressed within beta cells of the islets, only the insulin 2 gene is expressed within thymic medullary epithelial cells. It is likely that the dramatic effect of the insulin 2 gene knockout is secondary to lack of negative selection of anti-insulin autoreactive T cells within the thymus. This is analogous to the increased thymic expression of proinsulin messenger RNA with the VNTR of man associated with decreased diabetes risk (*38*).

INNATE IMMUNITY

Multiple abnormalities/differences of immune function have been documented in NOD mice and may contribute to disease pathogenesis (39). There is a deficiency of natural killer (NK) T cells and stimulation of NK T cells with glycolipids decreases the development of diabetes (40–42). NK cell activity level in NOD mice is lower than in C57BL/6 mice. In NOD NK cells, NKG2D (an activating receptor of human NK cells)-dependent cytotoxicity and cytokine production were decreased because of receptor modulation (43). NK cell-mediated cytotoxicity is reduced compared with other strains (44, 45). In contrast, NK cells are associated with more destructive forms of pancreatic islet autoimmunity (46). The cells in aggressive infiltrates had a higher level of NK-associated genes expressed at both the protein and the transcript level. The proportion and numbers of NK cells in the islet infiltrate, and the timing of their entry, correlated with the aggressivity of the lesion. Depletion and blockade of NK cell function significantly reduced the rate of development and penetrance of diabetes (46). In addition, when compared with C57BL/6 and BALB/c mice, bone marrow precursor cells in NOD mice have several myeloid differentiation abnormalities (42).

ADAPTIVE IMMUNITY

B Lymphocytes

Both B lymphocytes and autoantibodies contribute to the development of diabetes though transfer of diabetes by immunoglobulin from NOD mice has not been demonstrated. Genetic elimination of B lymphocytes prevents diabetes (47), and NOD mice lacking transplacental transfer of "autoantibodies" (e.g., non-NOD foster mothers) have a greatly decreased development of diabetes (48). Of note, rituximab, an anti-CD20 monoclonal antibody that depletes B lymphocytes (but not plasma cells), blocks the development of diabetes of NOD mice engineered to express the human CD20 molecule (49). Results of an initial trial of rituximab in patients with recent onset diabetes delays c-peptide loss.

The precise mechanism by which B lymphocytes contribute to diabetes pathogenesis is unknown, but a leading hypothesis is that of presentation of islet autoantigens to T lymphocytes. High levels of autoantibodies reacting with insulin are present in NOD mice, appearing as early as 3–4 weeks of age reaching peak levels several weeks thereafter, and then usually declining by the onset of overt hyperglycemia (50, 51). The loss of such autoantibodies does not simply correlate with loss of islet beta cells in that the NOR mouse that develops insulitis with relatively little beta-cell destruction follows a similar time course of expression of insulin autoantibodies (51).

T Lymphocytes

Both CD4 and CD8 T lymphocytes are essential for the spontaneous development of diabetes of NOD mice. Paradoxically CD8 T cells are particularly important early in the process that leads to diabetes (*52, 53*). Multiple target peptides of both CD4 and CD8 T-cell clones have been defined including insulin peptides (CD4 insulin peptide B:9-23; CD8 insulin peptide B:15-22), IGRP 206-214, and GAD peptide (glutamic acid decarboxylase) (*54, 55*). Tetramers are available reacting with both CD8 T cells recognizing insulin B:15-22 peptide and IGRP 206-214. IGRP reactive T cells are present in peripheral blood of NOD mice during the prodrome preceding overt diabetes and are the majority of CD8 islet infiltrating T lymphocytes. Affinity maturation of the T-cell receptor of IGRP reactive T cells as mice progress to diabetes has been described (*56*). T cells reacting with GAD are of interest as both the T-cell clones and anti-GAD T-cell receptor transgenes are protective rather than pathogenic (*57*). There is very little GAD within islets of mice in contrast to human islets, where GAD is expressed in beta and non-beta cells. Nevertheless, it is assumed that there is sufficient GAD (potentially GAD67 rather than GAD65) to allow NOD T cells to target GAD of islets and protect from diabetes (*58*).

Though anti-IGRP T cells are a very prominent component of islet reactive T cells, eliminating the immune response to IGRP does not alter progression to diabetes of NOD mice (*59*). In general, eliminating immune responses to many different islet target molecules does not prevent diabetes, including IGRP, GAD65, IA-2 alpha, and IA-2 beta. In contrast (as mentioned above), knocking out the insulin 1 gene prevents the great majority of NOD mice from developing diabetes. In addition, inducing tolerance to proinsulin with a transgene that leads to widespread proinsulin expression in antigen presenting cells (I-E promoter driving proinsulin expression) completely prevents the development of diabetes and the appearance of IGRP reactive T cells (*59, 60*). Induction of tolerance to insulin even prevents the development of diabetes of mice with a transgene recognizing IGRP leading to the hypothesis that the immune response to insulin is "upstream" of the immune response to IGRP (*60*).

Nakayama and coworkers have further explored the immune response to insulin with the creation of NOD mice lacking both the insulin 1 and the insulin 2 genes. To prevent "metabolic" diabetes in these mice, an insulin 2 transgene driving the islet expression of proinsulin was introduced. The proinsulin transgene encoded a proinsulin molecule with a single amino acid mutation at position 16 (alanine substituted for tyrosine). This mutation was chosen in that it eliminated the ability of the insulin B:9-23 peptide to stimulate proliferation of clones recognizing this peptide. The mice with a mutation in a single amino acid residue of insulin fail to develop diabetes and most lack the expression of insulin autoantibodies and insulitis (*61, 62*). Such studies have led to the hypothesis that insulin, and in particular the B:9-23 peptide of insulin, is a primary islet autoantigen of the NOD mouse (*20*).

The targeted autoantigens of many T-cell clones are just being defined. One of the most studied of these is the chromogranin autoantigen recognized by the BDC 2.5 T-cell clone (*63*). The BDC 2.5 diabetogenic T-cell clone was produced by Dr. Haskins and coworkers. A T-cell receptor transgenic mouse produced by Mathis and coworkers from this T-cell clone has been extensively studied (*64*). These studies have provided evidence that the activation of anti-islet T cells first occurs in the pancreatic lymph node (*65*), and T cells with the same receptor can be utilized to both cause and prevent diabetes, and FoxP3 positive regulatory BDC 2.5 T lymphocytes can prevent diabetes.

Vignali and coworkers have evaluated a large series of T-cell receptor retrogenics (*63*). These mice are produced with retroviral transfer of specific T-cell receptors into bone marrow cells that are transplanted into immunodeficient NOD.SCID mice. Retrogenic T-cell receptors reacting with insulin result in diabetes, while similar retrogenics recognizing GAD did not (*63*). In addition, retrogenic T-cell receptors derived from clones recognizing multiple targets also induced diabetes (BDC 10.1>BDC 2.5>NY4.1>BDC 6.9).

REGULATORY T CELLS IN NOD MICE

Regulatory T cells, termed Tregs, co-express a number of cell surface markers including CD4, CD25, CD62L^{hi}, CTLA4, and GITR and lack IL-7 receptors. CD4$^+$CD25$^+$ Tregs expressing FoxP3 cells have been shown to be essential for controlling autoimmunity in NOD mice by suppressing pathogenic T cells. The development of insulitis in NOD mice has been related to the balance between effector cells and Tregs. Tregs functional potency and intrapancreatic proliferative potential declines with age, in turn augmenting diabetogenic response and disease susceptibility (*66*). Tregs are present in infiltrates of islets in NOD mice for weeks to months before the onset of overt diabetes. Transfer experiments demonstrate that Treg cells can suppress the development of diabetes of inhibition on effector cells (*67*). Depletion of the CD62L^{hi} Treg population is followed by a loss of suppression and results in exacerbated T cell-mediated destruction of insulin-producing islet cells (*68*).

The transcription factor Foxp3 is currently the most specific marker for natural CD4$^+$ Treg cells (*69*). In mice, null mutations of Foxp3 cause massive lymphoproliferation and widespread inflammatory infiltration of organs. Fontenot et al. (*70*) reported that adoptive transfer of Treg cells into neonatal scurfy mutant mice prevented disease and all of the CD4⁺CD25⁺ Treg cells in the recipient mice were derived from the Foxp3+ donor. Benoist and coworkers crossed the Foxp3 scurfy mutation onto NOD mice having the BDC 2.5 T-cell receptor transgene (*71*). These mice with a single T-cell receptor targeting islets do not develop the widespread autoimmunity of FoxP3 mutant mice but do develop insulitis. In this model, the absence of Treg cells did not augment the initial activation or phenotypic characteristics of effector T cells in the draining lymph nodes, nor accelerate the onset of T-cell infiltration of the pancreatic islets. However, insulitis was immediately destructive with rapid progression to overt diabetes. Microarray analysis revealed that Treg cells in the insulitic lesion adopted a gene expression pattern different from that in lymph nodes, whereas Treg cells in draining or irrelevant lymph nodes appeared very similar. Thus, Treg cells are hypothesized to primarily impinge on autoimmune diabetes by reining in destructive T cells inside the islets.

There is evidence that Treg development, peripheral maintenance, and suppressive function can be dependent on antigen specificity. Antigen-specific Tregs were expanded in vitro using IL-2 and beads coated with recombinant peptide bound to I-A^{g7} and anti-CD28 monoclonal antibodies (*72*). The expanded antigen-specific Tregs expressed regulatory cell surface markers and cytokines. The expanded Tregs were capable of bystander suppression both in vitro and in vivo. Importantly, the islet peptide specific Tregs were more efficient than polyclonal Tregs in suppressing autoimmune diabetes. Tang and coworkers (*73*) expanded BDC 2.5/NOD T cells ex vivo with IL-2 and produced a Treg population that expressed the unique BDC 2.5 TCR specificity. These Tregs suppressed diabetes at remarkably low cell numbers when cotransferred with diabetogenic cells and even reversed new-onset diabetes in NOD mice. Furthermore, insulin-specific Tregs produced by active immunization could effectively suppress diabetes in a transfer model (*74*). It has been suggested that antigen-specific Tregs mediate immunosuppression in the context of T-cell activation (*75*). Tregs directly interacted with dendritic cells bearing islet antigen and the dendritic cell-expanded, islets-specific Tregs restored normoglycemia in diabetic NOD mice. Therefore, dendritic cells may play an important role in vivo in suppression of autoimmunity.

HUMANIZED MICE

The NOD mouse with its natural deficiency of NK T cells was combined with a common gamma chain knockout (to block cytokine signaling) and Rag mutation (to eliminate T lymphocytes).

This mouse (NOG) accepts transplantation of human stem cells to develop mice accepting human cells to develop a humanized immune system. The introduction of human CD34 stem cells derived from cord blood into these mice can result in a subset of mice expressing human T and B lymphocytes. These mice can reject islet transplants when human lymphocytes are injected directly into allogenic transplants (76, 77). As these models are improved, they will likely allow more precise study of the human immune system than is possible directly in man.

"IMMUNOLOGIC HOMUNCULUS" HYPOTHESIS

Irun Cohen coined the term immunologic homunculus to suggest that the hierarchy of risk for specific autoimmune disorders (some common and some rare) may be "hard-wired" in the immune system. We have been pursuing the hypothesis that there is a primary autoantigen for the development of autoimmune diabetes of the NOD mouse, and this antigen is insulin, and in particular the insulin B chain, B:9-23 peptide (20, 78). Given the large number of autoantigens recognized by T lymphocytes of NOD mice, and the existence of T-cell clones or T-cell receptor mice that recognize these antigens and cause diabetes, other investigators have postulated that there may be no primary autoantigen, rather recognition of multiple redundant islet molecules. The results of inducing tolerance to insulin and knocking out of insulin genes (including changing a single amino acid of insulin B16Y to B16A and preventing NOD diabetes) suggest that an immune response to insulin is crucial (61).

In that recognition of insulin peptide B:9-23 is such a prominent target of the autoimmunity of NOD mice, the question arises as to why? We believe that such recognition is primarily driven by an "accident" of nature. A common T-cell receptor alpha chain (TRAV5D-4) sequence facilitates the development of T cells reacting with the insulin B:9-23 peptide. The T-cell clones that Wegmann et al. originally isolated from islets of NOD mice had conservation of V alpha and J alpha chain utilization, but no conservation of the N region of the alpha chain and of beta chain (79). When just TRAV5D-4 transgenic or retrogenic alpha gene segment (from clones BDC 12-4.1 or BDC 12-4.4) are utilized to produce mice only capable of expressing these alpha chains, but utilizing endogenous beta chains, insulin autoimmunity is readily induced, with high levels of insulin autoantibodies (50). The hypothesis that such a V alpha chain sequence facilitates the development of insulin/islet autoimmunity would suggest that all mice would have an increased susceptibility to autoimmune diabetes, given ubiquitous expression of the alpha chain or related sequences in mice. Though V alpha chains with the TRAV5D-4*04 sequence are a substrate for autoimmunity, genetic polymorphism altering maintenance of tolerance is also crucial. Thus, we hypothesize that for the NOD mouse, presentation of insulin peptide B:9-23 to commonly generated T-cell receptors containing the V alpha sequence TRAV5D-4*04 sets the stage for the development of insulin autoimmunity given the inability of this animal to adequately maintain tolerance. We believe that analogous primary autoantigens and high-risk T-cell receptor motifs are present in patients developing type 1A diabetes given the dramatic restriction of HLA class II genotypes in patients [e.g., approximately 30% of patients have the genotype (DR3/4-DQ2/8)] and the observation that 80% of children with the IPEX syndrome (FoxP3 mutation) develop type 1 diabetes, often with onset in the first days of life (*80*).

THE NOD AS A PRECLINICAL MODEL

Though understanding of the immunopathogenesis of the NOD mouse is incomplete, it has served as a model to test multiple therapies that have also been studied in man either to halt beta-cell destruction after the onset of type 1A diabetes or to prevent beta-cell destruction prior to hyperglycemia. The studied therapies can be divided into those that are "antigen" specific, immunosuppressive, or immunomodulatory. Multiple antigens when administered to NOD mice can prevent diabetes and studies in man of oral insulin and GAD65 immunization are most advanced. A recent trial has provided preliminary data that the injection of GAD65 in alum may delay loss of C-peptide in patients with new onset diabetes (*81*). A trial of oral insulin, but not injected insulin, though failing to influence progression to diabetes in the group as a whole, provided preliminary data (subset analysis) of potential benefit for autoantibody positive relatives expressing higher levels of insulin autoantibodies. Trialnet is conducting a study to direct the ability of oral insulin to delay progression in insulin antibodies positive relatives.

In NOD mice, monoclonal antibodies to both T and B lymphocytes have long-lasting effects, and modified anti-CD3 antibodies are now in clinical trials. The anti-CD3 mechanism of action likely combines rapid reduction of T lymphocytes and inflammation followed by the induction of T-cell regulation (*8, 82*). Combination therapies are also being actively studied (*83*). A difficulty with the NOD mouse model may relate to the relative ease of prevention of diabetes, though it is harder to reverse diabetes and few therapies eliminate all insulitis (*4, 84*). Models such as the insulin 2 knockout NOD mouse, where most therapies effective in regular NOD mice fail to protect, may provide a more robust indication of potential efficacy of preventative therapies.

CONCLUSIONS

The NOD mouse model and hundreds of derivative strains have become major tools for the study of the immunopathogenesis of type 1A diabetes. Being inbred, the original strain represents a single genetic "individual" with dramatic insulitis preceding diabetes onset. There is progressive destruction of beta cells, but not all mice progress to diabetes, and multiple interventions readily prevent disease. It is now clear that multiple interventions can also reverse hyperglycemia of NOD mice. How many of such interventions will ultimately be applicable in man with appropriate adjustment of dose and timing is currently unknown. Nevertheless, caution in extrapolating to man will always be important. Fundamental questions are currently unanswered, such as whether a single-antigenic peptide such as insulin B:9-23 recognized by a conserved set of non-stringent T-cell receptors underlies disease pathogenesis. This hypothesis postulates many secondary target autoantigens, each dispensable for disease progression. If there are such key targets in man is unknown, though similar to the NOD mouse, there is autoimmunity to multiple autoantigens. The realization that islet autoimmunity, similar to many other autoimmune disorders, is critically dependent upon regulatory T cells provides an important additional avenue for testing therapeutics in the NOD mouse and eventually man.

ACKNOWLEDGMENT

This work is supported by grants from the National Institutes of Health (DK55969), the NIH Autoimmunity Prevention Center (2U19A1050864), the Diabetes Endocrine Research Center grant from the National Institute of Diabetes and Digestive and Kidney Diseases (P30 DK57516), the American Diabetes Association, the Juvenile Diabetes Foundation (1-2006-16 and 4-2007-1056), the Brehm coalition and the Children's Diabetes Foundation. Li Zhang is supported by a fellowship grant from the Juvenile Diabetes Foundation (3-2008-107) and an ADA postdoctoral fellowship (7-06-MN-17).

REFERENCES

1. Yang Y, Santamaria P. Lessons on autoimmune diabetes from animal models. Clin Sci (Lond). 2006; 110:627–639.
2. Anderson MS, Bluestone JA. The NOD mouse: a model of immune dysregulation. Annu Rev Immunol. 2005; 23:447–485.
3. Chatenoud L, Bach JF. Regulatory T cells in the control of autoimmune diabetes: the case of the NOD mouse. Int Rev Immunol. 2005; 24:247–267.
4. Shoda LK, Young DL, Ramanujan S, Whiting CC, Atkinson MA, Bluestone JA, Eisenbarth

GS, Mathis D, Rossini AA, Campbell SE, Kahn R, Kreuwel HT. A comprehensive review of interventions in the NOD mouse and implications for translation. Immunity. 2005; 23:115–126.
5. Braley-Mullen H, Sharp GC, Medling B, Tang H. Spontaneous autoimmune thyroiditis in NOD.H-2h4 mice. J Autoimmun. 1999; 12:157–165.
6. Bour-Jordan H, Thompson HL, Bluestone JA. Distinct effector mechanisms in the development of autoimmune neuropathy versus diabetes in nonobese diabetic mice. J Immunol. 2005; 175:5649–5655.
7. Salomon B, Rhee L, Bour-Jordan H, Hsin H, Montag A, Soliven B, Arcella J, Girvin AM, Miller SD, Bluestone JA. Development of spontaneous autoimmune peripheral polyneuropathy in b7-2-deficient nod mice. J Exp Med. 2001; 194:677–684.
8. Chatenoud L, Bluestone JA. CD3-specific antibodies: a portal to the treatment of autoimmunity. Nat Rev Immunol. 2007; 7:622–632.
9. Roep BO. Are insights gained from NOD mice sufficient to guide clinical translation? Another inconvenient truth. Ann N Y Acad Sci. 2007; 1103:1–10.
10. Serreze DV, Gaskins HR, Leiter EH. Defects in the differentiation and function of antigen presenting cells in NOD/Lt mice. J Immunol. 1993; 150:2534–2543.
11. Hattori M, Buse JB, Jackson RA, Glimcher L, Dorf ME, Minami M, Makino S, Moriwaki K, Korff M, Kuzuya H, Imura H, Seidman JG, Eisenbarth GS. The NOD mouse: recessive diabetogenic gene within the major histocompatibility complex. Science. 1986; 231:733–735.
12. Fujisawa T, Ikegami H, Noso S, Yamaji K, Nojima K, Babaya N, Itoi-Babaya M, Hiromine Y, Kobayashi M, Makino S, Ogihara T. MHC-linked susceptibility to type 1 diabetes in the NOD mouse: further localization of Idd16 by subcongenic analysis. Ann N Y Acad Sci. 2006; 1079:118–121.
13. Todd JA, Acha-Orbea H, Bell JI, Chao N, Fronek Z, Jacob CO, McDermott M, Sinha AA, Timmerman L, Steinman L, McDevitt HO. A molecular basis for MHC class II associated autoimmunity. Science. 1988; 240:1003–1009.
14. Todd JA, Bell JI, McDevitt HO. A molecular basis for genetic susceptibility to insulin dependent diabetes mellitus. Trends Genet. 1988; 4:129–134.
15. Corper AL, Stratmann T, Apostolopoulos V, Scott CA, Garcia KC, Kang AS, Wilson IA, Teyton L. A structural framework for deciphering the link between I-Ag7 and autoimmune diabetes. Science. 2000; 288:505–511.
16. Kanagawa O, Shimizu J, Unanue ER. The role of I-A^{g7} b chain in peptide binding and antigen recognition by T cells. Int Immunol. 1998; 9:1523–1526.
17. Suri A, Unanue ER. The murine diabetogenic class II histocompatibility molecule I-A(g7): structural and functional properties and specificity of peptide selection. Adv Immunol. 2005; 88:235–265.
18. Levisetti MG, Lewis DM, Suri A, Unanue ER. Weak proinsulin peptide-major histocompatibility complexes are targeted in autoimmune diabetes in mice. Diabetes. 2008; 57:1852–1860.
19. Levisetti MG, Suri A, Petzold SJ, Unanue ER. The insulin-specific T cells of nonobese diabetic mice recognize a weak MHC-binding segment in more than one form. J Immunol. 2007; 178:6051–6057.
20. Homann D, Eisenbarth GS. An immunologic homunculus for type 1 diabetes. J Clin Invest. 2006; 116:1212–1215.
21. Moriyama H, Abiru N, Paronen J, Sikora K, Liu E, Miao D, Devendra D, Beilke J, Gianani R, Gill RG, Eisenbarth GS. Evidence for a primary islet autoantigen (preproinsulin 1) for insulitis and diabetes in the nonobese diabetic mouse. Proc Natl Acad Sci U S A. 2003; 100:10376–10381.
22. Boulard O, Damotte D, Deruytter N, Fluteau G, Carnaud C, Garchon HJ. An interval tightly linked to but distinct from the h2 complex controls both overt diabetes (idd16) and chronic experimental autoimmune thyroiditis (ceat1) in nonobese diabetic mice. Diabetes. 2002; 51:2141–2147.
23. Aoki CA, Borchers AT, Ridgway WM, Keen CL, Ansari AA, Gershwin ME. NOD mice and autoimmunity. Autoimmun Rev. 2005; 4:373–379.
24. Chen YG, Silveira PA, Osborne MA, Chapman HD, Serreze DV. Cellular expression requirements for inhibition of type 1 diabetes by a dominantly protective major histocompatibility complex haplotype. Diabetes. 2007; 56:424–430.
25. Reifsnyder PC, Li R, Silveira PA, Churchill G, Serreze DV, Leiter EH. Conditioning the genome identifies additional diabetes resistance loci in Type I diabetes resistant NOR/Lt mice. Genes Immun. 2005; 6:528–538.
26. Inoue K, Ikegami H, Fujisawa T, Noso S, Nojima K, Babaya N, Itoi-Babaya M, Makimo S, Ogihara T. Allelic variation in class I K gene as candidate for a second component of

MHC-linked susceptibility to type 1 diabetes in non-obese diabetic mice. Diabetologia. 2004; 47:739–747.
27. Leiter EH. Nonobese diabetic mice and the genetics of diabetes susceptibility. Curr Diab Rep. 2005; 5:141–148.
28. Pomerleau DP, Bagley RJ, Serreze DV, Mathews CE, Leiter EH. Major histocompatibility complex-linked diabetes susceptibility in NOD/Lt mice: subcongenic analysis localizes a component of Idd16 at the H2-D end of the diabetogenic H2(g7) complex. Diabetes. 2005; 54:1603–1606.
29. Hamilton-Williams EE, Serreze DV, Charlton B, Johnson EA, Marron MP, Mullbacher A, Slattery RM. Transgenic rescue implicates beta2-microglobulin as a diabetes susceptibility gene in nonobese diabetic (NOD) mice. Proc Natl Acad Sci U S A. 2001; 98:11533–11538.
30. Yamanouchi J, Rainbow D, Serra P, Howlett S, Hunter K, Garner VE, Gonzalez-Munoz A, Clark J, Veijola R, Cubbon R, Chen SL, Rosa R, Cumiskey AM, Serreze DV, Gregory S, Rogers J, Lyons PA, Healy B, Smink LJ, Todd JA, Peterson LB, Wicker LS, Santamaria P. Interleukin-2 gene variation impairs regulatory T cell function and causes autoimmunity. Nat Genet. 2007; 39(3):329–337.
31. Bluestone JA. Is CTLA-4 a master switch for peripheral T cell tolerance? J Immunol. 1997; 158:1989–1993.
32. Hunter K, Rainbow D, Plagnol V, Todd JA, Peterson LB, Wicker LS. Interactions between Idd5.1/Ctla4 and other type 1 diabetes genes. J Immunol. 2007; 179:8341–8349.
33. Lenschow DJ, Herold KC, Rhee L, Patel B, Koons A, Qin HY, Fuchs E, Singh B, Thompson CB, Bluestone JA. CD28/B7 regulation of Th1 and Th2 subsets in the development of autoimmune diabetes. Immunity. 1996; 5:285–293.
34. Bergman ML, Cilio CM, Penha-Goncalves C, Lamhamedi-Cherradi SE, Lofgren A, Colucci F, Lejon K, Garchon HJ, Holmberg D. CTLA-4−/− mice display T cell-apoptosis resistance resembling that ascribed to autoimmune-prone non-obese diabetic (NOD) mice. J Autoimmun. 2001; 16:105–113.
35. Burton PR, Clayton DG, Cardon LR, Craddock N, Deloukas P, Duncanson A, Kwiatkowski DP, McCarthy MI, Ouwehand WH, Samani NJ, Todd JA, Donnelly P, Barrett JC, Davison D, Easton D, Evans DM, Leung HT, Marchini JL, Morris AP, Spencer CC, Tobin MD, Attwood AP, Boorman JP, Cant B, Everson U, Hussey JM, Jolley JD, Knight AS, Koch K, Meech E, Nutland S, Prowse CV, Stevens HE, Taylor NC, Walters GR, Walker NM, Watkins NA, Winzer T, Jones RW, McArdle WL, Ring SM, Strachan DP, Pembrey M, Breen G, St Clair D, Caesar S, Gordon-Smith K, Jones L, Fraser C, Green EK, Grozeva D, Hamshere ML, Holmans PA, Jones IR, Kirov G, Moskivina V, Nikolov I, O'donovan MC, Owen MJ, Collier DA, Elkin A, Farmer A, Williamson R, McGuffin P, Young AH, Ferrier IN, Ball SG, Balmforth AJ, Barrett JH, Bishop TD, Iles MM, Maqbool A, Yuldasheva N, Hall AS, Braund PS, Dixon RJ, Mangino M, Stevens S, Thompson JR, Bredin F, Tremelling M, Parkes M, Drummond H, Lees CW, Nimmo ER, Satsangi J, Fisher SA, Forbes A, Lewis CM, Onnie CM, Prescott NJ, Sanderson J, Matthew CG, Barbour J, Mohiuddin MK, Todhunter CE, Mansfield JC, Ahmad T, Cummings FR, Jewell DP, Webster J, Brown MJ, Lathrop MG, Connell J, Dominiczak A, Marcano CA, Burke B, Dobson R, Gungadoo J, Lee KL, Munroe PB, Newhouse SJ, Onipinla A, Wallace C, Xue M, Caulfield M, Farrall M, Barton A, Bruce IN, Donovan H, Eyre S, Gilbert PD, Hilder SL, Hinks AM, John SL, Potter C, Silman AJ, Symmons DP, Thomson W, Worthington J, Dunger DB, Widmer B, Frayling TM, Freathy RM, Lango H, Perry JR, Shields BM, Weedon MN, Hattersley AT, Hitman GA, Walker M, Elliott KS, Groves CJ, Lindgren CM, Rayner NW, Timpson NJ, Zeggini E, Newport M, Sirugo G, Lyons E, Vannberg F, Hill AV, Bradbury LA, Farrar C, Pointon JJ, Wordsworth P, Brown MA, Franklyn JA, Heward JM, Simmonds MJ, Gough SC, Seal S, Stratton MR, Rahman N, Ban M, Goris A, Sawcer SJ, Compston A, Conway D, Jallow M, Newport M, Sirugo G, Rockett KA, Bumpstead SJ, Chaney A, Downes K, Ghori MJ, Gwilliam R, Hunt SE, Inouye M, Keniry A, King E, McGinnis R, Potter S, Ravindrarajah R, Whittaker P, Widden C, Withers D, Cardin NJ, Davison D, Ferreira T, Pereira-Gale J, Hallgrimsdo'ttir IB, Howie BN, Su Z, Teo YY, Vukcevic D, Bentley D, Brown MA, Compston A, Farrall M, Hall AS, Hattersley AT, Hill AV, Parkes M, Pembrey M, Stratton MR, Mitchell SL, Newby PR, Brand OJ, Carr-Smith J, Pearce SH, McGinnis R, Keniry A, Deloukas P, Reveille JD, Zhou X, Sims AM, Dowling A, Taylor J, Doan T, Davis JC, Savage L, Ward MM, Learch TL, Weisman MH, Brown M. Association scan of 14,500 nonsynonymous SNPs in four diseases identifies autoimmunity variants. Nat Genet. 2007; 39:1329–1337.
36. Barratt BJ, Payne F, Lowe CE, Hermann R, Healy BC, Harold D, Concannon P, Gharani N, McCarthy MI, Olavesen MG, McCormack

R, Guja C, Ionescu-Tirgoviste C, Undlien DE, Ronningen KS, Gillespie KM, Tuomilehto-Wolf E, Tuomilehto J, Bennett ST, Clayton DG, Cordell HJ, Todd JA. Remapping the Insulin Gene/IDDM2 Locus in Type 1 Diabetes. Diabetes. 2004; 53:1884–1889.

37. Thebault-Baumont K, Dubois-LaForgue D, Krief P, Briand JP, Halbout P, Vallon-Geoffroy K, Morin J, Laloux V, Lehuen A, Carel JC, Jami J, Muller S, Boitard C. Acceleration of type 1 diabetes mellitus in proinsulin 2-deficient NOD mice. J Clin Invest. 2003; 111:851–857.

38. Pugliese A, Zeller M, Fernandez A, Zalcberg LJ, Bartlett RJ, Ricordi C, Pietropaolo M, Eisenbarth GS, Bennett ST, Patel DD: The insulin gene is transcribed in the human thymus and transcription levels correlate with allelic variation at the INS VNTR-IDDM2 susceptibility locus for type I diabetes. Nat Genet. 1997; 15:293–297.

39. Shultz LD, Schweitzer PA, Christianson SW, Gott B, Schweitzer IB, Tennent B, McKenna S, Mobraaten L, Rajan TV, Greiner DL. Multiple defects in innate and adaptive immunologic function in NOD/LtSz-scid mice. J Immunol. 1995; 154:180–191.

40. Laloux V, Beaudoin L, Jeske D, Carnaud C, Lehuen A. NK T cell-induced protection against diabetes in V alpha 14-J alpha 281 transgenic nonobese diabetic mice is associated with a Th2 shift circumscribed regionally to the islets and functionally to islet autoantigen. J Immunol. 2001; 166:3749–3756.

41. Peng RH, Paek E, Xia CQ, Tennyson N, Clare-Salzler MJ. Heightened interferon-alpha/beta response causes myeloid cell dysfunction and promotes T1D pathogenesis in NOD mice. Ann N Y Acad Sci. 2006; 1079:99–102.

42. Nikolic T, Bunk M, Drexhage HA, Leenen PJ. Bone marrow precursors of nonobese diabetic mice develop into defective macrophage-like dendritic cells in vitro. J Immunol. 2004; 173:4342–4351.

43. Ogasawara K, Hamerman JA, Hsin H, Chikuma S, Bour-Jordan H, Chen T, Pertel T, Carnaud C, Bluestone JA, Lanier LL. Impairment of NK cell function by NKG2D modulation in NOD mice. Immunity. 2003; 18:41–51.

44. Carnaud C, Gombert J, Donnars O, Garchon H, Herbelin A. Protection against diabetes and improved NK/NKT cell performance in NOD.NK1.1 mice congenic at the NK complex. J Immunol. 2001; 166:2404–2411.

45. Poulton LD, Smyth MJ, Hawke CG, Silveira P, Shepherd D, Naidenko OV, Godfrey DI, Baxter AG. Cytometric and functional analyses of NK and NKT cell deficiencies in NOD mice. Int Immunol. 2001; 13:887–896.

46. Poirot L, Benoist C, Mathis D. Natural killer cells distinguish innocuous and destructive forms of pancreatic islet autoimmunity. Proc Natl Acad Sci U S A. 2004; 101:8102–8107.

47. Serreze DV, Fleming SA, Chapman HD, Richard SD, Leiter EH, Tisch RM. B lymphocytes are critical antigen-presenting cells for the initiation of T cell-mediated autoimmune diabetes in nonobese diabetic mice. J Immunol. 1998; 161:3912–3918.

48. Greeley SA, Katsumata M, Yu L, Eisenbarth GS, Moore DJ, Goodarzi H, Barker CF, Naji A, Noorchashm H. Elimination of maternally transmitted autoantibodies prevents diabetes in nonobese diabetic mice. Nat Med. 2002; 8:399–402.

49. Hu CY, Rodriguez-Pinto D, Du W, Ahuja A, Henegariu O, Wong FS, Shlomchik MJ, Wen L. Treatment with CD20-specific antibody prevents and reverses autoimmune diabetes in mice. J Clin Invest. 2007; 117:3857–3867.

50. Kobayashi M, Jasinski J, Liu E, Li M, Miao D, Zhang L, Yu L, Nakayama M, Eisenbarth GS. Conserved T cell receptor alpha-chain induces insulin autoantibodies. Proc Natl Acad Sci U S A. 2008; 105:10090–10094.

51. Abiru N, Yu L, Miao D, Maniatis AK, Liu E, Moriyama H, Eisenbarth GS. Transient insulin autoantibody expression independent of development of diabetes: comparison of NOD and NOR strains. J Autoimmun. 2001; 17:1–6.

52. DiLorenzo TP, Serreze DV. The good turned ugly: immunopathogenic basis for diabetogenic CD8+ T cells in NOD mice. Immunol Rev. 2005; 204:250–263.

53. DiLorenzo TP, Lieberman SM, Takaki T, Honda S, Chapman HD, Santamaria P, Serreze DV, Nathenson SG. During the early prediabetic period in NOD mice, the pathogenic CD8(+) T-cell population comprises multiple antigenic specificities. Clin Immunol. 2002; 105:332–341.

54. Lieberman SM, Takaki T, Han B, Santamaria P, Serreze DV, DiLorenzo TP. Individual nonobese diabetic mice exhibit unique patterns of CD8+ T cell reactivity to three islet antigens, including the newly identified widely expressed dystrophia myotonica kinase. J Immunol. 2004; 173:6727–6734.

55. Lieberman SM, DiLorenzo TP. A comprehensive guide to antibody and T-cell responses in type 1 diabetes. Tissue Antigens. 2003; 62:359–377.

56. Han B, Serra P, Yamanouchi J, Amrani A, Elliott JF, Dickie P, DiLorenzo TP, Santamaria

57. Kim SK, Tarbell KV, Sanna M, Vadeboncoeur M, Warganich T, Lee M, Davis M, McDevitt HO. Prevention of type I diabetes transfer by glutamic acid decarboxylase 65 peptide 206-220-specific T cells. Proc Natl Acad Sci U S A. 2004; 101:14204–14209.
58. Gebe JA, Unrath KA, Yue BB, Miyake T, Falk BA, Nepom GT. Autoreactive human T-cell receptor initiates insulitis and impaired glucose tolerance in HLA DR4 transgenic mice. J Autoimmun. 2008; 30:197–206.
59. Krishnamurthy B, Dudek NL, McKenzie MD, Purcell AW, Brooks AG, Gellert S, Colman PG, Harrison LC, Lew AM, Thomas HE, Kay TW. Responses against islet antigens in NOD mice are prevented by tolerance to proinsulin but not IGRP. J Clin Invest. 2006; 116:3258–3265.
60. West J, Logan RF, Card TR, Smith C, Hubbard R. Fracture risk in people with celiac disease: a population-based cohort study. Gastroenterology. 2003; 125:429–436.
61. Nakayama M, Abiru N, Moriyama H, Babaya N, Liu E, Miao D, Yu L, Wegmann DR, Hutton JC, Elliott JF, Eisenbarth GS. Prime role for an insulin epitope in the development of type 1 diabetes in NOD mice. Nature. 2005; 435:220–223.
62. Nakayama M, Beilke JN, Jasinski JM, Kobayashi M, Miao D, Li M, Coulombe MG, Liu E, Elliott JF, Gill RG, Eisenbarth GS. Priming and effector dependence on insulin B:9-23 peptide in NOD islet autoimmunity. J Clin Invest. 2007; 117:1835–1843.
63. Burton AR, Vincent E, Arnold PY, Lennon GP, Smeltzer M, Li CS, Haskins K, Hutton J, Tisch RM, Sercarz EE, Santamaria P, Workman CJ, Vignali DA. On the pathogenicity of autoantigen-specific T-cell receptors. Diabetes. 2008; 57:1321–1330.
64. Hansson T, Dahlbom I, Rogberg S, Nyberg BI, Dahlstrom J, Anneren G, Klareskog L, Dannaeus A. Antitissue transglutaminase and antithyroid autoantibodies in children with Down syndrome and celiac disease. J Pediatr Gastroenterol Nutr. 2005; 40:170–174.
65. Hoglund P, Mintern J, Waltzinger C, Heath W, Benoist C, Mathis D. Initiation of autoimmune diabetes by developmentally regulated presentation of islet cell antigens in the pancreatic lymph nodes. J Exp Med. 1999; 189:331–339.
66. Tritt M, Sgouroudis E, d'Hennezel E, Albanese A, Piccirillo CA. Functional waning of naturally occurring CD4+ regulatory T-cells contributes to the onset of autoimmune diabetes. 2008; Diabetes 57:113–123.
67. Hutchings PR, Cooke A. The transfer of autoimmune diabetes in NOD mice can be inhibited or accelerated by distinct cell populations present in normal splenocytes taken from young males. J Autoimmun. 1990; 3:175–185.
68. Lepault F, Gagnerault MC. Characterization of peripheral regulatory CD4+ T cells that prevent diabetes onset in nonobese diabetic mice. J Immunol. 2000; 164:240–247.
69. Fontenot JD, Rudensky AY. A well adapted regulatory contrivance: regulatory T cell development and the forkhead family transcription factor Foxp3. Nat Immunol. 2005; 6:331–337.
70. Fontenot JD, Gavin MA, Rudensky AY. Foxp3 programs the development and function of CD4+CD25+ regulatory T cells. Nat Immunol. 2003; 4:330–336.
71. Chen Z, Herman AE, Matos M, Mathis D, Benoist C. Where CD4+CD25+ T reg cells impinge on autoimmune diabetes. J Exp Med. 2005; 202:1387–1397.
72. Masteller EL, Warner MR, Tang Q, Tarbell KV, McDevitt H, Bluestone JA. Expansion of functional endogenous antigen-specific CD4+CD25+ regulatory T cells from nonobese diabetic mice. J Immunol. 2005; 175:3053–3059.
73. Tang Q, Henriksen KJ, Bi M, Finger EB, Szot G, Ye J, Masteller EL, McDevitt H, Bonyhadi M, Bluestone JA. In vitro-expanded antigen-specific regulatory T cells suppress autoimmune diabetes. J Exp Med 2004; 199:1455–1465.
74. Mukherjee R, Chaturvedi P, Qin HY, Singh B. CD4+CD25+ regulatory T cells generated in response to insulin B:9-23 peptide prevent adoptive transfer of diabetes by diabetogenic T cells. J Autoimmun. 2003; 21:221–237.
75. Billiard F, Litvinova E, Saadoun D, Djelti F, Klatzmann D, Cohen JL, Marodon G, Salomon BL. Regulatory and effector T cell activation levels are prime determinants of in vivo immune regulation. J Immunol. 2006; 177:2167–2174.
76. King M, Pearson T, Shultz LD, Leif J, Bottino R, Trucco M, Atkinson M, Wasserfall C, Herold K, Mordes JP, Rossini AA, Greiner DL. Development of new-generation HU-PBMC-NOD/SCID mice to study human islet alloreactivity. Ann N Y Acad Sci. 2007; 1103:90–93.
77. Pearson T, Greiner DL, Shultz LD. Creation of "humanized" mice to study human immunity. Curr Protoc Immunol 2008 Chapter 15:Unit 15.21.

78. Wegmann DR, Norbury-Glaser M, Daniel D. Insulin-specific T cells are a predominant component of islet infiltrates in pre-diabetic NOD mice. Eur J Immunol. 1994; 24:1853–1857.
79. Simone E, Daniel D, Schloot N, Gottlieb P, Babu S, Kawasaki E, Wegmann D, Eisenbarth GS. T cell receptor restriction of diabetogenic autoimmune NOD T cells. Proc Natl Acad Sci USA. 1997; 94:2518–2521.
80. Ochs HD, Gambineri E, Torgerson TR. IPEX, FOXP3 and regulatory T-cells: a model for autoimmunity. Immunol Res. 2007; 38:112–121.
81. Ludvigsson J, Faresjo M, Hjorth M, Axelsson S, Cheramy M, Pihl M, Vaarala O, Forsander G, Ivarsson S, Johansson C, Lindh A, Nilsson NO, Aman J, Ortqvist E, Zerhouni P, Casas R. GAD Treatment and insulin secretion in recent-onset type 1 diabetes. N Engl J Med. 2008; 359(18):1909–1920.
82. Herold KC, Gitelman SE, Masharani U, Hagopian W, Bisikirska B, Donaldson D, Rother K, Diamond B, Harlan DM, Bluestone JA. A single course of anti-CD3 monoclonal antibody hOKT3{gamma}1(Ala-Ala) results in improvement in C-peptide responses and clinical parameters for at least 2 years after onset of type 1 diabetes. Diabetes. 2005; 54:1763–1769.
83. Bresson D, Togher L, Rodrigo E, Chen YL, Bluestone JA, Herold KC, von Herrath M. Anti-CD3 and nasal proinsulin combination therapy enhances remission from recent-onset autoimmune diabetes by inducing Tregs. Journal of Clinical Investigation. 2006; 116:1371–1381.
84. Roep BO, Atkinson M, von Herrath M. Satisfaction (not) guaranteed: re-evaluating the use of animal models of type 1 diabetes. Nat Rev Immunol. 2004; 4:989–997.

Chapter 13

Virus-Induced Type 1 Diabetes in the Rat

Travis R. Wolter and Danny Zipris

Summary

Evidence from epidemiological studies suggests that the mechanism of type 1 diabetes (T1D) involves environmental factors and viral infections, in particular. Data establishing a direct link between microbial infections and diabetes and demonstrating how viruses lead to disease onset in humans are currently lacking. Rat models of diabetes have recently emerged as powerful experimental tools for examining the role of pathogens in disease mechanisms. Studies conducted in the biobreeding diabetes-resistant (BBDR) and LEW1.WR1 rats show that infection with a parvovirus, designated Kilham rat virus (KRV), leads to islet inflammation and diabetes in a portion of infected animals via mechanisms that involve upregulation of the innate immune system. Indeed, KRV acts as a TLR9 agonist triggering a robust proinflammatory response in pancreatic lymph nodes of infected animals; inflammation that correlates with disease onset and involves the upregulation of a vast array of proinflammatory cytokines and chemokines. Data from the BBDR rat also show that innate immune system activation prior to virus infection induces a dramatic increase in the incidence of diabetes and precipitates disease induced by virus titers that are otherwise nondiabetogenic. The exact role of the innate immune system in virus-induced diabetes is not yet clear; however, it is postulated to involve tipping the balance between autoreactive T lymphocytes and regulatory T cells. Collectively, the available data underscore the opposing roles that the innate immune system plays in recognizing and eliminating invading pathogens and at the same time, under some circumstances, promoting autoimmunity against pancreatic islets.

Key Words: Type 1 diabetes, Parvovirus, Kilham rat virus, Pancreatic islets, Biobreeding diabetes-resistant rat, LEW1.WR1 rat, Autoimmunity, Toll-like receptor, Innate immunity, Inflammation, T regulatory cells

TYPE 1 DIABETES

Type 1 diabetes (T1D) is a T-cell-mediated organ-specific autoimmune disease that results from a specific reaction against islet beta cells (*1*). The disease affects primarily young children (*2*) and is thought to involve in some cases a slow and progressive loss of insulin secretion (*3*). The knowledge about mechanisms triggering islet destruction is limited; however, emerging data indicate that islet beta cell death is associated with pancreatic infiltration of immune cells, including CD8 and CD4 T cells, B lymphocytes, macrophages, and dendritic cells (DCs) (4).

THE BIOBREEDING AND LEW1.WR1 RAT MODELS OF DIABETES

There are two inbred strains of BB rats, the diabetes-prone BB (BBDP) and diabetes-resistant BB (BBDR) strains, and rats of both sexes develop diabetes with characteristics similar to the human disease (5, 6). The BBDP rat is highly deficient of T lymphocytes due to a mutation in the gene encoding the mitochondrial membrane protein Ian4 (7). This animal develops spontaneous disease between 55 and 110 days of age, and the transfer of spleen cells from normal MHC compatible to young BBDP rats can prevent the autoimmune process (8). Unlike BBDP, BBDR rats have normal levels and function of circulating T cells (6, 9), and spontaneous diabetes does not occur in viral antibody-free BBDR rats (10). However, islet inflammation, diabetes, and severe ketosis occur in nearly 100% of animals upon upregulation of the innate immune system with Poly(I:C) plus depletion of regulatory ART2+ T cells (see Table 13.1) (10) or following virus infection (see Fig. 13.1) (11). The disease in the BBDR rat is thought to be immune mediated, and one of the main observations supporting this hypothesis is that the transfer of lymph nodes from diabetic animals to RT1^u MHC compatible T-cell deficient WAG nu/nu rats can lead to disease onset (12).

Another useful animal model in studying the role of the environment in diabetes is the LEW1.WR1 rat. This animal has normal levels and function of T lymphocytes (13). Unlike the BBDR rat, there are reports that ~2% of both male and female rats develop spontaneous disease between the ages of 49 and 86 days in viral antibody-free environment (13). The LEW1.WR1 rat has a higher degree of disease penetrance compared with that of BBDR rats as evidenced by the finding that depletion of regulatory ART2.1+ cells by itself can induce diabetes (13). As seen in the BBDR rat, KRV infection leads to diabetes characterized by selective loss of islet beta cells, glycosuria, ketonuria, and polyuria in the LEW1.WR1 rat (10, 13).

KILHAM RAT PARVOVIRUS AND DIABETES INDUCTION

KRV is an environmentally ubiquitous rat virus that belongs to the family of *Parvoviridea*, a group of small single-stranded DNA viruses with an average genome size of 5 kbp encapsulated by

Table 13.1
KRV- and TLR-Induced Diabetes in Rat Models of Diabetes

Strain	MHC (RT1 haplotype A, B/D, C)	Method of diabetes induction	Endogenous TLR pathways involved in diabetes	Exogenously activated TLRs	Effect of exogenous TLR activation on diabetes	References
BBDR	RT1$^{u/u/u}$	Virus infection	TLR9	–	–	(40, 45)
		Virus infection plus TLR upregulation	TLR9	TLR2, TLR3, TLR4, TLR7/8, or TLR9	Exacerbation	(40, 45)
		TLR upregulation	–	TLR3 (high doses of TLR ligand)	De novo induction	(57)
		TLR upregulation plus ART2.1 cell depletion	–	TLR3	De novo induction	(67)
LEW.1R1	RT1$^{u/u/a}$	Spontaneous in a small portion of animals in virus-free antibody environment	Unknown	–	–	(17, 58)
		Virus infection	TLR9?	–	De novo induction?	(10)
		Virus infection plus TLR upregulation	TLR9?	TLR3	Exacerbation	(13)
Wistar Furth	RT1$^{u/u/u}$	TLR upregulation		TLR3	De novo induction	Ref. (17) and unpublished observations
PVG.RT1^u	RT1$^{u/u/u}$	TLR upregulation	–	TLR3	De novo induction	(10, 17)
WAG	RT1$^{u/u/u}$	TLR upregulation	–	TLR3	De novo induction	(17)
BBDP	RT1$^{u/u/u}$	Spontaneous	Unknown	–	–	(8)
		TLR upregulation	–	TLR3	Exacerbation	(56, 68)
		TLR upregulation	–	TLR3	Prevention (low dose)	(54)

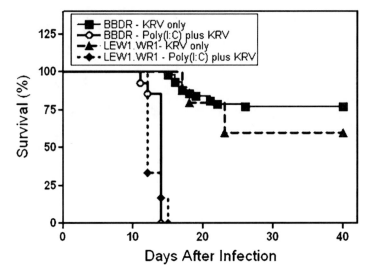

Fig. 13.1 Kaplan Meier analysis of diabetes in BBDR and LEW1.WR1 rats treated with KRV and purified TLR agonists plus KRV. Groups of BBDR and LEW1.WR1 rats 22–25 days were injected with 1×10^7 PFU of KRV only, or 1-3 µg/g body weight of Poly(I:C) on three consecutive days, followed by infection with 1×10^7 PFU of KRV. Animals were tested for diabetes and disease was defined as the presence of a plasma glucose concentration >250 mg/dl (11.1 mM/L) on two consecutive days. The incidence of diabetes in rats injected with TLR agonists plus KRV was significantly higher than in animals treated with KRV only ($p < 0.05$ using the log rank test). Animals administered with 1–3 µg/g body weight of Poly(I:C) only did not develop diabetes.

protein in an icosahedral nonenveloped particle (*14*). This virus group infects several animal species, including rodents (*15*) and humans (*16*). KRV, H-1, and the recently described rat parvovirus-1 (RPV-1, formerly designated orphan parvovirus) are the three autonomous parvoviruses that infect rats (*15*). KRV encodes three overlapping structural proteins, VP1, VP2, and VP3, and two overlapping nonstructural proteins, NS1 and NS2 (*15*). Infection with KRV leads to insulitis, islet destruction, and diabetes in BBDR and LEW1.WR1, but not in other rat strains (Table 13.1) (*10, 17*). H-1 parvovirus is a close homolog of KRV; H-1 and KRV VP proteins are ~80% homologous, whereas their NS proteins are 100% homologous. Infection of BBDR rats with H-1 with or without pretreatment with Poly(I:C) does not lead to diabetes (*18*).

Susceptibility to virus-induced diabetes is dependent on the presence of class I A^u and class II B/D^u expressed in BBDR, LEW1.WR1, and PVG.RT1^u rats (*10, 17*). The RT1^u haplotype, however, is not sufficient for diabetes development, as Wistar Furth rats express RT1^u, but are resistant to KRV-induced diabetes. Infection of PVG.R8 (A^a B/D^u C^u), PVG.R23 (A^u B/D^a C^a), and Lewis (A^l B/D^l C^l) rats with KRV does not lead to disease onset (Table 13.1) (*10*). Depletion of regulatory ART2.1+ T cells in conjunction with virus infection increases the incidence of diabetes in BBDR and LEW1.WR1, but not PVG.RT1^u or other rats (Table 13.1)

(*10, 17*). Disease triggered by KRV is T-cell-mediated since islet destruction is prevented by a treatment with antibodies directed against the T-cell receptor, CD5, and CD8 (*10, 17*), and the transfer of spleen cells from virus-infected BBDR rats to class II^u compatible rats adoptively transfer insulitis and diabetes (*10, 17*).

PARVOVIRUSES AND AUTOIMMUNITY IN HUMANS

There are currently two members of the *Parvoviridea* family known to be pathogenic in humans (*19*). Parvovirus B19 was identified in 1974 in human sera (*20*), and bocavirus was found in 2005 in the respiratory tract of children (*21*). Parvovirus B19 is a small nonenveloped icosahedral virus composed of only two capsid proteins and a single-stranded linear 5.6 kbp DNA genome (*22*). The two structural capsid proteins, VP1 (83 kDa) and VP2 (58 kDa), are encoded by overlapping reading frames (*23, 24*). VP2, the major constituent of the B19 capsid (90% of the 60 proteins that make up the capsid are composed of VP2), is contained within VP1 but lacks the 227 amino acid residues from the N-terminus. VP1 contains a domain that interacts with the cellular receptor, while VP2 is involved in recognition by neutralizing antibodies (*25*).

There is no evidence linking parvovirus infection with T1D in humans. However, there are reports that human parvovirus B19 is associated with inflammatory autoimmune diseases such as acute myocarditis (*26, 27*), rheumatoid arthritis (*25*), systemic lupus erythematosus (*28*), Sjögren's syndrome, and a series of other autoimmune disorders (*25*). Infection with B19 was linked with the appearance of elevated levels of autoantibodies against nuclear antigens and double-stranded DNA (*25*), and it was postulated that disease mechanisms involve STAT-3-induced upregulation of proinflammatory cytokines (*29*).

HUMORAL AND CELLULAR IMMUNITY TO KRV IN THE BBDR RAT

Both KRV and the homologous H-1 parvovirus induce similar levels of adaptive immune responses; the potential role of these responses in diabetes in the BBDR rat is currently unknown. BBDR rats infected with either KRV or H-1 develop a robust humoral immune response by day 14 following infection (*30*). Infection with H-1 generates Abs that cross-react only minimally with KRV, whereas infection with KRV generates Abs with no cross-reactivity with H-1 (*30*). Because of the complete homology in the NS sequence between KRV and H-1, these observations may imply that antibodies induced in the BBDR rat against KRV recognize different epitopes expressed in the VP region.

Both KRV and H-1 induce anti-KRV CD8+IFN-γ+ cells in the spleen and peripheral blood from BBDR rats that are CD4−TCRab+ and NKR-P1A+30. These virus-specific T cells are detectable by day 11 following virus infection and cross-react with each other (30).

KRV-INDUCED TREG DOWN-MODULATION

There is increasing evidence from animal models of T1D that CD4+CD25+FoxP3+ natural T regulatory (nTreg) cells play a key role in the development of autoimmune diabetes (30–39). In the BBDR rat, CD4+CD25+FoxP3+ Treg cells comprise ~8% of CD4+ T cells in the spleen and in pancreatic lymph nodes (30), and as observed in the mouse, they express high levels of CD62L (30) and FoxP3, are anergic (30), are capable of suppressing CD4+ effector T cell functions in vitro (30), and block diabetes upon transfer to prediabetic rat recipients (36–38).

CD4+CD25+FoxP3+ were implicated in the mechanism of virus-induced diabetes in the BBDR rat (30, 40, 41). It was suggested that virus infection induces an alteration in the balance between T effector and Treg cells. Infection of BBDR rats with KRV, but not the nondiabetogenic H-1 virus, leads to a reduction of ~50% in the proportion of CD4+CD25+FoxP3+ nTreg cells in the spleen of prediabetic-infected animals following infection (our unpublished data) (30). The association between virus-induced Treg downmodulation and autoimmunity is consistent with reports that microbial infections lead to a reduction in Treg cells in humans (42, 43), and a link between virus-induced Treg downmodulation and autoimmunity was demonstrated in humans with chronic hepatitis C infections (44). Data demonstrating how KRV modulates nTreg cells are still lacking. It can be postulated that the effects of KRV exerted on Treg cells are mediated directly by viral cytotoxicity, or virus-induced TLR upregulation (45, 46), or indirectly through cytokines produced by DCs (47, 48).

THE ROLE OF TLR PATHWAYS IN KRV-INDUCED DIABETES

The innate immune system senses the presence of pathogens via TLRs that recognize structurally conserved molecules expressed by microbes and designated pathogen-associated molecular patterns (PAMPs) expressed by microbes (49–51). The binding of PAMPs to TLRs expressed by B lymphocytes, DCs, and macrophages leads to the expression of proinflammatory cytokines and chemokines, including TNF-α, IL-1, IL-6, IL-12, and CXCL-10, in addition to a maturation program that includes upregulation of MHC molecules and costimulatory molecules on the cell surface of DCs, thereby enhancing their capability to present antigens to T cells (*52, 53*).

Recent data provide support for the involvement of TLR-induced innate immune upregulation in the autoimmune process leading to KRV-induced diabetes in genetically susceptible BBDR rats (*40*). Indeed, it was evident that treating BBDR and LEW1.WR1 rats with different purified agonists of TLRs or heat-killed *Escherichia coli* and *Staphylococcus aureus* that express natural TLR ligands synergizes with KRV infection to increase the incidence of diabetes from ~25–40% in animals treated with virus only to 50–100% in animals pretreated with TLR agonists, depending on the injected TLR ligand (Table 13.1) (*40*). TLR upregulation by itself with doses that in conjunction with KRV exacerbate diabetes does not result in autoimmune diabetes, underscoring the key role of virus infection in disease mechanisms. Virus infection and TLR-induced innate upregulation can also induce diabetes in rat strains other than BBDR and LEW1.WR1 rats, and susceptibility to diabetes is dependent on the expression of MHC Class II^u (Table 13.1) (*17*).

The role of the innate immune system in the mechanism of virus-induced disease is further evident by the observation that injecting BBDR rats with Poly(I:C) precipitates diabetes by virus titers that by themselves are nondiabetogenic (*40*). Finally, KRV itself acts as a TLR9 agonist to induce innate immune responses in vitro in plasmacytoid DCs (pDCs), but not myeloid DCs (mDCs) and B lymphocytes, and in vivo in pancreatic lymph nodes (*40, 45*).

Innate immune upregulation can also lead to diabetes prevention; administration of Poly(I:C) to BBDP rats blocks disease via mechanisms that could involve protective cytokines and regulatory T cells (Table 13.1) (*54*), as was previously reported in the NOD mouse (*55*). High Poly(I:C) doses, however, exacerbate disease development in BBDP rats (Table 13.1) (*56, 57*).

TLR upregulation with or without elimination of regulatory ART2.1+ T cells precipitates autoimmune diabetes in rat strains that do not typically develop spontaneous disease or are not susceptible to the development of virus-induced diabetes (*17, 58*). For example, repeated injections of relatively high doses of Poly(I:C) induce diabetes in WF, WAG, and PVG rats (*17, 58*), with PVG rats the most susceptible to disease induction (*13, 17, 58, 59*). The induction of disease by Poly(I:C) is observed in rat strains expressing Class II^u molecules and is not evident in animals expressing Class II^a or Class II^c (*17*), findings that are compatible with the central role that Class II antigens play in conferring susceptibility to human diabetes (*4, 60*).

TLR signaling pathways were recently implicated in various autoimmune disorders in mouse models (reviewed in *61*). For example, TLR2 and TLR9 were implicated in arthritis, whereas TLR4 and TLR9 were suggested to be involved in the course of experimental allergic encephalomyelitis. Endogenous upregulation of TLR9 pathways was recently linked with the pathogenesis of systemic lupus erythematosus in both humans and animal models of the disease.

The mechanism whereby TLR upregulation leads to diabetes is thought to involve activation of macrophages and CD8$^+$ T cells as well as elevated expression levels of Class I molecules in pancreatic islets (*17*), as previously reported for spontaneous disease in BBDP and KRV-induced disease in BBDR rats (*5, 6, 41, 62*). The disease also correlates with elevated expression of endothelial ICAM-1 and VCAM-1 and infiltration of macrophages and T cells into the pancreatic interstitium (*17*).

KRV-INDUCED PROINFLAMMATORY PATHWAYS IN THE BBDR RAT

The mechanism by which KRV triggers diabetes remains unresolved. It is postulated that proinflammatory responses induced by KRV in pancreatic lymph nodes of BBDR rats are linked with the autoimmune process leading to islet cell death (*40*). This is compatible with the observation that downmodulation of inflammation with chloroquine, an immunosuppressant agent, correlates with reduced diabetes incidence in the BBDR rat (*45*). Recent DNA microarray analyses conducted by us revealed that KRV, but not the homologous H-1 parvovirus, induces profound alterations in the global gene expression profile in pancreatic lymph nodes (Table 13.2 and our unpublished observations). It was observed that KRV induces transcripts for a vast array of proinflammatory chemokines and cytokines, including CXCL-9, CXCL-10, CXCL-11, IL-1α, IL-1β, IL-6, the p40 subunit of IL-12 and IL-23, and IL-18, and genes associated with interferon upregulation and signaling, such as IRF7, STAT-1, and STAT-2 (Table 13.2). The exact role of this proinflammatory reaction in the mechanism of diabetes is not yet clear; however, it could be associated with the upregulation of autoreactive T lymphocytes (*40*). Our microarray results are compatible with previous reports that IL-1β is upregulated in PBMCs from patients with T1D (*63*) and sera from newly diagnosed patients can induce the expression of members of the IL-1 cytokine superfamily in PBMCs from healthy subjects (*64*).

On the basis of the available data, we propose a model for virus-induced diabetes in the rat. This model envisions that infection of BBDR rats with KRV results in TLR-mediated

Table 13.2
DNA Microarray Analysis of Pancreatic Lymph Nodes from KRV-Infected BBDR Rats Groups of Three BBDR Rats 22–25 Days of Age were Left Untreated, or Administered with 1 × 10⁷ PFU of KRV (*40*)

Gene name	Gene function	References	Fold increase
Chemokines			
Chemokine (C–X–C motif) ligand 11 (CXCL-11)	Recruitment of activated T cells	(*69*)	58.1
Chemokine (C–X–C motif) ligand 10 (CXCL-10)	Recruitment of T and NK cells, macrophages, and dendritic cells	(*70*)	31.3
Chemokine (C–X–C motif) ligand 9 (CXCL-9)	T-cell chemoattractant	(*71*)	31.1
Chemokine (C–C motif) ligand 7 (CCL7)	Chemoattractant for monocytes, NK cells, and T cells	(*72*)	8.6
Chemokine (C–C motif) ligand 5 (CCL5)	Chemotactic for T cells, monocytes, eosinophils, and basophils	(*73*)	7.8
Chemokine (C–C motif) receptor 5 (CCR5)	Chemokine receptor expressed on T cells, monocytes, dendritic cells, and NK cells; binds CCL3, CCL4, and CCL5	(*74*)	7.7
Chemokine (C–C motif) ligand 9 (CCL9)	Chemotactic for T lymphocytes	(*75*)	5.5
Chemokine (C motif) ligand 1 (XCL1)	Chemotactic for T cells	(*76*)	3.9
Chemokine (C–C motif) ligand 13 (CCL2)	Attracts memory T cells, macrophages, and dendritic cells	(*77, 78*)	3.5
Cytokines			
Interleukin 1 receptor antagonist (IL-1ra)	Blocks IL-1α/β functions	(*79*)	75.8
Interleukin 1 alpha (IL-1α)	Proinflammatory cytokine; induces Th17 cells; activates both innate and adaptive immune systems	(*80, 81*)	4.3
Interleukin 6 (IL-6)	Induces Th17 cells; regulates innate and adaptive immune activities	(*82, 83*)	4
Interleukin 1 beta (IL-1β)	Proinflammatory cytokine; induces Th17 cells; activates both innate and adaptive immune systems	(*80, 81*)	3.1

(continued)

Table 13.2 (continued)

Gene name	Gene function	References	Fold increase
Interferon pathways			
Interferon gamma (IFN-γ)	Upregulation of Th1 and suppression of Th2 responses; promotes leukocyte migration, antigen presentation via induction of MHC molecules and NK function	(84)	13.6
Interferon regulatory factor 7 (IRF7)	Induces type I interferons	(85)	12.9
Signal transducer and activator of transcription 1 (STAT-1)	Mediation of IFN-α/β and IFN-γ biological activities	(86)	3.7
Signal transducer and activator of transcription 2 (STAT-2)	Mediation of IFN-α/β and IFN-γ biological activities	(86)	2.9

Pancreatic lymph nodes were recovered from animals on day 5 following virus infection. Total RNA was extracted and used for the DNA microarray analysis. Values shown are the fold increase in the expression level of the indicated gene in lymph nodes from KRV-infected rats relative to the expression in control uninfected animals. The p values for all the indicated genes are lower than 0.05

upregulation of proinflammatory cytokines and chemokines in the microenvironment of pancreatic lymph nodes. This proinflammatory response in conjunction with Treg downmodulation induces the recruitment and upregulation of islet-specific autoreactive T cells, leading to islet destruction and diabetes (Fig. 13.2) (45).

GENES INVOLVED IN KRV-INDUCED T1D

Diabetes susceptibility in BBDP and BBDR rats involves the expression of MHC Class II *RT1 B/D* region (*Iddm1*), and the presence of at least one *RT1 B/D^u* allele is required for disease development (65). In addition to *Iddm1*, diabetes in the BBDP rat is strongly linked with *Iddm2* that is a *Gimap5* mutation on chromosome 4 responsible for a T-cell lymphopenia (66), *Iddm3* on chromosome 2, and *Iddm24* on chromosome 8 (66). As shown in Table 13.1, the expression of a class II *RT1 B/D^u* haplotypes confers disease susceptibility in rat strains other than BBDP and BBDR rats (10, 17).

Data from the BBDR rat indicate that in addition to *Iddm1*, other background genes are required for diabetes induced by KRV. Blankenhorn et al. demonstrated that *Iddm4* on chromosome 4 is an obligatory requirement for diabetes induced by a treatment with Poly(I:C) plus ART2.1 depletion (58). However, for diabetes induced by Poly(I:C) plus KRV infection, *Iddm4* was

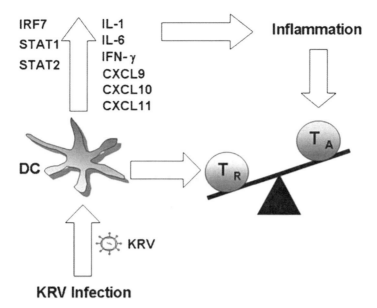

Fig. 13.2 Postulated mechanism of KRV-induced diabetes in the BBDR rat. Infection of BBDR rats with KRV leads to upregulation of the innate immune system in pancreatic lymph nodes, resulting in the expression of a vast array of proinflammatory cytokines and chemokines, including IL-1, IL-6, IFN-γ, CXCL-9, CXCL-10, and CXCL-11, as well as genes involved in interferon induction and signaling, such as IRF7, STAT-1, and STAT-2. This, in conjunction with down-modulation of nTreg cells lead to the upregulation of autoreactive T cells culminating in islet inflammation and destruction. *DC* dendritic cells, T_A T autoreactive, T_R T regulatory.

not sufficient and additional gene locus designated *Iddm20* on chromosome 17 was necessary (*58*).

SUMMARY

Rat models of T1D have proven to be a promising experimental tool in studying the role of the environment in diabetes mechanisms. Data obtained so far support the notion that interactions between microbes and innate immune genes play a key role in the induction of islet-reactive T cells. Future studies will be needed to identify innate immune pathways directly involved in the course of diabetes and mechanisms whereby they lead to islet cell destruction. Proinflammatory molecules identified to be linked with initiating autoimmunity against islets may be targeted to prevent disease in genetically susceptible individuals.

ACKNOWLEDGMENT

Our studies are supported by grants 1-2006-745, 1-2007-584, and 5-2008-224 from the Juvenile Diabetes Research Foundation.

REFERENCES

1. Eisenbarth GS. Update in type 1 diabetes. J Clin Endocrinol Metab 2007;92:2403–2407.
2. Kyvik KO, Nystrom L, Gorus F, Songini M, Oestman J, Castell C, Green A, Guyurs E, Ionescu-Tirgoviste C, McKinney PA, Michalkova D, Ostrauskas R, Raymond NT. The epidemiology of type 1 diabetes mellitus is not the same in young adults as in children. Diabetologia 2004;47:377–384.
3. Srikanta S, Ganda OP, Jackson RA, Gleason RE, Kaldany A, Garovoy MR, Milford EL, Carpenter C, Soeldner JS, Eisenbarth GS. Type I diabetes mellitus in monozygotic twins: chronic progressive beta cell dysfunction. Ann Intern Med 1983;99:320–326.
4. Gianani R, Eisenbarth GS. The stages of type 1A diabetes. Immunol Rev 2005;204:232–249.
5. Crisa L, Greiner DL, Mordes JP, MacDonald RG, Handler ES, Czech MP, Rossini AA. Biochemical studies of RT6 alloantigens in BB/Wor and normal rats. Evidence for intact unexpressed RT6a structural gene in diabetes-prone BB rats. Diabetes 1990;39:1279–1288.
6. Rossini AA, Handler ES, Mordes JP, Greiner DL. Human autoimmune diabetes mellitus: lessons from BB rats and NOD mice – Caveat emptor. Immunol Immunopathol Clin 1995;74:2–9.
7. Hornum L, Romer J, Markholst H. The diabetes-prone BB rat carries a frameshift mutation in Ian4, a positional candidate of Iddm1. Diabetes 2002;51:1972–1979.
8. Whalen BJ, Mordes JP, Rossini AA. The BB rat as a model of human insulin-dependent diabetes mellitus. Curr Protoc Immunol 2001 May;Chapter 15:Unit 15.3.
9. Greiner DL, Rossini AA, Mordes JP. Translating data from animal models into methods for preventing human autoimmune diabetes mellitus: caveat emptor and primum non nocere. Clin Immunol 2001;100:134–143.
10. Ellerman KE, Richards CA, Guberski DL, Shek WR, Like AA. Kilham rat triggers T-cell-dependent autoimmune diabetes in multiple strains of rat. Diabetes 1996;45:557–562.
11. Guberski DL, Thomas VA, Shek WR, Like AA, Handler ES, Rossini AA, Wallace JE, Welsh RM. Induction of type I diabetes by Kilham's rat virus in diabetes-resistant BB/Wor rats. Science 1991;254:1010–1013.
12. McKeever U, Mordes JP, Greiner DL, Appel MC, Rozing J, Handler ES, Rossini AA. Adoptive transfer of autoimmune diabetes and thyroiditis to athymic rats. Proc Natl Acad Sci U S A 1990;87:7618–7622.
13. Mordes JP, Guberski DL, Leif JH, Woda BA, Flanagan JF, Greiner DL, Kislauskis EH, Tirabassi RS. LEW.1WR1 rats develop autoimmune diabetes spontaneously and in response to environmental perturbation. Diabetes 2005;54:2727–2733.
14. Brown DD, Salzman LA. Sequence homology between the structural proteins of Kilham rat virus. J Virol 1984;49:1018–1020.
15. Jacoby RO, Ball-Goodrich LJ, Besselsen DG, McKisic MD, Riley LK, Smith AL. Rodent parvovirus infections. Lab Anim Sci 1996;46:370–380.
16. Cherry JD. Parvovirus infections in children and adults. Adv Pediatr 1999;46:245–269.
17. Ellerman KE, Like AA. Susceptibility to diabetes is widely distributed in normal class IIu haplotype rats. Diabetologia 2000;43:890–898.
18. Kato H, Takeuchi O, Sato S, Yoneyama M, Yamamoto M, Matsui K, Uematsu S, Jung A, Kawai T, Ishii KJ, Yamaguchi O, Otsu K, Tsujimura T, Koh CS, Reis e Sousa C, Matsuura Y, Fujita T, Akira S. Differential roles of MDA5 and RIG-I helicases in the recognition of RNA viruses. Nature 2006;441:101–105.
19. Aslanidis S, Pyrpasopoulou A, Kontotasios K, Doumas S, Zamboulis C. Parvovirus B19 infection and systemic lupus erythematosus: activation of an aberrant pathway? Eur J Intern Med 2008;19:314–318.
20. Cossart YE, Cant B, Field AM, Widdows D. Parvovirus-like particles in human sera. Lancet 1975;305:72–73.
21. Allander T, Tammi MT, Eriksson M, Bjerkner A, Tiveljung-Lindell A, Andersson BR. Cloning of a human parvovirus by molecular screening of respiratory tract samples. Proc Natl Acad Sci U S A 2005;102:12891–12896.
22. Berns KI. Parvoviridae: the viruses and their replication. In: Fields BN, Knipe DM, Howley PM, eds. Fields Virology. Philadelphia, PA: Lippincott-Raven, 1996:2173–2197.
23. Cotmore SF, McKie VC, Anderson LJ, Astell CR, Tattersall P. Identification of the major structural and nonstructural proteins encoded by human parvovirus B19 and mapping of their genes by procaryotic expression of isolated genomic fragments. J Virol 1986;60:548–557.
24. Ozawa K, Ayub J, Hao YS, Kurtzman G, Shimada T, Young N. Novel transcription map for the B19 (human) pathogenic parvovirus. J Virol 1987;61:2395–2406.

25. Tsay GJ, Zouali M. Unscrambling the role of human parvovirus B19 signaling in systemic autoimmunity. Biochem Pharmacol 2006;72: 1453–1459.
26. Bultmann BD, Klingel K, Sotlar K, Bock CT, Baba HA, Sauter M, Kandolf R. Fatal parvovirus B19-associated myocarditis clinically mimicking ischemic heart disease: an endothelial cell-mediated disease. Hum Pathol 2003;34: 92–95.
27. Schowengerdt KO, Ni J, Denfield SW, Gajarski RJ, Bowles NE, Rosenthal G, Kearney DL, Price JK, Rogers BB, Schauer GM, Chinnock RE, Towbin JA. Association of parvovirus B19 genome in children with myocarditis and cardiac allograft rejection: diagnosis using the polymerase chain reaction. Circulation 1997;96:3549–3554.
28. Nesher G, Rubinow A, Sonnenblick M. Efficacy and adverse effects of different corticosteroid dose regimens in temporal arteritis: a retrospective study. Clin Exp Rheumatol 1997;15:303–306.
29. Duechting A, Tschope C, Kaiser H, Lamkemeyer T, Tanaka N, Aberle S, Lang F, Torresi J, Kandolf R, Bock CT. Human parvovirus B19 NS1 protein modulates inflammatory signaling by activation of STAT3/PIAS3 in human endothelial cells. J Virol 2008;82:7942–7952.
30. Zipris D, Hillebrands JL, Welsh RM, Rozing J, Xie JX, Mordes JP, Greiner DL, Rossini AA. Infections that induce autoimmune diabetes in BBDR rats modulate CD4+CD25+ T cell populations. J Immunol 2003;170:3592–3602.
31. Gregori S, Giarratana N, Smiroldo S, Adorini L. Dynamics of pathogenic and suppressor T cells in autoimmune diabetes development. J Immunol 2003;171:4040–4047.
32. Pop SM, Wong CP, Culton DA, Clarke SH, Tisch R. Single cell analysis shows decreasing FoxP3 and TGF{beta}1 coexpressing CD4+CD25+ regulatory T cells during autoimmune diabetes. J Exp Med 2005;201: 1333–1346.
33. Tang Q, Henriksen KJ, Bi M, Finger EB, Szot G, Ye J, Masteller EL, McDevitt H, Bonyhadi M, Bluestone JA. In vitro-expanded antigen-specific regulatory T cells suppress autoimmune diabetes. J Exp Med 2004;199: 1455–1465.
34. Tarbell KV, Yamazaki S, Olson K, Toy P, Steinman RM. CD25+ CD4+ T cells, expanded with dendritic cells presenting a single autoantigenic peptide, suppress autoimmune diabetes. J Exp Med 2004;199: 1467–1477.
35. You S, Belghith M, Cobbold S, Alyanakian MA, Gouarin C, Barriot S, Garcia C, Waldmann H, Bach JF, Chatenoud L. Autoimmune diabetes onset results from qualitative rather than quantitative age-dependent changes in pathogenic T-cells. Diabetes 2005;54:1415–1422.
36. Holm TL, Lundsgaard D, Markholst H. Characteristics of rat CD4+CD25+ T cells and their ability to prevent not only diabetes but also insulitis in an adoptive transfer model in BB rats. Scan J Immunol 2006;64:17–29.
37. Lundsgaard D, Holm TL, Hornum L, Markholst H. In vivo control of diabetogenic T-cells by regulatory CD4+CD25+ T-cells expressing Foxp3. Diabetes 2005;54: 1040–1047.
38. Poussier P, Ning T, Murphy T, Dabrowski D, Ramanathan S. Impaired post-thymic development of regulatory CD4+25+ T cells contributes to diabetes pathogenesis in BB rats. J Immunol 2005;174:4081–4089.
39. Hillebrands JL, Whalen B, Visser JTJ, Koning J, Bishop KD, Leif J, Rozing J, Mordes JP, Greiner DL, Rossini AA. A regulatory CD4+ T cell subset in the BB rat model of autoimmune diabetes expresses neither CD25 nor Foxp3. J Immunol 2006;177:7820–7832.
40. Zipris D, Lien E, Xie JX, Greiner DL, Mordes JP, Rossini AA. TLR activation synergizes with Kilham rat virus infection to induce diabetes in BBDR rats. J Immunol 2005;174: 131–142.
41. Chung YH, Jun HS, Son M, Bao M, Bae HY, Kang Y, Yoon JW. Cellular and molecular mechanism for Kilham rat virus-induced autoimmune diabetes in DR-BB rats. J Immunol 2000;165:2866–2876.
42. Smyk-Pearson S, Golden-Mason L, Klarquist J, Burton J, Tester I, Wang C, Culbertson N, Vandenbark A, Rosen H. Functional suppression by FoxP3+CD4+CD25high regulatory T cells during acute hepatitis C virus infection. J Infect Dis 2008;197:46–57.
43. Zhou Y. Regulatory T cells and viral infections. Front Biosci 2008;13:1152–1170.
44. Boyer O, Saadoun D, Abriol J, Dodille M, Piette JC, Cacoub P, Klatzmann D. CD4+CD25+ regulatory T-cell deficiency in patients with hepatitis C-mixed cryoglobulinemia vasculitis. Blood 2004;103:3428–3430.
45. Zipris D, Lien E, Nair A, Xie JX, Greiner DL, Mordes JP, Rossini AA. TLR9-signaling pathways are involved in Kilham rat virus-induced autoimmune diabetes in the biobreeding diabetes-resistant rat. J Immunol 2007;178: 693–701.

46. Chiffoleau E, Heslan JM, Heslan M, Louvet C, Condamine T, Cuturi MC. TLR9 ligand enhances proliferation of rat CD4+ T cell and modulates suppressive activity mediated by CD4+ CD25+ T cell. Int Immunol 2007;19: 193–201.
47. Liu G, Zhao Y. Toll-like receptors and immune regulation: their direct and indirect modulation on regulatory CD4+ CD25+ T cells. Immunology 2007;122:149–156.
48. Pasare C, Medzhitov R. Toll pathway-dependent blockade of CD4+CD25+ T cell-mediated suppression by dendritic cells. Science 2003; 299:1033–1036.
49. Barton GM, Medzhitov R. Toll-like receptors and their ligands. Curr Top Microbiol Immunol 2002;270:81–92.
50. Lien E, Ingalls RR. Toll-like receptors. Crit Care Med 2002;30:S1–S11.
51. Medzhitov R, Janeway C Jr. Innate immunity. N Engl J Med 2000;343:338–344.
52. Janeway Jr CA, Medzhitov R. Innate immune recognition. Annu Rev Immunol 2002;20: 197–216.
53. Medzhitov R. Toll-like receptors and innate immunity. Nat Rev Immunol 2001;1: 135–145.
54. Sobel DO, Goyal D, Ahvazi B, Yoon JW, Chung YH, Bagg A, Harlan DM. Low dose poly I:C prevents diabetes in the diabetes prone BB rat. J Autoimmun 1998;11:343–352.
55. Sobel DO, Ahvazi B. Alpha-interferon inhibits the development of diabetes in NOD mice. Diabetes 1998;47:1867–1872.
56. Ewel CH, Sobel DO, Zeligs BJ, Bellanti JA. Poly I:C accelerates development of diabetes mellitus in diabetes-prone BB rat. Diabetes 1992;41:1016–1021.
57. Thomas VA, Woda BA, Handler ES, Greiner DL, Mordes JP, Rossini AA. Altered expression of diabetes in BB/Wor rats by exposure to viral pathogens. Diabetes 1991;40:255–258.
58. Blankenhorn EP, Rodemich L, Martin-Fernandez C, Leif J, Greiner DL, Mordes JP. The rat diabetes susceptibility locus Iddm4 and at least one additional gene are required for autoimmune diabetes induced by viral infection. Diabetes 2005;54:1233–1237.
59. Hornum L, Lundsgaard D, Markholst H. PolyI:C induction of diabetes is controlled by Iddm4 in rats with a full regulatory T cell pool. Ann N Y Acad Sci 2007;1110:65–72.
60. Aly TA, Ide A, Jahromi MM, Barker JM, Fernando MS, Babu SR, Yu L, Miao D, Erlich HA, Fain PR, Barriga KJ, Norris JM, Rewers MJ, Eisenbarth GS. Extreme genetic risk for type 1A diabetes. Proc Natl Acad Sci U S A 2006;103:14074–14079.
61. Marshak-Rothstein A. Toll-like receptors in systemic autoimmune disease. Nat Rev Immunol 2006;6:823–835.
62. Mordes JP, Bortell R, Blankenhorn EP, Rossini AA, Greiner DL. Rat models of type 1 diabetes: genetics, environment, and autoimmunity. ILAR J 2004;45:278–291.
63. Kaizer EC, Glaser CL, Chaussabel D, Banchereau J, Pascual V, White PC. Gene expression in peripheral blood mononuclear cells from children with diabetes. J Clin Endocrinol Metab 2007;92:3705–3711.
64. Wang X, Jia S, Geoffrey R, Alemzadeh R, Ghosh S, Hessner MJ. Identification of a molecular signature in human type 1 diabetes mellitus using serum and functional genomics. J Immunol 2008;180:1929–1937.
65. Colle E, Fuks A, Guttmann RD, Seemayer TA. Genetic susceptibility to the development of spontaneous insulin-dependent diabetes mellitus in the rat. Transplant Proc 1990;22: 2572–2573.
66. Wallis RH, Wang K, Dabrowski D, Marandi L, Ning T, Hsieh E, Paterson AD, Mordes JP, Blankenhorn EP, Poussier P. A novel susceptibility locus on rat chromosome 8 affects spontaneous but not experimentally induced type 1 diabetes. Diabetes 2007;56:1731–1736.
67. Greiner DL, Mordes JP, Handler ES, Angelillo M, Nakamura N, Rossini AA. Depletion of RT6.1+ T lymphocytes induces diabetes in resistant biobreeding/Worcester (BB/W) rats. J Exp Med 1987;166:461–475.
68. Sobel DO, Newsome J, Ewel CH, Bellanti JA, Abbassi V, Creswell K, Blair O. Poly I:C induces development of diabetes mellitus in BB rat. Diabetes 1992;41:515–520.
69. Cole KE, Strick CA, Paradis TJ, Ogborne KT, Loetscher M, Gladue RP, Lin W, Boyd JG, Moser B, Wood DE, Sahagan BG, Neote K. Interferon-inducible T cell alpha chemoattractant (I-TAC): a novel non-ELR CXC chemokine with potent activity on activated T cells through selective high affinity binding to CXCR3. J Exp Med 1998;187:2009–2021.
70. Dufour JH, Dziejman M, Liu MT, Leung JH, Lane TE, Luster AD. IFN-{gamma}-inducible protein 10 (IP-10; CXCL10)-deficient mice reveal a role for IP-10 in effector T cell generation and trafficking. J Immunol 2002; 168:3195–3204.
71. Liao F, Rabin RL, Yannelli JR, Koniaris LG, Vanguri P, Farber JM. Human Mig chemokine: biochemical and functional characterization. J Exp Med 1995;182:1301–1314.
72. Jia T, Serbina NV, Brandl K, Zhong MX, Leiner IM, Charo IF, Pamer EG. Additive roles for MCP-1 and MCP-3 in CCR2-mediated

recruitment of inflammatory monocytes during listeria monocytogenes infection. J Immunol 2008;180:6846–6853.
73. Dairaghi DJ, Soo KS, Oldham ER, Premack BA, Kitamura T, Bacon KB, Schall TJ. RANTES-induced T cell activation correlates with CD3 expression. J Immunol 1998;160: 426–433.
74. Schroder C, Pierson RN III, Nguyen BN, Kawka DW, Peterson LB, Wu G, Zhang T, Springer MS, Siciliano SJ, Iliff S, Ayala JM, Lu M, Mudgett JS, Lyons K, Mills SG, Miller GG, Singer II, Azimzadeh AM, DeMartino JA. CCR5 blockade modulates inflammation and alloimmunity in primates. J Immunol 2007;179:2289–2299.
75. Zhao X, Sato A, Dela Cruz CS, Linehan M, Luegering A, Kucharzik T, Shirakawa AK, Marquez G, Farber JM, Williams I, Iwasaki A. CCL9 is secreted by the follicle-associated epithelium and recruits dome region Peyer's patch CD11b+ dendritic cells. J Immunol 2003;171:2797–2803.
76. Kennedy J, Kelner GS, Kleyensteuber S, Schall TJ, Weiss MC, Yssel H, Schneider PV, Cocks BG, Bacon KB, Zlotnik A. Molecular cloning and functional characterization of human lymphotactin. J Immunol 1995;155:203–209.
77. Carr MW, Roth SJ, Luther E, Rose SS, Springer TA. Monocyte chemoattractant protein 1 acts as a T-lymphocyte chemoattractant. Proc Natl Acad Sci U S A 1994;91:3652–3656.
78. Xu LL, Warren MK, Rose WL, Gong W, Wang JM. Human recombinant monocyte chemotactic protein and other C–C chemokines bind and induce directional migration of dendritic cells in vitro. J Leukoc Biol 1996;60: 365–371.
79. Arend WP. Interleukin-1 receptor antagonist. Adv Immunol 1993;54:167–227.
80. Sutton C, Brereton C, Keogh B, Mills KHG, Lavelle EC. A crucial role for interleukin (IL)-1 in the induction of IL-17-producing T cells that mediate autoimmune encephalomyelitis. J Exp Med 2006;203:1685–1691.
81. Sims JE. IL-1 and IL-18 receptors, and their extended family. Curr Opin Immunol 2002;14:117–122.
82. Park H, Li Z, Yang XO, Chang SH, Nurieva R, Wang YH, Wang Y, Hood L, Zhu Z, Tian Q, Dong C. A distinct lineage of CD4 T cells regulates tissue inflammation by producing interleukin 17. Nat Immunol 2005;6:1133–1141.
83. Jones SA. Directing transition from innate to acquired immunity: defining a role for IL-6. J Immunol 2005;175:3463–3468.
84. Boehm U, Klamp T, Groot M, Howard JC. Cellular responses to interferon-gamma. Annu Rev Immunol 1997;15:749–795.
85. Honda K, Yanai H, Negishi H, Asagiri M, Sato M, Mizutani T, Shimada N, Ohba Y, Takaoka A, Yoshida N, Taniguchi T. IRF-7 is the master regulator of type-I interferon-dependent immune responses. Nature 2005;434: 772–777.
86. Baccala R, Kono DH, Theofilopoulos AN. Interferons as pathogenic effectors in autoimmunity. Immunol Rev 2005;204:9–26.

Chapter 14

Autoimmune Pathology of Type 1 Diabetes

Roberto Gianani and Mark Atkinson

Summary

A seeming majority of research articles pertaining to Type 1 diabetes (T1D) begin by noting that the disorder results from an autoimmune destruction of the insulin-secreting pancreatic β cells. This concept finds its basis in decades-old observations that at the symptomatic onset of T1D, a chronic inflammatory infiltrate affecting primarily the insulin-containing islets is present in most subjects. This infiltrate consists predominantly of T-lymphocytes, with lesser numbers of B-lymphocytes and macrophages. Apoptotic β cells, enhanced β cell expression of Fas, T-lymphocyte expression of Fas-L, hyperexpression of class I MHC on all endocrine cells in insulin-containing islets, and interferon α production by β cells are also noteworthy occurrences often seen with this lesion. The subsequent observation of islet cell autoantibodies in the serum of patients with T1D led to its definition as an autoimmune disease (Type 1A diabetes). In this chapter, we will review the pathology of Type 1A diabetes and discuss its possible pathogenesis on the basis of evidence obtained from pancreatic specimens. Finally, we will briefly discuss nonautoimmune forms of T1D.

Key Words: Type 1 diabetes, Pancreatic pathology, Insulitis, Beta cell apoptosis, Regeneration, Nonautoimmune forms of Type 1 diabetes

INTRODUCTION

Before discussing the pathology of Type 1 diabetes (T1D), it is important to accurately define the disease; given that this term is often used with widely different meaning by clinicians having a different level of expertise within this field. The official typology of diabetes describes the existence of two main forms of primary diabetes (i.e., not secondary to other diseases as hemochromatosis or endocrine disturbances); T1D and Type 2 diabetes (T2D). In actuality, the distinction between the two forms of diabetes is not always clear cut, because we do not know the precise biological mechanisms underlying these conditions. At a more fundamental level, it remains unclear whether T1D (or even more so T2D) represents just one disease or a syndrome resulting from multiple disease processes.

For the purpose of this chapter, T1D will be defined as a disease accompanied with beta cell loss, exceeding 80% of normal beta cell mass (defined as the average beta cell mass of nondiabetic controls) after 5 years of diagnosed disease. This definition, albeit somehow arbitrary, is based on the observation that T1D does not usually develop in animal models until at least 80% of the beta cell mass is destroyed. According to this definition, a subset of patients with a clinical history of T2D (i.e., diabetes treatable with oral agents in subjects with high BMI and high level of C-peptide) might eventually develop T1D because of beta cell loss. This pathological transition would be marked clinically by the onset of insulin dependence. Beta cell loss in patients with T2D is believed to be caused by glucose toxicity, amylin deposition, and/or a combination of both. This subset of T2D patients will be defined as having T1D secondary to Type 2 disease.

Much of what we understand regarding the pathogenesis of T1D has been derived from the analysis of serum and peripheral blood lymphocytes from patients with the disorder. Indeed, from these tissue sources, evidence of both humoral as well as cell-mediated autoimmunity to islet cell antigens was noted. The genes forming susceptibility to the disease were also identified from leukocytes. Support for the concept that environment influences cause T1D emanated from serological observations suggesting that at clinical presentation, T1D patients were more likely to possess enteroviral RNA (as well as antibodies suggestive of recent enteroviral infection). Analysis of serum C-peptide demonstrated that nearly all T1D patients continue to secrete insulin for variable periods following disease onset, indicating that even though the patient may present with an apparent acute illness, a complete β cell functional decline extends over a long period of time. These provide just a few examples of the unquestionable value that blood-based studies have provided for T1D research. However, given that T1D is a disorder of the immune system that targets pancreatic β cells, it is also valuable to consider how studies of the pancreas in patients with or at increased risk for the disease, contributed to our understanding of its pathogenesis.

THE CONUNDRUM OF EVALUATING HUMAN PANCREAS

Clearly, the reason studies of peripheral blood have predominated in T1D research relates to the fact that investigations of the pancreas in those with the disease are limited by the difficulty of obtaining a suitable tissue. Historically, the most common source of pancreatic specimens from subjects with T1D has involved retrospective collections of pancreata obtained at autopsy from individuals who died at or near the time of their disease diagnosis (*1, 2*). This approach is hampered by several significant limitations; the pancreatic tissues might be subject to a degree of autolysis, and furthermore these samples are most often formalin fixed and paraffin embedded, a facet that restricts the range of investigative techniques available. These factors, combined with limited pancreatic sampling, poor knowledge of clinical histories, and little access to modern assessments of either β cell function (e.g., C-peptide and insulin use) or metabolic control (e.g., HbA1C), significantly limit, from a historical perspective, the range of potential correlative information that could have been gleaned from studies on these otherwise highly valuable pancreata.

This situation has, however, been subject to a variety of changes that have and will, with time, dramatically improve our understanding of pancreatic pathology, as it relates to T1D. Among these newer approaches, investigators have performed laparoscopic pancreatic biopsies on T1D patients with recent diagnosis of their disease (*3*). While controversial with respect to its risk versus reward potential, and subject to question both in terms of its ethics and practicality, this protocol does, in fact, overcome many of the aforementioned limitations. The method of collection is, however, hampered by a significant disadvantage related to sampling bias, wherein the biopsies are exceedingly small (i.e., 20–30 mg). Also in the mid-1990s, studies suggestive of a "viral superantigen" in pancreata removed at the time of organ donation from patients who died due to severe diabetic ketoacidosis at clinical onset of T1D (*4*), inspired many investigators to step up efforts to obtain pancreatic tissue from this source. This process not only allowed for removal of the pancreas for research studies immediately after death but also overcame additional limitations related to tissue preparation, quantity, and storage. Other methods recently developed to obtain more optimal pancreata include sampling of organs from T1D patients undergoing pancreatectomy for islet tumors or other pancreatic diseases. Pancreatic tissue has also been sought from islet autoantibody positive organ donors deemed to be at increased risk for the development of T1D (*5, 6*). These methods, when combined with modern assessments of metabolic activity, β cell development, and immune function (as well as the potential future for in vivo imaging), should allow for major improvements in our understanding of the human pancreas in T1D.

WHAT IS "INSULITIS?"

The proverbial "hallmark" study of the pancreas in T1D, both in terms of patient cases and depth of description, was that published in the journal, "Diabetes" in 1965 by Gepts (*1*). This established two morphological factors that clearly distinguished what we now refer to as T1D from those of T2D. In cases of T1D, a reduction of β cells was demonstrated, with many islets being completely devoid of them. We would note, parenthetically, that this study pre-dated the technique of immunohistochemistry, so strictly speaking, the cells were not proven to be insulin secreting. Furthermore, a chronic inflammatory cell infiltrate affecting islets, termed "insulitis," was also noted in these subjects. Neither of these phenomena was observed in pancreata of those with T2D (*7*). Furthermore, Gept's observation of pancreatic insulitis in 15 of 22 cases of recent onset (i.e., less than 6 months of clinical duration) T1D led him to hypothesize that the β cells were undergoing destruction by either viral infection or through a self-directed immune (i.e., autoimmune) process. Interestingly, a wide body of evidence acquired in the ensuing 40 years has supported, to some degree, both of these early suggestions regarding disease pathogenesis.

Alongside noting a potential autoimmune basis for T1D, similar early studies provided many other valuable insights. Among those, in subjects having T1D for more than 5 years, a majority of the remaining islets were noted as insulin deficient, containing a normal complement of the other hormone-secreting cells (i.e., glucagon-secreting α cells, somatostatin-secreting δ cells, and pancreatic polypeptide-secreting PP cells) (these islets devoid of insulin-producing cells are referred as pseudoatrophic islets) (*8*). Thus, the disorder clearly represents a disease involving the selective loss of β cells. It is important to emphasize that these historical studies also suggested the natural history of β cell loss represented a variable response, subject to marked heterogeneity in both the degree as well as the patterns of destruction.

Three forms of islet were noted in pancreases of recent onset T1D patients. First, approximately 70% of the islets in recent onset T1D pancreata displayed complete insulin absence (pseudoatrophic islets) (i.e., similar to those observed in T1D patients with prolonged disease). Second, approximately 20% of insulin-containing islets, as opposed to only 1% of insulin-deficient islets, were inflamed (i.e., insulitis) (*1, 2*). Third, in many pancreases, noninflamed insulin-containing islets that appeared essentially normal were present. Thus, within a given pancreas, near the time of clinical presentation, there are islets where the β cells have been destroyed, islets where the β cells are being destroyed, and islets where the β cells are yet to be destroyed (i.e., insulin-deficient islets, inflamed islets, and normal islets, respectively).

THE PANCREAS BEFORE AND AFTER CLINICAL ONSET OF T1D

An important point is that the pancreas before clinical presentation, at clinical presentation, and for a few years after clinical presentation may be qualitatively similar, with all three types of islet present, although in vastly variable proportions (9). For example, one study noted that insulitis affecting insulin-containing islets could be observed in T1D cases up to 6 years following clinical presentation and in such a pancreas, approximately 95% of islets were insulin deficient (2). By contrast, in a prediabetic-T1D pancreas, less than 4% of islets were noted as insulin deficient, yet insulitis was present (10). Pathologic examinations would suggest that clinical presentation occurs when approximately two-thirds of the islets are insulin deficient (2). The importance of this lies in the fact that if the pathogenesis of T1D within the pancreas involves progression from a normal insulin-containing islet to an inflamed insulin-containing islet, and then to an insulin-deficient islet, then the mechanisms involved may be studied in pancreases obtained at clinical presentation, as all three islet types are usually present in such organs (11). Recent evidence suggests that a large number of individuals (up to 88%) with T1D preserve some beta cells even decades after the onset of the disease (12). If these data are correct, they challenge the fundamental assumption that long standing T1D is characterized by total beta cell loss. However, extreme caution is necessary in interpreting these data. The study describing the conservation of beta cells has utilized autopsy specimens and therefore the description of subjects as having T1D relies exclusively on clinical records. Thus, there is the possibility that individuals found to maintain beta cells many years, after the onset of the disease might have been misclassified as having T1D (while in actuality had T2D even though these patient were diagnosed in childhood). Furthermore, it is also possible that individuals with preserved beta cells after long standing T1D might represent nonautoimmune forms of this disease (hence referred to as nonType 1A T1D. Previous studies (as well as our own preliminary evidence from the Network for Pancreatic Organ Donors with Diabetes (nPOD) obtained pancreata of patients with Type 1A diabetes) have suggested that only very few patients with autoimmune diabetes preserve a residual, (albeit reduced) beta cell mass, several years after disease onset. In this case, the surviving beta cells show a characteristic lobular distribution with some areas of the pancreas containing residual beta cells and others containing only islets without a beta cell. The available evidence suggests that maintenance of beta cell mass is a rare event in Type 1A diabetes, and autopsy study suggesting otherwise can probably be explained by the initial misclassification of cases as representing Type 1A diabetes.

To clarify this issue, it will be important to study the pancreatic pathology (with respect to beta cell maintenance and pattern of beta cell loss) in individuals with long-standing diabetes characterized at onset as Type 1A (on the basis of the presence of islet cell autoantibodies). For many years, investigators have not considered it practical or ethical to obtain pancreatic biopsies from living subjects at increased risk for developing T1D. To address this problem, recent investigations have attempted to collect pancreatic tissue from organ donors with serological evidence of islet autoimmunity, a subset of whom would presumably have developed T1D had they survived. For this purpose, the T1D research community, including a consortium of investigators organized in Belgium (5) as well as the (nPOD (http://www.jdrfnpod.org), has developed large programs to screen asymptomatic organ donors for islet autoantibodies. These efforts to study "prediabetic" pancreases should aid in addressing three questions that are of primary importance to this disease. First, is β cell destruction a chronic progressive process that slowly occurs over a long time period in subjects with autoimmunity or does it represent a fairly acute process? Second, does β cell regeneration occur in concert with β cell destruction in subjects with islet autoimmunity? Third and finally, what role (if any) does viral infection within β cells play in subjects with ongoing islet autoimmunity?

The available evidence supports the notion that there are several degrees of islet autoimmunity, which can be associated with insulitis and phenotyped by the number of autoantibodies for which a subject is positive. The Belgium Organ Donor consortium retrospectively analyzed pancreatic tissue from 1,507 organ donors, identifying 62 individuals as positive for islet autoantibodies (i.e., ICA, GAD, IA-2, or insulin antibodies) (5). Insulitis, defined in this study as more than five inflammatory cells per islet section, was detected in only two cases, both of which were positive for three autoantibodies. It is important to note that only three of the 62 subjects were positive for three autoantibodies, while the remaining 59 were positive for only one autoantibody. One caveat of this study is that only a relatively small quantity of pancreas was sampled; hence the potential exists that the prevalence of insulitis was underestimated due to under-sampling of focal areas subject to islet inflammation. A second study involving the analysis of pancreas obtained from an organ donor identified as positive for IA-2 antibodies also failed to detect insulitis, this, despite numerous sections of pancreas being subject to examination (6). With these two efforts, it is feasible to speculate that subjects possessing only one autoantibody will not show significant insulitis, as the degree of immunity does not reach a threshold reflective of widespread islet infiltration. It is also possible that secondary events (e.g., viral islet infection, endocrine stress, etc.) are necessary to trigger full-blown islet mononuclear cell infiltration, even in the presence of established islet autoimmunity.

SIX KEY FEATURES OF β CELL-CONTAINING ISLETS IN HUMAN T1D AT CLINICAL PRESENTATION

Beyond the important issues of the natural history of islet inflammation, islet hormone expression, and the percentage of viable β cells resident to the pancreas in those with T1D are issues related to the insulitis lesion itself (Fig. 14.1). While the number of studies addressing this issue is somewhat limited, subject to methodological variation, and have marked differences in their patient numbers (Table 14.1), we do believe that a series of characteristics of the insulitis lesion can be considered as "likely representative" and hence, key features in this disease.

Feature 1: Cells Composing the Insulitis Lesion

A case report in the mid-1980s was the first of what to date, still represents only a handful (Table 14.1) of investigations involving immunohistochemistry, seeking to define the nature of the inflammatory infiltrate composing the insulitis lesion (13). This effort was noteworthy in its defining the lesion as one predominantly formed of both T- and B-lymphocytes, with macrophages being largely inconspicuous. Furthermore, this study noted a majority of the lymphocytes were cytotoxic in their phenotype rather than helper (i.e., CD8+ > CD4+) T-lymphocytes. Since the publication of this study, subsequent reports have supported the observation

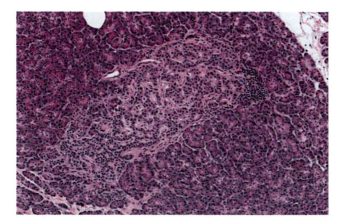

Fig. 14.1 Insulitis in recent onset human T1D. H&E (obtained the nPOD program with permission). Note the numerous lymphocytes infiltration accumulating at the edge of the islet (arrow).

Table 14.1
Literature Involving Immunohistochemical Review of the Histologic Features of Pancreatic Inflammation in Human Type 1 Diabetes

Reference (number)	Cases	CD8/CD4/Mac	β Cell apoptosis	Class I MHC in insulin-containing islets	Class II MHC β cells	FAS	FAS-L	ICAM-1	Cytokine presence	Cytokine absence
Bottazzzo (16)	1	CD8 > CD4 > macs		+++	+					
Foulis	37	Lymph > macs		+++	++				IFN-γ, IFN-α	
Hanafusa (6, 18, 20)	29	CD3 > macs > CD4	Not detected	+++	Rare + (1/29)	++β Cells	−β Cells, + lymph	−β Cells, + endo T	IFN-γ	IL-4
Stassi (19)	2	CD4 > CD8 and macs	Not detected			+β Cells, +α cells	−β Cells, + lymph			Perforin
Hanninen	1	CD8 > CD4 > macs	Present on FAS+ β cells	+++	−			−β Cells, + endo T		
Somoza	1	CD3 > macs		+++	+ (Including α)			+β Cells, + endo T	Perforin, IL-6, IFN-alpha and IFN-beta	IL-1, 2, 4, 10; TNF-α, IFN-γ

that macrophages represent a minor population within the infiltrate in T1D. Specifically, in a study of 87 affected islets obtained from 12 autopsy pancreases from subjects with T1D, the ratio of lymphocytes to macrophages was 10:1, while the average number of lymphocytes per inflamed islet section studied was 85 (*14*). With this background, it was quite surprising that a study of pancreatic biopsies failed to observe evidence of insulitis in T1D patients, even in the pancreases of four subjects noted to contain residual β cells (*3*). The significance of this finding was somewhat blurred, however, when subsequent studies by the same investigators did in fact note insulitis (*15*). One factor that may have contributed to this apparent discrepancy is that for the latter study, the definition of insulitis was given as an islet infiltrated by more than two inflammatory cells per histological section.

Feature 2: Fas Expression

At least two studies have investigated the expression of Fas and its cognate ligand Fas-L, in T1D insulitis (*16, 17*). Both studies suggested Fas-positive endocrine cells were present in islets affected by insulitis (Fig. 14.2) but interestingly, not in uninflamed islets. Islets in pancreata obtained from healthy controls did not express Fas. Furthermore, the latter of the two studies (i.e., Moriwaki et al.) demonstrated that while a majority of β cells were Fas positive, a significant number of α cells also expressed this molecule. Infiltrating lymphocytes were Fas-L positive, while islet endocrine cells were Fas-L negative. These observations have led to the hypothesis that cytokines such as interferon γ, tumor necrosis factor α, or interleukin 1, each of which induce Fas expression by islet endocrine cells in vitro, could be released during insulitis, resulting in similar outcomes in vivo. Under one scenario, it could be posited that Fas-L-positive infiltrating cells in islets undergoing inflammation would destroy Fas-positive β cells.

Feature 3: β Cell Apoptosis

While still limited in number, more studies have attempted to identify evidence of β cell apoptosis (Fig. 14.3) in human T1D pancreata than those evaluating the expression of Fas/Fas-L. The results have, however, been mixed, starting with the observation that no apoptotic β cells were found in pancreatic biopsies of T1D patients performed in Japanese patients (*17*). This finding was contrasted (somewhat dramatically) by other studies that noted marked numbers of β cells undergoing apoptosis using TUNEL staining methods, albeit in autopsy-based specimens (*12*).

Feature 4: Aberrant β Cell Expression of Class II MHC

Among the most surprising and at the time of their initial description, controversial findings of pancreatic insulitis were efforts noting MHC class II expression by β cells. At that time, investigators hypothesized that this seemingly aberrant class II expression could lead to their presenting self-antigens, eventually resulting in autoimmunity (*18*). Class II MHC expression by islet endocrine

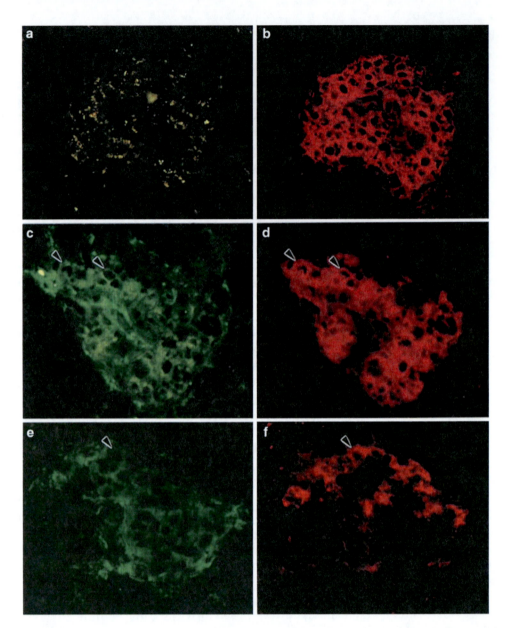

Fig. 14.2 Pancreas sections of a control subject (**a, b**) and a recent onset Type I diabetic patient (**c–f**) were stained with anti-Fas antibody (*green;* **a, c, e**) and antiinsulin (*red;* **b, d**) and antiglucagon antibody (*red;* **f**) (400×). Fas is positive in the islet of a Type I diabetic patient (**c, e**), but not in the islet of the control subject (**a**). Double immunostaining of Fas-stained sections with antiinsulin (**b, d**) and antiglucagon (**f**) antibodies (*red*) shows that Fas-positive cells are mostly insulin-positive cells and partly glucagon-positive cells. Representative double-positive cells are indicated by *arrowheads*. Reproduced with permission from (*17*).

cells was shown in pancreata from 21 out of 23 cases of recent onset T1D (*18*). In this study, aberrant expression of class II MHC was observed in 12% of insulin-containing islets, with double stains showing its confinement to β cells (i.e., not present in α, δ, or PP cells). Further validating this notion, the phenomenon

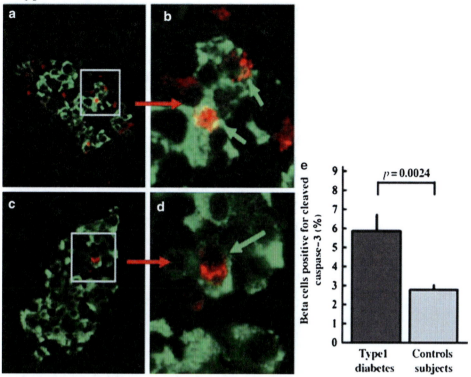

Fig. 14.3 Examples of islets in a patient with Type 1 diabetes (a) and a nondiabetic autopsy control subject (c) stained for insulin (*green*) and cleaved caspase-3 (for apoptosis; *red*) and imaged at 200× magnification. Panels **b** and **d** show inserts taken from these images at higher magnification. *Arrows* indicate apoptosis in beta cells (*green*). *Right* panels indicate the frequency of apoptosis in beta cells (**e**), determined in four patients with Type 1 diabetes and eight nondiabetic autopsy control subjects. Data are presented as means ± SEM (one-way ANOVA). Reproduced with permission from (*12*).

was noted in pancreatic biopsies of two Japanese T1D patients (*19*). Interestingly, one-half of the islets in which β cells expressed class II MHC showed no evidence of inflammation, raising the possibility that within a given islet, this abnormality preceded insulitis. In other words, it represented an early stage in the natural history of islet inflammation (*18*). Validating the unique nature of this observation, β cells expressing class II MHC were not observed in 95 pancreases obtained from nonT1D subjects having a variety of disorders including T2D, chronic pancreatitis, cystic fibrosis, graft versus host disease, and enteroviral pancreatitis (*18*). However, in the time since these early observations, subsequent investigations have noted that in addition to class II MHC, an antigen-presenting cell must also express costimulatory molecules (e.g., CD80 and CD86) in order to successfully present antigen to T-lymphocytes. This latter concept does, in part, call into question the pathogenic relevance of aberrant β cell expression of class II MHC.

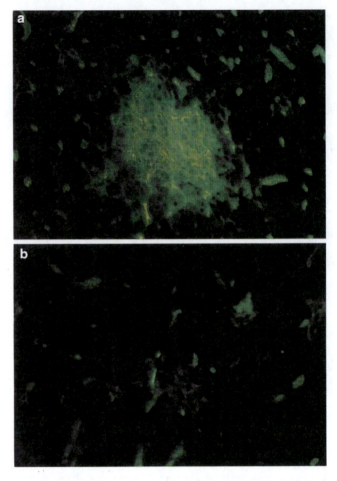

Fig. 14.4 Expression of MHC class I antigens is increased in an islet from a 26-year-old subject with Type 1 diabetes of 1 year duration. Normal control pancreas shows only faint expression of MHC class I antigens in islet cells and weak one in endothelial cells (**b**; 200×). Reproduced with permission from (*12, 15*).

Feature 5: Hyperexpression of Class I MHC by Insulin-Containing Islets

Cytotoxic CD8+ T-lymphocytes, which are by most accounts (Table 14.1) the dominant immune cell type in insulitis, recognize antigen when it is presented in association with class I MHC by a target cell. Hyperexpression of class I MHC by the target cell would be considered a positive step toward enhancing this engagement. A phenomenon unique to T1D is hyperexpression of class I MHC (by all endocrine cells) in insulin-containing islets (Fig. 14.4) (*18*). Indeed, in one study, 92% of insulin-containing islets hyperexpressed class I MHC, in contrast to only 1% of insulin-deficient islets. Furthermore, the phenomenon was not observed within islets in any of the aforementioned 95 "controls." As far as the mechanisms underlying this observation, MHC class I hyperexpression of islet endocrine cells has been induced in vitro by the interferons α, β, and γ (*20*). In T1D pancreata, 40% of the lymphocytes in the insulitis infiltrate expressed interferon γ; hence, one could speculate that the hyperexpression of class I MHC might represent a secondary event, following the induction of insulitis (14). However, even when whole islets in multiple serial sections were examined, over one-half of the insulin-containing islets that hyperexpressed class I MHC failed to reveal evidence of insulitis. Therefore, an alternate view has emerged that the hyperexpression of class I MHC by insulin-containing islets precedes insulitis.

Comparison of class I hyperexpression and aberrant class II expression by β cells demonstrated that in all situations, islets subject to the latter phenomenon also hyperexpressed class I MHC. The reverse setting, however, did not hold, in that 73% of islets that hyperexpressed class I MHC showed no evidence of aberrant class II MHC expression on β cells. Taken collectively, hyperexpression of class I MHC appears to be an earlier event in the natural history of insulitis than class II MHC expression by β cells. Finally, it should also be noted that α and δ cells hyperexpressed class I MHC when they were in immediate association with β cells within insulin-containing islets of T1D pancreata, but not when they were physically separated from β cells in insulin-deficient islets (14). This observation raised the mechanistic possibility that release of Type 1 interferon by β cells causes this hyperexpression via a paracrine effect.

Feature 6: β cell Expression of Interferon α

A final noteworthy observation from pancreata of those with T1D is that β cells, but not α, δ, or PP cells, express interferon α. In one study, all 28 pancreases obtained from patients with recent onset T1D demonstrated this phenomenon (18). Importantly, this expression was closely related to class I MHC hyperexpression. Beta cells expressing interferon α were noted in 94% of islets that hyperexpressed class I MHC, but were seen in only 0.2% of islets that did not hyperexpress this complex. Furthermore, among 80 control pancreases that have been subjected to this form of analysis, β cells expressed interferon α in only four cases, those where Coxsackie B viral pancreatitis was evident, but not in other pancreatic diseases (14).

It has to be admitted that the great majority of patients studied in autopsy series of T1D died of severe ketoacidosis. This has raised the question of whether these immunological phenomena observed in the insulitis lesion are, in fact, the consequences of such a metabolic derangement. An important contribution to this debate has been made by a study analyzing pancreatic biopsies on metabolically well-controlled T1D patients, some 2 months after clinical diagnosis (21). The nature of the insulitis infiltrate, islet FAS expression, and the phenomena of aberrant class II expression by β cells and hyperexpression of class I MHC by insulin-containing islets have all been shown to be the same in the biopsies as has been described by others in autopsy patients dying of ketoacidosis.

REGENERATION IN THE PANCREAS OF HUMAN T1D: FACT OR FICTION?

The oft-quoted notion portending "β cell extinction" did not develop without some basis of fact. This list would include an absolute loss in C-peptide for most T1D patients, lack of spontaneous remissions from disease, and histological examinations suggesting that a healthy islet cell mass is not readily evident in long-standing disease. However, this concept has recently been challenged by the concept of pancreatic β cell regeneration (22). This challenge, to a large extent, was derived from a recent study that performed immunocytochemical detection of insulin-producing cells in pancreata obtained from subjects with a T1D duration of 4–67 years (12). The pancreases were also examined for many features including inflammation, periductal fibrosis, as well as β cell apoptosis and replication. The study reported, in contrast to the established dogma, that 88% of T1D patients had insulin-producing cells, and this feature was unrelated to disease duration or age at death (12). Having said this, it should also be pointed out that the beta cell mass in these 42 cases was only 2.3% of that of normal control pancreases. β Cell apoptosis was studied in the four T1D patients who had sufficient β cell mass for calculation, and 6% of β cells were noted to express the apoptosis marker, cleaved caspase 3. This is a remarkably high figure, given the transient nature of apoptotic cells, and would imply an extremely high turnover of β cells to provide a stable long-term population. However, no insulin- containing cells in these four pancreases expressed the proliferation marker Ki-67. Thus, doubt has to be expressed about the observed rate of apoptosis reported.

The same group also studied the pancreas of an 89-year-old patient with recent onset T1D who had undergone a distal pancreatectomy for the removal of pancreatic intraepithelial neoplasia (12). The tumor-free tissue showed a reduced fractional β cell area, islet infiltration with CD3+ positive T-lymphocytes and macrophages, increased β cell apoptosis, and a marked increase in β cells undergoing replication (i.e., Ki67+ β cells). This publication was followed up by that group (23) examining autopsy pancreata from nine T1D patients (age 11.5–38 years) who died of ketoacidosis and whose disease was less than 3 years in duration. They reported a "surprisingly" modest increase in β cell apoptosis, as assessed by the TUNEL technique, and no evidence of β cell regeneration. It is possible that the crucial difference between the two situations is represented by the fact that in the first setting, the single patient had developed T1D very late in life, possibly as a result of a protracted struggle between the forces of β cell destruction (i.e., lymphocytes and macrophages) and the forces of regeneration (i.e., β cell replication). These reports exemplify the difficulties involved in the study of the pancreas in human T1D and form the basis wherein rodent models of pancreatic β cell regeneration are often subject to investigation. However, great caution must be considered when extending findings of β cell regeneration from animal models to human T1D. Until then, examinations of many more human cases are required to substantiate the concept of β cell regeneration since as for now, it remains an unproven concept for human T1D.

NON-AUTOIMMUNE FORMS OF T1D

While the majority of cases of T1D are thought to be autoimmune, there are known forms of nonautoimmune T1D. As discussed earlier, we do not know whether a nonidentified form of nonautoimmune T1D (apart from T1D resulting from a clinical history of T2D) accounts for a major subset of the disease. However, it has been shown that approximately 15% of subjects with clinically diagnosed T1D lack islet autoantibodies at the onset of the disease (24). Furthermore a subset of these antibody negative (with the obvious caveat that they can be defined as negative) only for the four islet autoantigens we currently measure namely insulin, GAD65, IA-2 and ZnT8 (25, 26) subjects also lack the DR3 or DR4 alleles often associated with the autoimmune form of diabetes (25). It is thus conceivable that at least some of these antibody-negative subjects with T1D have a not-yet characterized nonautoimmune form of T1D. In addition to this potential but yet-not unproven form of nonautoimmune Type 1, there are well characterized forms of nonautoimmune T1D. In the following sections, we will describe the following forms of nonautoimmune T1D:

1. T1D secondary to a clinical history of T2D.
2. T2D secondary to persistent hyperinsulinemic hypoglycemia of infancy.
3. Monogenic forms of T1D.

T1D Secondary to a Clinical History of T2D

T2D, the most common form of diabetes in humans, is probably a heterogeneous syndrome characterized by multiple processes leading to functional defects of insulin action. Several investigators have showed that in T2D, there is also a progressive loss of β cell mass, which in some cases results in insulin dependence (27). In relation to Type 1A diabetes, it is important to know whether this can be distinguished on the basis of pancreatic pathology from long-lasting T2D with severe beta cell loss. β Cell loss in T2D is generally attributed to apoptosis triggered by glucose toxicity and/or amylin deposition. An autopsy study from Rahier and coworkers has shown that β cell mass was on an average 24% lower in the group of T2D subjects in comparison with BMI-matched nondiabetic controls, after 1–5 years of overt diabetes (*27*). This degree of β cell loss is much milder than the one observed after similar duration of Type 1A diabetes. However, due to the progressive nature of the beta cell loss in T2D, it is conceivable that patients with longer duration of T2D might have a more severe beta cells loss. In these cases, there maybe some diagnostic confusion with the rare patients with Type 1A diabetes preserving a β cell mass. As described earlier, the absence of pseudo-atrophic islets and islets of "lobular," distribution of surviving β cells (as well as the presence of amylin-derived amyloid (easily identifiable by Congo Red Stain)), should allow distinction between the pathology of long-standing T2D and Type 1A diabetes.

T1D Secondary to Persistent Hyperinsulinemic Hypoglycemia of Infancy (PHHI)

Persistent Hyperinsulinemic Hypoglycemia of Infancy (PHHI) is a rare genetic disorder often caused by mutations in either the sulfonylurea receptor (SUR1) or the inward-rectifying potassium channel (Kir6.2), two subunits of the Beta cell KATP channel (*28*). Patients with PHHI often have to undergo a partial pancreatectomy to control otherwise untreatable hypoglycemia. Later in life, these patients develop diabetes mellitus that requires insulin treatment, although it is rarely associated with ketoacidosis. While there is no pathological description of the pancreas in diabetes secondary to PHHI, the evidence suggests that diabetes in these individuals is caused by a combination of partial pancreatectomy and increased rate of β cell apoptosis. Kassem and coworkers (*28*) have demonstrated that patients with PHHI have an increased rate of both proliferation and apoptosis of β cells, which they hypothesize eventually results in a net loss of β cells, as evidenced by the gradual decline of their C-peptide levels. Takashi and coworkers have generated transgenic mice expressing a dominant-negative form of the KATP channel subunit Kir6.2 (Kir6.2G132S, substitution of glycine with serine at position 132) in pancreatic β cells. Kir6.2G132S transgenic mice develop hypoglycemia with hyperinsulinemia in neonates and hyperglycemia with hypoinsulinemia and decreased β cell population in adults (*29*). The pattern of β cell loss in these is represented by a global decline in β cell population, but without any islets with complete β cell loss (i.e., the presence of pseudoatrophic islets) (We termed this pattern B β cell loss). This differs from the pattern of beta cell loss of both human Type 1A diabetes and the non obese diabetic mouse (NOD, an animal model of human Type 1A (*25*)), which are characterized by either total or subtotal β cell loss with numerous pseudoatrophic islets (we termed these pattern A β cell loss).

Monogenic Forms of T1D

Recently, it has become apparent that childhood diabetes is heterogeneous. In addition to the most common autoimmune diabetes, T2D, secondary diabetes, maturity onset diabetes of the young, and rare syndromic forms of diabetes such as Wolfram syndrome and Alstrom syndrome have been identified in children (*30*). In some cases, these rare forms of diabetes can clinically present as T1D, but they are distinguishable from Type 1A by lack of autoantibodies. Neonatal diabetes mellitus, defined as insulin-requiring hyperglycemia within the first month of life, is a rare disorder that is usually associated with intrauterine growth retardation (*30*).

Neonatal diabetes is a heterogeneous disease that can be either transient or permanent. Well-defined forms of permanent neonatal diabetes include diabetes associated with intrauterine growth restriction, mutation in insulin promoter factor 1 (*30*), mutation of the proinsulin molecule (*31*), and activating mutations of SUR (*32*). Neonatal diabetes caused by severe glucokinase deficiency is associated with severe hyperglycemia requiring insulin treatment (*33*). There are currently no data on the pancreatic pathology in patients with neonatal diabetes due to glucokinase deficiency but due to the nature of the physiological defect (i.e., inability to couple insulin secretion with extracellular glucose levels), it is likely that these patients have a normal β cell mass. This situation constitutes a typical example on how clinically defined T1D can be due to a functional defect rather than a loss of β cell mass.

CONCLUSIONS

We believe a strong case has been presented that much more in the way of research involving human pancreas in T1D should be performed, with emphasis on elucidating the etiology of the process underlying the activation of the immune system, the natural history of β cell loss, and questions related to β cell regeneration. Address of these areas should not only improve our understanding of the natural history of T1D, but in addition, address the question of why the disorder develops. The definition of heterogeneity in the pathology of T1D might lead to the characterization of yet undefined forms of diabetes with nonautoimmune pathogenesis representing a sizable portion of islet autoantibody negative cases. This possibility is strengthened by the existence of rare forms of T1D (or beta cell loss secondary to the primary metabolic derangement observed in most cases of T2D) characterized by nonautoimmune beta cell loss. An improved understanding of events within the pancreas should also provide information relevant to the design of novel therapeutics capable of preventing β cell destruction in the different forms of T1D.

REFERENCES

1. Gepts W. Pathologic anatomy of the pancreas in juvenile diabetes mellitus. Diabetes 1965;14: 619–633.
2. Foulis AK, Liddle CN, Farquharson JA, Richmond JA, Weir RS. The histopathology of the pancreas in Type 1 (insulin-dependent) diabetes mellitus: a 25-year review of deaths in patients under 20 years of age in the United Kingdom. Diabetologia 1986;29:267–274.
3. Hanafusa T, Miyazaki A, Miyagawa J, Tamura S, Inada M, Yamada K, et al. Examination of islets in the pancreas biopsy specimens from newly diagnosed type 1 (insulin-dependent) diabetic patients. Diabetologia 1990;33: 105–111.
4. Conrad B, Weidmann E, Trucco G, Rudert WA, Behboo R, Ricordi C, et al. Evidence for superantigen involvement in insulin-dependent diabetes mellitus aetiology. Nature 1994;371: 351–355.
5. In't Veld P, Lievens D, De Grijse J, Ling Z, Van der Auweea B, Pipeleers-Marichal M, et al. Screening for insulitis in adult autoantibody-positive organ donors. Diabetes 2007; 56:2400–2404.
6. Gianani R, Putnam A, Still T, Yu L, Miao D, Gill RG, et al. Initial results of screening of nondiabetic organ donors for expression of islet autoantibodies. J Clin Endocrinol Metab 2006;91:1855–1861.
7. Clark A, Wells CA, Buley ID, Cruickshank JK, Vanhegan RI, Matthews DR, et al. Islet amyloid, increased A-cells, reduced B-cells and exocrine fibrosis: quantitative changes in the pancreas in type 2 diabetes. Diabetes Res 1988;9(4):151–159.
8. Foulis AK, Stewart JA. The pancreas in recent-onset type 1 (insulin-dependent) diabetes mellitus: insulin content of islets, insulitis and associated changes in the exocrine acinar tissue. Diabetologia 1984;26:456–461.
9. Foulis AK. In type 1 diabetes, does a noncytopathic viral infection of insulin-secreting B-cells initiate the disease process leading to their autoimmune destruction? Diabet Med 1989;6:666–674.
10. Foulis AK, Jackson RA, Farquharson MA. The pancreas in idiopathic Addison's disease – a search for a prediabetic pancreas. Histopathology 1988;12:481–490.
11. Daaboul J, Schatz D. Overview of prevention and intervention trials for type 1 diabetes. Rev Endocr Metab Disord 2003;4:317–323.
12. Meier JJ, Bhushan A, Butler PC. Sustained beta cell apoptosis in patients with long-standing type 1 diabetes: indirect evidence for islet regeneration? Diabetologia 2008;48(11): 2221–2228.
13. Bottazzo GF, Dean BM, McNally JM, MacKay EH, Swift PG, Gambe DR. In situ characterization of autoimmune phenomena and expression of HLA molecules in the pancreas in diabetic insulitis. N Engl J Med 1985;313: 353–360.
14. Foulis AK, McGill M, Farquharson MA. Insulitis in type 1 (insulin-dependent) diabetes mellitus in man – macrophages, lymphocytes, and interferon-gamma containing cells. J Pathol 1991;165:97–103.
15. Itoh N, Hanafusa T, Miyazaki A, Miyagawa J, Yamagata K, Yamamoto K, et al. Mononuclear cell infiltration and its relation to the expression of major histocompatibility complex antigens and adhesion molecules in pancreas biopsy specimens from newly diagnosed insulin-dependent diabetes mellitus patients. J Clin Invest 1993;92:2313–2322.
16. Stassi G, De Maria R, Trucco G, Rudert W, Test R, Galluzzo A, et al. Nitric oxide primes pancreatic beta cells for Fas-mediated destruction in insulin-dependent diabetes mellitus. J Exp Med 1997;186:1193–1200.
17. Moriwaki M, Itoh N, Miyagawa J, Yamamoto K, Imagawa K, Yamagata K, et al. Fas and Fas ligand expression in inflamed islets in pancreas sections of patients with recent-onset Type I diabetes mellitus. Diabetologia 1999;42: 1332–1340.
18. Foulis AK, Farquharson MA, Meager A. Immunoreactive alpha-interferon in insulin-secreting beta cells in type 1 diabetes mellitus. Lancet 1987;2:1423–1427.
19. Imagawa A, Hanafusa T, Itoh N, Miyagawa J, Nakajima H, Namba M, et al. Islet-infiltrating T lymphocytes in insulin-dependent diabetic patients express CD80 (B7-1) and CD86 (B7-2). J Autoimmun 1996;9:391–396.
20. Pujol-Borrell R, Todd I, Doshi M, Gray D, Feldmann M, Bottazzo GF. Differential expression and regulation of MHC products in the endocrine and exocrine cells of the human pancreas. Clin Exp Immunol 1986;65:128–139.
21. Imagawa A, Hanafusa T, Tamura S, Moriwaki M, Itoh N, Yamamoto K, et al. Pancreatic biopsy as a procedure for detecting in situ autoimmune phenomena in type 1 diabetes. Diabetes 2001;50:1269–1271.
22. Atkinson MA, Rhodes CJ. Pancreatic regeneration in type 1 diabetes: dreams on a deserted islet? Diabetologia 2005;48:2200–2202.

23. Butler AE, Galasso R, Mejer JJ, Basu R, Rizza RA, Butler PC. Modestly increased beta cell apoptosis but no increased beta cell replication in recent-onset type 1 diabetic patients who died of diabetic ketoacidosis. Diabetologia 2007;50:2323–2331.
24. Wang J, Miao D, Babu S, Yu J, Barker J, Klingensmith G, et al. Prevalence of autoantibody-negative diabetes is not rare at all ages and increases with older age and obesity. J Clin Endocrinol Metab 2007;92:88–92.
25. Gianani R, Eisenbarth GS. The stages of type 1A diabetes. Immunol Rev 2005;204:232–249.
26. Wenzlau JM, Juhl K, Yu L, Moua O, Sarkar SA, Gottlieb P, et al. The cation efflux transporter ZnT8 (Slc30A8) is a major autoantigen in human type 1 diabetes. Proc Natl Acad Sci 2007;104:17040–17045.
27. Rahier J, Guiot Y, Goebbels RM, Sempoux C, Henquin JC. Pancreatic B-cell mass in European subjects with type 2 diabetes. Diabetes Obes Metab 2008;10(4):32–42.
28. Kassem S, Ariel I, Thornton PS, Sheimberg I, Glaser B. Beta-cell proliferation and apoptosis in the developing normal human pancreas and in hyperinsulinism of infancy. Diabetes 2000;49:1325–1333.
29. Leibowitz G, Glaser B, Higazi AA, Salameh M, Cerasi E, Landau H. Hyperinsulinemic hypoglycemia of infancy (nesidioblastosis) in clinical remission: high incidence of diabetes mellitus and persistent beta-cell dysfunction at long-term follow-up. J Clin Endocrinol Metab 1995;80(2):386–396.
30. Njolstad PR, Sovk O, Cuesta-Munoz A, Bjorkaug L, Massa O, Barbetti F, et al. Neonatal diabetes mellitus due to complete glucokinase deficiency. N Engl J Med 2008;344:1588–1592.
31. Colombo C, Porzio O, Liu M, Massa O, Vasta M, Salardi S, et al. Seven mutations in the human insulin gene linked to permanent neonatal/infancy-onset diabetes mellitus. J Clin Invest 2008;118(6):2148–2156.
32. Tarasov AI, Girard CA, Larkin B, Tammaro P, Flanagan SE, Ellard S, et al. Functional analysis of two Kir6.2 (KCNJ11) mutations, K170T and E322K, causing neonatal diabetes. Diabetes Obes Metab 2007;9(Suppl 2):46–55.
33. Rubio-Cabezas O, Diaz-Gonzales F, Aragones A, Argente J, Campos-Barros A. Permanent neonatal diabetes caused by a homozygous nonsense mutation in the glucokinase gene. Pediatr Diabetes 2008;9(3 Pt 1):245–249.

Chapter 15

Genetics of Type 1 Diabetes

Immunoendocrinology: Scientific and Clinical Aspects

Aaron Michels, Joy Jeffrey, and George S. Eisenbarth

Key Words: Major histocompatibility complex, Autoimmune regulator gene, FoxP3, Human leukocyte antigens, Insulin gene, Genomewide association studies

INTRODUCTION

By the American Diabetes Association Classification, Type 1A Diabetes is the immune-mediated form of diabetes, while Type 1B represents nonimmune-mediated forms of diabetes with beta-cell destruction leading to absolute insulin deficiency (1). There are additional forms of insulin-dependent diabetes with defined etiologies ("Other Specific Types of Diabetes:" genetic, hormonal, and environmental). Finally, type 2 diabetes is, overall, the most common form of diabetes and is characterized by insulin resistance and less beta-cell loss. Even in children, it is important to identify individuals who do not have type 1A diabetes with estimates that approximately 1.5% of children presenting with diabetes have monogenic forms of diabetes. Several monogenetic forms of diabetes are reported to be better treated with sulfonylurea therapy than insulin (e.g., mutations of the ATP-sensitive beta cell selective potassium channels and HNF-1alpha mutations) (2), and diabetes due to glucokinase mutations require no therapy at all. Approximately, one half of permanent neonatal diabetes is due to either mutations of the proinsulin gene that leads to beta-cell loss (similar to the Akita mouse (3)) or Kir6.2/SUR1 mutations (4).

This chapter will deal almost exclusively with genetics of the polygenic forms of immune-mediated diabetes. There are instructive animal models and humans with predominantly "monogenic" forms of immune-mediated diabetes resulting from mutations of the *FoxP3* gene or the *AIRE* gene (AutoImmune REgulator) that will be discussed in other chapters. These autoimmune syndromes with diabetes, IPEX (Immune Dysfunction, Polyendocrinopathy, Enteropathy, X-linked: *FoxP3* mutation) and APS-1 (Autoimmune Polyendocrine Syndrome Type 1: *AIRE* mutation), illustrate how readily immune-mediated diabetes develops when regulatory T cells or central tolerance mechanisms are deficient (5).

Primarily, genetic polymorphisms contributing to the familial aggregation and inheritance of diabetes risk in animal models and humans will be discussed given the autoimmune (T cell mediated) nature of the disease, although the genetic mechanisms generating T-cell diversity/targeting are likely essential disease determinants. The crucial specific molecular mediators of the disease are very likely T-cell receptors recognizing peptides of islet beta cells. Prior to programmed genetic recombination of T-cell receptor genes, these genes do not apparently differ between individuals and thus do not contribute to genetically determined familial aggregation of disease. We have evidence for the nonobese diabetic (NOD) mouse model that specific alpha chains of the T-cell receptor combine with multiple T-cell receptor beta chains to recognize a "primary" insulin peptide (6–8). Thus, as the technology for sequencing large numbers (tens of thousands) of T-cell receptors is now feasible (9), analysis of somatically generated T-cell receptor sequence diversity may contribute to both disease prediction and understanding of pathogenesis. The hypothesis we favor for the frequent occurrence of immune-mediated diabetes in animal models and humans is that polymorphisms of multiple genes influencing immune function (regulation of central and peripheral tolerance along with innate immunity) control the probability that T lymphocytes (CD4 and CD8) with frequently generated T-cell receptors will target islet peptides. The timing and penetrance of antiislet autoimmunity can be influenced by environmental factors. Direct evidence for the importance of the environment is the remarkable increase in the incidence of type 1A diabetes. The disorder, similar to other immune-mediated diseases, such as asthma, is doubling approximately every 20 years (10). Nevertheless, type 1A diabetes almost always develops in the setting of genetic susceptibility best defined at present with analysis of polymorphisms of HLA alleles (11). Though there have been dramatic advances in our understanding of the genetics of this disease over the past decade, more remains to be discovered.

ANIMAL MODELS

The pathogenesis of the animal models of type 1A diabetes will be covered in more detail in accompanying chapters. The most intensively studied spontaneous models are the NOD mouse and the BioBreeding (BB) rat, and for both, though genetic polymorphisms are key determinants of disease, environmental factors can either induce or suppress diabetes. For both the animal models, multiple genetic polymorphisms on multiple different chromosomes determine disease penetrance with class II immune response genes, the key determinants of risk, similar to humans. For the NOD mouse, lack of the DR-like molecule (I-E) due to a common mouse polymorphism and presence of a specific sequence of I-A (namely I-A^{g7}) are essential for susceptibility (*12, 13*). The susceptible MHC haplotype of the BB rat is termed RT1-U, and multiple "normal" rat strains with the RT1-U haplotype can be induced to develop diabetes with the administration of agents that suppress regulation or activate innate immunity (*14*). These MHC polymorphisms are not enough to lead to autoimmune diabetes, as congenic strains with the NOD MHC (I-E null with I-A^{g7}) on other murine genetic backgrounds do not develop insulin autoantibodies, insulitis, or diabetes (*15*). The diabetes-associated class II genes most likely contribute to diabetes pathogenesis by the islet peptides they present and influence thymic T-cell development. Most of the polygenic genetic controls on development of diabetes can be bypassed by increasing precursor frequency (e.g., transgenic (*16–19*) and retrogenic mice (*20*)) of T cells with specific receptors targeting islet peptides as long as the appropriate presenting MHC alleles are present (*21*). Both susceptible MHC alleles and a lack of suppressive alleles are needed for disease risk. This appears directly analogous to humans, where multiple high-risk genotypes have been identified, and multiple class II-associated haplotypes can provide dominant protection (*11*).

In humans, the next most important locus after the MHC contributing to diabetes risk is the insulin locus, and, in particular, polymorphisms associated with differential expression of insulin in the thymus (*22*). Mouse strains do not differ in terms of their insulin genes and both rats and mice have two insulin genes. However, genetic manipulation of the proinsulin/insulin genes either accelerates or prevents diabetes in NOD mice. The insulin 2 gene of the NOD mouse is expressed in both islets and thymus while the insulin 1 gene is expressed only within islets. A knockout of the insulin 1 gene prevents almost all diabetes, while a knockout of the insulin 2 gene greatly accelerates the development of diabetes (*23*). Knocking out both insulin genes and restoring insulin synthesis with a mutated insulin gene (B16 tyrosine replaced with alanine producing a B:9-23 insulin peptide not recognized by a dominant T-cell response) prevents diabetes (6). Inducing "tolerance" to proinsulin similarly prevents all diabetes and abrogates a common immune response to the islet molecule IGRP (islet-specific glucose-6-phosphatase catalytic subunit-related protein), (24) implying that the immune response to insulin is "upstream" of the T-cell response to IGRP.

Multiple other genes and loci, both for the NOD mouse and the BB rat, influencing diabetes susceptibility have been identified. The BB rat strain has a mutation of a gene, *gimap/ian*, that disrupts normal T-cell development (25) such that BB rats are severely lymphopenic despite developing autoimmune diabetes (26, 27). This mutation induces lymphopenia and autoimmune diabetes in an autosomal recessive manner (28). The BB-DR strain (BB rat-Diabetes Resistant) lacking this mutation is not lymphopenic and does not spontaneously develop diabetes, but can be induced to develop diabetes with activation of innate immunity as occurs with infection with the Kilham rat virus (see accompanying chapter) (14). The different "diabetogenic" loci of the NOD mouse can differentially influence immune phenotypes, such as expression of insulin autoantibodies and/or progression to diabetes (29). A single nucleotide polymorphism (SNP) of cytotoxic T lymphocyte-associated antigen 4 (CTLA4) of mice is associated with higher expression of the ligand-independent form of CTLA4 (unable to bind to its "receptor" B7.1/B7.2) and is associated with protection from diabetes (30). Decreasing CTLA4 expression with RNA interference accelerates development of insulitis and diabetes (31), and subtle decreases of IL2 (putative idd3 gene) expression are associated with autoimmunity, presumably through influence on regulatory T cells that are dependent upon IL2 signaling (32).

Inbred rat and mouse strains are not diallelic at any locus and thus are fundamentally genetically different from humans, where even monozygotic twins are diallelic at tens of thousands of loci. Such genetic homogeneity probably influences the ease with which diabetes can be prevented in the NOD mouse. In this strain, multiple relatively nonspecific factors can prevent disease, though it is more difficult to reverse diabetes, and more difficult to eliminate insulitis. As mentioned above, the NOD mouse lacking the insulin 2 genes has a more aggressive disease course, and many nonspecific factors (e.g., complete Freund's adjuvant) are unable to prevent diabetes in this model.

TYPE 1A DIABETES OF MAN

Descriptive Genetics

In the United States, with a population of 300 million, there are approximately 1.5 million individuals with type 1 diabetes, and of

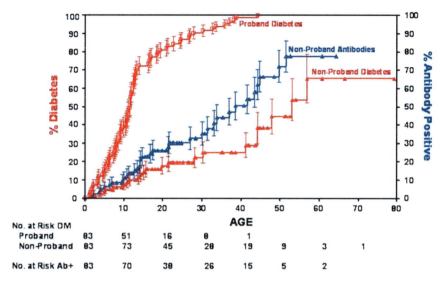

Fig. 15.1 Progression to diabetes of initially discordant monozygotic twin siblings of patients with type 1 diabetes, illustrating progressive conversion to diabetes. More than 80% of this cohort became concordant for expression of antiislet autoantibodies (from Teaching Slides www.barbaradaviscenter.org). Modified from (*34*).

these, approximately 170,000 are less than age 20 (18 million with diagnosed diabetes overall). Approximately 1/300 individuals from the general population develop type 1A diabetes compared with 1/20 siblings of patients with type 1A diabetes (Lambda-s approximately 15). Risk of an identical twin developing diabetes with long-term follow-up is greater than 60% (Fig. 15.1), and a recent analysis from our twin series indicates that there is no age at which an initially discordant monozygotic twin is no longer at risk (*33*).

In contrast to monozygotic twins of patients with type 1A diabetes, initially discordant dizygotic twins are less often positive for antiislet autoantibodies and at no greater level of positivity than nontwin siblings (*34*). Offspring of a father with type 1A diabetes have a greater risk compared with offspring of a mother (*35*).

The Major Histocompatibility Complex

The primary determinant of type 1A diabetes risk are genes within or linked to the Major Histocompatibility Complex and in particular class II HLA alleles, such as DQ, DR, and DP (for an explanation of HLA nomenclature see Chap. 1). There is a spectrum of risk, which is easiest to define for specific DR and DQ alleles by analyzing transmission of HLA DR/DQ haplotypes from parents to children with type 1A diabetes. Under the null hypothesis of no influence on risk, transmission to their diabetic offspring of specific alleles from parents heterozygous for HLA alleles should be 50:50. Instead as shown in Fig. 15.2, there is a hierarchy of distorted transmission (not 50:50), going from almost 90% to almost no transmission of specific HLA-DQ alleles from heterozygous parents (for this analysis, the alternative HLA DQ allele of the parent was not high risk DQ8 (DQA1*0301/

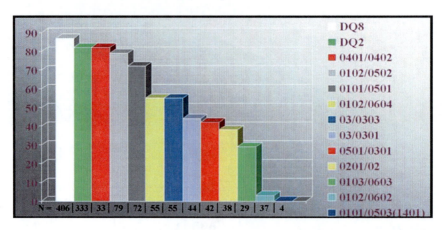

Fig. 15.2 Transmission of DQ alleles from heterozygous parents, second haplotype not DQ2 or DQ8, to diabetic children from the Human Biological Data Interchange (HBDI) Series. The HBDI is a repository for DNA from 276 families with type 1A diabetes. From Teaching Slides www.barbaradaviscenter.org.

DQB1*0302) and DQ2 (DQA1*0501/DQB1*0201) alleles). A recent manuscript by Erlich and coworkers analyzing the large family data set of the Type 1 Diabetes Genetics Consortium (*11*) has documented the differential risk associated with specific DR and DQ alleles, specific haplotypes (combinations of DR and DQ alleles on the same chromosome), and most important specific genotypes (combinations of both haplotypes, one inherited from each parent). The three most protective haplotypes with extreme odds ratios of less than 0.03 were DRB1*1401-DQA1 *0101-DQB1*0503, DRB1*1501-DQA1*0102-DQB1*0602, and DRB1*0701-DQA1*0201-DQB1*0303.

High-risk haplotypes in this large study are also similar to those shown in Fig. 15.2 and, of note, DRB1*0801-DQB1*0401-DQB1*0402 is a moderately high-risk haplotype (odds ratio 1.25). Despite being high risk, this haplotype has aspartic acid at position 57 of DQ beta chain (often this amino acid is referred to as "protective" with only analysis of common Caucasian DQ beta alleles), as does the related high-risk Asian DQ haplotype DQA1*0301-DQB1*0401, and has the third highest transmission as seen in Fig. 15.2.

The most common protective haplotype (DRB1*1501-DQA1*0102-DQB1*0602) is present in approximately 20% of the general US population and 1% of children with type 1A diabetes. The etiology of dominant protection is not yet understood. The highest risk common genotype (Genotype = two HLA haplotypes with one inherited from each parent) consists of DR3/4-DQ2/8 (DRB1*0301-DQA1*0501-DQB1*0201/ DRB1*0401-DQA1*0301-DQB1*0302). This genotype is present in 2.4% of children born in Denver, Colorado and approximately 30% of children developing type 1A diabetes. The excess risk encoded by "being heterozygous" for these haplotypes may relate to the trans-encoded DQ molecule (DQA and DQB encoded by different chromosomes) that can form in DR3/4 heterozygous individuals, namely, DQA1*0501-DQB1*0302 for this genotype (*11*).

In addition to DQ effects on risk, DRB1*04 alleles influence risk and in particular the DRB1*0403 allele is protective. DP also influences risk, and for the high-risk DR3/4-DQ2/8 genotype, absence of both DRB1*0403 and DPB1*0402 leads to a cumulative risk of activating antiislet autoimmunity of approximately 1/5 in the general population (*36*). Furthermore, siblings of patients with type 1A diabetes, who have the high-risk DR3/4-DQ2/8 genotype and share both HLA haplotypes identical by descent with their proband, had an 80% risk of expressing antiislet autoantibodies and 60% risk for diabetes by age 18 in the DAISY study (Fig. 15.3) (*37*). If this extreme risk is confirmed, it will allow trials to be designed for diabetes prevention prior to the appearance of antiislet autoantibodies in these high-risk siblings. Such an extreme risk implies that for this common HLA genotype, environmental factors contributing to diabetes are likely to be ubiquitous. If prediction of an 80% genetic risk at birth can be determined, rare essential environmental factors are unlikely.

Given the MHC data reviewed above, a number of groups are pursuing the identification of additional genes contributing to diabetes risk within or linked to the MHC. We have reported a locus telomeric of the UBD gene several million base pairs away from DR and DQ alleles (*38*). HLA molecules such as HLA-A24 (*39*) and HLA-B39 (*40, 41*) may have independent influences but the existence of frequent MHC haplotypes, where all SNPs for several million base pairs across the MHC are identical, will make pinpointing specific causal polymorphisms difficult (*42, 43*).

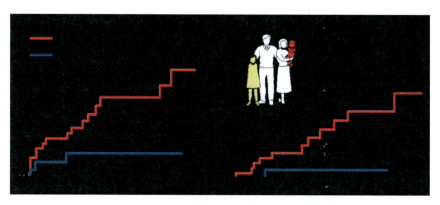

Fig. 15.3 Haplotype sharing survival curves from the DAISY study. Shown is progression to antiislet autoimmunity and type 1A diabetes in DR3/4-DQ8 siblings stratified by the number of HLA haplotypes shared with their proband siblings (from Teaching Slides www.barbaradaviscenter.org). From (*37*). *HR* hazard ratio, *CI* confidence interval.

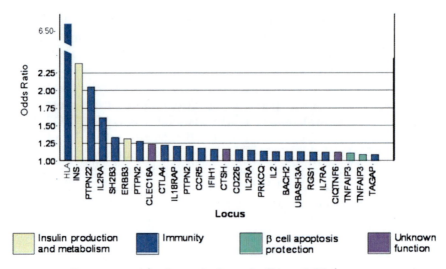

Genome-wide Associations in Type 1 Diabetes

Fig. 15.4 Summary of subsets of confirmed loci from whole-genome screens associated with type 1A diabetes and their odds ratio (from Teaching Slides www.barbaradaviscenter.org). Modified from Concannon P et al., Genetics of type 1A diabetes, N J Engl Med. 2009; 360:1646. *HLA* human leukocyte antigen, *INS* insulin, *PTPN22* protein tyrosine phosphatase nonreceptor 22, *IL2RA* interleukin-2 receptor alpha chain, also known as CD 25, *ERBB3e* an unidentified gene at 12q, *PTPN2* protein tyrosine phosphatase nonreceptor 2, *KIAA 0350* a lectin-like gene, *CTLA 4* cytotoxic T lymphocyte-associated antigen 4.

In general, we believe there remain major genetic influences within the MHC to define.

Nonmajor Histocompatibility Complex Genes

Several genetic loci were discovered with candidate gene approaches (insulin and PTPN22), but most recent genetic loci contributing to diabetes risk were defined with analysis of thousands of SNPs in large populations, including the recent Genome Wide Association Studies. Figure 15.4 illustrates odds ratios for a number of replicated loci. The unique influence of the class II HLA genes is obvious as well as the relatively small (less than 1.3) odds ratios of the more recently defined loci.

The Insulin Gene (Chromosome 11p)

Bell and coworkers originally described the association of polymorphisms 5 (variable nucleotide tandem repeats) to the proinsulin gene for type 1A diabetes (*44*). Those proinsulin genes with the greatest number of repeats were associated with both greater expression of minute amounts of insulin message within the thymus and decreased risk of diabetes (*45, 46*). In animal models, variation in thymic insulin is associated with antiinsulin autoimmunity (*47*) and the putative mechanism of the AIRE gene, also "controlling" thymic insulin message expression, contend for a general role of genes controlling thymic insulin in influencing disease risk. Relatively small differences in insulin message have measurable effects on the development of autoimmunity and diabetes.

PTPN22 (Chromosome 1p13)

The specific association of a single amino-acid change of the lymphocyte PTPN22 tyrosine phosphatase nonreceptor 22 (R620W: Arginine for Tryptophan) with autoimmunity was first discovered with a candidate gene approach by Bottini and coworkers (*48*). This same polymorphism has subsequently been associated with a series of autoimmune disorders, most notably rheumatoid arthritis (*49*). The amino acid change leads to a gain of function, enhancing suppression of T-cell receptor signaling (*50*). It is not clear why decreasing T-cell receptor signaling would enhance autoimmunity, but it can be hypothesized that deficient negative selection of thymic autoreactive T cells may be involved.

CTLA4 (Chromosome 2q31)

Similar to PTPN22, CTLA4 is a negative regulator of T-lymphocyte activation. The CTLA4 molecule, when it is induced on a T lymphocyte, interacts with its ligand on an antigen-presenting cell and mediates a negative signal to downregulate T-cell activation, proliferation, and differentiation. There are several polymorphisms of the CTLA4 locus that are associated with type 1A diabetes at both the 3 promoter (-319C>T) and 5 untranslated region (+6230G>A) (*51*), and the protective 5 polymorphism (protective for diabetes and thyroid autoimmunity) (*52*) is associated with higher levels of mRNA of the soluble isoform of CTLA4.

IL2RA (Il2 Receptor Alpha Chain-CD25- Chromosome 10p15-p14)

Regulatory T cells are dependent upon IL2 signaling through the IL2 receptor, and thus, subtle disruption of this pathway can enhance development of autoimmunity. Type 1A diabetes risk is associated with two SNPs of the IL2 receptor alpha region (*53*) and associated with lower levels of circulating IL2RA itself (*54*). Graves' disease is associated with these SNPs in a similar manner, while multiple sclerosis is associated with different IL2RA SNPs.

Additional Loci

With recent technology (Genome Wide Association Studies) and repositories of DNA from tens of thousands of patients with type 1A diabetes and controls, additional loci with strong statistical evidence of association with type 1A diabetes have been identified as shown in Table 15.1 (*55*). In general, the diabetes-associated loci are related to immunologic function, and type 2 diabetes loci have not been implicated (*56–61*). A number of the loci are interesting given the potential immunologic pathways such as the Interferon-Induced Helicase that may relate to association with innate immunity (*62*), and KIAA 0350, a presumed lectin-like gene (*63*). Interferon alpha therapy has been associated with both the de novo appearance of antiislet autoantibodies and development of diabetes (*64*).

It is estimated that there will be 50 or more loci identified within the next few years associated with type 1A diabetes with further analysis of Genome Wide Association Studies. It is unlikely that outside the MHC any new loci contributing to diabetes risk with odds ratios greater than 1.5 will be discovered (*30*). Most of

Table 15.1
Loci from Genome Wide Association Studies Contributing to Type 1A Diabetes Risk

Study	Initial sample size	Replication sample size	Region	Gene(s)	OR [95% CI]	P-value
Hakonarson et al. (58)	563 cases, 1,146 controls, 483 trios	549 families, 1,092 individuals from 364 trios	12q13.2	RAB5B, SUOX, IKZF4, ERBB3, CDK2	1.25 [1.12–1.40]	9×10^{-10}
Hakonarson et al. (63)	561 cases, 1,143 controls, 467 trios	1,333 individuals in 549 families; 390 trios	16p13.13	KIAA0350	1.54 [1.32–1.79]	7×10^{-11}
WTCCC. June 07, 2007 Nature.	1,963 cases, 2,938 controls	4,000 cases, 5,000 controls, 2,997 trios	12q24.13 12q13.2 16p13.13 12p13 4q27	SH2B3,LNK,TRAFD1, PTPN1ERBB3 KIAA0350 None Reported None Reported	1.34 [1.16–1.53] 1.34 [1.17–1.54] 1.19 [0.97–1.45] 1.49 [1.28–1.73] 1.26 [1.11–1.42]	$2 \times 10^{-14} 1 \times 10^{-11}$ 5×10^{-7} 7×10^{-7} 3×10^{-6}
Todd et al. (61)	1,963 cases, 2,938 controls	4,000 cases, 5,000 controls, 2,997 trios	12q13.2 16p13.13 12q24.13 18p11.21 18q22.2	ERBB3KIAA0350 C12orf30 PTPN2 CD226	1.28 [1.21–1.35] 1.23 [1.16–1.30] 1.22 [1.15–1.28] 1.30 [1.22–1.40] 1.16 [1.10–1.22]	2×10^{-20} 3×10^{-18} 2×10^{-16} 1×10^{-14} 1×10^{-8}

[a]Modified from (55)

the familial aggregation of type 1A diabetes apparently remains unexplained given the low odds ratios for the newly defined loci. This may indicate that very many uncommon mutations/polymorphisms might contribute to disease risk, in addition to the relatively common polymorphisms currently identified.

Combinatorial Analysis

Given the large number of non-MHC loci identified with odds ratios less than 1.5, disease prediction has not dramatically improved. Analysis of HLA, Insulin, PTPN22, and CTLA4 jointly found no influence on ROC curve area (a measure of predictive sensitivity and specificity) when adding these additional polymorphisms to HLA-defined risk (65). This, in part, occurs because of the relatively low frequency of individuals with multiple different high-risk non-MHC polymorphisms even in a study of approximately 1,700 patients with type 1A diabetes combined with the dominant influence of HLA alleles on risk.

Gene/Environment

The alarming increase in risk of type 1A diabetes over the past 60 years in many developed countries suggests that environmental factors increasing diabetes risk have been introduced or factors decreasing risk have been removed. There is no evidence that this "epidemic" of increasing type 1A diabetes has leveled off in Finland (10), and in particular, the incidence of diabetes in children developing the disease prior to age 5 is increasing. Though the Hygiene Hypothesis ascribes increasing immune disorders to decreased infectious burden of Western populations(66), there is no consensus as to which of multiple environmental factors are important. There is a report of low vitamin D levels in Scandinavia and of polymorphisms of vitamin D-metabolizing enzyme SNPs (O.R. approximately 1.1) associated with diabetes. A large prospective study of islet autoimmunity has failed to confirm an association of autoimmunity risk with serum alpha and gamma-tocopherol concentrations (67). Multiple additional dietary environmental factors including timing of the introduction of cereals, omega-3 fatty acid levels, and neonatal exposure to bovine milk products have been implicated in diabetes risk (68–71). Epigenetic influences secondary to dietary factors such as hypermethylation (71) potentially associated with dietary supplements are likely to be evaluated in individuals with genetic susceptibility, especially given the observation that discordance of methylation of monozygotic twins increases with age (73).

CONCLUSIONS

Though less than 90% of patients developing type 1A diabetes have a first-degree relative with the disease, almost all patients express one or more HLA DR/DQ alleles associated with the disease (e.g., 90% DR3 and or DR4). In general, as the incidence of type 1A diabetes has increased the proportion of patients with the highest risk DR3/4 genotype has decreased (74). This suggests that the environment is becoming more permissive for the development of type 1A diabetes, particularly for individuals with moderate-risk HLA alleles (75). At present, gene–environment interactions are poorly defined. Large prospective environmental studies are underway, such as the NIH Teddy study, where more than 300,000 newborns are being HLA-typed to identify a subgroup of newborn children at high risk. It is now possible to measure four antiislet autoantibodies that precede the development of diabetes in genetically susceptible children, including the latest discovered, the ZnT8 (Zinc transporter), expressed in islet beta cells (76). A polymorphism of the ZnT8 gene is associated with a specific epitope of the molecule recognized by islet autoantibodies. For the subset of patients whose antibodies recognize a single epitope, the epitope recognized is the one they express, with either tryptophan or arginine at amino acid 325 of the ZnT8 (77). This is consistent with true autoimmunity to ZnT8, not molecular mimicry, as the specific autoantigenic sequence is the target of an immune response. As illustrated by the autoantibodies targeting ZnT8, it is likely that with improved genetic knowledge, genetic polymorphisms will be found to influence not only disease risk but also many intermediate aspects of pathogenesis. At present, we have only a partial understanding of the genetics of type 1A diabetes, but we suspect this understanding is likely to increase as the critical MHC locus is further defined and phenotypic characterization improves.

REFERENCES

1. Diagnosis and classification of diabetes mellitus. Diabetes Care. 2008;31(Suppl 1):S55–S60.
2. Murphy R, Ellard S, Hattersley AT. Clinical implications of a molecular genetic classification of monogenic beta-cell diabetes. Nat Clin Pract Endocrinol Metab. 2008;4:200–213.
3. Liu M, Hodish I, Rhodes CJ, Arvan P. Proinsulin maturation, misfolding, and proteotoxicity. Proc Natl Acad Sci USA. 2007;104:15841–15846.
4. Gloyn AL, Pearson ER, Antcliff JF, Proks P, Bruining GJ, Slingerland AS, et al. Activating mutations in the gene encoding the ATP-sensitive potassium-channel subunit Kir6.2 and permanent neonatal diabetes. N Engl J Med. 2004;350:1838–1849.
5. Eisenbarth GS, Gottlieb PA. Autoimmune polyendocrine syndromes. N Engl J Med. 2004;350:2068–2079.
6. Nakayama M, Abiru N, Moriyama H, Babaya N, Liu E, Miao D, et al. Prime role for an insulin epitope in the development of type 1 diabetes in NOD mice. Nature. 2005;435: 220–223.
7. Kobayashi M, Jasinski J, Liu E, Li M, Miao D, Zhang L, et al. Conserved T cell receptor alpha-chain induces insulin autoantibodies. Proc Natl Acad Sci USA. 2008;5: 10090–10094.
8. Homann D, Eisenbarth GS. An immunologic homunculus for type 1 diabetes. J Clin Invest. 2006;116:1212–1215.

9. Palacios G, Druce J, Du L, Tran T, Birch C, Briese T, et al. A new arenavirus in a cluster of fatal transplant-associated diseases. N Engl J Med. 2008;358:991–998.
10. Harjutsalo V, Sjoberg L, Tuomilehto J. Time trends in the incidence of type 1 diabetes in Finnish children: a cohort study. Lancet. 2008; 371:1777–1782.
11. Erlich H, Valdes AM, Noble J, Carlson JA, Varney M, Concannon P et al. HLA DR-DQ haplotypes and genotypes and type 1 diabetes risk: analysis of the type 1 diabetes genetics consortium families. Diabetes. 2008; 57: 1084–1092.
12. Hattori M, Buse JB, Jackson RA, Glimcher L, Dorf ME, Minami M, et al. The NOD mouse: recessive diabetogenic gene within the major histocompatibility complex. Science. 1986; 231:733–735.
13. Todd JA, Bell JI, McDevitt HO. HLA-DQB gene contributes to susceptibility and resistance to insulin-dependent diabetes mellitus. Nature. 1987;329:599–604.
14. Zipris D, Lien E, Nair A, Xie JX, Greiner DL, Mordes JP, et al. TLR9-signaling pathways are involved in Kilham rat virus-induced autoimmune diabetes in the biobreeding diabetes-resistant rat. J Immunol. 2007;178:693–701.
15. Wicker LS, Miller BJ, Fischer PA, Pressey A, Peterson LB. Genetic control of diabetes and insulitis in the nonobese diabetic mouse. Pedigree analysis of a diabetic H-2nod/b heterozygote. J Immunol. 1989;142:781–784.
16. Katz JD, Wang B, Haskins K, Benoist C, Mathis D. Following a diabetogenic T cell from genesis through pathogenesis. Cell. 1993;74:1089–1100.
17. Han B, Serra P, Yamanouchi J, Amrani A, Elliott JF, Dickie P, et al. Developmental control of CD8 T cell-avidity maturation in autoimmune diabetes. J Clin Invest. 2005;115:1879–1887.
18. Du W, Wong FS, Li MO, Peng J, Qi H, Flavell RA, et al. TGF-beta signaling is required for the function of insulin-reactive T regulatory cells. J Clin Invest. 2006;116:1360–1370.
19. DiLorenzo TP, Lieberman SM, Takaki T, Honda S, Chapman HD, Santamaria P, et al. During the early prediabetic period in NOD mice, the pathogenic CD8(+) T-cell population comprises multiple antigenic specificities. Clin Immunol. 2002;105:332–341.
20. Burton AR, Vincent E, Arnold PY, Lennon GP, Smeltzer M, Li CS, et al. On the pathogenicity of autoantigen-specific T-cell receptors. Diabetes. 2008;57:1321–1330.
21. Jasinski JM, Yu L, Nakayama M, Li MM, Lipes MA, Eisenbarth GS, et al. Transgenic insulin (B:9-23) T-cell receptor mice develop autoimmune diabetes dependent upon RAG genotype, H-2g7 homozygosity, and insulin 2 gene knockout. Diabetes. 2006;55:1978–1984.
22. Chentoufi AA, Binder NR, Berka N, Abunadi T, Polychronakos C. Advances in type I diabetes associated tolerance mechanisms. Scand J Immunol. 2008;68:1–11.
23. Moriyama H, Abiru N, Paronen J, Sikora K, Liu E, Miao D, et al. Evidence for a primary islet autoantigen (preproinsulin 1) for insulitis and diabetes in the nonobese diabetic mouse. Proc Natl Acad Sci USA. 2003;100: 10376–10381.
24. Krishnamurthy B, Mariana L, Gellert SA, Colman PG, Harrison LC, Lew AM, et al. Autoimmunity to both proinsulin and IGRP is required for diabetes in nonobese diabetic 8.3 TCR transgenic mice. J Immunol. 2008; 180:4458–4464.
25. Hornum L, Romer J, Markholst H. The diabetes-prone BB rat carries a frameshift mutation in Ian4, a positional candidate of Iddm1. Diabetes. 2002;51:1972–1979.
26. Kupfer R, Lang J, Williams-Skipp C, Nelson M, Bellgrau D, Scheinman RI. Loss of a gimap/ian gene leads to activation of NF-kappaB through a MAPK-dependent pathway. Mol Immunol. 2007;44:479–487.
27. MacMurray AJ, Moralejo DH, Kwitek AE, Rutledge EA, Van Yserloo B, Gohlke P, et al. Lymphopenia in the BB rat model of type 1 diabetes is due to a mutation in a novel immune-associated nucleotide (Ian)-related gene. Genome Res. 2002;12:1029–1039.
28. Jackson R, Rassi N, Crump A, Haynes BF, Eisenbarth GS. The BB diabetic rat. Profound T-cell lymphocytopenia. Diabetes. 1981;30: 887–889.
29. Robles DT, Eisenbarth GS, Dailey NJM, Peterson LB, Wicker LS. Insulin autoantibodies are associated with islet inflammation but not always related to diabetes progression in NOD congenic mice. Diabetes. 2002;52: 882–886.
30. Rainbow DB, Esposito L, Howlett SK, Hunter KM, Todd JA, Peterson LB, et al. Commonality in the genetic control of type 1 diabetes in humans and NOD mice: variants of genes in the IL-2 pathway are associated with autoimmune diabetes in both species. Biochem Soc Trans. 2008;36:312–315.
31. Chen Z, Stockton J, Mathis D, Benoist C. Modeling CTLA4-linked autoimmunity with RNA interference in mice. Proc Natl Acad Sci USA. 2006;103:16400–16405.
32. Yamanouchi J, Rainbow D, Serra P, Howlett S, Hunter K, Garner VE, et al. Interleukin-2 gene variation impairs regulatory T cell function

and causes autoimmunity. Nat Genet. 2007;39:329–337.
33. Redondo MJ, Fain PR, Krischer JP, Yu L, Cuthbertson D, Winter WE, et al. Expression of beta-cell autoimmunity does not differ between potential dizygotic twins and siblings of patients with type 1 diabetes. J Autoimmun. 2004;23:275–279.
34. Redondo MJ, Jeffrey J, Fain PR, Eisenbarth GS, Orban T. Concordance for islet autoimmunity among monozygotic twins. N Engl J Med. 2008;359:2849–2850.
35. Bonifacio E, Pfluger M, Marienfeld S, Winkler C, Hummel M, Ziegler AG. Maternal type 1 diabetes reduces the risk of islet autoantibodies: relationships with birthweight and maternal HbA(1c). Diabetologia. 2008;51:1245–1252.
36. Baschal EE, Aly TA, Babu SR, Fernando MS, Yu L, Miao D, et al. HLA-DPB1*0402 protects against type 1A diabetic autoimmunity in the highest risk DR3-DQB1*0201/DR4-DQB1*0302 DAISY population. Diabetes. 2007;56:2405–2409.
37. Aly TA, Ide A, Jahromi MM, Barker JM, Fernando MS, Babu SR, et al. Extreme genetic risk for type 1A diabetes. Proc Natl Acad Sci USA. 2006;103:14074–14079.
38. Aly TA, Baschal EE, Jahromi MM, Fernando MS, Babu SR, Fingerlin TE, et al. Analysis of single nucleotide polymorphisms identifies major type 1A diabetes locus telomeric of the major histocompatibility complex. Diabetes. 2008;57:770–776.
39. Nakanishi K, Kobayashi T, Murase T, Nakatsuji T, Inoko H, Tsuji K, et al. Association of HLA-A24 with complete beta-cell destruction in IDDM. Diabetes. 1993;42:1086–1093.
40. Nejentsev S, Reijonen H, Adojaan B, Kovalchuk L, Sochnevs A, Schwartz EI, et al. The effect of HLA-B allele on the IDDM risk defined by DRB1*04 subtypes and DQB1*0302. Diabetes. 1997;46:1888–1892.
41. Nejentsev S, Howson JM, Walker NM, Szeszko J, Field SF, Stevens HE, et al. Localization of type 1 diabetes susceptibility to the MHC class I genes HLA-B and HLA-A. Nature. 2007;450:887–892.
42. Bilbao JR, Calvo B, Aransay AM, Martin-Pagola A, Perez DN, Aly TA, et al. Conserved extended haplotypes discriminate HLA-DR3-homozygous Basque patients with type 1 diabetes mellitus and celiac disease. Genes Immun. 2006;7:550–554.
43. Aly TA, Eller E, Ide A, Gowan K, Babu SR, Erlich HA, et al. Multi-SNP analysis of MHC region: remarkable conservation of HLA-A1-B8-DR3 haplotype. Diabetes. 2006;55:1265–1269.
44. Bell GI, Horita S, Karam JH. A polymorphic locus near the human insulin gene is associated with insulin-dependent diabetes mellitus. Diabetes. 1984;33:176–183.
45. Vafiadis P, Bennett ST, Todd JA, Nadeau J, Grabs R, Goodyer CG, et al. Insulin expression in human thymus is modulated by INS VNTR alleles at the IDDM2 locus. Nat Genet. 1997;15:289–292.
46. Pugliese A, Zeller M, Fernandez A, Zalcberg LJ, Bartlett RJ, Ricordi C, et al. The insulin gene is transcribed in the human thymus and transcription levels correlate with allelic variation at the INS VNTR-IDDM2 susceptibility locus for type I diabetes. Nat Genet. 1997;15:293–297.
47. Chentoufi AA, Polychronakos C. Insulin expression levels in the thymus modulate insulin-specific autoreactive T-cell tolerance: the mechanism by which the IDDM2 locus may predispose to diabetes. Diabetes. 2002;51:1383–1390.
48. Bottini N, Musumeci L, Alonso A, Rahmouni S, Nika K, Rostamkhani M, et al. A functional variant of lymphoid tyrosine phosphatase is associated with type I diabetes. Nat Genet. 2004;36:337–338.
49. Lee AT, Li W, Liew A, Bombardier C, Weisman M, Massarotti EM, et al. The PTPN22 R620W polymorphism associates with RF positive rheumatoid arthritis in a dose-dependent manner but not with HLA-SE status. Genes Immun. 2005;6:129–133.
50. Vang T, Congia M, Macis MD, Musumeci L, Orru V, Zavattari P, et al. Autoimmune-associated lymphoid tyrosine phosphatase is a gain-of-function variant. Nat Genet. 2005;37:1317–1319.
51. Anjos SM, Tessier MC, Polychronakos C. Association of the cytotoxic T lymphocyte-associated antigen 4 gene with type 1 diabetes: evidence for independent effects of two polymorphisms on the same haplotype block. J Clin Endocrinol Metab. 2004;89:6257–6265.
52. Ueda H, Howson JM, Esposito L, Heward J, Snook H, Chamberlain G, et al. Association of the T-cell regulatory gene CTLA4 with susceptibility to autoimmune disease. Nature. 2003;423:506–511.
53. Qu HQ, Montpetit A, Ge B, Hudson TJ, Polychronakos C. Toward further mapping of the association between the IL2RA locus and type 1 diabetes. Diabetes. 2007;56:1174–1176.
54. Lowe CE, Cooper JD, Brusko T, Walker NM, Smyth DJ, Bailey R, et al. Large-scale genetic fine mapping and genotype-phenotype associations implicate polymorphism in the IL2RA region in type 1 diabetes. Nat Genet. 2007;39:1074–1082.
55. Hindorff LA, Junkins HA, Hall PN, Mehta JP, Manolio TA. A catalog of published genome-wide

associationstudies.www.genome.gov/26525384. Accessed September 1, 2008.
56. Field SF, Howson JM, Smyth DJ, Walker NM, Dunger DB, Todd JA. Analysis of the type 2 diabetes gene, TCF7L2, in 13,795 type 1 diabetes cases and control subjects. Diabetologia. 2007;50:212–213.
57. Field SF, Howson JM, Walker NM, Dunger DB, Todd JA. Analysis of the obesity gene FTO in 14,803 type 1 diabetes cases and controls. Diabetologia. 2007;50:2218–2220.
58. Hakonarson H, Qu HQ, Bradfield JP, Marchand L, Kim CE, Glessner JT, et al. A novel susceptibility locus for type 1 diabetes on Chr12q13 identified by a genome-wide association study. Diabetes. 2008;57:1143–1146.
59. Concannon P, Onengut-Gumuscu S, Todd JA, Smyth DJ, Pociot F, Bergholdt R et al. A human type 1 diabetes susceptibility locus maps to chromosome 21q22.3. Diabetes. 2008;57:2858–2861.
60. Burton PR, Clayton DG, Cardon LR, Craddock N, Deloukas P, Duncanson A, et al. Association scan of 14,500 nonsynonymous SNPs in four diseases identifies autoimmunity variants. Nat Genet. 2007;39:1329–1337.
61. Todd JA, Walker NM, Cooper JD, Smyth DJ, Downes K, Plagnol V, et al. Robust associations of four new chromosome regions from genome-wide analyses of type 1 diabetes. Nat Genet. 2007;39:857–864.
62. Smyth DJ, Cooper JD, Bailey R, Field S, Burren O, Smink LJ, et al. A genome-wide association study of nonsynonymous SNPs identifies a type 1 diabetes locus in the interferon-induced helicase (IFIH1) region. Nat Genet. 2006;38:617–619.
63. Hakonarson H, Grant SF, Bradfield JP, Marchand L, Kim CE, Glessner JT, et al. A genome-wide association study identifies KIAA0350 as a type 1 diabetes gene. Nature. 2007;448:591–594.
64. Schreuder TC, Gelderblom HC, Weegink CJ, Hamann D, Reesink HW, Devries JH, et al. High incidence of type 1 diabetes mellitus during or shortly after treatment with pegylated interferon alpha for chronic hepatitis C virus infection. Liver Int. 2008;28:39–46.
65. Bjornvold M, Undlien DE, Joner G, Dahl-Jorgensen K, Njolstad PR, Akselsen HE, et al. Joint effects of HLA, INS, PTPN22 and CTLA4 genes on the risk of type 1 diabetes. Diabetologia. 2008;51:589–596.
66. Bach JF. The effect of infections on susceptibility to autoimmune and allergic diseases. N Engl J Med. 2002;347:911–920.
67. Uusitalo L, Nevalainen J, Niinisto S, Alfthan G, Sundvall J, Korhonen T, et al. Serum alpha- and gamma-tocopherol concentrations and risk of advanced beta cell autoimmunity in children with HLA-conferred susceptibility to type 1 diabetes mellitus. Diabetologia. 2008;51:773–780.
68. Virtanen SM, Kenward MG, Erkkola M, Kautiainen S, Kronberg-Kippila C, Hakulinen T, et al. Age at introduction of new foods and advanced beta cell autoimmunity in young children with HLA-conferred susceptibility to type 1 diabetes. Diabetologia. 2006;49:1512–1521.
69. TRIGR Study Group. Study design of the Trial to Reduce IDDM in the Genetically at Risk (TRIGR). Pediatr Diabetes. 2007;8:117–137.
70. Norris JM, Barriga K, Klingensmith G, Hoffman M, Eisenbarth GS, Erlich H, et al. Timing of cereal exposure in infancy and risk of islet autoimmunity. The Diabetes Autoimmunity Study in the Young (DAISY). JAMA. 2003;290:1713–1720.
71. Norris JM, Yin X, Lamb MM, Barriga K, Seifert J, Hoffman M, et al. Omega-3 polyunsaturated fatty acid intake and islet autoimmunity in children at increased risk for type 1 diabetes. JAMA. 2007;298:1420–1428.
72. Waterland RA, Jirtle RL. Transposable elements: targets for early nutritional effects on epigenetic gene regulation. Mol Cell Biol. 2003;23:5293–5300.
73. Fraga MF, Ballestar E, Paz MF, Ropero S, Setien F, Ballestar ML, et al. Epigenetic differences arise during the lifetime of monozygotic twins. Proc Natl Acad Sci USA. 2005;102:10604–10609.
74. Vehik K, Hamman RF, Lezotte D, Norris JM, Klingensmith GJ, Rewers M, et al. Trends in high-risk HLA susceptibility genes among Colorado youth with type 1 diabetes. Diabetes Care. 2008;31:1392–1396.
75. Hermann R, Knip M, Veijola R, Simell O, Laine AP, Akerblom HK, et al. Temporal changes in the frequencies of HLA genotypes in patients with type 1 diabetes-indication of an increased environmental pressure? Diabetologia. 2003;46:420–425.
76. Wenzlau JM, Juhl K, Yu L, Moua O, Sarkar SA, Gottlieb P, et al. The cation efflux transporter ZnT8 (Slc30A8) is a major autoantigen in human type 1 diabetes. Proc Natl Acad Sci USA. 2007;104:17040–17045.
77. Wenzlau JM, Liu Y, Yu L, Moua O, Fowler KT, Rangasamy S, et al. A common non-synonymous single nucleotide polymorphism in the SLC30A8 gene determines ZnT8 autoantibody specificity in type 1 diabetes. Diabetes. 2008;57:2693–2697.

Chapter 16

Epidemiology of Type 1 Diabetes

Molly M. Lamb and Jill M. Norris

Summary

Type 1 diabetes is thought to be caused by both genetic and environmental factors, each of which accounts for approximately 50% of a person's risk. The incidence of type 1 diabetes is increasing around the world, and evidence suggests that changing environmental factors may be responsible for the observed increase. Viral infections, nutritional exposures, perinatal factors, childhood growth, and other environmental factors have been explored as potential risk factors for type 1 diabetes. In this chapter, we describe the epidemiology of type 1 diabetes, outline the incidence trends of the disease, and present the latest evidence regarding the genetic and environmental risk factors for type 1 diabetes.

Key Words: Type 1 diabetes, Islet autoimmunity, Incidence, Genetic risk factors, Environmental risk factors, Viral infections, Nutrition, Growth, Toxins, Psychosocial stress

Type 1A diabetes (T1DM) is an autoimmune disease that accounts for approximately 10% of all cases of diabetes. While about 60% of individuals with T1DM develop the disease in adulthood, T1DM is also one of the most common chronic diseases in childhood. The complications of this disease are both microvascular (nephropathy, retinopathy, and neuropathy) and macrovascular (cardiovascular disease). T1DM is the leading cause of blindness, limb amputation, and end-stage renal disease, and increases a person's risk of early death. There is no cure for T1DM, but the disease is treatable. Management of T1DM involves regular blood glucose monitoring and insulin injections, as well as frequent doctor visits for early detection and treatment of complications.

Epidemiologic research aimed at identifying genetic risk factors and environmental triggers for T1DM offers hope that we may one day be able to delay or prevent the development of T1DM. Large prospective cohort studies are identifying factors that increase or decrease risk for T1DM, and clinical trials are testing possible interventions designed to delay or prevent the initiation of the autoimmune disease process.

NATURAL HISTORY OF TYPE 1 DIABETES

T1DM is an autoimmune disease that results from Th1-mediated destruction of the pancreatic beta cells. Beta-cell loss progresses at different rates, but the steady loss of beta cells may eventually lead to absolute insulin deficiency and development of T1DM (Fig. 16.1). As beta-cell loss progresses, the body undergoes a number of biologic changes. Insulin secretion is reduced, followed by a loss of pulsatile insulin secretion, hyperglycemia, and impaired glucose tolerance (*1*). Rising hemoglobin A1c levels and increased insulin resistance have also been observed prior to T1DM onset (*2, 3*).

The autoimmune attack on the pancreatic beta cells can be detected years before clinical onset of T1DM via presence of any of the four following autoantibodies in the blood: Islet cell (ICA), insulin (IAA), protein tyrosine phosphatase (IA2), and glutamic acid decarboxylase (GAD65) (Fig. 16.1). Islet autoimmunity (IA) is an asymptomatic condition that has been described in a number of different ways, but most researchers define IA as the presence of ICA, IAA, IA2, and/or GAD65, which indicates that an individual is experiencing an autoimmune reaction targeting the pancreas (*4*).

IA typically precedes the development of T1DM, and children who develop autoantibodies at very young age progress to T1DM more rapidly than children who develop autoantibodies at older age (*4*). The number of autoantibodies also predicts future T1DM disease risk. A person who persistently tests posi-

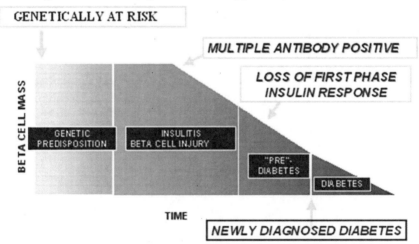

Fig. 16.1 Stages in development of type 1 diabetes (*1*).

tive for multiple autoantibodies is at a much higher risk of developing T1DM than a person with a single detectable autoantibody (5). However, autoantibodies may be transiently positive (5), and there are not yet enough longitudinal data to determine if all people who develop autoantibodies will eventually develop T1DM (4, 6). While not 100% predictive of future T1DM development, IA serves as a very useful intermediate end point when studying the autoimmune disease process and potential risk factors for T1DM.

While subclinical IA may be present for years prior to the presentation of clinical symptoms, the onset of T1DM is generally acute. Symptoms of T1DM include increased thirst (polydipsia) and urination (polyuria), constant hunger, sudden weight loss, blurred vision, and extreme fatigue. The criteria used for T1DM diagnosis include symptoms of polydipsia and/or polyuria, random glucose >200 mg/dl, and/or hemoglobin A1c >7%. Younger children often present with more severe symptoms at diagnosis due to communication barriers as well as more rapid, and often more complete, beta-cell loss. Rapid identification of symptoms and initiation of insulin therapy may prevent onset of diabetic ketoacidosis (DKA), a critical condition that can be fatal if not recognized and treated promptly.

PREVALENCE AND INCIDENCE

In the United States, T1DM affects approximately 1 in 300 children and 1 in 100 adults, with approximately 30,000 new cases developing each year (7). Worldwide, the incidence of T1DM varies widely. Finland has the highest recorded incidence of T1DM, at 42.9 new cases per 100,000 persons per year (8), while Venezuela reports the lowest incidence, at 0.1 new cases per 100,000 persons per year (9) (Fig. 16.2). However, T1DM case reporting is often incomplete, and many countries do not record T1DM incidence at all (Fig. 16.3). These factors make it difficult to estimate the burden and describe trends of T1DM worldwide, especially in the developing world.

T1DM incidence varies by race, gender, and age. T1DM incidence is highest in Europe or populations of European descent (9). Consistent with global trends, T1DM incidence in the US is highest in non-Hispanic whites, followed by lower rates in African Americans, Hispanics, and Asian/Pacific Islanders, with the lowest rates in American Indians (10). T1DM incidence does not vary by gender in young children, but beginning around the age of puberty, more boys than girls develop T1DM. This pattern is especially noticeable in high-risk populations (9). In terms of age, T1DM incidence peaks around the age of puberty (10) in both boys and girls (Fig. 16.4).

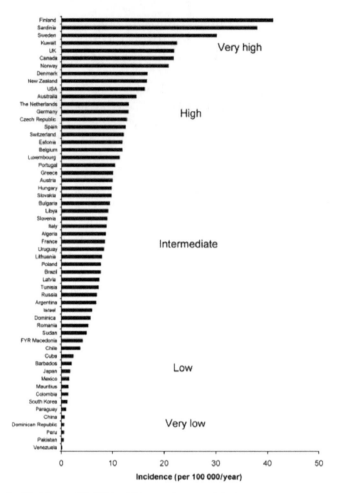

Fig. 16.2 Age-standardized incidence of T1DM in children under age 14 (*11*).

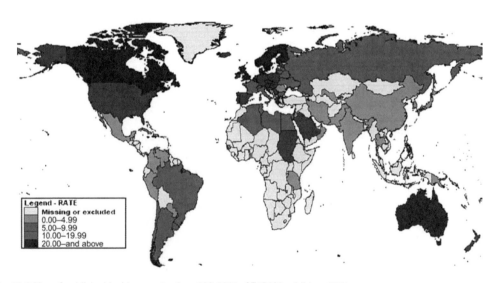

Fig. 16.3 Map of published incidence rates (per 100,000) of T1DM in children (*54*).

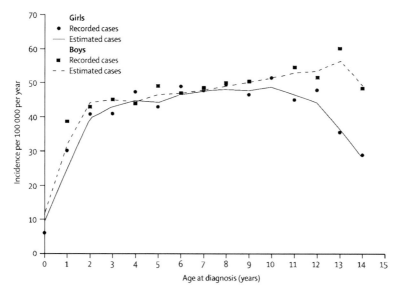

Fig. 16.4 T1DM incidence by age in childhood (*8*).

The incidence of T1DM has been steadily increasing around the world in recent decades, with an average annual increase in incidence of 2.8% (*11*). Countries with both low and high T1DM prevalences have seen increases in T1DM incidence in recent years. T1DM incidence increases have been observed in both genders and all races (*12*). Notably, the strongest increases in incidence have been observed in the youngest age groups (*8, 9, 11, 13, 14*). This trend toward the younger age groups has sparked a debate as to whether there is a true increase in T1DM incidence or simply a downward shift in age at T1DM onset, perhaps resulting from increasing exposure to early environmental triggers for the disease (*8, 15*).

TYPE 1 DIABETES ETIOLOGY

Genetic Risk Factors for Type 1 Diabetes

T1DM is a complex chronic disease that is caused by a combination of genetic and environmental factors. It is estimated that genetics account for up to 50% of T1DM risk. A family history of T1DM increases a person's risk of developing the disease, and paternal diabetes conveys more disease risk to the offspring than maternal diabetes (*16*). However, while a family history is a strong risk factor for T1DM, the great majority of those who develop T1DM (~85%) do not have a family history of the disease (*16*).

A number of genes that predispose a person to T1DM have been identified thus far. The most prominent are the Human Leukocyte Antigen (HLA) genes found in the Major Histocompatibility

Complex on chromosome 6p21 (*7, 16*). These HLA genes encode proteins involved in the immune response, and account for an estimated 50% of the genetic susceptibility to T1DM.

Other genes have also been identified (*16*), such as the insulin (INS) gene on chromosome 11p15, which is involved in regulating insulin expression, and the CTLA-4 gene on chromosome 2q33, which acts as a negative regulator of T-cell function. Together, these two genes are estimated to account for 15% of genetic T1DM risk (*17*). Additional replicated type 1 diabetes candidate genes include PTPN22, IL2RA, and IFIH (*18*). Ongoing research is using progressively more sophisticated techniques to identify, and describe the function of, other genes that may contribute to T1DM risk.

While strong genetic factors that increase T1DM risk have been identified, recent research indicates that HLA genes are not responsible for the increases in T1DM incidence observed around the world (*19–22*). The proportion of persons with T1DM who carry the high-risk HLA genotype is actually falling, and many researchers have suggested that increasing environmental pressures may explain this and the recent rapid rise in T1DM incidence worldwide (*15, 23, 24*).

Environmental Risk Factors for Type 1 Diabetes

Decades of research conducted in both animals and humans has led to the identification of many potential environmental risk factors for T1DM. This research is providing important insights on the environmental risk factors for T1DM, as well as giving researchers an idea as to possible biologic mechanisms. The environmental risk factors explored thus far include viral infections, infant diet (lack of breast-feeding, timing of introduction of cow's milk and cereals, and low vitamin D intake), childhood diet (high nitrate intake, low omega-3 fatty acids intake), rapid growth and weight gain in infancy and childhood, psychological stress in childhood, and factors related to a complicated birth or high-risk pregnancy.

Armed with the ability to identify persons at increased genetic risk for T1DM, researchers have been following cohorts of genetically high-risk children for the development of the intermediate outcome of islet autoimmunity and the final outcome of T1DM to identify the environmental triggers for T1DM. The longest-running of these prospective cohort studies is BABY-DIAB, based in Germany, which has been following children of T1DM parents since 1989 (*25*). The Diabetes Autoimmunity Study in the Young (DAISY), based in Denver, Colorado, has been following children with high-risk HLA genotypes or family history of T1DM since 1993 (*26*), and the Finnish Diabetes Prediction and Prevention Project (DIPP) began following high-risk newborns in 1994 (*27*). Much of the data presented in the remainder of this chapter is drawn from these studies, and thus pertains mostly to children at increased genetic risk of T1DM. In addition, most of the results published by these studies thus far pertain to development of IA, an intermediate step in the autoimmune disease process that is highly predictive of T1DM development.

Viruses

The relationship between viral infections and T1DM development appears to be complex. While some evidence suggests that viral infections protect against T1DM development, other evidence implies that viral infections may trigger the initiation of the autoimmune process or the precipitation of T1DM.

Research suggests that contracting at least two viral infections in the first year of life protects against T1DM development, as does day-care attendance in the first year of life (considered a proxy for increased exposure to viral infections) and not being the first-born child (later born children are exposed to viral infections brought home by older siblings) (*6, 28*). These findings and research in mice has led to the development of the "Hygiene Hypothesis". This hypothesis proposes that viral infections and other illnesses stimulate, and thus "train", the immune system (*28*). A child that is not exposed to a wide variety of foreign particles and pathogens may have an incompletely developed immune system that is predisposed to autoimmunity. Thus, *decreasing* the number of viral infections in early childhood may *increase* risk of T1DM in genetically susceptible individuals.

Contrary to the research supporting the Hygiene Hypothesis, a substantial body of research in both mice and humans indicates that viral infections may increase T1DM risk. Viral infections appear to be able to impact T1DM risk at all stages of early life, from the prenatal period through childhood. A variety of viruses, including enteroviruses, mumps, rubella (notably congenital rubella), rotavirus, parvovirus, and cytomegalovirus (CMV), have been associated with increased T1DM risk thus far (*24, 29, 30*).

Furthermore, indirect support for the role of viral infections in increasing T1DM risk can be found in the temporal and spatial patterns of T1DM incidence. T1DM develops more frequently in winter months than in summer months, and the increase in viral infections during the winter months is often used as an explanation for this association (*23*). Worldwide, T1DM incidence is higher in countries that are further from the equator (Fig. 16.3), where the winters are colder and some viral infections are more common. Correspondingly, greater variations in temperature between winter and summer seasons are correlated with greater variability of incidence throughout the year (*9*).

A variety of biologic mechanisms have been proposed to describe how viral infections may trigger beta-cell attack and/or precipitate T1DM development. Proposed mechanisms include direct cytolysis of virus-infected beta cells, molecular mimicry (where activated T-cells cross-react with islet antigens), induction of autoimmune responses to "altered self-antigens" as a result of increased beta-cell antigenicity, loss of regulatory T-cells, and bystander activation of autoreactive T-cells (described in detail in (*29*)).

Nutrition

A number of nutritional factors have been explored for association with islet autoimmunity and T1DM, including vitamin D, dietary toxins such as nitrosamines and bafilomycin, long-chain omega-3 fatty acids, and cow's milk and cereal (timing of introduction in infancy). Vitamin D can be obtained either endogenously (via skin exposure to sunlight) or exogenously (from food or supplements). The observation that T1DM incidence increases in the winter months has led to the hypothesis that lower vitamin D may be responsible for greater T1DM incidence in the darker/colder months of the year, especially in those countries further away from the equator (*23*). Epidemiologic studies in humans on vitamin D supplementation in infancy have offered initial support for the protective effect of vitamin D (*31, 32*), although this has not been confirmed in the cohort studies of islet autoimmunity. Prospective data on vitamin D levels are necessary to explore mechanism, dosing, and relevant timing related to the association between vitamin D and type 1 diabetes.

Earlier introduction of cow's milk and shorter breast-feeding duration have long been suspected of influencing IA initiation and T1DM development. Many case–control and prospective cohort studies have been conducted (*33*). Breast-feeding duration is closely linked to timing of cow's milk exposure in infants. Shorter breast-feeding duration (exclusive and total) has been shown to increase the risk of developing autoantibodies (*34*) and has been associated with increased T1DM risk (*35*). However, the effect is small, and none of the prospective cohort studies have found an association between early introduction of cow's milk and islet autoimmunity (*36–38*).

A variety of other dietary exposures in infancy have been explored for association with later IA risk. Dietary gluten has been linked to diabetes in animal studies (*32*), and human studies have shown that timing of cereal exposure in infancy can affect IA risk. Exposure to cereals too early (0–3 months of age) (*38, 39*) or too late (>7 months of age) (*39*) may increase IA risk. Other infant dietary factors such as early introduction of fruits, berries, and root vegetables (*37*) have been associated with increased IA risk.

Long-chain omega-3 fatty acids have anti-inflammatory effects in the body and have been shown to reduce diabetes risk in animal models. Low levels of omega-3 fatty acids consumption in infancy (*40*) and childhood (*41*) have been associated with increased risk of T1DM and IA, respectively. Additional studies replicating these results and exploring the potential biologic mechanism underlying the protective effect of omega-3 fatty acids are needed.

Dietary toxins, such as N-nitroso compounds, nitrates, and nitrites, as well as bafilomycin, have also been explored for association with T1DM. N-nitroso compounds, nitrates, and nitrites, most commonly found in processed meat and beer products, as well as in vegetables such as potatoes, cabbages, and carrots, appear to convey risk for T1DM in both the fetal and childhood periods (reviewed in (*32*)). Similarly, research in mice has suggested that bafilomycin, a toxin found in root vegetables such as potatoes, is diabetogenic when exposure occurs in fetal life and infancy. However, DAISY showed that increased maternal consumption of root vegetables during pregnancy (as reported on a food frequency questionnaire) did not increase the risk of IA in the child (*42*). Further research needs to be conducted on these potentially diabetogenic dietary toxins to define their association with different stages in the autoimmune disease process, and to better understand their biologic mechanism.

Childhood Obesity and Rapid Growth Rate

Childhood obesity is rising in parallel with T1DM incidence. The overload hypothesis (*43*) suggests that the high insulin demand on the beta cell that results from the accelerated growth and weight gain of today's youth make the beta cells vulnerable to autoimmune attack and apoptosis. Similarly, the accelerator hypothesis postulates that insulin resistance caused by excess weight gain may accelerate beta-cell apoptosis in individuals at genetic risk (*44*). Both obesity and rapid growth rate are known to decrease insulin sensitivity (which "stresses" the beta cells), and have been associated with T1DM development (*45–48*), albeit inconsistently. A number of studies are currently testing the overload and accelerator hypotheses, and the results are still controversial.

Psychosocial Stress

Psychological stress in early childhood increases insulin resistance, which may increase demand on the beta cells, and may also have a direct impact on the immune system. Either mechanism has the potential to contribute to the induction or progression of autoimmunity. Currently, there are only a handful of studies that have examined the role of stressful life events in the development of IA and T1DM. The results thus far are quite controversial, and there are only few significant results. The first of the two reviews concludes that stressful life events do not play a role in the development of T1DM (*49*), while the second, the more recent review, concludes that psychological stress may influence the development of both IA and T1DM (*50*).

Perinatal Factors

The autoimmune disease process may have its roots in the earliest stages of human life, and a number of perinatal factors have been shown to increase T1DM risk. Greater maternal age at delivery, blood-type incompatibility between the mother and child, preeclampsia, maternal infections during gestation, large birth size, lower gestational age, earlier birth order, and complicated delivery (*24, 51, 52*) have been associated with increased T1DM risk, while complicated delivery and increasing maternal age have been associated with increased IA risk (*53*). This is a relatively new area of research, and the results of studies on this topic thus far are not consistent. Biologic mechanisms explaining these findings are not well understood, although researchers hypothesize that many of these factors stress the fetal immune system.

CONCLUSION

The incidence of T1DM is steadily increasing in populations around the world, and changing environmental pressures are likely to be responsible for this trend. Large prospective studies and intervention trials are providing valuable data that may lead to better understanding of the etiology of this serious chronic disease. While there are not yet any interventions proven to delay or prevent the development of T1DM, epidemiologic research will continue to identify risk factors for T1DM, and define their underlying biologic mechanisms. Such knowledge may eventually give researchers and clinicians the tools to reduce the burden of this serious chronic disease.

REFERENCES

1. Type 1 Diabetes: Molecular, Cellular, and Clinical Immunology. Online Edition version 3.0. http://www.uchsc.edu/misc/diabetes/books/type1/type1_ch12.html. Accessed January 19, 2009.
2. Stene LC, Barriga K, Hoffman M, et al. Normal but increasing hemoglobin A1c levels predict progression from islet autoimmunity to overt type 1 diabetes: Diabetes Autoimmunity Study in the Young (DAISY). Pediatr Diabetes 2006;7(5):247–253.
3. Bingley PJ, Mahon JL, Gale EA, European Nicotinamide Diabetes Intervention Trial Group. Insulin resistance and progression to type 1 diabetes in the European Nicotinamide Diabetes Intervention Trial (ENDIT). Diabetes Care 2008;31(1):146–150.
4. Achenbach P, Bonifacio E, Koczwara K, Ziegler AG. Natural history of type 1 diabetes. Diabetes 2005;54(Suppl 2):S25–S31.
5. Taplin CE, Barker JM. Autoantibodies in type 1 diabetes. Autoimmunity 2008;41(1):11–18.
6. Kishiyama CM, Chase HP, Barker JM. Prevention strategies for type 1 diabetes. Rev Endocr Metab Disord 2006;7(3):215–224.
7. Jahromi MM, Eisenbarth GS. Cellular and molecular pathogenesis of type 1A diabetes. Cell Mol Life Sci 2007;64(7–8):865–872.
8. Harjutsalo V, Sjöberg L, Tuomilehto J. Time trends in the incidence of type 1 diabetes in Finnish children: a cohort study. Lancet 2008;371(9626):1777–1782.
9. Soltesz G, Patterson CC, Dahlquist G, EURODIAB Study Group. Worldwide childhood type 1 diabetes incidence – what can we learn from epidemiology? Pediatr Diabetes 2007;8(Suppl 6):6–14.
10. Writing Group for the SEARCH for Diabetes in Youth Study Group. Incidence of diabetes in youth in the United States. J Am Med Assoc 2007;297(24):2716–2724.
11. DIAMOND Project Group. Incidence and trends of childhood Type 1 diabetes worldwide 1990–1999. Diabet Med 2006;23(8):857–866.

12. Karvonen M, Viik-Kajander M, Moltchanova E, Libman I, LaPorte R, Tuomilehto J. Incidence of childhood type 1 diabetes worldwide. Diabetes Mondiale (DiaMond) Project Group. Diabetes Care 2000;23(10):1516–1526.
13. Vehik K, Hamman RF, Lezotte D, et al. Increasing incidence of type 1 diabetes in 0- to 17-year-old Colorado youth. Diabetes Care 2007;30(3):503–509.
14. Chong JW, Craig ME, Cameron FJ, et al. Marked increase in type 1 diabetes mellitus incidence in children aged 0–14 yr in Victoria, Australia, from 1999 to 2002. Pediatr Diabetes 2007;8(2):67–73.
15. Gale EA. Spring harvest? Reflections on the rise of type 1 diabetes. Diabetologia 2005;48(12):2445–2450.
16. Redondo MJ, Eisenbarth GS. Genetic control of autoimmunity in type I diabetes and associated disorders. Diabetologia 2002;45(5):605–622.
17. Anjos S, Polychronakos C. Mechanisms of genetic susceptibility to type I diabetes: beyond HLA. Mol Genet Metab 2004;81(3):187–195.
18. Ounissi-Benkalha H, Polychronakos C. The molecular genetics of type 1 diabetes: new genes and emerging mechanisms. Trends Mol Med 2008;14(6):268–275.
19. Fourlanos S, Varney MD, Tait BD, et al. The rising incidence of type 1 diabetes is accounted for by cases with lower risk HLA genotypes. Diabetes Care 2008;31(8):1546–1549.
20. Vehik K, Hamman RF, Lezotte D, et al. Trends in high-risk HLA susceptibility genes among Colorado youth with type 1 diabetes. Diabetes Care 2008;31(7):1392–1396.
21. Hermann R, Knip M, Veijola R, et al. Temporal changes in the frequencies of HLA genotypes in patients with type 1 diabetes–indication of an increased environmental pressure? Diabetologia 2003;46(3):420–425.
22. Gillespie KM, Bain SC, Barnett AH, et al. The rising incidence of childhood type 1 diabetes and reduced contribution of high-risk HLA haplotypes. Lancet 2004;364(9446):1699–1700.
23. Knip M, Veijola R, Virtanen SM, Hyoty H, Vaarala O, Akerblom HK. Environmental triggers and determinants of type 1 diabetes. Diabetes 2005;54(Suppl 2):S125–S136.
24. Peng H, Hagopian W. Environmental factors in the development of type 1 diabetes. Rev Endocr Metab Disord 2006;7(3):149–162.
25. Roll U, Christie MR, Füchtenbusch M, Payton MA, Hawkes CJ, Ziegler AG. Perinatal autoimmunity in offspring of diabetic parents. The German Multicenter BABY-DIAB study: detection of humoral immune responses to islet antigens in early childhood. Diabetes 1996;45(7):967–973.
26. Rewers M, Bugawan TL, Norris JM, et al. Newborn screening for HLA markers associated with IDDM: diabetes autoimmunity study in the young (DAISY). Diabetologia 1996;39(7):807–812.
27. Kupila A, Muona P, Simell T, et al. Feasibility of genetic and immunological prediction of type I diabetes in a population-based birth cohort. Diabetologia 2001;44(3):290–297.
28. Feillet H, Bach JF. On the mechanisms of the protective effect of infections on type 1 diabetes. Clin Dev Immunol 2004;11(3–4):191–194.
29. van der Werf N, Kroese FG, Rozing J, Hillebrands JL. Viral infections as potential triggers of type 1 diabetes. Diabetes Metab Res Rev 2007;23(3):169–183.
30. Akerblom HK, Vaarala O, Hyoty H, Ilonen J, Knip M. Environmental factors in the etiology of type 1 diabetes. Am J Med Genet 2002;115(1):18–29.
31. Zipitis CS, Akobeng AK. Vitamin D supplementation in early childhood and risk of type 1 diabetes: a systematic review and meta-analysis. Arch Dis Child 2008;93(6):512–517.
32. Virtanen SM, Knip M. Nutritional risk predictors of beta cell autoimmunity and type 1 diabetes at a young age. Am J Clin Nutr 2003;78(6):1053–1067.
33. Simpson M, Norris JM. Early-life diet and risk of type 1 diabetes. In: Dabelea D, Klingensmith GJ, eds. Epidemiology of Pediatric and Adolescent Diabetes. New York: Informa Healthcare USA, 2008.
34. Holmberg H, Wahlberg J, Vaarala O, Ludvigsson J, ABIS Study Group. Short duration of breast-feeding as a risk-factor for beta-cell autoantibodies in 5-year-old children from the general population. Br J Nutr 2007;97(1):111–116.
35. Malcova H, Sumnik Z, Drevinek P, Venhacova J, Lebl J, Cinek O. Absence of breast-feeding is associated with the risk of type 1 diabetes: a case-control study in a population with rapidly increasing incidence. Eur J Pediatr 2006;165(2):114–119.
36. Norris JM, Beaty B, Klingensmith G, et al. Lack of association between early exposure to cow's milk protein and beta-cell autoimmunity. Diabetes Autoimmunity Study in the Young (DAISY). JAMA 1996;276(8):609–614.
37. Virtanen SM, Kenward MG, Erkkola M, et al. Age at introduction of new foods and advanced beta cell autoimmunity in young children with

HLA-conferred susceptibility to type 1 diabetes. Diabetologia 2006;49(7):1512–1521.
38. Ziegler AG, Schmid S, Huber D, Hummel M, Bonifacio E. Early infant feeding and risk of developing type 1 diabetes-associated autoantibodies. JAMA 2003;290(13): 1721–1728.
39. Norris JM, Barriga K, Klingensmith G, et al. Timing of initial cereal exposure in infancy and risk of islet autoimmunity. JAMA 2003;290(13):1713–1720.
40. Stene LC, Joner G, Norwegian Childhood Diabetes Study Group. Use of cod liver oil during the first year of life is associated with lower risk of childhood-onset type 1 diabetes: a large, population-based, case-control study. Am J Clin Nutr 2003;78(6):1128–1134.
41. Norris JM, Yin X, Lamb MM, et al. Omega-3 polyunsaturated fatty acid intake and islet autoimmunity in children at increased risk for type 1 diabetes. JAMA 2007;298(12):1420–1428.
42. Lamb MM, Myers MA, Barriga K, Zimmet PZ, Rewers M, Norris JM. Maternal diet during pregnancy and islet autoimmunity in offspring. Pediatr Diabetes 2008;9(2):135–141.
43. Dahlquist G. Can we slow the rising incidence of childhood-onset autoimmune diabetes? The overload hypothesis. Diabetologia 2006;49(1): 20–24.
44. Wilkin TJ. The accelerator hypothesis: weight gain as the missing link between type I and type II diabetes. Diabetologia 2001;44(7):914–922.
45. Blom LG, Persson LA, Dahlquist G. A high linear growth is associated with an increased risk of childhood diabetes mellitus. Diabetologia 1992;35(6):528–533.
46. Hypponen E, Virtanen SM, Kenward MG, Knip M, Akerblom HK. Obesity, increased linear growth, and risk of type 1 diabetes in children. Diabetes Care 2000;23(12):1755–1760.
47. Pundziute-Lycka A, Persson LA, Cedermark G, et al. Diet, growth, and the risk for type 1 diabetes in childhood: a matched case-referent study. Diabetes Care 2004;27(12): 2784–2789.
48. EURODIAB Substudy 2 Study Group. Rapid early growth is associated with increased risk of childhood type 1 diabetes in various European populations. Diabetes Care 2002; 25(10):1755–1760.
49. Cosgrove M. Do stressful life events cause type 1 diabetes? Occup Med 2004;54(4): 250–254.
50. Sepa A, Ludvigsson J. Psychological stress and the risk of diabetes-related autoimmunity: a review article. Neuroimmunomodulation 2006;13(5–6):301–308.
51. Haynes A, Bower C, Bulsara MK, Finn J, Jones TW, Davis EA. Perinatal risk factors for childhood type 1 diabetes in Western Australia – a population-based study (1980–2002). Diabet Med 2007;24(5):564–570.
52. Larsson K, Elding-Larsson H, Cederwall E, et al. Genetic and perinatal factors as risk for childhood type 1 diabetes. Diabetes Metab Res Rev 2004;20(6):429–437.
53. Stene LC, Barriga K, Norris JM, et al. Perinatal factors and development of islet autoimmunity in early childhood: the diabetes autoimmunity study in the young. Am J Epidemiol 2004;160(1):3–10.
54. Soltész G, Patterson C, Dahlquist G. Global trends in childhood Type 1 diabetes. In: International Diabetes Federation. Diabetes Atlas Third Edition. Brussels: IDF, 2006: 154–190.

Chapter 17

Natural History of Type 1 Diabetes

Spiros Fourlanos, Leonard C. Harrison, and Peter G. Colman

Key Words: Islet autoantibodies, Diabetes prediction, Type 1 diabetes, Intravenous glucose tolerance test, Islet autoantibodies, Insulin resistance

Type 1 diabetes is a chronic autoimmune disease occurring in genetically predisposed individuals. Much interest has focused on the identification of susceptibility and protective genes. Genome-wide linkage analyses using the Type 1 diabetes, Genetics Consortium and three other datasets have confirmed that approximately 40% of the familial aggregation of type 1 diabetes can be attributed to allelic variation of HLA loci in the major histocompatibility locus on chromosome 6p21 (*1*). Also, *INS* (chromosome 11p15), *CTLA4* (chromosome 2q33), and *PTPN22* (chromosome 1p13) have clearly been demonstrated as susceptibility loci and nine further non-HLA linked regions show linkage with type 1 diabetes (*1*).

Prior to the discovery of circulating pancreatic islet-cell antibodies (ICAs), it was believed type 1 diabetes had an acute pathogenesis, given its dramatic sudden clinical onset. It is now recognized that acute metabolic decompensation is usually the final stage in a relatively slow autoimmune disease process that erodes insulin secretory capacity of the pancreatic beta cells over years. This was revealed by a landmark longitudinal study of ICAs in monozygotic twins and triplets, which demonstrated a long preclinical period during which immunological markers of diabetes were present without hyperglycemia (*2*). In this study, ICAs were detected in a twin and triplet, 5 and 8 years, respectively, before the onset of clinical diabetes.

A preclinical phase, during which β-cell autoimmunity can be detected but metabolism remains normal, described in numerous studies, forms the basis for attempts designed to preserve beta-cell function and prevent type 1 diabetes. Several type 1 diabetes natural history studies have evaluated insulin secretion throughout the preclinical period using the first phase insulin response

(FPIR) in an intravenous glucose tolerance test (IVGTT). Individuals with islet autoantibodies and a FPIR less than the first percentile inevitably progress to diabetes; some studies have shown progressive falls in FPIR over time, although this is not universal. There is still debate as to whether the finding of a low FPIR adds significant predictive information to the presence of multiple autoantibodies (3). At diagnosis, there is profound impairment of insulin production, but recent studies suggest greater than expected reserves of insulin production may be present in some cases at diagnosis. Residual β-cell function is of great significance. Those with higher levels of residual insulin secretion appear to benefit the most from therapeutic attempts to reduce β-cell damage after diagnosis. In addition, the Diabetes Control and Complications Trial clearly showed that those with measurable residual insulin secretion achieved better metabolic control and less chronic complications over time (4).

This review will focus on recent developments in measuring islet autoantibodies and β-cell function in diagnosing prediabetes, in the significance of the metabolic variable, in insulin resistance, in the development of type 1 diabetes and in the changing genetic risk landscape.

CHANGING GENETIC PROFILE CONFIRMS ENVIRONMENTAL INFLUENCE

Recent studies have demonstrated an increase in type 1 diabetes in those with lower risk susceptibility genes (5–7). The shift in the genetic profile of type 1 diabetes in the last 50 years cannot be attributed to a change in the gene pool and is the evidence for emerging environmental influences promoting the development of type 1 diabetes in people with varying degrees of genetic risk. In the United Kingdom and Finland, it has been shown that cohorts of people with type 1 diabetes diagnosed since 1980 have a lower proportion of highest risk HLA genotypes (DR3,4; DQ2,8) compared with cohorts diagnosed before 1965. In addition to these Northern Hemisphere reports, a contemporary Southern Hemisphere (Australian) study has identified a similar changing pattern with cases of lower risk HLA class II genotypes rapidly increasing over the last five decades in parallel with the rising incidence of type 1 diabetes (7), illustrating that the contribution of HLA genes has broadened to involve children with lower genetic risk of diabetes who in previous eras would not have developed diabetes.

While it is generally believed that environmental factors play a role in triggering the autoimmune process, which ultimately leads to destruction of the islet beta-cell mass, these remain poorly characterized and may be changing over time. The environmental risk determinants, which have been most studied, are viral infections (mainly enteroviruses) and early infant feeding (exclusive breast feeding vs. early introduction of cow's milk). More recently, other environment-associated risk factors for type 1 diabetes have received attention including insulin resistance (*8*), weight gain (*9*), and lack of vitamin D supplementation (*10, 11*).

ISLET CELL ANTIBODIES AND BEYOND

The initial studies describing the preclinical phase of type 1 diabetes used the labour-intensive ICA immunofluorescence assay (*2, 12*). Shortly after, Palmer et al. described the presence of insulin autoantibodies (IAA) in patients with newly diagnosed diabetes prior to treatment with exogenous insulin (*13*). Quickly, it became clear that relatives with the combination of ICA and IAA were more likely to develop diabetes than those without it (*14, 15*). The identification of antibodies to glutamic acid decarboxylase (GAD) (*16*) and tyrosine phosphatase-like insulinoma antigen-2 (IA-2) (*17*) allowed the development of much simpler assays to track the events occurring in the preclinical phase of type 1 diabetes. However, the greatest boost in understanding the natural history of type 1 diabetes has been the utilization of these assays in first-degree relatives of people with type 1 diabetes followed from birth (*18–21*). These BABYDIAB studies have been remarkably concordant in demonstrating the first antibody to develop in infants is usually IAA with the second, most commonly, being GAD Ab. Most infants who progress to diabetes will develop multiple autoantibodies prior to diagnosis. The longest running prospective study, the German BABYDIAB study, has made a number of important observations. Children who develop antibodies within the first year of life are those who most often develop multiple antibodies and progress to type 1 diabetes in childhood (*22*).

TITER, IGG SUBCLASS, AND AFFINITY OF ANTIBODIES: ADDITIONAL PREDICTORS

One of the major recent developments in the antibody prediction arena has been the observation that stratification for risk of type 1 diabetes appears dependent on characteristics of islet autoantibodies such as titer, IgG subclass, and affinity. In an analysis of sera of first-degree relatives of patients with type 1 diabetes from the Bart's Oxford (BOX) and Munich Family Studies, those found to be positive for at least one of GADA, IA-2A, or IAA (n = 180 of whom 59 developed diabetes during follow up) were tested for end titer, IgG subclass, and epitope specificity (23). GAD antibody epitope specificities were classified as GAD65-NH$_2$ terminal (residues 1–100), GAD65-MID (residues 235–442), GAD65-COOH-terminal (residues 436–585), and/or GAD67. IA-2/IA-2β antibody epitopes were classified as IA-2-JM (residues 605–682), IA-2-PTP-specific (unique to IA-2 PTP domain), IA-2/IA-2β-PTP-cross-reactive, and IA-2β-PTP specific. For IAA and IA-2, but not GAD antibodies, titer was predictive of risk. In terms of subclass analysis, no relationship was found with subclass in GADAb-positive relatives, whereas for IA-2-positive relatives, the risk was higher in those with IgG2, IgG3, or IgG4 IA-2 antibodies. In the IAA-positive relatives, the risk was higher in those with IgG2, IgG3, or IgG4 IAA. One possible hypothesis to explain these observations is that titer is the primary marker of diabetes risk and that multiple IgG subclasses are markers of high-titer responses. Analysis of epitopes showed no association between GAD antibody epitope reactivity and the risk of diabetes; however, in the IA-2 antibody-positive relatives, type 1 diabetes risk was higher in those with antibodies to IA-2β. These observations have recently been confirmed using the large European Nicotinamide Diabetes Intervention Trial (ENDIT) cohort (24).

The affinity of antibody binding has also been examined as a determinant of progression to type 1 diabetes in the Munich BABYDIAB cohort (25). In this study, IAA affinity was measured from the first IAA-positive sample obtained. There was a wide range of IAA affinity observed, but notably high affinity was associated with HLA DRB1*04 and young age of IAA appearance, and identified a cohort more likely to develop both multiple autoantibodies and diabetes. This observation has been confirmed in the Karlsburg Type 1 diabetes Risk Study of a Normal Childhood population (26). In this study, which screened 11,840 school children for IAA, GADAb, IA2Ab, and ICA, IAA affinity was also found to be higher in children who developed multiple autoantibodies or diabetes. On the basis of these relatively large studies, it appears that affinity of IAA may be an extremely useful marker of diabetes risk in islet autoantibody-positive people in the general population as well as in relatives of type 1 diabetes patients.

ZINC TRANSPORTER: A NEW ANTIGEN TARGET IN TYPE 1 DIABETES

Recently, a new antigenic target, the β-cell specific zinc transporter isoform 8 (ZnT8) has been identified in type 1 diabetes using a multidimensional analysis of microarray data (27). ZnT8 is a member of a large family of cation efflux proteins, which play a critical role in exporting Zn, Co, Fe, Mn, and Cd ions from cells (28). Using a C-terminal construct spanning amino acids 268–

369 of the molecule, a robust and sensitive antibody assay (sensitivity 50%, specificity and 98% for type 1 diabetes) has been reported. Using this assay, ~30% of patients with newly diagnosed type 1 diabetes negative for GADAb, IA2Ab, and IAA were found to be positive. Analysis in terms of reactivity with other autoantibodies demonstrates a weak correlation of ZnT8 antibodies with IA2Ab, but not with IAA or GADAb. These findings have led to the conclusion that antibodies to ZnT8 are an independent marker of type 1 diabetes. Use of the ZnT8 antibody assay in the DAISY study (20) showed that antibodies appeared usually many years before disease and frequently appeared by 3 years of age. ZnT8 antibodies usually appear later than GADAb and IAA in prediabetes, although there is no strict order. Interestingly, the autoreactive B-lymphocyte repertoire is restricted to a few ZnT8 epitopes and is truly self-reactive as opposed to arising as a bystander response to a foreign antigen (29). Excitingly, the combined measurement of ZnT8 antibodies, GADAb, IA2Ab, and IAA, leads to a detection rate of greater than 96% at disease onset in Caucasian populations. The ZnT8 antibody assay has now been successfully set up in a number of labs and a preliminary workshop (presented at the 9th International Congress of the Immunology of Diabetes Society, Miami, Florida, 2007) showed excellent concordance between laboratories. It is hoped that the use of this new autoantibody assay will enhance studies seeking to identify individuals with preclinical type 1 diabetes within families and in the general population.

β-CELL DESTRUCTION AND DYSFUNCTION

Based on autopsy studies at diagnosis of type 1 diabetes, approximately only 15% of residual β-cell mass remains (30). A temporary remission from insulin dependence may occur in up to one in four patients, within the first year of diagnosis, attributed to β-cell "rest" from insulin treatment. Ongoing autoimmune destruction eventually results in complete loss of β-cell mass in long-standing type 1 diabetes (31). In a large autopsy series reported by Foulis et al. (32), insulitis was present in 78% of subjects with recent-onset (less than 1 year) diabetes, and insulitis was present in only 1% of insulin-deficient islets supporting the concept of immunologically mediated destruction of pancreatic islet β cells (33). Interestingly, some individuals with recent onset had no evidence of insulitis in at least 40% of their insulin-positive islets, and some individuals with long-standing diabetes (up to 9 years post-diagnosis) possessed islets without evidence of insulitis. In another autopsy series of long-standing type 1 diabetes, 88% of patients had insulin-positive islets but overall had markedly reduced β-cell mass compared with control subjects (*34*). The number of β cells was not related to duration of diabetes but was higher in individuals with lower blood glucose (*34*). Hence, autopsy studies suggest that β-cell mass may be greater than anticipated in some cases of type 1 diabetes at and after diagnosis.

Quantifying β-cell mass has proven to be challenging in established type 1 diabetes and especially difficult in preclinical diabetes, given the limited access to human pancreas tissue and ethical concerns about pancreas biopsy for research. With the problems of assessing β-cell mass, the role of metabolic testing for β-cell function has become important in understanding the pathogenesis of type 1 diabetes. In preclinical type 1 diabetes, dynamic stimulation testing with an IVGTT has been the most widely used and validated test of β-cell function. The IVGTT allows calculation of the FPIR, defined as the sum of the first and third minute blood-insulin levels post-stimulation, which is a relatively early marker for loss of β-cell function in preclinical diabetes (*35, 36*). The IVGTT has been used extensively, given its safety in children, ease of implementation, and validated reproducibility (*37*).

Declining FPIR has been demonstrated in individuals within months of seroconversion for islet autoantibodies (*38*), and in people positive for multiple islet autoantibody, specificities is highly predictive for the development of type 1 diabetes. This finding has been consistent in multiple natural history studies of type 1 diabetes across several continents (Europe, North America, and Australia), including ICARUS (*39*), DPT-1 (*40*), ENDIT (*41*), and the Melbourne Pre-Diabetes Family Study (*37*). The 5-year risk of diabetes in ICA-positive relatives of people with type 1 diabetes is 85% if the FPIR is <50 mU/L (i.e., less than the first percentile), 48% if the FPIR 50–100 mU/L, and 17% if the FPIR >100 mU/L (*39*). However, the rate of decline in FPIR is recognized to be highly variable across individuals. A spectrum of longitudinal β-cell function profiles is evident including some cases with constant slow decline, others with stepwise decline over years, less fortunate cases with a rapid decline over months, and other cases with no decline (*42*).

Individuals with clinical diabetes have a very low FPIR and other dynamic stimulation tests such as the mixed meal test and glucagon stimulation test for measurement of stimulated C-peptide have been adopted to assess residual β-cell function post-diagnosis. A large study of dynamic stimulation testing for β-cell function in type 1 diabetes coordinated by TrialNet USA determined the mixed meal stimulation test had the best reproducibility and sensitivity for assessing residual β-cell function (*43*). Age of onset and glycemic control seem to be important moderators of residual beta-cell function. In adult-onset classical type 1 diabetes and latent autoimmune diabetes in adults (LADA), there is greater β-cell function than juvenile-onset type 1 diabetes at diagnosis (*44, 45*). Also, intensive insulin therapy aiming for tighter glycemic control in type 1 diabetes sustains endogenous insulin production (*4, 46*).

Loss of β-cell function can be due to either β-cell destruction (presumed to be due to apoptosis) or β-cell dysfunction (impaired responsiveness to glucose stimulation). In preclinical type 1 diabetes, it is assumed that loss of β-cell function is mainly indicative of β-cell destruction. However, in late preclinical type 1 diabetes, β cells may respond poorly to stimulation with glucose compared with glucagon or arginine, suggesting "dysfunction" prior to complete loss of function (*47*). A significant period of β-cell dysfunction before destruction offers a greater window of opportunity for intervention to salvage β cells. Future novel pancreas biopsy or β-cell imaging techniques may allow more accurate quantification of β cells in humans, and in combination with metabolic testing, help dissect the question of destruction vs. dysfunction.

INSULIN RESISTANCE IN PRE-CLINICAL TYPE 1 DIABETES

Glucose disposal and prevailing glycemia are determined not only by insulin secretion but also insulin action (*48*). In contrast to type 2 diabetes, impaired insulin action or insulin resistance had not been considered previously to play a major role in the pathogenesis of type 1 diabetes. The "accelerator hypothesis" (*49*) proposed "three processes which variably accelerate the loss of beta cells through apoptosis: constitution, insulin resistance and autoimmunity," and stimulated interest in the potential role for insulin resistance in the pathogenesis of type 1 diabetes. It proposed a model for diabetes pathogenesis whereby excess body weight contributes to insulin resistance resulting in rising blood glucose, which accelerates β-cell apoptosis in all individuals and induces β-cell "immunogens" in a subset of individuals genetically predisposed to islet autoimmunity, i.e., to type 1 diabetes (*49*). The molecular process in the accelerator hypothesis is based on animal studies which suggest hyperglycemia leads to β-cell apoptosis, which, in turn, induces immune responses to autoreactive antigens in apoptotic cells presented to dendritic cells (*50, 51*). Currently, there are no longitudinal data demonstrating that insulin resistance measured from birth (i.e., prior to the development of islet autoantibodies) triggers or increases the likelihood of developing islet autoimmunity.

The well-documented rise of obesity (*52*), in parallel with the increasing incidence of type 1 diabetes (*53*), also prompted investigation of the role of obesity and insulin resistance in the pathogenesis of type 1 diabetes. Evidence has accumulated in the last decade that insulin resistance influences progression to clinical diabetes in islet autoantibody-positive individuals. Given plasma glucose is determined by the interplay of insulin secretion and insulin action, insulin resistance would be expected to lead to an earlier appearance of hyperglycemia when β-cell function is compromised by pancreatic insulitis, thereby unmasking clinical diabetes.

Three large prospective studies, in Australia, the United States, and Europe, have recently shown that markers of insulin resistance independently predict progression to type 1 diabetes in individuals with islet autoantibodies. They demonstrate a subtle metabolic disturbance characterized by increased insulin resistance in relation to β-cell function, which increases over time to diabetes, indicating progressive dysregulation of the relationship between insulin action and insulin secretion. The significance of these findings lies in the fact that the most rapid progressors can be identified early even when metabolic parameters such as fasting glucose and insulin, and FPIR, are still within the normal ranges.

Use of the validated basal insulin resistance index, HOMA-IR (54), in large natural history type 1 diabetes studies has facilitated investigating insulin resistance in preclinical diabetes. This is an important consideration because invasive techniques for directly measuring insulin resistance via clamp studies are not feasible or ethically acceptable in longitudinal studies involving children.

In the Melbourne Pre-Diabetes Family Study (8), 104 first-degree relatives of type 1 diabetes probands identified as islet antibody positive were followed for a median of 4 years. Progressors had a higher ratio of insulin resistance to insulin secretion at baseline. The HOMA-IR/FPIR ratio was an independent predictor of progression to diabetes. A recent substudy of the North American Diabetes Prevention Trial-1 (DPT-1) divided a cohort of 356 individuals with preclinical type 1 diabetes into moderate-risk ($n=186$) and high-risk ($n=170$) groups (55). In a multivariate analysis, HOMA-IR and the ratio of FPIR to HOMA-IR were significantly independently associated with development of type 1 diabetes in both groups. In DPT-1, the hazard ratio for HOMA-IR was 2.70 in the moderate-risk population and 1.83 for the high-risk population, suggesting that insulin resistance could have a greater contribution to diabetes in those with lower risk of developing type 1 diabetes. An analysis of 213 islet autoantibody-positive subjects in the ENDIT found that HOMA-IR was an independent predictor of diabetes in subjects with low FPIR [≤10th percentile] ($p=0.025$), but not in those with preserved FPIR (56). These findings suggest that insulin resistance may be a more critical factor when beta-cell function is already significantly affected.

Insulin resistance in individuals with islet autoimmunity could have a genetic-constitutional basis or be secondary to the autoimmune disease process itself. It is likely that insulin resistance is closely linked to an individual's physical constitution in preclinical type 1 diabetes because adiposity in children and adolescents, in general, accounts for approximately 50% of the variance seen in insulin sensitivity (*57*). Numerous cross-sectional studies have identified higher bodyweight in children at diagnosis of type 1 diabetes compared to age and sex-matched controls (*58–61*), consistent with insulin resistance having a role in the pathogenesis of type 1 diabetes. In addition, a Finnish longitudinal study found that a 10% increment in weight percentile was associated with a 50–60% increase in the risk for developing type 1 diabetes before 3 years of age and 20–40% increase from 3 to 10 years of age (*62*), and the Australian BabyDiab Study found that increased bodyweight percentiles were associated with increased risk of developing islet autoantibodies (*9*). As more natural history data are obtained in genetically predisposed children, through studies such as the TEDDY study (*63*), detailed analyses of the relationship between insulin resistance and adiposity and their relationship to the development of islet autoimmunity will become available. Alternatively, insulin resistance may reflect a more aggressive form of autoimmune disease mediated, for example, by immunoinflammatory factors that also mediate beta-cell destruction, e.g., TNF-α and IL-6 (*64, 65*).

IMPAIRED GLUCOSE TOLERANCE

Declining FPIR is the first measure of deteriorating β-cell function and is then accompanied by declining stimulated C-peptide with impaired oral glucose tolerance (IGT) and/or impaired fasting glycemia (IFG), prior to the onset of overt diabetes (*66, 67*). Given that hyperglycemia can occur due to deficits in insulin secretion and/or insulin action, one can appreciate that with declining β-cell function an increase in insulin resistance will exacerbate the hyperglycemia. It is likely that insulin-resistant individuals present earlier with overt diabetes for any given loss of β-cell mass. Furthermore, an increase in plasma glucose secondary to insulin resistance could augment islet inflammation and beta-cell death. Glucose has been shown to induce the proinflammatory cytokine IL-1 beta in islets (*68*), to upregulate expression of the Fas death receptor (*69*) and autoantigens (*70, 71*) in beta cells and to induce beta-cell apoptosis (*72*).

Raised awareness of diabetes among children is prompting more screening for diabetes at early ages. Children detected with incidental IFG in the presence of islet autoimmunity (i.e., islet autoantibody positive) have higher risk for developing type 1 diabetes (*73*). Such children have been shown to have a lower FPIR and higher frequency of type 1 diabetes risk alleles HLA DR3 and DR4 compared to normoglycemic children. Thus, children with subtle hyperglycemia, such as impaired fasting glycemia (i.e., fasting blood glucose >6.0 mmol/L), might warrant screening for islet autoantibodies and more detailed metabolic testing. Also with the advent of large-scale natural history studies and type 1 diabetes prevention trials, there is increasing recognition of a subgroup of type 1 diabetes characterized by a lack of diabetes symptoms but fulfilling the metabolic criteria for diagnosis of diabetes (74). Interestingly, prediabetic children followed to diabetes compared with community cases have been shown to have less hospitalizations and in general a milder clinical onset and lower insulin requirement in the first year after diagnosis (75).

SUMMARY

Strong evidence demonstrates that in addition to loss of β-cell function, increased insulin resistance predicts progression to type 1 diabetes in individuals with preexisting islet autoimmunity. Multiple pathophysiological pathways may lead to the clinical presentation of type 1 diabetes; hyperglycemia can be due to a combined deficit of insulin secretion and insulin action. This would partly explain the rising incidence of type 1 diabetes in an increasingly "obesogenic" environment and account for the recent change in genetic profile of type 1 diabetes.

A role for insulin resistance in the pathogenesis of type 1 diabetes implies that interventions to reduce insulin resistance may at least delay or possibly prevent progression to type 1 diabetes in some "at-risk" individuals. Improved prediction using markers of β-cell function and insulin resistance could enhance appropriate selection of subjects for intervention trials to prevent clinical disease.

REFERENCES

1. Concannon P, Erlich HA, Julier C, Morahan G, Nerup J, Pociot F, Todd JA, Rich SS. Type 1 diabetes: evidence for susceptibility loci from four genome-wide linkage scans in 1,435 multiplex families. Diabetes 2005;54:2995–3001.
2. Srikanta S, Ganda OP, Eisenbarth GS, Soeldner JS. Islet-cell antibodies and beta-cell function in monozygotic triplets and twins initially discordant for type I diabetes mellitus. N Engl J Med 1983;308:322–325.
3. Sherry NA, Tsai EB, Herold KC. Natural history of beta-cell function in type 1 diabetes. Diabetes 2005;54(Suppl 2):S32–S39.
4. The Diabetes Control and Complications Trial Research Group. Effect of intensive therapy on residual beta-cell function in patients with type 1 diabetes in the diabetes control and complications trial. A randomized, controlled trial. Ann Intern Med 1998;128:517–523.
5. Hermann R, Knip M, Veijola R, Simell O, Laine AP, Akerblom HK, Groop PH, Forsblom C, Pettersson-Fernholm K, Ilonen J. Temporal changes in the frequencies of HLA genotypes in patients with type 1 diabetes – indication of an increased environmental pressure? Diabetologia 2003;46:420–425.
6. Gillespie KM, Bain SC, Barnett AH, Bingley PJ, Christie MR, Gill GV, Gale EA. The rising incidence of childhood type 1 diabetes and reduced contribution of high-risk HLA haplotypes. Lancet 2004;364:1699–1700.
7. Fourlanos S, Varney MD, Tait BD, Morahan G, Honeyman MC, Colman PG, Harrison LC. The rising incidence of type 1 diabetes is

8. Fourlanos S, Narendran P, Byrnes GB, Colman PG, Harrison LC. Insulin resistance is a risk factor for progression to type 1 diabetes. Diabetologia 2004;47:1661–1667.
9. Couper JJ, Beresford S, Hirte C, Baghurst PA, Pollard A, Tait BD, Harrison LC, Colman PG. Weight gain in early life predicts risk of islet autoimmunity in children with a first-degree relative with type 1 diabetes. Diabetes Care 2009;32:94–99.
10. Stene LC, Ulriksen J, Magnus P, Joner G. Use of cod liver oil during pregnancy associated with lower risk of type I diabetes in the offspring. Diabetologia 2000;43:1093–1098.
11. Hypponen E, Laara E, Reunanen A, Jarvelin MR, Virtanen SM. Intake of vitamin D and risk of type 1 diabetes: a birth-cohort study. Lancet 2001;358:1500–1503.
12. Gorsuch AN, Spencer KM, Lister J, McNally JM, Dean BM, Bottazzo GF, Cudworth AG. Evidence for a long prediabetic period in type I (insulin-dependent) diabetes mellitus. Lancet 1981;2:1363–1365.
13. Palmer JP, Asplin CM, Clemons P, Lyen K, Tatpati O, Raghu PK, Paquette TL. Insulin antibodies in insulin-dependent diabetics before insulin treatment. Science 1983;222:1337–1339.
14. Vardi P, Dib SA, Tuttleman M, Connelly JE, Grinbergs M, Radizabeh A, Riley WJ, Maclaren NK, Eisenbarth GS, Soeldner JS. Competitive insulin autoantibody assay. Prospective evaluation of subjects at high risk for development of type I diabetes mellitus. Diabetes 1987;36:1286–1291.
15. Atkinson MA, Maclaren,NK, Riley WJ, Winter WE, Fisk DD, Spillar RP. Are insulin autoantibodies markers for insulin-dependent diabetes mellitus? Diabetes 1986;35:894–898.
16. Baekkeskov S, Aanstoot HJ, Christgau S, Reetz A, Solimena M, Cascalho M, Folli F, Richter-Olesen H, De Camilli P. Identification of the 64K autoantigen in insulin-dependent diabetes as the GABA-synthesizing enzyme glutamic acid decarboxylase. Nature 1990;347:151–156.
17. Rabin DU, Pleasic SM, Shapiro JA, Yoo-Warren H, Oles J, Hicks JM, Goldstein DE, Rae PM. Islet cell antigen 512 is a diabetes-specific islet autoantigen related to protein tyrosine phosphatases. J Immunol 1994;152:3183–3188.
18. Ziegler AG, Hillebrand B, Rabl W, Mayrhofer M, Hummel M, Mollenhauer U, Vordemann J, Lenz A, Standl E. On the appearance of islet associated autoimmunity in offspring of diabetic mothers: a prospective study from birth. Diabetologia 1993;36:402–408.
19. Kupila A, Muona P, Simell T, Arvilommi P, Savolainen H, Hamalainen AM, Korhonen S, Kimpimaki T, Sjoroos M, Ilonen J, et al. Feasibility of genetic and immunological prediction of type I diabetes in a population-based birth cohort. Diabetologia 2001;44:290–297.
20. Rewers M, Bugawan TL, Norris JM, Blair A, Beaty B, Hoffman M, McDuffie RS, Jr, Hamman RF, Klingensmith G, Eisenbarth GS, et al. Newborn screening for HLA markers associated with IDDM: Diabetes Autoimmunity Study in the Young (DAISY). Diabetologia 1996;39:807–812.
21. Colman PG, Steele C, Couper JJ, Beresford SJ, Powell T, Kewming K, Pollard A, Gellert S, Tait B, Honeyman M, et al. Islet autoimmunity in infants with a type I diabetic relative is common but is frequently restricted to one autoantibody. Diabetologia 2000;43:203–209.
22. Achenbach P, Bonifacio E, Koczwara K, Ziegler AG. Natural history of type 1 diabetes. Diabetes 2005;54(Suppl 2):S25–S31.
23. Achenbach P, Warncke K, Reiter J, Naserke HE, Williams AJ, Bingley PJ, Bonifacio E, Ziegler AG. Stratification of type 1 diabetes risk on the basis of islet autoantibody characteristics. Diabetes 2004;53:384–392.
24. Achenbach P, Bonifacio E, Williams AJ, Ziegler AG, Gale EA, Bingley PJ. Autoantibodies to IA-2beta improve diabetes risk assessment in high-risk relatives. Diabetologia 2008;51:488–492.
25. Achenbach P, Koczwara K, Knopff A, Naserke H, Ziegler AG, Bonifacio E. Mature high-affinity immune responses to (pro)insulin anticipate the autoimmune cascade that leads to type 1 diabetes. J Clin Invest 2004;114:589–597.
26. Schlosser M, Koczwara K, Kenk H, Strebelow M, Rjasanowski I, Wassmuth R, Achenbach P, Ziegler AG, Bonifacio E. In insulin-autoantibody-positive children from the general population, antibody affinity identifies those at high and low risk. Diabetologia 2005;48:1830–1832.
27. Wenzlau JM, Juhl K, Yu L, Moua O, Sarkar SA, Gottlieb P, Rewers M, Eisenbarth GS, Jensen J, Davidson HW, et al. The cation efflux transporter ZnT8 (Slc30A8) is a major autoantigen in human type 1 diabetes. Proc Natl Acad Sci USA 2007;104:17040–17045.
28. Wenzlau JM, Hutton JC, Davidson HW. New antigenic targets in type 1 diabetes. Curr Opin Endocrinol Diabetes Obes 2008;15:315–320.

29. Wenzlau JM, Liu Y, Yu L, Moua O, Fowler KT, Rangasamy S, Walters J, Eisenbarth GS, Davidson HW, Hutton JC. A common nonsynonymous single nucleotide polymorphism in the SLC30A8 gene determines ZnT8 autoantibody specificity in type 1 diabetes. Diabetes 2008;57:2693–2697.
30. Wrenshall GA, Bogoch A, Ritchie RC. Extractable insulin of pancreas; correlation with pathological and clinical findings in diabetic and nondiabetic cases. Diabetes 1952;1:87–107.
31. Martin P, Tindall H, Harvey JN, Handley TM, Chapman C, Davies JA. Glomerular and tubular proteinuria in type 1 (insulin-dependent) diabetic patients with and without retinopathy. Ann Clin Biochem 1992;29:2665–2270.
32. Foulis AK, Liddle CN, Farquharson MA, Richmond JA, Weir RS. The histopathology of the pancreas in type 1 (insulin-dependent) diabetes mellitus: a 25-year review of deaths in patients under 20 years of age in the United Kingdom. Diabetologia 1986;29:267–274.
33. Willcox A, Richardson SJ, Bone AJ, Foulis AK, Morgan NG. Analysis of islet inflammation in human type 1 diabetes. Clin Exp Immunol 2009;155:173–181.
34. Meier JJ, Bhushan A, Butler AE, Rizza RA, Butler PC. Sustained beta cell apoptosis in patients with long-standing type 1 diabetes: indirect evidence for islet regeneration? Diabetologia 2005;48:2221–2228.
35. Bingley PJ, Colman P, Eisenbarth GS, Jackson RA, McCulloch DK, Riley WJ, Gale EA. Standardization of IVGTT to predict IDDM. Diabetes Care 1992;15:1313–1316.
36. Srikanta S, Ganda OP, Gleason RE, Jackson RA, Soeldner JS, Eisenbarth GS. Pre-type I diabetes. Linear loss of beta cell response to intravenous glucose. Diabetes 1984;33:717–720.
37. Colman PG, McNair P, Margetts H, Schmidli RS, Werther GA, Alford FP, Ward GM, Tait BD, Honeyman MC, Harrison LC. The Melbourne Pre-Diabetes Study: prediction of type 1 diabetes mellitus using antibody and metabolic testing. Med J Aust 1998;169:81–84.
38. Keskinen P, Korhonen S, Kupila A, Veijola R, Erkkila S, Savolainen H, Arvilommi P, Simell T, Ilonen J, Knip M, et al. First-phase insulin response in young healthy children at genetic and immunological risk for type I diabetes. Diabetologia 2002;45:1639–1648.
39. Bingley PJ. Interactions of age, islet cell antibodies, insulin autoantibodies, and first-phase insulin response in predicting risk of progression to IDDM in ICA+ relatives: the ICARUS data set. Islet Cell Antibody Register Users Study. Diabetes 1996;45:1720–1728.
40. Chase HP, Cuthbertson DD, Dolan LM, Kaufman F, Krischer JP, Schatz DA, White NH, Wilson DM, Wolfsdorf J. First-phase insulin release during the intravenous glucose tolerance test as a risk factor for type 1 diabetes. J Pediatr 2001;138:244–249.
41. Bingley PJ, Gale EA, European Nicotinamide Diabetes Intervention Trial (ENDIT) Group. Progression to type 1 diabetes in islet cell antibody-positive relatives in the European Nicotinamide Diabetes Intervention Trial: the role of additional immune, genetic and metabolic markers of risk. Diabetologia 2006;49:881–890.
42. McCulloch DK, Klaff LJ, Kahn SE, Schoenfeld SL, Greenbaum CJ, Mauseth RS, Benson EA, Nepom GT, Shewey L, Palmer JP. Nonprogression of subclinical beta-cell dysfunction among first-degree relatives of IDDM patients. 5-yr follow-up of the Seattle Family Study. Diabetes 1990;39:549–556.
43. Greenbaum CJ, Mandrup-Poulsen T, McGee PF, Battelino T, Haastert B, Ludvigsson J, Pozzilli P, Lachin JM, Kolb H. Mixed-meal tolerance test versus glucagon stimulation test for the assessment of beta-cell function in therapeutic trials in type 1 diabetes. Diabetes Care 2008;31:1966–1971.
44. Karjalainen J, Salmela P, Ilonen J, Surcel HM, Knip M. A comparison of childhood and adult type I diabetes mellitus. N Engl J Med 1989;320:881–886.
45. Gottsater A, Landin-Olsson M, Fernlund P, Lernmark A, Sundkvist G. Beta-cell function in relation to islet cell antibodies during the first 3 yr after clinical diagnosis of diabetes in type II diabetic patients. Diabetes Care 1993;16:902–910.
46. Linn T, Ortac K, Laube H, Federlin K. Intensive therapy in adult insulin-dependent diabetes mellitus is associated with improved insulin sensitivity and reserve: a randomized, controlled, prospective study over 5 years in newly diagnosed patients. Metabolism 1996;45:1508–1513.
47. Soeldner JS, Srikanta S, Eisenbarth GS, Gleason RE. Pre-hyperglycaemic diabetes mellitus. Clin Chem 1986;32:B7–B18.
48. Kahn SE, Prigeon RL, McCulloch DK, Boyko EJ, Bergman RN, Schwartz MW, Neifing JL, Ward WK, Beard JC, Palmer JP, et al. Quantification of the relationship between

insulin sensitivity and beta-cell function in human subjects. Evidence for a hyperbolic function. Diabetes 1993;42(11):1663–1672.
49. Wilkin TJ. The accelerator hypothesis: weight gain as the missing link between type I and type II diabetes. Diabetologia 2001;44:914–922.
50. Koyama M, Wada R, Sakuraba H, Mizukami H, Yagihashi S. Accelerated loss of islet beta cells in sucrose-fed Goto-Kakizaki rats, a genetic model of non-insulin-dependent diabetes mellitus. Am J Pathol 1998;153:537–545.
51. Bar-On H, Ben-Sasson R, Ziv E, Arar N, Shafrir E. Irreversibility of nutritionally induced NIDDM in Psammomys obesus is related to beta-cell apoptosis. Pancreas 1999;18:259–265.
52. Hedley AA, Ogden CL, Johnson CL, Carroll MD, Curtin LR, Flegal KM. Prevalence of overweight and obesity among US children, adolescents, and adults, 1999–2002. JAMA 2004;291:2847–2850.
53. Onkamo P, Vaananen S, Karvonen M, Tuomilehto J. Worldwide increase in incidence of Type I diabetes – the analysis of the data on published incidence trends. Diabetologia 1999;42:1395–1403.
54. Matthews DR, Hosker JP, Rudenski AS, Naylor BA, Treacher DF, Turner RC. Homeostasis model assessment: insulin resistance and beta-cell function from fasting plasma glucose and insulin concentrations in man. Diabetologia 1985;28:412–419.
55. Xu P, Cuthbertson D, Greenbaum C, Palmer JP, Krischer JP. Role of insulin resistance in predicting progression to type 1 diabetes. Diabetes Care 2007;30:2314–2320.
56. Bingley PJ, Mahon JL, Gale EA. Insulin resistance and progression to type 1 diabetes in the European Nicotinamide Diabetes Intervention Trial (ENDIT). Diabetes Care 2008;31:146–150.
57. Caprio S. Insulin resistance in childhood obesity. J Pediatr Endocrinol Metab 2002;15(Suppl 1):487–492.
58. Baum JD, Ounsted M, Smith MA. Weight gain in infancy and subsequent development of diabetes mellitus in childhood. Lancet 1975;2:866.
59. Johansson C, Samuelsson U, Ludvigsson J. A high weight gain early in life is associated with an increased risk of type 1 (insulin-dependent) diabetes mellitus. Diabetologia 1994;37:91–94.
60. Kibirige M, Metcalf B, Renuka R, Wilkin TJ. Testing the accelerator hypothesis: the relationship between body mass and age at diagnosis of type 1 diabetes. Diabetes Care 2003;26:2865–2870.
61. Knerr I, Wolf J, Reinehr T, Stachow R, Grabert M, Schober E, Rascher W, Holl RW. The 'accelerator hypothesis': relationship between weight, height, body mass index and age at diagnosis in a large cohort of 9,248 German and Austrian children with type 1 diabetes mellitus. Diabetologia 2005;48:2501–2504.
62. Hypponen E, Virtanen SM, Kenward MG, Knip M, Akerblom HK. Obesity, increased linear growth, and risk of type 1 diabetes in children. Diabetes Care 2000;23:1755–1760.
63. TEDDY Study Group. The Environmental Determinants of Diabetes in the Young (TEDDY) Study: study design. Pediatr Diabetes 2007;8:286–298.
64. Yoon KH, Ko SH, Cho JH, Lee JM, Ahn YB, Song KH, Yoo SJ, Kang MI, Cha BY, Lee KW, et al. Selective beta-cell loss and alpha-cell expansion in patients with type 2 diabetes mellitus in Korea. J Clin Endocrinol Metab 2003;88:2300–2308.
65. Campbell IL, Harrison LC. Molecular pathology of type 1 diabetes. Mol Biol Med 1990;7:299–309.
66. Sosenko JM, Palmer JP, Greenbaum CJ, Mahon J, Cowie C, Krischer JP, Chase HP, White H, Buckingham B, Herold KC, et al. Patterns of metabolic progression to type 1 diabetes in the Diabetes Prevention Trial-Type 1. Diabetes Care 2006;29:643–649.
67. Barker JM, McFann K, Harrison LC, Fourlanos S, Krischer J, Cuthbertson D, Chase HP, Eisenbarth GS, DPT-1 Study Group. Pre-type 1 diabetes dysmetabolism: maximal sensitivity achieved with both oral and intravenous glucose tolerance testing. J Pediatr Endocrinol Metab 2007;150:31–36.
68. Maedler K, Sergeev P, Ris F, Oberholzer J, Joller-Jemelka HI, Spinas GA, Kaiser N, Halban PA, Donath MY. Glucose-induced beta cell production of IL-1beta contributes to glucotoxicity in human pancreatic islets. J Clin Invest 2002;110:851–860.
69. Maedler K, Spinas GA, Lehmann R, Sergeev P, Weber M, Fontana A, Kaiser N, Donath MY. Glucose induces beta-cell apoptosis via upregulation of the Fas receptor in human islets. Diabetes 2001;50:1683–1690.
70. Aaen K, Rygaard J, Josefsen K, Petersen H, Brogren CH, Horn T, Buschard K. 1990. Dependence of antigen expression on functional state of beta-cells. Diabetes 1990;39:697–701.

71. Björk E, Kämpe O, Karlsson FA, Pipeleers DG, Andersson A, Hellerström C, Eizirik DL. Glucose regulation of the autoantigen GAD65 in human pancreatic islets. J Clin Endocrinol Metab 1992;75:1574–1576.

72. Donath MY, Gross DJ, Cerasi E, Kaiser N. Hyperglycemia-induced beta-cell apoptosis in pancreatic islets of Psammomys obesus during development of diabetes. Diabetes 1999;48: 738–744.

73. Lorini R, Alibrandi A, Vitali L, Klersy C, Martinetti M, Betterle C, d'Annunzio G, Bonifacio E, Pediatric Italian Study Group of Prediabetes. Risk of type 1 diabetes development in children with incidental hyperglycemia: a multicenter Italian study. Diabetes Care 2001;24:1210–1216.

74. Greenbaum CJ, Cuthbertson D, Krischer JP, Disease Prevention Trial of Type I Diabetes Study Group. Type I diabetes manifested solely by 2-h oral glucose tolerance test criteria. Diabetes 2001;50:470–476.

75. Barker JM, Barriga KJ, Yu L, Miao D, Erlich HA, Norris JM, Eisenbarth GS, Rewers M, Diabetes Autoimmunity Study in the Young. Prediction of autoantibody positivity and progression to type 1 diabetes: Diabetes Autoimmunity Study in the Young (DAISY). J Clin Endocrinol Metab 2004;89: 3896–3902.

Chapter 18

Immunotherapy of Type-1 Diabetes: Immunoprevention and Immunoreversal

Frank Waldron-Lynch and Kevan C. Herold

Summary

Type-1A diabetes (T1D) is characterized by a progressive insidious loss of self-tolerance to pancreatic islet beta cells resulting in their destruction and the development of overt hyperglycemia. Immunotherapy aims either to reverse the autoimmune process thereby preventing the development of the disease (immunoprevention) or to intervene at clinical diagnosis of type-1 diabetes and preserve residual b cell function (immunoreversal). Murine models and clinical studies of patients with type-1 diabetes have provided insights into the immunopathogenesis of type-1 diabetes and have led to the development of immunomodulatory therapeutic strategies. Recent clinical trials of anti-CD3 monoclonal antibody (mAbs) and glutamic acid decarboxylase (GAD) peptide have proven successful in attenuating loss of insulin production. Current individual clinical trials are investigating the use of anti-CD3 mAb, GAD, Rituximab, and Abatacept to maintain insulin responses. These trials will lay the groundwork for future studies in which more complete metabolic correction and immunologic tolerance will be restored, possibly with the use of combinations of therapies.

Key Words: Type-1 diabetes, Immunotherapy, Anti-CD3 monoclonal antibody, Glutamic acid decarboxylase, Rituximab, Abatacept

INTRODUCTION

Type-1A diabetes (T1D) is one of the most common chronic autoimmune conditions, characterized by autoimmune destruction of pancreatic beta cells (b cells) leading to insulin deficiency and hyperglycemia at clinical onset in genetically susceptible individuals (*1*). Despite improvement in outcomes in recent years, patients with type-1 diabetes remain with a reduced life expectancy of 10–15 years due to macrovascular and microvascular complications (*2*). A great deal of clinical and experimental evidence has demonstrated that there is a loss of self-tolerance to pancreatic b cells with the emergence of autoreactive immune cells. Immunomodulatory therapy aims to restore self-tolerance and downregulate autoimmune responses to pancreatic islets and restore euglycemia (*3*).

Current therapy in type-1 diabetes involves replacement of insulin and has been incrementally optimized over the last 87 years with the development of insulin analogs, education programs, glucose monitoring, and cardiovascular risk factor modification to improve outcomes (*4*). The Diabetes Control and Complication Trial (DCCT) demonstrated that intensive glycemic control reduced microvascular complications, with the aim of therapy to normalize glucose levels (*5–7*). Despite these advances, most patients are unable to achieve euglycemia with the main limiting factor being hypoglycemia (*8*). In practice, the average hemoglobin A1c level in most pediatric diabetes clinics exceeds 8%, a level that was achieved by the "standard" control group of the DCCT in which the risk of significant eye disease exceeded 80% over 7 years. However, patients in the DCCT who had residual beta cell function as measured by C-peptide responses (>0.20 nmol/l) had a reduced rate of microvascular complications, and hypoglycemia was the main limiting factor of intensive insulin treatment (*9*). The preservation of C-peptide responses has, therefore, been deemed to be an appropriate outcome measure of immunomodulatory trials designed to maintain pancreatic beta-cell function (*10*).

While complete reversal of the metabolic abnormalities is the ultimate goal, clinical evidence, primarily from the DCCT, has identified the significance of residual insulin production, even if it is not sufficient to restore normal metabolic control in the absence of exogenous insulin. In the DCCT, a stimulated C-peptide level of greater than 0.2 pmol/ml was associated with improved glycemic control, reduced hypoglycemia, and even reduced rates of development of long-term complications. More recently, Steffes et al. have reported that participants in the DCCT with sustained C-peptide levels of at least 0.2 pmol/ml had a two- to fourfold reduced rate of severe hypoglycemia during the first 6 years of the DCCT (*9*).

IMMUNOPATHOGENESIS: MURINE MODELS, T-CELLS, B LYMPHOCYTES, INNATE IMMUNE SYSTEM

The rationale for human trials in T1D has largely been derived from studies in rodent models of the disease, most commonly the nonobese diabetic (NOD) mouse, because a large animal model is not available. These studies have generated evidence that there is failure of tolerance of T cells to self-antigens (*11*) and have provided essential preclinical data on the effects of immune modulatory therapies. Both CD4+ (T helper) and CD8+ T Cell (T cytotoxic) subsets are required for the development of Type-1 diabetes in this model (*12*). Autoreactive CD4+ and CD8+ T cells that may recognize endogenous insulin as an antigen when presented on major histocompatibility complex (MHC) class II and I molecules, respectively, by antigen-presenting cells (APC), or alternatively pancreatic b cells themselves (*13*) are the trigger for a cascade of cellular and humoral immune responses that result in β-cell destruction. CD4+ Th1 (proinflammatory) cells play a pivotal role in activation of other CD4+ and CD8+ T cells and the creation of a proinflammatory cytokine environment that leads to further amplification of the immune response with resultant destruction of pancreatic β cells (*14*). With a limited number of approaches, such as transfer of antigen-specific regulatory T cells, anti-CD3 mAb, or immunization with complete Freund's adjuvant, this process may be reversed in the NOD mice with cure of diabetes (*15*).

The role of B lymphocytes in the pathogenesis of type-1 diabetes has also been investigated in the NOD mouse (*16*). Although B cells are not absolutely required for the adoptive transfer of type-1 diabetes from NOD mice into immune-deficient NOD/scid mice, B lymphocytes clearly play a role in the initiation of insulitis and activation and propagation of autoreactive T-cells after the loss of self-tolerance (*17, 18*). It is thought that their importance lies in their function as APCs rather than their production of antibodies, since even nonantibody-secreting B cells can restore development of diabetes in B cell-deficient mice (*19–22*).

The innate immune system also plays a key role in induction of diabetes in the NOD mice. The initial cellular infiltrates are predominantly composed of cells of the innate immune system (*23*). Both natural killer (NK) cells and macrophages shape the pancreatic islet inflammatory environment and subsequent recruitment of adaptive immune cells by cytokine secretion and cell–cell interactions (*24*). NK cells are thought to produce interferon gamma (IFNg) that results in a Th1 predominant islet microenvironment that accelerates the recruitment of islet-specific CD4+ T cells (*25, 26*). Macrophages participate cooperatively with T cells to destroy pancreatic β-cells (*27*). Macrophages via the production of proinflammatory cytokines interleukin-1 (IL-1), tumor necrosis factor α (TNFα), interleukin-8 (IL-8), and interleukin-12 (IL-12) amplify T cell responses and may cause direct pancreatic beta-cell dysfunction (*28*). Recent evidence has suggested that Toll-like receptors (TLR) that recognize pattern recognition motifs (PAM) that are found on cells of innate immune system may have a direct role in susceptibility of the NOD mouse to diabetes by modification of the composition of distal gut microflora. However, it is important to note that in

NOD mice lacking functional TLR pathways may still develop diabetes via an antiislet-mediated T-cell response (*24, 29*). Interestingly, the lesions of human insulitis, found in individuals who have succumbed at the time of diagnosis, show a heavy infiltration of macrophages and NK cells, which differ from the lesions that are seen in newly diabetic NOD mice (*30, 31*). These observations highlight the limitations of the current rodent models.

IMMUNO-PATHOGENESIS: HUMAN DATA, PREDICTION OF DEVELOPMENT, T-CELL ISLET INFILTRATES

Nevertheless, the studies in preclinical models have largely shaped our understanding of type-1 diabetes in humans (*32*). Longitudinal studies of genetically susceptible individuals have demonstrated that the development of autoimmunity may occur very early in life within months of birth, many years prior to any overt disease (*33, 34*). As in mice, genetic susceptibility is largely related to inheritance of the MHC genes, i.e., most importantly to HLA-DR and DQ haplotypes located within the MHC on chromosome 6p21 (*35*). Evidence from prediabetic subjects suggests that the primary autoimmune response may be a T cell-mediated response directed at insulin (*36*). The finding that type-1 diabetes could develop in a patient with X-linked agammaglobulinemia suggests that the primary role of B lymphocytes as APCs and initiators of the autoimmune response could be bypassed although data from the ongoing trial of anti-CD20 mAb will establish the requirements for these cells in the late stages of the disease (*37*).

Insulin antibodies may be detected in susceptible individuals from 6 to 12 months of age onward, predating the development of type-1 diabetes by up to 10 years (*33, 38*). With the progression of autoimmunity, there is an evolution of autoantibody responses with the emergence of antibodies to glutamic acid decarboxylase 65 (GAD65) and tyrosine phosphatases, insulin antibody-2 (IA-2) and IA-2β (*39, 40*). The risk of diabetes appears to be related to the number of positive autoantibodies suggesting that the progression of the disease is associated with spreading of the autoantigenic repertoire (*41, 42*). In the Diabetes Prevention Trial-Type1 (DPT-1), single antibody-positive individuals had approximately a 6% 5-year risk of development of type-1 diabetes, while those with four antibodies positive had a greater than 60% 5-year risk of diagnosis (*41*). During the later stages of autoimmune pancreatic β-cells destruction, prior to clinical diagnosis of type-1 diabetes, metabolic abnormalities may be detected (*43*). By combining metabolic and autoantibody tests, it is possible now to predict with a 90% certainty the 6-year risk of development of type-1 diabetes in young relatives of patients with type-1 diabetes (*44–46*). These observations have important implications for the design of clinical trials. The extraordinarily high risk of disease in the autoantibody+ relatives with metabolic abnormalities suggests that the disease process is active. Their metabolic condition differs from those with overt T1D only in time.

In newly diagnosed patients with type-1 diabetes, a mononuclear infiltrate in the islet (insulitis) of CD4+ T cells, CD8+ T cells, B lymphocytes, and macrophages are found on pancreatic biopsy (*47*). In human insulitis, CD8+ T cells have been found to predominate, in frequency, followed by macrophages. Increased expression of MHC class I molecules by pancreatic β-cells is also observed (*31*). A recent report showed a predominance of NK cells within the islet infiltrates, with evidence of viral inclusion bodies in their pancreatic β cells suggesting a role for viral infection – a notion that has neither been proven nor refuted but suggested by the heightened expression of TNF-α and MHC class I molecules (*30, 47*).

IMMUNOMODULATION: IMMUNOPREVENTION VS. IMMUNOREVERSAL

From our understanding of the immunopathogenesis of type-1 diabetes in human and murine models, it is possible to identify potential targets and time points during the disease process to intervene and potentially reverse autoimmunity. The optimal strategy would be to intervene prior to the development of symptomatic type-1 diabetes and reverse the autoimmune process, thereby preventing the development of disease entirely (immunoprevention). The second strategy involves intervening at the time of onset of type-1 diabetes and preserving residual b-cell function (immunoreversal) – this approach is largely supported by the clinical significance of the residual C-peptide that can be found at diagnosis (*3*). Both strategies are complementary and aim to induce remission from autoimmunity by reestablishment of tolerance. Tolerance refers to establishing a state in which autoimmunity is curtailed without the need for continuous immunosuppression. However, additional therapies may be required to expand β-cell mass and to maintain remission to prevent the reemergence of autoimmunity (*48*).

Immunoprevention trials of type-1 diabetes involve the identification of genetically susceptible individuals with evidence of the emergence of islet autoimmunity as demonstrated by autoantibodies (*49*). Since the rate of positive screening autoantibodies among first-degree relatives is about 3.5%, screening of a large number (50,000–100,000) relatives of type-1 patients, depending on risk category, is needed to identify a sufficient sample size for Phase II prevention studies. This requirement limits the number of immunoprevention trials that may be undertaken at any one time (*44*).

It is postulated that the immune response leading to T1D is limited at its initiation but then diversifies through intra and intermolecular epitope spreading. Therefore, antigen-specific therapies are particularly well suited for prevention trials, since these agents are considered low risk for adverse events and therefore have an acceptable risk profile in asymptomatic individuals (*50*). The equipoise of trials aimed at immunoprevention and immune intervention reflects a dynamic between the risks of the intervention, the certainty of diagnosis, and the efficacy and duration of the treatment.

At the time of presentation with hyperglycemia, the autoimmune repertoire is thought to be diverse. Therefore, an immune modulator with nonantigen-specific effects might be considered most suitable, and such agents have been evaluated in this setting. However, it is also important to note that the regulatory effects of even antigen-specific cells, such as regulatory T cells, may not be antigen specific. Through bystander suppression, polyclonal cells may be inhibited (*51*).

ANTIGEN SPECIFIC IMMUNO-MODULATION

Mechanisms

Antigen-specific approaches aim to reestablish tolerance by modifying responses to key specific antigens involved in initiating and spreading the autoimmune response (*52*). Studies in animal models have shown that the modified cells have regulatory properties and can inhibit the autoreactive T-cells (*53, 54*). Tregs may act by direct cell–cell contact or, more likely, by producing a local tolergenic microenvironment by the release of regulatory cytokines that affect the functional phenotype of other cells: a process termed "infectious tolerance" (*53, 54*). A similar mechanism has been suggested for orally administered antigens. Orally administered antigens induce Th2-like cytokines such as IL-4 and IL-10 and Th3 (TGF-β+) antigen-specific cells (*55*). In addition, CD4+CD25+ regulatory cells and latency-associated peptide+ T cells that have regulatory function may be induced. Intranasal antigens may also induce immune modulatory cells. A modified proinsulin peptide (removing the Class I binding motif) induced antigen-specific regulatory T cells and prevented diabetes in the NOD mouse after a single intranasal dose (*56*). The specificity of the response avoids the side effects of systemic immunosuppression though care needs to be taken in the selection of tolergen epitopes, since they may induce effector T cells rather than Tregs and have been found to exacerbate diabetes in the NOD mouse (*57*). To date insulin, GAD65, and DiaPep277 trials in humans have been largely based on murine data, limited human pilot trials, and detection of human autoantibodies to antigen (*58–61*).

Insulin

Insulin was identified as a prime candidate as an immunoprevention agent, given the evidence of its ability to cure type-1 diabetes in rodent models of type-1 diabetes (*60, 62*). Mechanistically, it is also very attractive as a target since the proposed primary antigen in type-1 diabetes inhibition of immune response to this epitope would prevent the subsequent development of autoimmunity (*63*). A pilot trial showed that administration of parenteral insulin to first-degree relatives of patients with T1D significantly reduced the progression to diabetes (*61*), and formed the basis for the larger DPT-1. Other studies had suggested that orally administered antigens might have immune modulatory effects. Zhang et al. postulated that when antigen was presented by cells of the intestinal mucosa, antigen-specific regulatory T cells were induced that inhibited responses through a TGF-β dependent mechanism (*60*). Both parenteral and oral routes of antigen administration were tested in the DPT-1.

To recruit sufficient numbers of subjects, 84,228 first and second-degree relatives were screened for type-1-associated antibodies, genetic susceptibility, and metabolic derangement. From this group, depending on the 5-year risk of diabetes, individuals were randomized to a parenteral trial in which subcutaneous insulin was compared with placebo, or an oral trial in which oral insulin was compared with placebo. At the conclusion of the study, there was no difference between the rate of progression of diabetes between the insulin-treated groups and the control (*64*). Overall, the oral insulin trial, which recruited subjects with a lower 5-year risk of the disease, also did not show an effect on progression of the disease. However, a subsequent subgroup analysis demonstrated a treatment effect on the oral insulin-treated group with high antiinsulin titers (*65*).

Recently, a second large trial investigating the use of nasal insulin to prevent diabetes in children with high-risk HLA genotypes and autoantibodies has been concluded. In this trial, 116,720 consecutively born infants and 3,430 of their siblings were screened to identify 11,225 and 1,574, respectively, who had increased risk of the development of diabetes. Two hundred and twenty-four infants and 40 siblings were randomized in a blinded fashion to receive intranasal insulin or placebo. The trial was discontinued early since intranasal insulin did not delay or prevent the development of type-1 diabetes (*66*).

Despite the heroic efforts of the investigators in the insulin prevention trials, neither has been able to demonstrate that administration of insulin modifies the progression of autoimmunity in type-1 diabetes. The failure of insulin to reverse autoimmunity may relate to several factors. In the rodent models of type-1 diabetes, insulin was administered to extremely young animals between 2 and 4 weeks old without an evidence of autoimmunity (*60, 62, 67*), while in both the DPT and the Finnish study, participants were older (DPT median 11.2, Finnish study range 2–11.2 years) and had already developed autoantibodies (*64, 66*). In retrospect, it appeared that commencing treatment after multiple autoantibodies had emerged was too late to reverse autoimmunity. Second, the original studies of the NOD mouse had demonstrated that the dose of insulin used was critical to prevent diabetes (*68*). However, the dose of insulin used in the DPT was five- to sevenfold less than the equivalent dose used in the mice (*50*). Similarly, the insulin dose selected for the Finnish study, though much higher than that of the DPT, was based on estimated physiological requirement rather the optimal doses found in mice to reverse autoimmunity (*66*). Finally, the insulin used in the Finnish study did not contain preproinsulin, which contains diabetogenic epitopes (*69*).

While both of these trials have not had a positive outcome, they have been useful in defining the direction of future immunoprevention and antigen-specific trials. These trials have demonstrated the importance of understanding the action of insulin as a tolergen at a mechanistic level in humans. Unfortunately, the trials determined neither if the dose of insulin used induced a tolergenic response by measurement of autoantibody responses nor the characterization of T-cell populations as the trial proceeded. Currently, a phase II trial is underway to examine the effect of mucosal insulin on autoantibody negative children at high risk of development of type-1 diabetes and to determine the optimal insulin dose that will elicit an immune response (*70*). In another trial, insulin has been administered in a targeted fashion to genetically susceptible individuals with positive insulin antibodies based on the subgroup analysis from the DPT-1 (*71*).

Another approach to modify immune responses to antigens is with an "altered peptide ligand," which has been shown to alter the phenotype of the antigen-specific response (*72*). Studies in the NOD mouse showed that a subcutaneous injection of NBI-6024 to NOD mice administered either before or after the onset of diabetes substantially delayed the onset or reduced the incidence of disease (*73*). In a clinical trial, Alleva et al. found that a modified insulin B9-23 peptide (NBI 6024) T cell responds to the modified peptide after commencing six injections with the altered peptide. Higher IL-5 responses to the altered peptide were seen after 25 weeks; however, higher IFN-γ responses were also seen after 14 weeks in the treated subjects. The results from a larger clinical trial are pending (*74*).

Glutamic Acid Decarboxylase 65

GAD is the enzyme responsible for the production of the inhibitory neurotransmitter γ-amino butyric (GABA) from glutamate found in neurons and pancreatic β-cells, where it may function in a paracrine manner (*5*). The GAD65 isoform of the protein has been identified as a major autoantigen in type-1 diabetes and the neurological disease Stiff Man Syndrome (*76, 77*). In patients with type-1 diabetes and at-risk individuals, both autoreactive CD4+ T cells and autoantibodies to GAD65 are found (*78*). As previously discussed, anti-GAD antibodies may be used to predict the risk of development of type-1 diabetes (*41*).

In murine preclinical studies, small amounts of GAD65 administered by oral, intrathymic, and subcutaneous routes were demonstrated to prevent the development diabetes (*79, 80*). Mechanistically, GAD65 treatment induced a shift in CD4+ T cell population from Th1 (cellular) to Th2 (humoral) response (*81*). In addition, GAD65 was found to induce a Treg population that restored tolerance and prevented the reemergence of autoimmunity (*82*). A dose finding phase II human trial in patients, with latent autoimmune diabetes in adulthood (LADA),who were anti-GAD antibody positive found that a 20 μg dose of GAD increased fasting and stimulated C-peptide levels 24 weeks after commencing the treatment with two doses of GAD65 in alum, with no serious adverse reactions. The 20 μg dose of GADA was found to increase the relative proportion of CD4+CD25+ T cells in the peripheral blood. The titer of anti-GAD65 antibodies was increased in the group that received 500 μg dose even though the stimulated C-peptide levels were decreased in that group (*83*).

Recently, an immunoreversal trial was reported where two 20 μg doses of GAD (Day 1 and 30) were administered to type-I diabetes patients, positive for GAD antibodies and had residual C-peptide responses, within 18 months of diagnosis. The primary end point was a change in fasting C-peptide at 15 months. The treated subjects and the controls were then followed for another 15 months of observation. There was a progressive decline in C-peptide from baseline with no change in C-peptide levels observed between study groups at the primary end point. However, at 30 months C-peptide levels were significantly improved only in the group treated within 6 months of diagnosis. The treatment with GAD was associated with an initial increase in anti-GAD antibody followed by a progressive decline. This decline in antibody was concurrent with the induction cells expressing FOXP3 and TGF-β, suggesting the presence of a Treg population (*84*). Based on this data, large-scale trial of GAD antigen for immunoreversal of type-1 diabetes is now in progress in Europe (NCT00723411) and the United States (NCT00751842) (*85*).

Diapep 277

In human and murine models of type-I diabetes, Diapep 277 (corresponding to positions 437–460 of the human heat shock protein 60 (HSP60)) has been found to be an immunodominant epitope (*58*). In rodent models, Diapep 277 administration has been shown to prevent type-1 diabetes when combined with dietary modifications (*59*). HSP60 has been found to be expressed on the membrane of pancreatic β-cell insulin secretory granules (*86, 87*). Immunologically, Diapep277 was considered to induce a phenotypic change in T-cell responses, from a Th1 response to a Th2 response (*88*). However, a more recent study has suggested that Diapep 277 may immunomodulate T cells via the TLR2 receptor found on the cells of the innate immune system (*89*). Human trials to reverse diabetes at the time of diagnosis have demonstrated that the effect of Diapep 277 is dose dependent. In three studies published, C-peptide responses were only preserved in treated subjects as compared with controls with the 2.5 mg dose (administered at 1–10 months) (*90–92*). This effect also appears to be age related. Diapep277 was not found to be effective when administered to young children (*93*).

NONANTIGEN SPECIFIC IMMUNO-MODULATION

Mechanisms

Nonantigen-specific approaches aim to suppress immune responses to pancreatic β-cells to modify the total or individual components of the immune system. The indications and timing of the use of these agents is largely determined by their specificity and side effect profile in a risk/benefit assessment. A nonspecific agent with a benign side effect profile is suitable for an immunoprevention trial, while those that are highly specific with limited side effects have been considered suitable for immunotherapy trials at the time of diagnosis of type-1 diabetes (*94*). An important consideration is the need for repeated administration of these agents. The safety concerns of long-term broad immune suppression render this approach generally unacceptable to most investigators, particularly if the end result were not to be a complete reversal of disease. Thus, the ability to achieve immunologic tolerance, i.e., short administration of an agent with lasting immunologic effects even after the agent is withdrawn, has become the goal of therapies. Anti-CD3 antibody has been suggested to achieve this goal by potentially inducing a population of regulatory T cells (*95, 96*).

The European Nicotinamide Diabetes Intervention Trial (ENDIT) was a prevention trial based on the notion that the toxic effects of the immune response on β cells could be attenuated by nicotinamide, a hypothesis that was supported by preclinical studies (*64, 97*). The trial failed to achieve its primary outcome of prevention of diabetes onset. The basis for the clinical failure of this intervention, like the negative findings from the DPT-1, is not known – one plausible explanation is that the immune response is diversified and robust at the time of presentation, and any successful intervention will need to be sufficiently potent and broad.

SYSTEMIC IMMUNO-SUPPRESSION: CYCLOSPORINE, AZATHIOPRINE, PREDNISONE

Initial trials with immunosuppressive agents that were used in organ transplantation provided definitive evidence that type-1 diabetes in human is an autoimmune disease that could be treated by immunomodulation (*98–100*). Subsequent studies found that other nonspecific T cell immunosuppressive protocols with prednisone and azathioprine could induce immunoreversal and lower insulin requirement at onset of type-1 diabetes (*101*). However, the remission induced was limited to the duration of the treatment with the reemergence of autoimmunity once treatment was discontinued (*102*). Furthermore, cyclosporine induced nephrotoxicity, while azathioprine was found to be ineffective when used as a single agent (*103, 104*). These findings combined with the fact that prednisone causes insulin resistance, thereby accelerating the development of type-1 diabetes, have precluded their clinical use (*105*). More recent studies have concentrated on combining generalized immunosuppression with mycophenolate mofetil with a specific immunomodulating agent using daclizumab (anti-CD25/interleukin 2 receptor antibody) (*49*). Unfortunately, this more "benign" approach to immune modulation was not successful in attenuating the loss of C-peptide responses in new-onset T1D (*106*).

BIOLOGICAL IMMUNO-MODULATORS

Anti-CD3 mAbs

The anti-CD3(OKT3) mAb was the first monoclonal antibody to be licensed for clinical practice to treat solid organ allograft rejection in humans (*107, 108*). Though successful in reversing and preventing acute rejection, their use was associated with a cytokine release syndrome due to the murine Fc portion of the molecule interacting with Fc receptors on macrophages (*109, 110*). This limited OKT3s therapeutic potential resulting in it being superseded by other immunosuppressive agents for acute allograft rejection (*111*). To minimize the mitogenic potential of anti-CD3 mAbs, humanized CD3-specfic Fc-modified Mabs were produced to decrease their potential to bind Fc receptors (*112*). Two of these antibodies, hOKT3γ1 Ala-Ala (Teplizumab) (a FcR nonbinding, humanized version of OKT3) and chAglyCD3 (Otelixizumab) (aglycosylated FcR nonbinding anti-CD3 mAb) have been used to treat patients with type-1 diabetes (*113, 114*). Chatenoud et al. showed that treatment of NOD mice at the time of diagnosis with hyperglycemia induced a lasting remission of the disease – a brief course of treatment with either whole of F(ab')2 fragments of anti-CD3 mAb induced immunologic tolerance and established normal blood sugar levels even in mice with hyperglycemia (*115*). The effects were lasting – hyperglycemia did not recur after the acute effects of mAb treatment, such as TCR modulation, had resolved. Moreover, even in the ~20% of animals that did not respond to drug treatment, syngeneic islet grafts were not destroyed showing that the metabolic and immunologic effects of drug treatment could be differentiated. The immunomodulation of T-cells in the NOD mouse occurs in two consecutive phases. The first is of short duration at the initiation of treatment and involves the depletion of pathogenic T cells with a transient Th2 polarization. The second is permanent and occurs after treatment with the restoration of tolerance to pancreatic β-cell by the induction of a population of Tregs (*95, 116–118*). The therapeutic effectiveness of anti-CD3 antibody is dependent on the emergence of autoimmunity and was less effective in young NOD mice compared with older animals (*117*). The induction of Tregs results in an antigen-specific effect leading to no impairment of T-cell responses to foreign antigens after treatment (*119*). The overall result is reversal of the autoimmunity without the need for recurrent administration of anti-CD3 (*115*). These unique properties of tolerance induction without persistent immunosuppression have led to the clinical translation of these findings (*120*).

Anti-CD3 antibodies act by binding the T cell receptor-CD3 complex. They do induce T cell receptor signals, but the magnitude and outcomes of the signal are different from activation after FcR binding anti-CD3 antibody (*121*). Studies with human cells have shown that overall, there is reduced cytokine release and greater induction of IL-10 and reduced production of IFN-γ on a molar basis when compared to FcR binding anti-CD3 mAb.

The first human trial of single anti-CD3 treatment (hOKT3γ1 Ala-Ala) in recent-onset type-1 diabetes demonstrated that a single course of treatment led to improvement in C-peptide response for up to 2 years post-diagnosis. C-peptide responses were stable on average after 1 year – at 2 years, patient's C-peptide responses had declined but remained significantly higher than in the untreated group. The treated patients also had improved metabolic control with lower HbA1c and reduced insulin usage (*122, 123*). A study with anti-CD3 (chAglyCD3) found that patients in the treated group at 18 months had maintained baseline insulin secretion and had lower exogenous insulin requirements. The greatest treatment effects were observed in patients in the upper ½ of insulin production rates at the time of study entry – a finding reminiscent of the improved responses to Cyclosporin A in those with the highest C-peptide levels. In this trial, a self-limiting reactivation of EBV was reported (*100, 124*).

In contrast to the murine data, the improvement in C-peptide responses and metabolic parameters was not permanent in the human trials (*117*). The basis for the decline in insulin production after 1 year is unclear but may relate to the development or reemergence of pathogenic T cells after initial clearance. Recently, a study of islet cell transplant patients found that long-term graft failure is related to the finding of autoreactive T cells after their initial depletion by immunosuppressive agents (*96, 125*).

Rituximab (Anti-CD20)

Rituximab (anti-CD20) antibody targets the CD20 transmembrane receptor that is found on all immature and mature B lymphocytes (*126*). Rituximab was originally licensed for the treatment of non-Hodgkin's B cell lymphomas in 1997. Rituximab binds the CD20 receptor and induces B cell depletion. Generally, it is well tolerated, and there is extensive clinical experience in its use (*127*). In autoimmune diseases, Rituximab in combination with systemic immunosuppressive agents has been used to successfully treat rheumatoid arthritis (RA) and, with questionable efficacy, systemic lupus erythematosis (SLE), though both the diseases relapse following the withdrawal of therapy indicating that the effects are immunosuppressive rather than tolergenic (*128, 129*).

The lack of a suitable anti-CD20 antibody in murine models limited the studies of B lymphocyte mechanisms involved in diabetes. However, the development of a mouse anti-CD20 antibody and a transgenic mouse expressing human CD20 has now facilitated the investigation (*130*). Treatment of NOD mice with B lymphocyte depleting anti-mouse CD-20 monoclonal antibody (mAbs) reversed diabetes in NOD mice though this treatment was most effective during the transition to overt diabetes at 9–15 weeks of age (*131*). At the onset of hyperglycemia, approximately 30% of mice could be rendered euglycemic with treatment producing a lasting tolerance with the induction Tregs and a novel population of B lymphocytes with regulatory properties (*131*). The direct action of Rituximab is related to decrease in activation of CD4+ and CD8+ T cells by a lack of antigen presentation by B cells and by inhibition of antigen presentation by macrophages and dendritic cells (*132*). In humans, a clinical trial of once-weekly Rituximab for 4 weeks in patients with recently diagnosed type-1 diabetes has completed enrolment with results awaited (*133*).

Abatacept (CTLA4-Ig)

Abatacept (Cytotoxic T-lymphocyte-associated protein 4-immunoglobulin/CTLA4-Ig) is a immunoglobulin fusion protein of the extracellular domain of CTLA4 and part of the Fc domain of IgG1 (*134*). CTLA4Ig binds the costimulatory ligands B7.1 and B7.2 (CD80/86), which provide a second signal, through CD28, needed for T cell activation. Activated T cells express CTLA4, but in these cells, CTLA-4 imparts a negative signal and is thought to inhibit T cell function possibly by reversing the TCR stop signal at the sites of antigen recognition (*135, 136*). In addition, regulatory T cells express CTLA4. CTLA4Ig is thought to act in humans by competing with CD28 for its ligands CD80/86 on APC's providing a costimulatory blockade to T cell effector activation (*137*).

Interestingly, polymorphisms of the CTLA-4 gene have been linked to susceptibility of type-1 diabetes in humans (*138*).

In humans, CTLA4Ig has been successfully used to treat psoriasis and RA (*139*). In RA, abatacept was used in combination with methotrexate and was superior to treatment with methotrexate alone in ameliorating symptoms and preventing structural damage. Based on these results, abatacept has been licensed for use in patients unresponsive to anti-TNF agents. Combination treatment with anti-TNF agents and abatacept is relatively contraindicated since there is an increase in serious infections without improvement in outcome (*140–142*). In the RA studies, abatacept was not tolergenic and required monthly administration to maintain optimal clinical effects (*143*). Preclinical studies with CTLA4Ig have been conflicting with regard to its effects on progression of disease in the NOD mouse. When administered to NOD mice of 6–8 weeks of age, human but not mouse CTLA4Ig attenuated development of diabetes (*144*). Diabetes was exacerbated when murine CTLA4Ig was administered during this age or expressed as a transgene in NOD mice. Likewise, administration of both anti-B7.1 and B7.2 antibodies exacerbated diabetes in this model (*144*). Interestingly, CD28-deficient NOD mice also develop accelerated diabetes, which has been shown to be due to an impairment in the development of naturally occurring CD4+ regulatory T cells (*145*).

A type-1 diabetes trial enrolling patients within 3 months of diagnosis has completed recruitment. These subjects will receive monthly infusions of CTLA4Ig or placebo to determine the response to treatment in preservation of C-peptide responses (*146, 147*).

COMBINATION THERAPIES

Even successful therapies including anti-CD3 mAb, GAD65, and others have failed to completely reverse the metabolic abnormalities of new-onset T1D or to cause permanent stability in C-peptide responses. It is likely, therefore, that a combination of agents will be required to achieve these goals. Multiple immunotherapies could be combined to produce immunoreversal and reestablish tolerance, although care need to be taken, since dominant tolerance requires the generation of de novo Tregs that may be inhibited by specific immunosuppressive therapies that block T-cell activation (*148*). Preclinical studies have suggested potential combinations. When nasal proinsulin peptide was administered with anti-CD3 mab in synergy, reversal of the disease was found to occur, and there was induction of antigen -pecific regulatory T cells that could transfer dominant tolerance (*149*). Similarly, immunomodulatory treatment could be combined with treatment to augment pancreatic β-cell mass. In the NOD mouse, sequential treatment of anti-CD3 followed by extendin-4 (GLP-1 receptor agonist) improved the rate of remission compared with anti-CD3 alone (*150*). Another potential therapeutic strategy would be to sequentially target the cells of the innate immune system followed by those of the adaptive to produce sustained remission of the autoimmunity. Proinflammatory cytokines, TNFα and IL1 β, are produced by macrophages and dendritic cells that infiltrate pancreatic beta cells in humans (*151*). These mediators create a proinflammatory environment leading to the recruitment and activation of autoreactive CD4+ and CD8+ T cells that propagate and maintain an autoreactive immune response to pancreatic beta cell self-antigens (*27, 52, 153*). In patients with type-1 diabetes, endogenous production of anti-inflammatory IL-1 receptor antagonist is associated with the preservation of beta cell function (*154*). A therapeutic option would be to treat patients with a limited course of anti-IL-1 therapy, similar to that previously used in type-2 diabetes to downregulate the proinflammatory innate immune response (*155*).

CONCLUSIONS

In recent years, considerable progress has been made in the understanding of the immunopathogenesis of type-1 diabetes by trials of immunomodulatory agents in patients. A key advance from the DPT-1 trial is the ability to predict the development of diabetes in genetically susceptible individuals (*156*). In the future, agents that have been previously considered only for recent-onset disease may be utilized in high-risk individuals prior to the onset of hyperglycemia (*3*).

New data has shown that the natural progression of the disease may be altered by immune modulators. To date, evidence from human studies indicates that a single course of administration of an agent therapy in type-1 diabetes is unlikely to produce a sustained remission from autoimmunity with adequate beta cell mass to ensure insulin independence (*157*). As the number of potential immunotherapeutic agents successfully used in other autoimmune disease continues to grow (Fig. 18.1), new combinations and approaches to drug administration will be tested (*158*). By trials of these agents in type-1 diabetes and studies of their effects in patients, we may gain a greater understanding of the key rate-limiting steps in the development of the chronic phase of type-1 diabetes and hyperglycemia (*59*). In addition, further understanding of human immune responses is likely, in the future, to identify the key therapeutic targets in man.

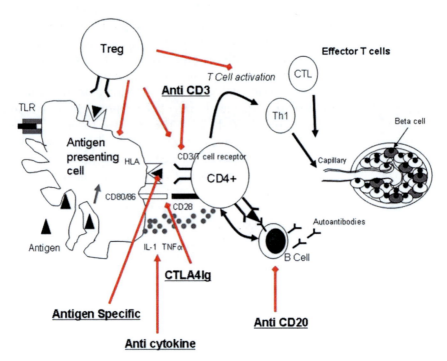

Fig. 18.1 Sites of immunmodulation in type 1 diabetes. An antigen presenting cell (APC) may be activated via a Toll-like receptor (TLR) and process a self-antigen (insulin or others), and present antigenic peptides by Class II MHC molecules to CD4+ T cells. CD8+ cells may directly recognize self-peptide displayed in the context of Class I MHC molecules on the surfaces of β cells. The development of autoimmunity may be inhibited by regulatory T cells (Tregs) that are able to prevent activation of autoreactive T cells, and these cells may also directly affect APCs. The release of proinflammatory cytokines Interleukin 1β (IL-1β) and Tumor Necrosis Factor (TNF) a may enhance antigen presentation and/or have direct cytotoxic effects on β cells. Each of these sites of immune activation may be targeted by therapies. Antigen-specific therapies may involve altered modes of T-cell activation and/or T-cell receptor ligands with weak affinity. Blockade of costimulation by CTLA4Ig may prevent T-cell activation, whereas anti-CD3 mAb may alter the activation of T cells to generate Tregs. Anti-CD20 mAb can deplete B lymphocytes. Finally, anticytokine reagents may prevent cell activation and/or the toxic effects of the soluble mediators on β cells.

REFERENCES

1. Daneman D. Type 1 diabetes. Lancet 2006;367:847–858.
2. Liu E, Eisenbarth GS. Type 1A diabetes mellitus-associated autoimmunity. Endocrinol Metab Clin North Am 2002;31:391–410, vii–viii.
3. Waldron-Lynch F, Herold K. Advances in type 1 diabetes therapeutics: immunomodulation and beta cell salvage. Endocrinol Metab Clin North Am 2009;38(2):303–317.
4. American Diabetes Association. Standards of medical care in diabetes–2008. Diabetes Care 2008;31(Suppl 1):S12–S54.
5. The effect of intensive treatment of diabetes on the development and progression of long-term complications in insulin-dependent diabetes mellitus. The Diabetes Control and Complications Trial Research Group. N Engl J Med 1993;329:977–986.
6. Nathan DM, Cleary PA, Backlund JY, et al. Intensive diabetes treatment and cardiovascular disease in patients with type 1 diabetes. N Engl J Med 2005;353:2643–2653.
7. Perkins BA, Ficociello LH, Silva KH, Finkelstein DM, Warram JH, Krolewski AS. Regression of microalbuminuria in type 1 diabetes. N Engl J Med 2003;348: 2285–2293.
8. Hypoglycemia in the Diabetes Control and Complications Trial. The Diabetes Control

and Complications Trial Research Group. Diabetes 1997;46:271–286.
9. Steffes MW, Sibley S, Jackson M, Thomas W. Beta-cell function and the development of diabetes-related complications in the diabetes control and complications trial. Diabetes Care 2003;26:832–836.
10. Palmer JP, Fleming GA, Greenbaum CJ, et al. C-peptide is the appropriate outcome measure for type 1 diabetes clinical trials to preserve beta-cell function: report of an ADA workshop, 21-22 October 2001. Diabetes 2004;53:250–264.
11. Yoshida K, Kikutani H. Genetic and immunological basis of autoimmune diabetes in the NOD mouse. Rev Immunogenet 2000;2:140–146.
12. DiLorenzo TP, Serreze DV. The good turned ugly: immunopathogenic basis for diabetogenic CD8+ T cells in NOD mice. Immunol Rev 2005;204:250–263.
13. Nakayama M, Abiru N, Moriyama H, et al. Prime role for an insulin epitope in the development of type 1 diabetes in NOD mice. Nature 2005;435:220–223.
14. Tremblau S, Penna G, Bosi E, Mortara A, Gately MK, Adorini L. Interleukin 12 administration induces T helper type 1 cells and accelerates autoimmune diabetes in NOD mice. J Exp Med 1995;181:817–821.
15. Tang Q, Henriksen KJ, Bi M, et al. In vitro-expanded antigen-specific regulatory T cells suppress autoimmune diabetes. J Exp Med 2004;199:1455–1465.
16. Silveira PA, Grey ST. B cells in the spotlight: innocent bystanders or major players in the pathogenesis of type 1 diabetes. Trends Endocrinol Metab 2006;17:128–135.
17. Chiu PP, Serreze DV, Danska JS. Development and function of diabetogenic T-cells in B-cell-deficient nonobese diabetic mice. Diabetes 2001;50:763–770.
18. Yang M, Charlton B, Gautam AM. Development of insulitis and diabetes in B cell-deficient NOD mice. J Autoimmun 1997;10:257–260.
19. Wong FS, Wen L, Tang M, et al. Investigation of the role of B-cells in type 1 diabetes in the NOD mouse. Diabetes 2004;53:2581–2587.
20. Noorchashm H, Lieu YK, Noorchashm N, et al. I-Ag7-mediated antigen presentation by B lymphocytes is critical in overcoming a checkpoint in T cell tolerance to islet beta cells of nonobese diabetic mice. J Immunol 1999;163:743–750.
21. Marino E, Grey ST. A new role for an old player: do B cells unleash the self-reactive CD8+ T cell storm necessary for the development of type 1 diabetes? J Autoimmun 2008;31:301–305.
22. De Aizpurua HJ, French MB, Chosich N, Harrison LC. Natural history of humoral immunity to glutamic acid decarboxylase in non-obese diabetic (NOD) mice. J Autoimmun 1994;7:643–653.
23. Morran MP, McInerney MF, Pietropaolo M. Innate and adaptive autoimmunity in type 1 diabetes. Pediatr Diabetes 2008;9:152–161.
24. Zipris D. Innate immunity and its role in type 1 diabetes. Curr Opin Endocrinol Diabetes Obes 2008;15:326–331.
25. Hill NJ, Van Gunst K, Sarvetnick N. Th1 and Th2 pancreatic inflammation differentially affects homing of islet-reactive CD4 cells in nonobese diabetic mice. J Immunol 2003;170:1649–1658.
26. Alba A, Planas R, Clemente X, et al. Natural killer cells are required for accelerated type 1 diabetes driven by interferon-beta. Clin Exp Immunol 2008;151:467–475.
27. Jun HS, Santamaria P, Lim HW, Zhang ML, Yoon JW. Absolute requirement of macrophages for the development and activation of beta-cell cytotoxic CD8+ T-cells in T-cell receptor transgenic NOD mice. Diabetes 1999;48:34–42.
28. Pearl-Yafe M, Kaminitz A, Yolcu ES, Yaniv I, Stein J, Askenasy N. Pancreatic islets under attack: cellular and molecular effectors. Curr Pharm Des 2007;13:749–760.
29. Wen L, Ley RE, Volchkov PY, et al. Innate immunity and intestinal microbiota in the development of Type 1 diabetes. Nature 2008;455:1109–1113.
30. Dotta F, Censini S, van Halteren AG, et al. Coxsackie B4 virus infection of beta cells and natural killer cell insulitis in recent-onset type 1 diabetic patients. Proc Natl Acad Sci U S A 2007;104:5115–5120.
31. Itoh N, Hanafusa T, Miyazaki A, et al. Mononuclear cell infiltration and its relation to the expression of major histocompatibility complex antigens and adhesion molecules in pancreas biopsy specimens from newly diagnosed insulin-dependent diabetes mellitus patients. J Clin Invest 1993;92:2313–2322.
32. von Herrath M, Sanda S, Herold K. Type 1 diabetes as a relapsing-remitting disease? Nat Rev Immunol 2007;7:988–994.
33. Barker JM, Barriga KJ, Yu L, et al. Prediction of autoantibody positivity and progression to type 1 diabetes: Diabetes Autoimmunity Study in the Young (DAISY). J Clin Endocrinol Metab 2004;89:3896–3902.

34. Roll U, Christie MR, Fuchtenbusch M, Payton MA, Hawkes CJ, Ziegler AG. Perinatal autoimmunity in offspring of diabetic parents The German Multicenter BABY-DIAB study: detection of humoral immune responses to islet antigens in early childhood. Diabetes 1996;45:967–973.
35. Erlich H, Valdes AM, Noble J, et al. HLA DR-DQ haplotypes and genotypes and type 1 diabetes risk: analysis of the type 1 diabetes genetics consortium families. Diabetes 2008;57:1084–1092.
36. Kent SC, Chen Y, Bregoli L, et al. Expanded T cells from pancreatic lymph nodes of type 1 diabetic subjects recognize an insulin epitope. Nature 2005;435:224–228.
37. Martin S, Wolf-Eichbaum D, Duinkerken G, et al. Development of type 1 diabetes despite severe hereditary B-lymphocyte deficiency. N Engl J Med 2001;345:1036–1040.
38. Verge CF, Gianani R, Kawasaki E, et al. Prediction of type I diabetes in first-degree relatives using a combination of insulin, GAD, and ICA512bdc/IA-2 autoantibodies. Diabetes 1996;45:926–933.
39. Yu L, Rewers M, Gianani R, et al. Antiislet autoantibodies usually develop sequentially rather than simultaneously. J Clin Endocrinol Metab 1996;81:4264–4267.
40. Yu L, Cuthbertson DD, Maclaren N, et al. Expression of GAD65 and islet cell antibody (ICA512) autoantibodies among cytoplasmic ICA+ relatives is associated with eligibility for the Diabetes Prevention Trial-Type 1. Diabetes 2001;50:1735–1740.
41. Bingley PJ, Bonifacio E, Williams AJ, Genovese S, Bottazzo GF, Gale EA. Prediction of IDDM in the general population: strategies based on combinations of autoantibody markers. Diabetes 1997;46:1701–1710.
42. Mahon JL, Sosenko JM, Rafkin-Mervis L, et al. The TrialNet Natural History Study of the Development of Type 1 Diabetes: objectives, design, and initial results. Pediatr Diabetes 2009;10(2):97–104.
43. Sosenko JM, Palmer JP, Greenbaum CJ, et al. Patterns of metabolic progression to type 1 diabetes in the diabetes prevention trial-type 1. Diabetes Care 2006;29:643–649.
44. Sherr J, Sosenko J, Skyler J, Herold K. Prevention of type 1 diabetes: the time has come. Nat Clin Pract Endocrinol Metab 2008;4:334–343.
45. Sosenko JM, Palmer JP, Greenbaum CJ, et al. Increasing the accuracy of oral glucose tolerance testing and extending its application to individuals with normal glucose tolerance for the prediction of type 1 diabetes: the diabetes prevention trial-type 1. Diabetes Care 2007;30:38–42.
46. Sosenko JM, Krischer JP, Palmer JP, et al. A risk score for type 1 diabetes derived from autoantibody-positive participants in the diabetes prevention trial-type 1. Diabetes Care 2008;31:528–533.
47. Foulis AK, McGill M, Farquharson MA. Insulitis in type 1 (insulin-dependent) diabetes mellitus in man–macrophages, lymphocytes, and interferon-gamma containing cells. J Pathol 1991;165:97–103.
48. Waldron-Lynch F, von Herrath M, Herold K. Towards a curative therapy in type 1 diabetes: remission of autoimmunity, maintenance and augmentation of B cell mass. Novartis Found Symp 2008;292:146–155.
49. Haller MJ, Gottlieb PA, Schatz DA. Type 1 diabetes intervention trials 2007: where are we and where are we going? Curr Opin Endocrinol Diabetes Obes 2007;14:283–287.
50. Staeva-Vieira T, Peakman M, von Herrath M. Translational mini-review series on type 1 diabetes: immune-based therapeutic approaches for type 1 diabetes. Clin Exp Immunol 2007;148:17–31.
51. Waldmann H, Cobbold SP, Fairchild P, Adams E. Therapeutic aspects of tolerance. Curr Opin Pharmacol 2001;1:392–397.
52. Fousteri G, Bresson D, von Herrath M. Rational development of antigen-specific therapies for type 1 diabetes. Adv Exp Med Biol 2007;601:313–319.
53. Cobbold SP, Nolan KF, Graca L, et al. Regulatory T cells and dendritic cells in transplantation tolerance: molecular markers and mechanisms. Immunol Rev 2003;196:109–124.
54. St Clair EW, Turka LA, Saxon A, et al. New reagents on the horizon for immune tolerance. Annu Rev Med 2007;58:329–346.
55. Winer S, Gunaratnam L, Astsatourov I, et al. Peptide dose, MHC affinity, and target self-antigen expression are critical for effective immunotherapy of nonobese diabetic mouse prediabetes. J Immunol 2000;165:4086–4094.
56. Martinez NR, Augstein P, Moustakas AK, et al. Disabling an integral CTL epitope allows suppression of autoimmune diabetes by intranasal proinsulin peptide. J Clin Invest 2003;111:1365–1371.
57. Graca L, Chen TC, Le Moine A, Cobbold SP, Howie D, Waldmann H. Dominant tolerance: activation thresholds for peripheral generation of regulatory T cells. Trends Immunol 2005;26:130–135.
58. Horvath L, Cervenak L, Oroszlan M, et al. Antibodies against different epitopes of heat-

58. shock protein 60 in children with type 1 diabetes mellitus. Immunol Lett 2002;80:155–162.
59. Brugman S, Klatter FA, Visser J, Bos NA, Elias D, Rozing J. Neonatal oral administration of DiaPep277, combined with hydrolysed casein diet, protects against type 1 diabetes in BB-DP rats. An experimental study. Diabetologia 2004;47:1331–1333.
60. Zhang ZJ, Davidson L, Eisenbarth G, Weiner HL. Suppression of diabetes in nonobese diabetic mice by oral administration of porcine insulin. Proc Natl Acad Sci U S A 1991;88:10252–10256.
61. Keller RJ, Eisenbarth GS, Jackson RA. Insulin prophylaxis in individuals at high risk of type I diabetes. Lancet 1993;341:927–928.
62. Bergerot I, Fabien N, Maguer V, Thivolet C. Oral administration of human insulin to NOD mice generates CD4+ T cells that suppress adoptive transfer of diabetes. J Autoimmun 1994;7:655–663.
63. Sercarz EE. Driver clones and determinant spreading. J Autoimmun 2000;14:275–277.
64. Diabetes Prevention Trial–Type 1 Diabetes Study Group. Effects of insulin in relatives of patients with type 1 diabetes mellitus. N Engl J Med 2002;346:1685–1691.
65. Skyler JS, Krischer JP, Wolfsdorf J, et al. Effects of oral insulin in relatives of patients with type 1 diabetes: The Diabetes Prevention Trial – Type 1. Diabetes Care 2005;28:1068–1076.
66. Näntö-Salonen K, Kupila A, Simell S, et al. Nasal insulin to prevent type 1 diabetes in children with HLA genotypes and autoantibodies conferring increased risk of disease: a double-blind, randomised controlled trial. Lancet 2008;372:1746–1755.
67. Polanski M, Melican NS, Zhang J, Weiner HL. Oral administration of the immunodominant B-chain of insulin reduces diabetes in a co-transfer model of diabetes in the NOD mouse and is associated with a switch from Th1 to Th2 cytokines. J Autoimmun 1997;10:339–346.
68. Bergerot I, Fabien N, Mayer A, Thivolet C. Active suppression of diabetes after oral administration of insulin is determined by antigen dosage. Ann N Y Acad Sci 1996;778:362–367.
69. Di Lorenzo TP, Peakman M, Roep BO. Translational mini-review series on type 1 diabetes: systematic analysis of T cell epitopes in autoimmune diabetes. Clin Exp Immunol 2007;148:1–16.
70. Achenbach P, Barker J, Bonifacio E, Pre PSG. Modulating the natural history of type 1 diabetes in children at high genetic risk by mucosal insulin immunization. Curr Diab Rep 2008;8:87–93.
71. Trialnet. The oral insulin for the prevention of type 1 diabetes study. In: 2008.
72. Sloan-Lancaster J, Allen PM. Altered peptide ligand-induced partial T cell activation: molecular mechanisms and role in T cell biology. Annu Rev Immunol 1996;14:1–27.
73. Alleva DG, Gaur A, Jin L, et al. Immunological characterization and therapeutic activity of an altered-peptide ligand, NBI-6024, based on the immunodominant type 1 diabetes autoantigen insulin B-chain (9-23) peptide. Diabetes 2002;51:2126–2134.
74. Alleva DG, Maki RA, Putnam AL, et al. Immunomodulation in type 1 diabetes by NBI-6024, an altered peptide ligand of the insulin B epitope. Scand J Immunol 2006;63:59–69.
75. Fenalti G, Rowley M. GAD65 as a prototypic autoantigen. J Autoimmun 2008;31(3): 228–232.
76. Baekkeskov S, Aanstoot HJ, Christgau S, et al. Identification of the 64K autoantigen in insulin-dependent diabetes as the GABA-synthesizing enzyme glutamic acid decarboxylase. Nature 1990;347:151–156.
77. Skorstad G, Hestvik AL, Vartdal F, Holmoy T. Cerebrospinal fluid T cell responses against glutamic acid decarboxylase 65 in patients with stiff person syndrome. J Autoimmun 2009;32(1):24–32.
78. Oling V, Marttila J, Ilonen J, et al. GAD65- and proinsulin-specific CD4+ T-cells detected by MHC class II tetramers in peripheral blood of type 1 diabetes patients and at-risk subjects. J Autoimmun 2005;25:235–243.
79. Tisch R, Yang XD, Singer SM, Liblau RS, Fugger L, McDevitt HO. Immune response to glutamic acid decarboxylase correlates with insulitis in non-obese diabetic mice. Nature 1993;366:72–75.
80. Tian J, Clare-Salzler M, Herschenfeld A, et al. Modulating autoimmune responses to GAD inhibits disease progression and prolongs islet graft survival in diabetes-prone mice. Nat Med 1996;2:1348–1353.
81. Tian J, Atkinson MA, Clare-Salzler M, et al. Nasal administration of glutamate decarboxylase (GAD65) peptides induces Th2 responses and prevents murine insulin-dependent diabetes. J Exp Med 1996;183: 1561–1567.
82. Tisch R, Liblau RS, Yang XD, Liblau P, McDevitt HO. Induction of GAD65-specific regulatory T-cells inhibits ongoing autoimmune diabetes in nonobese diabetic mice. Diabetes 1998;47:894–899.
83. Agardh CD, Cilio CM, Lethagen A, et al. Clinical evidence for the safety of GAD65 immunomodulation in adult-onset autoimmune

84. Ludvigsson J, Faresjo M, Hjorth M, et al. GAD treatment and insulin secretion in recent-onset type 1 diabetes. N Engl J Med 2008;359:1909–1920.
85. Ludvigsson J. Immune intervention at diagnosis–should we treat children to preserve beta-cell function? Pediatr Diabetes 2007;8(Suppl 6):34–39.
86. Brudzynski K, Martinez V, Gupta RS. Secretory granule autoantigen in insulin-dependent diabetes mellitus is related to 62 kDa heat-shock protein (hsp60). J Autoimmun 1992;5:453–463.
87. Brudzynski K, Cunningham IA, Martinez V. A family of hsp60-related proteins in pancreatic beta cells of non-obese diabetic (NOD) mice. J Autoimmun 1995;8:859–874.
88. Zanin-Zhorov A, Tal G, Shivtiel S, et al. Heat shock protein 60 activates cytokine-associated negative regulator suppressor of cytokine signaling 3 in T cells: effects on signaling, chemotaxis, and inflammation. J Immunol 2005;175:276–285.
89. Zanin-Zhorov A, Cahalon L, Tal G, Margalit R, Lider O, Cohen IR. Heat shock protein 60 enhances CD4+ CD25+ regulatory T cell function via innate TLR2 signaling. J Clin Invest 2006;116:2022–2032.
90. Raz I, Avron A, Tamir M, et al. Treatment of new-onset type 1 diabetes with peptide DiaPep277 is safe and associated with preserved beta-cell function: extension of a randomized, double-blind, phase II trial. Diabetes Metab Res Rev 2007;23:292–298.
91. Huurman VA, Decochez K, Mathieu C, Cohen IR, Roep BO. Therapy with the hsp60 peptide DiaPep277 in C-peptide positive type 1 diabetes patients. Diabetes Metab Res Rev 2007;23:269–275.
92. Schloot NC, Meierhoff G, Lengyel C, et al. Effect of heat shock protein peptide DiaPep277 on beta-cell function in paediatric and adult patients with recent-onset diabetes mellitus type 1: two prospective, randomized, double-blind phase II trials. Diabetes Metab Res Rev 2007;23:276–285.
93. Lazar L, Ofan R, Weintrob N, et al. Heat-shock protein peptide DiaPep277 treatment in children with newly diagnosed type 1 diabetes: a randomised, double-blind phase II study. Diabetes Metab Res Rev 2007;23:286–291.
94. Cernea S, Pozzilli P. New potential treatments for protection of pancreatic B-cell function in type 1 diabetes. Diabet Med 2008;25:1259–1267.
95. Bisikirska B, Colgan J, Luban J, Bluestone JA, Herold KC. TCR stimulation with modified anti-CD3 mAb expands CD8+ T cell population and induces CD8+CD25+ Tregs. J Clin Invest 2005;115:2904–2913.
96. Chatenoud L, Bluestone JA. CD3-specific antibodies: a portal to the treatment of autoimmunity. Nat Rev Immunol 2007;7:622–632.
97. Gale EA, Bingley PJ, Emmett CL, Collier T, European Nicotinamide Diabetes Intervention Trial Group. European Nicotinamide Diabetes Intervention Trial (ENDIT): a randomised controlled trial of intervention before the onset of type 1 diabetes. Lancet 2004;363:925–931.
98. Stiller CR, Dupre J, Gent M, et al. Effects of cyclosporine immunosuppression in insulin-dependent diabetes mellitus of recent onset. Science 1984;223:1362–1367.
99. Stiller CR, Dupre J, Gent M, et al. Effects of cyclosporine in recent-onset juvenile type 1 diabetes: impact of age and duration of disease. J Pediatr 1987;111:1069–1072.
100. Bougneres PF, Carel JC, Castano L, et al. Factors associated with early remission of type I diabetes in children treated with cyclosporine. N Engl J Med 1988;318:663–670.
101. Silverstein J, Maclaren N, Riley W, Spillar R, Radjenovic D, Johnson S. Immunosuppression with azathioprine and prednisone in recent-onset insulin-dependent diabetes mellitus. N Engl J Med 1988;319:599–604.
102. Bougneres PF, Landais P, Boisson C, et al. Limited duration of remission of insulin dependency in children with recent overt type I diabetes treated with low-dose cyclosporin. Diabetes 1990;39:1264–1272.
103. Cook JJ, Hudson I, Harrison LC, et al. Double-blind controlled trial of azathioprine in children with newly diagnosed type I diabetes. Diabetes 1989;38:779–783.
104. Parving HH, Tarnow L, Nielsen FS, et al. Cyclosporine nephrotoxicity in type 1 diabetic patients. A 7-year follow-up study. Diabetes Care 1999;22:478–483.
105. Bingley PJ, Mahon JL, Gale EA, European Nicotinamide Diabetes Intervention Trial Group. Insulin resistance and progression to type 1 diabetes in the European Nicotinamide Diabetes Intervention Trial (ENDIT). Diabetes Care 2008;31:146–150.
106. Rother KI, Wijewickrama RC, Digon BJ, et al. Effect of exenatide alone or in combination with daclizumab on endogenous insulin secretion in patients with long-standing type 1 diabetes. In: 68th Scientific Sessions of the American Diabetes Associations. 2008;471-P.
107. Cosimi AB, Burton RC, Colvin RB, et al. Treatment of acute renal allograft rejection with

OKT3 monoclonal antibody. Transplantation 1981;32:535–539.
108. Friend PJ, Hale G, Chatenoud L, et al. Phase I study of an engineered aglycosylated humanized CD3 antibody in renal transplant rejection. Transplantation 1999;68:1632–1637.
109. Abramowicz D, Schandene L, Goldman M, et al. Release of tumor necrosis factor, interleukin-2, and gamma-interferon in serum after injection of OKT3 monoclonal antibody in kidney transplant recipients. Transplantation 1989;47:606–608.
110. Chatenoud L, Ferran C, Reuter A, et al. Systemic reaction to the anti-T-cell monoclonal antibody OKT3 in relation to serum levels of tumor necrosis factor and interferon-gamma [corrected]. N Engl J Med 1989;320:1420–1421.
111. Chatenoud L. CD3-specific antibody-induced active tolerance: from bench to bedside. Nat Rev Immunol 2003;3:123–132.
112. Hirsch R, Bluestone JA, DeNenno L, Gress RE. Anti-CD3 F(ab')2 fragments are immunosuppressive in vivo without evoking either the strong humoral response or morbidity associated with whole mAb. Transplantation 1990;49:1117–1123.
113. Bolt S, Routledge E, Lloyd I, et al. The generation of a humanized, non-mitogenic CD3 monoclonal antibody which retains in vitro immunosuppressive properties. Eur J Immunol 1993;23:403–411.
114. Alegre ML, Peterson LJ, Xu D, et al. A non-activating "humanized" anti-CD3 monoclonal antibody retains immunosuppressive properties in vivo. Transplantation 1994;57:1537–1543.
115. Chatenoud L, Thervet E, Primo J, Bach JF. Anti-CD3 antibody induces long-term remission of overt autoimmunity in nonobese diabetic mice. Proc Natl Acad Sci U S A 1994;91:123–127.
116. Belghith M, Bluestone JA, Barriot S, Megret J, Bach JF, Chatenoud L. TGF-beta-dependent mechanisms mediate restoration of self-tolerance induced by antibodies to CD3 in overt autoimmune diabetes. Nat Med 2003;9:1202–1208.
117. Chatenoud L, Primo J, Bach JF. CD3 antibody-induced dominant self tolerance in overtly diabetic NOD mice. J Immunol 1997;158:2947–2954.
118. Herold KC, Burton JB, Francois F, Poumian-Ruiz E, Glandt M, Bluestone JA. Activation of human T cells by FcR nonbinding anti-CD3 mAb, hOKT3gamma1(Ala-Ala). J Clin Invest 2003;111:409–418.
119. Plain KM, Chen J, Merten S, He XY, Hall BM. Induction of specific tolerance to allografts in rats by therapy with non-mitogenic, non-depleting anti-CD3 monoclonal antibody: association with TH2 cytokines not anergy. Transplantation 1999;67:605–613.
120. Chatenoud L. The use of CD3-specific antibodies in autoimmune diabetes: a step toward the induction of immune tolerance in the clinic. Handb Exp Pharmacol 2008;181:221–236.
121. Smith JA, Tso JY, Clark MR, Cole MS, Bluestone JA. Nonmitogenic anti-CD3 monoclonal antibodies deliver a partial T cell receptor signal and induce clonal anergy. J Exp Med 1997;185:1413–1422.
122. Herold KC, Gitelman SE, Masharani U, et al. A single course of anti-CD3 monoclonal antibody hOKT3gamma1(Ala-Ala) results in improvement in C-peptide responses and clinical parameters for at least 2 years after onset of type 1 diabetes. Diabetes 2005;54:1763–1769.
123. Herold KC, Hagopian W, Auger JA, et al. Anti-CD3 monoclonal antibody in new-onset type 1 diabetes mellitus. N Engl J Med 2002;346:1692–1698.
124. Keymeulen B, Vandemeulebroucke E, Ziegler AG, et al. Insulin needs after CD3-antibody therapy in new-onset type 1 diabetes. N Engl J Med 2005;352:2598–2608.
125. Monti P, Scirpoli M, Maffi P, et al. Islet transplantation in patients with autoimmune diabetes induces homeostatic cytokines that expand autoreactive memory T cells. J Clin Invest 2008;118:1806–1814.
126. Martin F, Chan AC. B cell immunobiology in disease: evolving concepts from the clinic. Annu Rev Immunol 2006;24:467–496.
127. Molina A. A decade of rituximab: improving survival outcomes in non-Hodgkin's lymphoma. Annu Rev Med 2008;59:237–250.
128. Looney RJ. B cells as a therapeutic target in autoimmune diseases other than rheumatoid arthritis. Rheumatology (Oxford) 2005;44(Suppl 2):ii13–ii17.
129. Kazkaz H, Isenberg D. Anti B cell therapy (rituximab) in the treatment of autoimmune diseases. Curr Opin Pharmacol 2004;4:398–402.
130. Uchida J, Lee Y, Hasegawa M, et al. Mouse CD20 expression and function. Int Immunol 2004;16:119–129.
131. Hu CY, Rodriguez-Pinto D, Du W, et al. Treatment with CD20-specific antibody prevents and reverses autoimmune diabetes in mice. J Clin Invest 2007;117:3857–3867.
132. Xiu Y, Wong CP, Bouaziz JD, et al. B lymphocyte depletion by CD20 monoclonal antibody prevents diabetes in nonobese diabetic mice despite isotype-specific differences

in Fc gamma R effector functions. J Immunol 2008;180:2863–2875.
133. Rituximab. 2008. (Accessed at http://www.diabetestrialnet.org/patientinfo/studies/rituximab.htm.)
134. Vincenti F. Costimulation blockade in autoimmunity and transplantation. J Allergy Clin Immunol 2008;121:299–306.
135. Fife BT, Bluestone JA. Control of peripheral T-cell tolerance and autoimmunity via the CTLA-4 and PD-1 pathways. Immunol Rev 2008;224:166–182.
136. Schneider H, Downey J, Smith A, et al. Reversal of the TCR stop signal by CTLA-4. Science 2006;313:1972–1975.
137. Bluestone JA, St Clair EW, Turka LA. CTLA4Ig: bridging the basic immunology with clinical application. Immunity 2006;24:233–238.
138. Ueda H, Howson JM, Esposito L, et al. Association of the T-cell regulatory gene CTLA4 with susceptibility to autoimmune disease. Nature 2003;423:506–511.
139. Abrams JR, Lebwohl MG, Guzzo CA, et al. CTLA4Ig-mediated blockade of T-cell costimulation in patients with psoriasis vulgaris. J Clin Invest 1999;103:1243–1252.
140. Kremer JM, Dougados M, Emery P, et al. Treatment of rheumatoid arthritis with the selective costimulation modulator abatacept: twelve-month results of a phase iib, double-blind, randomized, placebo-controlled trial. Arthritis Rheum 2005;52:2263–2271.
141. Kremer JM, Genant HK, Moreland LW, et al. Effects of abatacept in patients with methotrexate-resistant active rheumatoid arthritis: a randomized trial. Ann Intern Med 2006;144:865–876.
142. Russell AS, Wallenstein GV, Li T, et al. Abatacept improves both the physical and mental health of patients with rheumatoid arthritis who have inadequate response to methotrexate treatment. Ann Rheum Dis 2007;66:189–194.
143. Kremer JM, Genant HK, Moreland LW, et al. Results of a two-year followup study of patients with rheumatoid arthritis who received a combination of abatacept and methotrexate. Arthritis Rheum 2008;58:953–963.
144. Lenschow DJ, Herold KC, Rhee L, et al. CD28/B7 regulation of Th1 and Th2 subsets in the development of autoimmune diabetes. Immunity 1996;5:285–293.
145. Salomon B, Lenschow DJ, Rhee L, et al. B7/CD28 costimulation is essential for the homeostasis of the CD4+CD25+ immunoregulatory T cells that control autoimmune diabetes. Immunity 2000;12:431–440.
146. Trialnet. CTLA4-Ig. In: 2008.
147. Shevach EM. Immunology. Regulating suppression. Science 2008;322:202–203.
148. Cobbold SP, Adams E, Graca L, et al. Immune privilege induced by regulatory T cells in transplantation tolerance. Immunol Rev 2006;213:239–255.
149. Bresson D, Togher L, Rodrigo E, et al. Anti-CD3 and nasal proinsulin combination therapy enhances remission from recent-onset autoimmune diabetes by inducing Tregs. J Clin Invest 2006;116:1371–1381.
150. Sherry NA, Chen W, Kushner JA, et al. Exendin-4 improves reversal of diabetes in NOD mice treated with anti-CD3 monoclonal antibody by enhancing recovery of beta-cells. Endocrinology 2007;148:5136–5144.
151. Uno S, Imagawa A, Okita K, et al. Macrophages and dendritic cells infiltrating islets with or without beta cells produce tumour necrosis factor-alpha in patients with recent-onset type 1 diabetes. Diabetologia 2007;50:596–601.
152. Kaizer EC, Glaser CL, Chaussabel D, Banchereau J, Pascual V, White PC. Gene expression in peripheral blood mononuclear cells from children with diabetes. J Clin Endocrinol Metab 2007;92:3705–3711.
153. Bilgic S, Aktas E, Salman F, et al. Intracytoplasmic cytokine levels and neutrophil functions in early clinical stage of type 1 diabetes. Diabetes Res Clin Pract 2008;79:31–36.
154. Pfleger C, Mortensen HB, Hansen L, et al. Association of IL-1ra and adiponectin with C-peptide and remission in patients with type 1 diabetes. Diabetes 2008;57:929–937.
155. Larsen CM, Faulenbach M, Vaag A, et al. Interleukin-1-receptor antagonist in type 2 diabetes mellitus. N Engl J Med 2007;356:1517–1526.
156. Skyler JS. Prediction and prevention of type 1 diabetes: progress, problems, and prospects. Clin Pharmacol Ther 2007;81:768–771.
157. Gandhi GY, Murad MH, Flynn DN, et al. Immunotherapeutic agents in type 1 diabetes: a systematic review and meta-analysis of randomized trials. Clin Endocrinol (Oxf) 2008;69:244–252.
158. Strand V, Kimberly R, Isaacs JD. Biologic therapies in rheumatology: lessons learned, future directions. Nat Rev Drug Discov 2007;6:75–92.
159. Feldmann M, Steinman L. Design of effective immunotherapy for human autoimmunity. Nature 2005;435:612–619.

Chapter 19

Latent Autoimmune Diabetes in Adults

Barbara M. Brooks-Worrell and Jerry P. Palmer

Key Words: Latent autoimmune diabetes, Islet autoimmunity, Autoimmune diabetes, Type 2 diabetes, Autoantibodies, GAD, Islet-reactive T cells, Adult-onset autoimmune diabetes, Insulin resistance, Beta cell function

INTRODUCTION

Diabetes mellitus is a heterogeneous disorder classified clinically into two types: type 1 and type 2 diabetes (1, 2). The diagnosis of type 1 vs. type 2 diabetes is usually made using criteria such as age at onset, abruptness of hyperglycemic symptoms, presence of ketosis, degree of obesity, and the perceived need for insulin replacement. Most type 1 diabetes patients are diagnosed in childhood or young adulthood before the age of 35 years and are considered to have an autoimmune disease. In contrast, type 2 diabetes occurs most commonly in adults and is considered nonautoimmune. However, in 1994, Zimmet et al. (3) introduced the term "latent autoimmune diabetes of adults" (LADA) to describe a subgroup of adult phenotypic type 2 diabetes patients positive for an autoantibody to glutamic acid decarboxylase (GAD) and those who present clinically without ketoacidosis and weight loss. The presence of GAD positivity in these phenotypic type 2 diabetes patients suggested that they had an autoimmune form of diabetes with immune-mediated beta cell dysfunction and damage as part of their disease process. As expected for an immune attack on the beta cells, these patients also became insulin dependent more rapidly than "classic" type 2 diabetes patients who were negative for islet autoantibodies (3). In this chapter, we will define LADA, compare this group of patients with both type 1 and type 2 diabetes, and discuss possible treatment approaches.

WHAT IS LATENT AUTOIMMUNE DIABETES OF ADULTS?

For a clinician, the definition of type 1, type 2 diabetes, and LADA is not always straightforward. The diagnosis of LADA is currently based on three criteria: adult age of onset (over the age of 35 years), the presence of circulating beta-cell autoantibodies, and the lack of insulin requirement for at least 6 months post-diagnosis. The presence of autoantibodies and islet-reactive T cells distinguishes LADA from type 2 diabetes and the lack of requirement for insulin distinguishes LADA from type 1 diabetes (*4–7*). LADA is estimated to encompass approximately 10–30% of adult Caucasian phenotypic type 2 diabetes patients (*4, 5, 8–10*). Recently, Cervin et al. (*11*) observed in a large cohort of LADA patients that the LADA patients share genetic features with both type 1 (HLA, INS VNTR, and PTPN22) and type 2 (TCF7L2) diabetes. These authors concluded that LADA is an admixture of both type 1 and type 2 diabetes, hence the term "double diabetes" was used to label LADA patients. Thus, over the years, autoantibody positive phenotypic type 2 diabetes or LADA has been labeled as slowly progressive type 1 diabetes (*12, 13*), Latent type 1 diabetes (*14, 15*), double diabetes (*11*), and type 1.5 diabetes (*10, 15, 16*).

Both T1DM and LADA are considered to be cell-mediated autoimmune diseases directed against the beta cells. A major question is whether LADA is a distinct form of autoimmune diabetes or just part of a phenotypic continuum with a similar disease pathogenesis as type 1 diabetes (*17*). Though both type 1 and LADA are autoimmune in nature, there are apparent similarities and differences at the genetic, autoantibody, and T-cell levels. Another important difference between type 1 and LADA is the timeline for the development of clinical disease. LADA has been hypothesized to be a more "slowly progressive" form of autoimmune disease compared to "classic" type 1 diabetes (*9, 18*). In other words, by definition, LADA patients do not develop clinical disease until later in life. However, the question remains as to whether LADA patients actually lose beta cell function more slowly post-diagnosis compared to classic T1DM and more quickly when compared with classic T2DM.

AUTOANTIBODIES

Autoantibodies in T1DM and LADA Patients

The presence of autoantibodies and islet-reactive T cells in both LADA and classic childhood type 1 diabetes provides strong evidence that the underlying disease process in both patient groups is autoimmune. However, differences in autoantibodies between LADA and type 1 diabetes suggest potential immunologic differences. All four of the most common islet autoantibodies (ICA, GAD, IA-2, IAA) are found in childhood type 1 diabetes with many patients being positive for multiple autoantibodies. In fact, positivity for an increasing number of islet autoantibodies is associated with a progressively greater risk of developing type 1 diabetes (*19–28*). Positivity for only one autoantibody (ICA or GAD) is characteristic of LADA patients (*1, 7, 10, 29–31*). Lohmann et al. (*32*) and van Deutekom et al. (*33*) reported that the clinical characteristic of LADA patients correlates with the titer and numbers of diabetes-associated autoantibodies. Van Deutekom et al. (*33*) observed that the simultaneous presence of multiple autoantibodies and/or a high titer of anti-GAD autoantibodies, compared with single and low-titer autoantibody, was associated with an early age of onset and low fasting C-peptide values, and had a high predictive value for future insulin requirement. Buzzetti et al. (*34*) also demonstrated that LADA patients could be characterized based on their GAD titer levels and HLA haplotype. Futhermore, LADA patients with high-titer anti-GAD autoantibodies or multiple autoantibodies have been reported to have a low prevalence of markers of the metabolic syndrome (high BMI, hypertension, and dyslipidemia), and a high prevalence of the diabetes high-risk haplotypes (*35, 36*). However, in a large study in the United Kingdom Prospective Diabetes Study (UKPDS), there were no associations observed between GAD autoantibody levels with disease progression or future insulin requirements (*37*).

Many researchers (*9–11, 31, 38, 39*) have demonstrated that glutamic acid decarboxylase autoantibodies (GADAb) and islet-cell autoantibodies (ICA) are much more common than insulin autoantibodies (IAA), insulinoma-associated antigen 2 (IA-2) autoantibodies, and zinc-transporter autoantibodies in LADA patients vs. type 1 patients. IA-2 autoantibodies, however, are more common in Japanese LADA patients (*31*). Wenzlau et al. (*38*) reported that ZnT8 autoantibodies were detected in up to 80% of new-onset T1D patients compared with <2% of controls, <3% of T2D patients, and up to 20% of patients with other autoimmune diseases.

Differences in the GAD autoantibody IgG subclasses also appear to exist in LADA patients when compared with type 1 diabetes patients. The IgG4 subclass of GAD autoantibodies have been demonstrated to be more frequent in LADA than in type 1 diabetic patients, implying a greater TH2 type or regulated immune response in LADA as compared to type 1 patients (*40*). In collaboration with Hampe and Lernmark (*41*), we investigated whether there are differences in epitope specificity of GAD autoantibody in LADA vs. type 1 diabetes patients. Using recombinant 35 S-GAD65/67 fusion proteins, we found that sera from over 90% of type 1 diabetes patients bound to the middle or COOH-terminal portion of GAD65, whereas only 65% of sera from LADA patients bound to these regions of

GAD65 autoantibody. In contrast, the NH2-terminal portion of GAD65 was recognized by 20% of LADA patients compared with only 5% of type 1 diabetes patients. We have also demonstrated similar results using GAD65-specific recombinant Fabs (*42*). Desai et al. (*37*) observed that GAD autoantibodies persist for 5 years following diagnosis of LADA, but levels and reactivity to different GAD65 epitopes are not associated with disease progression. To add further complexity to this topic, we have recently described a group of adult phenotypic type 2 diabetes patients who are autoantibody negative but present with T-cell responses to islet proteins (T-LADA) similar to antibody positive LADA patients (*43*). Discussion of islet reactive T cells in LADA patients is presented later in this chapter. Therefore, the use of autoantibodies alone to identify LADA patients could potentially miss a large percentage of autoantibody-negative LADA patients, T-LADAs.

One important issue to stress is the fact that autoantibodies used to categorize and identify LADA patients are islet autoantibodies originally identified in T1D patients. Therefore, there may be other islet autoantibodies specific to LADA patients that have not yet been identified which would classify them more accurately or differently. In support of this concept, Seissler et al. (*44*) demonstrated that GAD and IA-2 could block ICA staining in approximately 60% of sera from type 1 diabetes patients but in a much lower percentage of sera from LADA patients. These results suggest that autoantibodies to antigens other than GAD and IA-2 are more prevalent in LADA. These studies illustrate the important autoantibody differences between LADA and type 1 diabetes and suggests potential differences in pathogenesis. One hypothesis would be the possible loss of tolerance to different beta-cell antigens in LADA compared with type 1 diabetes, or a difference in the responding or regulatory populations between the different groups. However, the answer to these questions awaits further research.

Autoantibodies in T2DM and LADA

By definition, the presence or absence of autoantibodies distinguishes between patients with "classic" nonautoimmune type 2 diabetes vs. LADA (*4*). In a study we conducted in 125 adult phenotypic type 2 patients screened for autoantibodies, 36 (28.8%) of the 125 patients were positive for at least one autoantibody (*10*). This datum is shown in Fig. 19.1. Moreover, with the identification of autoantibody-negative LADA patients (T-LADA, (*43*)), the use of known autoantibodies to screen T2DM patients may need to be reevaluated. Other phenotypic, immunologic, clinical, and genetic identifiers may be needed to distinguish LADA patients from type 2 patients when a designation of LADA is considered, but the T2DM patient lacks known islet autoantibodies.

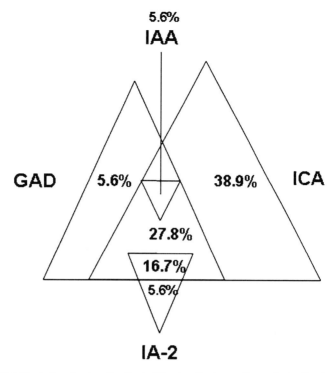

Fig. 19.1 Clustering of autoantibodies in 36 autoantibody-positive patients. *Numbers* (%) refer to the percentage of the 36 antibody-positive patients who were positive for the respective antibodies (*10*).

ISLET REACTIVE T CELLS

T Cell Responses to Islet Proteins in T1DM and LADA Patients

Islet-reactive T cells responding to multiple islet proteins have been found in LADA patients with and without autoantibodies (*5–7, 43*), type 1 diabetes patients (*45–50*), and subjects at risk of developing type 1 diabetes prior to development of clinical disease (*46*). Differences in islet proteins recognized by T cells from type 1 vs. LADA have been identified using multiple islet proteins (*5*). Figure 19.2 illustrates the percentage of type 1 and LADA patients with T cells responding to different human islet proteins (*5*). As illustrated in Fig. 19.2, there are some islet proteins that T cells from both type 1 and LADA diabetes patients appear to respond to equally (molecular weight 116, 97 and 60 kDa). However, there are also molecular weight regions that differentiate T-cell responses from type 1 vs. LADA patients (proteins in the molecular weight regions: 65–90 and 21–38 kDa). What immunological mechanisms are important in the delay and apparent differences in the pathogenesis of LADA vs. type 1 diabetes is not yet understood. Many of the above findings point to potential differences in immunological regulatory mechanisms.

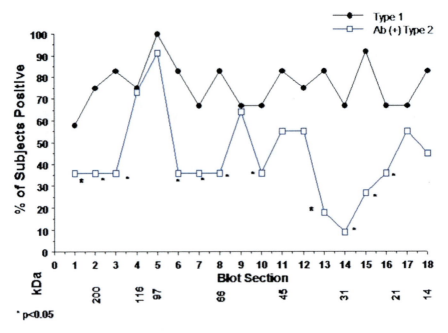

Fig. 19.2 T-cell responses of 12 type 1 diabetes patients (*closed circles*) and 11 autoantibody-positive type 2 patients (type 1.5 patients, *open squares*). The percentage of subjects responding to each molecular weight region is shown. A positive response is taken as SI > 2.0. Blot sections correspond to molecular weight regions >200 kDa (*1*) and <14 kDa (*18*). *p < 0.05 significant differences (*5*).

Immunoregulatory mechanisms function in normal subjects to maintain control of autoreactive T cells, which are present in normal individuals (*51–53*). Tolerance or protection against development of autoimmune disease can be mediated by several different mechanisms. These mechanisms include regulation or production of different cytokines and presence of different regulatory cell populations (*54*). Understanding the immunoregulatory mechanisms responsible for preventing breakdown of peripheral self-tolerance and avoiding the development of autoimmune disease has become a central issue in immunological research in the diabetes field. It is unclear, at this point, which of these mechanisms or combination of mechanisms will be important in the control of or protection against type 1 diabetes or in the apparent delay in presentation of LADA.

T-Cell Responses to Islets in T2DM and LADA Patients

By definition, classic type 2 diabetes is nonautoimmune. Therefore, type 2 diabetes patients should be devoid of both islet autoantibodies and islet-reactive T cells. T-LADA (*43*) patients have T cells reactive to islet proteins but are negative for ICA/GAD/IA-2 and IAA antibodies. Thus, assessing patients for T cell responses to islet proteins may help to more accurately distinguish LADA from type 2 patients especially if the LADA patients are autoantibody negative (T-LADA).

Recently, we observed the importance of assessing T-cell responses from T2DM patients to islet proteins by demonstrating that identifying type 2 diabetes patients with T cells response to islet proteins identified T2DM patients with a more severe beta-cell lesion compared to assessing islet autoantibodies alone (*55*). Identification of patients with a more severe beta-cell lesion may identify those patients progressing more rapidly toward the need for insulin replacement therapy.

GENETICS

Genetics in T1DM and LADA

LADA patients have been reported to be more commonly positive for HLA DR3 and DR4 and their associated DQb1 alleles 0201 and 0302, which have been linked to a predisposition to childhood type 1 diabetes (*31, 39, 56*). In contrast, the HLA DR2 and DQb1*0602, which has been associated with protection from childhood type 1 diabetes, has also been reported to be relatively common in LADA patients (*57*). The protection associated with DR2/DQb1*0602 may partially explain the age of onset of LADA vs. childhood T1DM. Hosszufalusi et al. (*31*) compared a group of LADA patients with control and adult type 1 diabetes patients. They reported that the HLA high-risk haplotype DR4-DQb1*0302 and the DR3/DR4-DQb1*0302 genotype were significantly more common in LADA patients compared with control subjects, whereas the frequencies were no different in LADA vs. adult-onset type 1 diabetes. An increased frequency of the cytotoxic T-lymphocyte antigen-4 (CTLA-4) genotype A/G has been observed in both type 1 diabetes and LADA, suggesting a similar role for this marker in both types of diabetes (*58*). Similar allelic variation in the insulin gene is also present in both type 1 and LADA. However, the relative risk associated with the one S/S genotype was significantly higher for LADA than for type 1 diabetes (*59*). Other non-HLA genetic differences between type 1 and LADA are seen in the major histocompatibility complex class I chain-related gene A (MICA) (*60, 61*) and an allelic polymorphism within the promoter region of the tumor necrosis factor-a (TNF-a) gene and the TNF2 allele (*62*). Recent genome-wide association studies demonstrated a link between the ZnT8 gene polymorphisms and type 2 diabetes, even though ZnT8 autoantibodies are rarely detected (*63–69*).

Recently, Wenzlau et al. (*70*) reported that a single polymorphic Arg325 encoding residue polymorphism in *SLC30A8* was associated with type 1 diabetes risk. Common variants in the TCF7L2 gene, in association with HLA-DQb1 genotyping, can distinguish GAD autoantibody-positive and GAD autoantibody-negative diabetes patients diagnosed between 15 and 34 years (*71*). However, the TCF7L2 gene variants do not distinguish between autoimmune and nonautoimmune diabetes patients diagnosed between the ages of 40 and 59 years suggesting that the disease pathogenesis in middle-aged (40–59 years) GAD autoantibody-positive patients is different from young (15–34 years) GAD autoantibody-positive diabetes patients (*71*).

Genetics in T2DM and LADA

HLA DR2 and DQb1*0602, which are protective for childhood type 1 diabetes, are rarely seen in T1DM patients. In contrast, HLA DR2 and DQb1*0602 are relatively common in LADA patients (*57*). Also, LADA patients share the same TCF7L2 genotype with type 2 diabetes (*11*). Thus, LADA patients appear to share genetic features common in both T1DM and T2DM patients.

BETA CELL FUNCTION

Beta cell dysfunction in LADA patients has been reported to be intermediate between type 1 diabetes patients and type 2 diabetes patients (*72–74*). LADA patients appear to have a faster decline in C-peptide levels compared to T2DM patients who show a more gradual decline (*31, 73, 74*). In comparison, a greater rate of decline in C-peptide has been reported in adult T1DM patients compared with LADA patients (*31, 75*). Differences in insulin secretion have also been observed between T1DM, LADA, and T2DM patients. Gottsater et al. (*75*) found that the level of insulin secretion in LADA was intermediate between type 1 and type 2 diabetes and that fasting and stimulated C-peptide were reduced in LADA compared with type 2 diabetes and healthy controls.

INSULIN RESISTANCE AND THE METABOLIC SYNDROME

Insulin resistance is an integral part of the pathophysiology of type 2 diabetes and is affected by many variables including age, BMI (body mass index), ethnicity, physical activity, and medications. When insulin resistance is assessed by the homeostasis model and is corrected for BMI, insulin resistance in LADA and type 2 diabetes patients does not differ (*76*). Furthermore, both LADA and type 2 diabetes patients were more insulin resistant than normal control subjects when corrected for BMI.

Increased body weight, central obesity, hypertension, and dyslipidemia is indicative of the metabolic syndrome. Most LADA patients are initially diagnosed as having type 2 diabetes, since they are indistinguishable phenotypically from T2DM patients. Some studies have reported a significantly lower mean BMI in LADA patients as compared to type 2 patients (*35, 77*), whereas other studies do not show a difference (*76*). However, the range of BMIs is often large with tremendous overlaps between LADA and T2DM patients (*10*). Fewer markers of the metabolic syndrome have been reported to be associated with LADA patients compared with T2DM patients (*35, 36*).

IMPORTANCE OF FAMILY HISTORY IN TYPE 1, TYPE 2, AND LADA

Family history of diabetes has been identified as a risk factor for the development of diabetes, both type 1 and type 2 (*4*). Familial clustering of diabetes is believed to be, in part, due to a combination of shared genetic and environmental factors. For both type 1 and type 2 diabetes, the risk of developing diabetes increases with increasing number of affected relatives (*71, 78, 79*). The results of the Nord-Trøndelag Health Study (*80*) showed that family history of diabetes, though the type of diabetes in the relatives was unknown, was also a strong risk factor for the development of LADA.

TREATMENT

LADA patients typically have a shorter duration of success utilizing diet or oral antidiabetic treatment therapies before requiring insulin therapy when compared with classic nonautoimmune T2DM patients. This treatment failure was initially noted when sulfonylureas were the only treatment option. Speculations have been presented regarding the value of thiazoledinediones in the treatment of LADA, not only because of their ability to improve insulin sensitivity but also because of their anti-inflammatory effect. If the decline in b-cell function is, in part, a result of T cell autoimmune destruction of the b-cells, then the addition of an anti-inflammatory medication may slow the decline in b-cell function. Recently, Rosiglitazone, a Thiazoledinedione with anti-inflammatory properties, has been reported to provide greater preservation of islet b-cell function in LADA patients compared to LADA patients treated with insulin alone during a 3 year follow-up (*81*). We have also recently observed diminished islet T-cell autoimmunity and preserved glucagon-stimulated C-peptide responses in T cell-positive T2DM patients treated with rosiglitazone compared with T cell-positive type 2 patients treated with glyburide. Kobayashi et al. (*82*) and Maruyama et al. (*83*) found that treatment of LADA patients with insulin resulted in better preservation of b-cell function compared to sulfonylureas. Further testing is needed to determine the best long-term treatment of autoimmune T2DM patients.

Another potential treatment for diabetes is antigen-specific immunomodulation. A randomized, double-blind, placebo-controlled, dose-finding, Phase IIa, GAD vaccine study in LADA patients demonstrated not only safety of the drug product, Diamyd, but also efficacy in preserving b-cell function in LADA patients (*84*). Based upon the apparent differences in the immune system recognition of the b-cell antigens between LADA and type 1 diabetes, different islet antigens might be more important for the autoimmune attack against the b-cells in type 1 diabetes compared to LADA. With that in mind, the success of antigen-based therapies may depend upon whether tolerance to the important islet antigens has been reinstated. Treatment with some antigens may be efficacious in both type 1 diabetes and LADA, whereas other antigens may be selectively effective in treating type 1 diabetes vs. LADA and vice versa.

CONCLUSIONS

The similarities between type 1 and LADA outlined in this chapter strongly suggest that LADA has an underlying autoimmune pathogenesis. The differences in autoantibody and T-cell recognition of islet proteins between type 1 diabetes patients and LADA, however, suggest important differences in the disease process between the two groups of patients. Research into identifying and quantifying specific cell populations involved in regulation or b-cell destruction will be an important area for future studies. The strongest evidence as to whether type 1 and LADA have similar autoimmune pathogenesis will most likely come from intervention protocols designed to halt the autoimmune process. If therapies are efficacious both in type 1 and LADA patients, these results would support the hypothesis that the two diseases are indistinguishable immunologically. However, if therapies are effective only in one or the other autoimmune group, these results would be supportive of the idea that LADA and type 1 diabetes constitute separate autoimmune processes. Then, the accurate identification and classification of patients would become clinically important so that they can be treated with the most efficacious regimen (personalized medicine).

REFERENCES

1. The Expert Committee on the Diagnosis and Classification of Diabetes Mellitus. Report of the expert committee on the diagnosis and classification of diabetes mellitus. Diabetes Care. 1997; 20: 1183–1197.
2. McCance DR, Hanson RL, Pettitt DF, Bennett PH, Hadden DR, Knowler WC: Diagnosing diabetes mellitus: do we need new criteria? Diabetologia. 1997; 40: 247–255.
3. Zimmet PZ. The pathogenesis and prevention of diabetes in adults: genes, autoimmunity, and demography. Diabetes Care. 1994; 18: 1050–1064.
4. Fourlanos S, Dotta F, Greenbaum CJ, Palmer JP, Rolandsson O, Colman PG, and Harrison LC. Latent auoimmune sdiabetes in adults (LADA) should be less latent. Diabetologia. 2005; 48: 2206–2212.

5. Brooks-Worrell BM, Juneja R, Minokadeh A, Greenbaum CJ, Palmer JP: Cellular immune response to human islet proteins in antibody-positive type 2 diabetic patients. Diabetes. 1999; 48: 983–988.
6. Mayer A, Fabien N, Gutowski MC, Dubois V, Gebuhrer L, Bienvenu J, Orgiazzi J, Madec AM. Contrasting cellular and humoral autoimmunity associated with latent autoimmune diabetes in adults. Eur J Endocrinol. 2007; 157: 53–61.
7. Zavala AV, Fabiano de Bruno LE, Cardoso AI, Mota AH, Capucchio M, Poskers E, Fanbeim L, Basabe JC. Cellular and humoral autoimmunity markers in type 2 (non-insulin-dependent) diabetic patients with secondary drug failure. Diabetologia. 1992; 35: 1159–1164.
8. Lohmann T, Seissler J, Verlohren H-J, Schroder S, Rotger J, Dahn K, Mortgenthaler N, Scherbaum WA. Distinct genetic and immunological features in patients with onset of IDDM before and after age 40. Diabetes Care. 1997; 20: 524–529.
9. Tuomi T, Groop LC, Zimmet PZ, Rowley MJ, Knowles W, Mackay IR. Antibodies to glutamic acid decarboxylase reveal latent autoimmune diabetes mellitus in adults with a non-insulin-dependent onset of diabetes. Diabetes. 1993; 42: 359–362.
10. Juneja R, Hirsch IB, Naik RG, Brooks-Worrell BM, Greenbaum CJ, Palmer JP. Islet cell antibodies and glutamic acid decarboxylase antibodies but not the clinical phenotype help to identify type 1 1/2 diabetes in patients presenting with type 2 diabetes. Metabolism. 2001; 50: 1008–1013.
11. Cervin C, Lyssenko V, Bakhtadze E, Lindholm E, Nilsson P, Tuomi T, Cilio CM, Groop L. Genetic similarities between latent autoimmune diabetes in adults, type 1 diabgetes, and type 2 diabetes. Diabetes. 2008; 57: 1433–1437.
12. Kobayashi T, Tamemoto K, Nakanishi K, Kato N, Okubo M, Kajio H, Sugimoto T, Murase T, Kosaka K. Immunogenetic and clinical characterization of slowly progressive IDDM. Diabetes Care. 1993; 16: 780–788.
13. Kobayashi T. Subtype of insulin-dependent diabetes mellitus (IDDM) in Japan: Slowly progressive IDDM – the clinical characteristics and pathogenesis of the syndrome. Diabetes Res Clin Prac. 1994; 24: S96–S99.
14. Groop L, Botazzo GF, Koniach D. Islet cell antibodies identify latent type 1 diabetes in patients aged 35–75 years at diagnosis. Diabetes. 1986; 35: 237–241.
15. Palmer JP, Hirsch IB. What's in a name: latent autoimmune diabetes of adults, type 1.5, adult-onset, and type 1 diabetes. Diabetes Care. 2003; 26: 536–538.
16. Juneja R, Palmer JP. Type 1 1/2 diabetes: Myth or reality? Autoimmunity. 1999; 29: 65–83.
17. Leslie RDG, Kolb H, Schloot NC, Buzzetti R, Mauricio D, De Leiva A, Yderstraede K, Sarti C, Thivolet C, Hadden D, Hunter S, Schernthaner G, Scherbaum W, Williams R, Pozzilli P. Diabetes classification: grey zones, sound and smoke: action LADA1. Diabetes Metab Res Rev. 2008; 24(7):511–519.
18. Alberti KG, Zimmet PZ. Definition, diagnosis and classification of diabetes mellitus and its complications. Part 1: Diagnosis and classification of diabetes mellitus: provisional report of a WHO consultation. Diabet med. 1998; 15: 539–553.
19. Verge CF, Gianani R, Kawasake I, Yu LP, Pietropaolo F, Chase HP, Eisenbarth GS. Number of autoantibodies (against insulin, GAD or ICA512/IA2) rather than particular autoantibody specificities determines risk of type 1 diabetes. J Autoimmun. 1996; 9: 370–383.
20. Verg CF, Gianani R, Kawasake E, Yu LP, Pietropaolo F, Jackson RA, Chase HP, Eisenbarth G. Prediction of type 1 diabetes in first-degree relatives using a combination of insulin, GAD, and ICA512bdc/IA-2 autoantibodies. Diabetes. 1996; 45: 926–933.
21. Krischer JP, Cuthbertson DD, Yu L, Orban T, MaclarenN, Jackson R, Winter WE, Schatz DA, Palmer JP, Eisenbarth GS, The Diabetes Prevention Trial-Type 1 Study Group. Screening strategies for the identification of multiple antibody-positive relatives of individuals with type 1 diabetes. J Clin Endocrinol Metabol. 2003; 88: 103–108.
22. Naserke HE, Ziegler A-G, Lampasona V, Bonifacio E. Early development and spreading of autoantibodies to epitopes of IA-2 and their association with progression to type 1 diabetes. J Immunol. 1998; 161: 6963–6969.
23. Kawasaki E, Yu L, Rewers MJ, Hutton JC, Eisenbarth GS. Definition of multiple ICA 512/phogrin autoantibody epitopes and detection of intramolecular epitope spreading in relatives of patients with type 1 diabetes. Diabetes. 1998; 47: 733–742.
24. Palmer JP. Predicting IDDM. Use of humoral immune markers. Diabetes Rev. 1993; 1: 104–115.
25. Greenbaum CJ, Brooks-Worrell BM, Palmer JP, Lernmark A. Autoimmunity and prediction of insulin dependent diabetes mellitus. In: Marshal SM, Home PD, editors. Diabetes Annual. Amsterdam, Elsevier Science, 1994; 8: 21–29.

26. Ziegler A-G, Hummel M, Schenker M, Bonifacio E. Autoantibody appearance and risk for development of childhood diabetes in offspring of parents with type 1 diabetes. The 2-year analysis of the German BABYDIAB study. Diabetes. 1999; 48: 460–468.
27. Bingley PJ, ICARUS Group. Interactions of age, islet cell antibodies, insulin autoantibodies, and first-phase insulin response in prediction risk of progression to IDDM in ICA+ relatives. The ICARUS data set. Diabetes. 1996; 45: 1720–1728.
28. Bingley PJ, Christie MR, Bonifacio E, Bonfanti R, Shattock M, Fonte M-T, Bottazzo G-F, Gale EAM. Combined analysis of autoantibodies improves prediction of IDDM in islet cell antibody-positive relatives. Diabetes. 1994; 43: 1304–1310.
29. Turner R, Stratton I, Horton V, Manley S, Zimmet P, Mackay IR, Shattock M, Bottazzo GF, Holman R. UKPDS 25: Autoantibodies to islet-cell cytoplasm and glutamic acid decarboxylase for prediction of insulin requirement in type 2 diabetes. Lancet. 1997; 350: 1288–1293.
30. Rowley MJ, Mackay IR, Chen Q-Y, Knowles WJ, Zimmet PZ. Antibodies to glutamic acid decarboxylase discriminate major types of Diabetes mellitus. Diabetes. 1992; 41: 548–551.
31. Hosszufalusi N, Yatay A, Rajczy K, Prohaszka Z, Pozsonyi E, Horvath L, Grosz A, Gero L, Madacxsy L, Romics L, Karadi I, Fust G, Panczel P. Similar genetic features and different islet cell autoantibody pattern of latent autoimmune diabetes in adults (LADA) compared with adult-onset type 1 diabetes with rapid progression. Diabetes Care. 2003; 26: 452–457.
32. Lohmann T, Kellner K, Verlohren HJ, Krug J, Steindorf J, Scherbaum WA, Seissler J. Titre and combination of ICA and autoantibodies to glutamic acid decarboxylase discriminate two clinically distinct types f latent autoimmune diabetes in adults (LADA). Diabetologia. 2001; 44: 1005–1010.
33. van Deutekom AW, Heine RJ, Simsek S. The islet autoantibody titers their clinical relevance in latent autoimmune diabetes in adults (LADA) and the classification of diabetes mellitus. Diabetic medicine. 2008; 25: 117–125.
34. Buzzetti R, Di Pietro S, Giaccari A, Petrone A, Locatelli M, Suraci C, Capizzi M, Arpi ML, Bazzigaluppi E, Dotta F, Fosi E, For the Non-Insulin Requiring Autoimmune Diabetes (NIRAD) Study Group. High titer of autoantibodies to GAD identifies a specific phenotype of adult-onset autoimmune diabetes. Diabetes Care. 2007; 30: 932–938.
35. Zinman B, Kahn SE, Hafner SM, O'Neill MC, Heise MA, Freed MI. Phenotypic characteristics of GAD antibody-positive recently diagnosed patients with type 2 diabetes in North America and Europe. Diabetes. 2004; 53: 3193–3200.
36. Tuoni T, Carlsson A, Li H, Isomaa B, Miettinen A, Nilsson A, Nissen M, Ehrnstrom B-O, Forsen B, Snickars B, Lahti K, Forsblom C, Saloranta C, Taskinen M-R, Groop LC. Clinical and genetic characteristics of type 2 diabetes with and without GAD antibodies. Diabetes. 1999; 48: 150–157.
37. Desai M, Cull CA, Horton VA, Christie MR, Bonifacio WE, Lampasona V, Bingley PJ, Levy JC, Mackay IR, Zimmet P, Holman RR, Clark A. GAD autoantibodies and epitope reactivities persist after diagnosis in latent autoimmune diabetes in adults but do not predict disease progression: UKPDS 77. Diabetologia. 2007; 50: 2052–2060.
38. Wenzlau JM, Moua O, Sarkar SA, Yu L, Rewers M, Eisenbarth GS, Davidson HW, Hutton JC. SIC30A8 is a major target of humoral autoimmunity in type 1 diabetes and a predictive marker in prediabetes. Immunology of Diabetes V: Ann NY Acad Sci. 2008; 1150: 256–259.
39. Murao S, Kondo S, Ohashi J, Fujii Y, Shimizu I, Fujiyama M, Ohno K, Takada Y, Nakai K, Yamane Y, Osawa H, Makino H. Anti-thyroid peroxidase antibody, IA-2 antibody, and fasting C-peptide levels predict beta cell failure in patients with latent autoimmune diabetes in adults (LADA)-A 5 year follow-up of the Ehime study. Diabetes Res Clin Pract. 2008; 38: 114–121.
40. Hillman M, Torn C, Thorgeirsson H, Thorgeirsson H, Landin-Olsson M. IgG4 subclass of glutamic acid decarboxylase antibody is more frequent in latent autoimmune diabetes in adults than in type 1 diabetes. Diabetologia. 2004; 47: 1984–1989.
41. Hampe CS, Kockum I, Landin-Olsson M, Torn C, Ortqvist E, Persson B, Rolandsson O, Palmer JP, Lernmark A. GAD65 antibody epitope patterns of type 1.5 diabetes patients are consistent with slow onset autoimmune diabetes. Diabetes Care. 2002; 25: 1481–1482.
42. Padoa CJ, Banga JP, Madec A-M, Ziegler M, Schlosser M, Ortqvist E, Kockum I, Palmer JP, Rolandsson O, Binder KA, Foote J, Luo D, Hampe CS. Recombinant Fab of human monoclonal antibodies specific to the middle epitope of GAD65 inhibit type 1 diabetes-specific GAD65abs. Diabetes. 2003; 52: 2689–2695.
43. Ismail H, Wotring M, Kimmie C, Au L, Palmer JP, Brooks-Worrell B. "T cell-positive antibody-negative" phenotypic type 2 patients,

a unique subgroup of autoimmune diabetes. Diabetes. 2007; 56(S1): A325.
44. Seissler J, DeSonnaville JJ, Morgenthaler NG, Steinbrenner H, Glawe D, Khoo-Morgenthaler UY, Lan MS, Notkins AL, Heine RJ, Scherbaum WA. Immunological heterogeneity in type 1 diabetes: Presence of distinct autoantibody patterns in patients with acute onset and slowly progressive disease. Diabetologia. 1998; 41: 891–897.
45. Brooks-Worrell BM, Starkebaum GA, Greenbaum C, Palmer JP. Peripheral blood mononuclear cells of insulin-dependent diabetic patients: Respond to multiple islet cell proteins. J Immunol. 1996; 157: 5668–5674.
46. Brooks-Worrell B, Gersuk VH, Greenbaum C, Palmer JPP. Intermolecular antigen spreading occurs during the preclinical period of human type 1 diabetes. J Immunol. 2007; 166: 5265–5270.
47. Roep BO, Kallan AA, Duinkerken G, Arden SD, Hutton JC, Bruining GJ, de Vries RR. T cell reactivity to beta-cell membrane antigens associated with beta cell destruction in IDDM. Diabetes 1995; 44: 278–283.
48. Roep BO, Arden DS, DeVries RRP, Hutton JC. T cell clones from a type 1 diabetic patient respond to insulin secretory granule proteins. Nature. 1990; 345: 632–634.
49. Roep BO. T cell responses to autoantigens in IDDM: The search for the Holy Grail. Diabetes. 1996; 45: 1147–1156.
50. Durinovic-Bello I, Hummel M, Ziegler A-G. Cellular immune response to diverse islet cell antigens in IDDM. Diabetes. 1996; 45: 795–800.
51. Goverman J, Brabb T, Paez A, Harrington C, von Dassow P. Initiation and regulation of CNS autoimmunity. Crit Rev Immunol. 1997; 17: 469–480.
52. Burns J, Rosenzwerg A, Zwerman B, Lisak RP. Isolation of myelin basic protein-reactive T cell lines from normal human blood. Cell Immunol. 1983; 81: 435–440.
53. Correle J, McMillian M, McCarthy K, Le T, Weiner LP. Isolation and characterization of autoreactive proteolipid protein-peptide specific T cell clones from multiple sclerosis patients. Neurology. 1995; 45: 1370–1378.
54. Homann D, and von Herrath M. Regulatory T cells and type 1 diabetes. Clinical Immunology. 2004; 112: 202–209.
55. Goel A, Chiu H, Felton J, Palmer JP, Brooks-Worrell B. T cell responses to islet antigens improves detection of autoimmune diabetes and identifies patients with more severe b-cell lesions in phenotypic type 2 diabetes. Diabetes. 2007; 56: 2110–2115.
56. Gleichmann H, Zorcher B, Greulick B. Correlation of islet cell antibodies and HLA-DR phenotypes with diabetes mellitus in adults. Diabetologia. 1984(Suppl); 27: 90–92.
57. Tuomi T, Carlsson A, Li H, Isomaa B, Miettinen A, Nilsson A, Nissen M, Ehrnstrom BO, Forsen B, Snickars B, Lahti K, Forsblom C, Saloranta C, Taskinen M, Groop L. Clinical and genetic characteristics of type 2 diabetes with and without GAD antibodies. Diabetes. 1999; 48: 150–157.
58. Cosentino A, Gambelunghe G, Tortoioli C, Falorni A. CTLA-4 gene polymorphism contributes to the genetic risk for latent autoimmune diabetes in adults. Ann NY Acad Sci. 2002; 958: 337–340.
59. Cerrone GE, Caputo M, Lopez AP, Gonzalez C, Massa C, Cedola N, Targovnik HM, Frechtel GD. Variable number of tandem repeats of the insulin gene determines susceptibility to latent autoimmune diabetes in adults. Mol Diagn. 2004; 8: 43–49.
60. Torn C, Gupta M, Zake LN, Sanjeevi CB, Landin-Olsson M. Heterozygosity for MICA 4.0/MiCA 5.1 and HLA DR3-DQ2/DR4-DQ8 are independent genetic risk factors for latent autoimmune diabetes in adults. Hum Immunol. 2003; 64: 902–909.
61. Sanjeevi CB, Gambelunghe G, Falorni A, Shtauvere-Brameus A, Kanungo A. Genetics of latent autoimmune diabetes in adults. Ann NY Acad Sci. 2002; 958: 107–111.
62. Vatay A, Rajczy K, Pozsonyi E, Horvath L, Grosz A, Gero L, Madacsy L, Romics L, Daradi I, Gust G, Panczel P. Differences in the genetic background of latent autoimmune diabetes in adults (LADA) and type 1 diabetes mellitus. Immunol Lett. 2002; 84: 109–115.
63. Sladek R, Rocheleau G, Rung J, Dina C, Shen L, Serre D, Boutin P, Vincent D, Belisle A, Hadjadj S, Balkau B, Heude B, Charpentier G, Hudson TJ, Montpetit A, Pshezhetsky AV, Prentki M, Posner BI, Balding DJ, Meyre D, Polychronakos C, Froguel P. A genome-wide association study identifies novel risk loci for type 2 diabetes. Nature. 2007; 445: 881–885.
64. Scott JL, Mohlke KL, Bonnycastle LL, Willer CJ, Li Y, Duren WL, Erdos Mr, Stringham HM, Chines PS, Jackson AU, Prokunina-Olsson L, Ding CJ, Swift AJ, Narisu N, Hu T, Prim R, Ziao R, Li XY, Conneely KN, Riebow NL, Sprau AG, Tong M, White PP, Hetrick KN, Barnhart MW, Bark CW, Goldstein JL, Watkins L, Ziang F, Saramies J, Buchanan TA, Watanabe RM, Valle TT, Kinnunen L, Abecasis GR, Pugh EW, Doheny KF, Bergman RN, Tuomilehto J, Collins FS, Boehnke M. A genome-wide association study of type 2

diabetes in Finns detects multiple susceptibility variants. Science. 2007; 316: 1341–1345.

65. Saxena R, Voight BF, Lyssenko V, Burtt NP, DeBakker PI, Chen H, Roix JJ, Kathiresan S, Hirschhorn JN, Daly MJ, Hughes TE, Groop L, Altshuler D, Almgren P, Florez JC, Meyer J, Ardlie K, Bengtsson Bostrom K, Isomaa B, Lettre G, Lindblad U, Lyon HN, Melander O, Newton-Cheh C, Nilsson P, Orho-Melander M, Rastam L, Speliotes EK, Taskinen MR, Tuomi T, Guiducci C, Berglund A, Carlson J, Gianniny L, Hackett R, Hall L, Holmkvist J, Laurila E, Sjogren M, Sterner M, Surti A, Svensson M, Svensson M, Tewhey R, Blumenstiel B, Parkin M, Defelice M, Barry R, Brodeur W, Camarata J, Chia N, Fava M, Gibbons J, Handsaker B, Healy C, Nguyen K, Gates C, Sougnez C, Gage D, Nizzari M, Gabriel SB, Chirn GW, Ma Q, Parikh H, Richardson D, Ricke D, Purcell S. Genome-wide association analysis identifies loci for type 2 diabetes and triglyceride levels. Science. 2007; 316: 1331–1336.

66. Zeggini E, Weedon MN, Lindgren CM, Frayling TM, Elliott KS, Lango H, Timpson NJ, Perry JR, Rayner NW, Freathy RM, Barrett JC, Shields B, Morris AP, Ellard S, Groves CJ, Harries LW, Marchini JL, Owen KR, Knight B, Cardon LR, Walker M, Hitman GA, Morris AD, Doney AS, McCarthy MI, Hattersley AT. Replication of genome-wide association signals in UK samples reveals risk loci for type 2 diabetes. Science. 2007; 36: 1336–1341.

67. Staiger H, Machicao F, Stefan N, Tschritter O, Thamer C, Kantartzis K, Schafer SA, Kirchhoff K, Fritsche A, Haring HU. Polymorphisms within novel risk loci for type 2 diabetes determine beta-cell function. PloS ONE. 2007; 2: 3832.

68. Kirchhoff K, Machicao F, Haupt A, Schafer SA, Tschritter O, Staiger H, Stefan N, Haring HU, Fritsche A. Polymorphisms in the TCF7L2, CDKAL1, and SLC30A8 genes are associated with impaired proinsulin conversion. Diabetologia. 2008; 51: 597–601.

69. Boesgaard TW, Zilinskaite J, Vanttinen M, Laakso M, Jansson PA, Hammarstedt A, Smith U, Stefan N, Fritsche A, Harin H, Hribal M, Sesti G, Zobel DP, Pedersen O, Hansen T. The common SLC30A8 Arg325Trp variant is associated with reduced first-phase insulin release in 846 non-diabetic offspring of type 2 diabetes patients: The EUGENE2 study. Diabetologia. 2008; 51: 816–820.

70. Wenzlau JM, Liu Y, Yu L, Moua O, Fowler KT, Rangasamy S, Walters J, Eisenbarth GS, Davidson HW, Hutton JC. A common non-synonymous single nucleotide polymorphism in the SLC30A8 gene determines ZnT8 autoantibody specificity in type 1 diabetes. Diabetes. 2008; 57: 2693–2697.

71. Grill V, Persson P-G, Carlsson S, Alvarsson M, Normal A, Svanstrom L, Efendic S, The Stockholm Diabetes Prevention Program Group. Family history of diabetes in middle-age Swedish men is a gender unrelated factor which associates with insulinopenia in newly diagnosed diabetes subjects. Diabetologia. 1999; 42: 15–23.

72. The Diabetes Control and Complications Trial Research Group. Effect of intensive therapy on residual b-cell function in patients with type 1 diabetes in the diabetes control and complications trial. Ann Intern Med. 1998; 128: 517–523.

73. Borg H, Gottsater A, Fernlund P, Sundkvist G. A 12-year prospective study of the relationship between islet antibodies and beta-cell function at and after the diagnosis in patients with adult-onset diabetes. Diabetes. 2002; 51: 1754–1762.

74. Torn C, Landin-Olsson M, Learnmark A, Palmer JP, Arnqvist HJ, Blohme G., Lithner F, Littorin B, Nystrom L, Schersten B, Sundkvist G, Wibell L, Ostman J. Prognostic factors for the course of beta cell function in autoimmune diabetes. J. Clin Endocrinol Metab. 2000; 85: 4619–4623.

75. Gottsater A, Landin-Olsson M, Fernlund P, Lernmark A, Sundkvist G. Beta cell function in relation to islet cell antibodies during the first 3 yr after clinical diagnosis of diabetes in type II diabetic patients. Diabetes Care. 1993; 16: 902–910.

76. Chiu HK, Tsai EC, Juneja R, Stoever J, Brooks-Worrell B, Goel A, Palmer JP. Equivalent insulin resistance in latent autoimmune diabetes in adults (LADA) and type 2 diabetes patients. Diabetes Res Clin Pract. 2007; 77: 237–244.

77. Davis TM, Zimmet P, Davis WA, Bruce DG, Fida S, Mackay IR. Autoantibodies to glutamic acid decarboxylase in diabetic atients from a multi-ethnic Australian community: The Fremantle Diabetes Study. Diabet Med. 2000; 17: 667–674.

78. Meigs JB, Cupples LA, Wilson PW. Parental transmission of type 2 diabetes: The Framingham Offspring Study. Diabetes. 2000; 49: 2201–2207.

79. Bonifacio E, Hummel M, Walter M, Schmid S, Ziegler AG. IDDM1 and multiple family history of type 1 diabetes combine to identify neonates at high risk for type 1 diabetes. Diabetes Care. 2004; 27: 2695–2700.

80. Carlsson S, Midthjell K, Grill V. Influence of family history of diabetes on incidence and prevalence of latent autoimmune diabetes of the adult: results from the Nord-Trøndelag Health Study. Diabetes Care. 2007; 30: 3040–3045.
81. Yang Z, Zhou A, Li X, Huang G, Lin J. Rosiglitazone perserves islet b-cell function of adult-onset latent autoimmune diabetes in 3 years follow-up study. Diabetes Res Clin Pract. 2009; 83: 54–60.
82. Kobayashi T, Nakanishi K, Murase T, Kosaka K. Small doses of subcutaneous insulin as a strategy for preventing slowly progressive beta-cell failure in islet cell antibody-positive patients with clinical features of NIDDM. Diabetes. 1996; 45: 622–626.
83. Maruyama T, Tanaka S, Shimada A, Funae O, Kasuga A, Kanatsuka A, Takei I, Yamada S, Harii N, Shimura H, Kobayashi T. Insulin intervention in slowly progressive insulin-dependent (type 1) diabetes mellitus. J Clin Endocrinol Metab. 2008; 93: 2115–2121.
84. Agardh CD, Cilio CM, Lethagan A, Lynch K, Leslie RD, Palmer M., Harris RA, Robertson JA, Lernmark A. Clinical evidence for the safety of GAD65 immunomodulation in adult-onset autoimmune diabetes. J Diabetes Complicat. 2005; 19: 238–246.

Chapter 20

Fulminant Type 1 Diabetes Mellitus

Akihisa Imagawa and Toshiaki Hanafusa

Summary

Established as a novel subtype of type 1 diabetes in Japan in the year 2000, fulminant type 1 diabetes is characterized by a rapid onset and an absence of diabetes-related antibodies. This disease has been mainly reported in East Asia, especially in Japan. The prevalence of fulminant type 1 diabetes among ketosis-onset type 1 diabetes was 19.4% in a Japanese nationwide survey. Both genetic and environmental factors are involved in the etiology of fulminant type 1 diabetes. The former includes, for example, HLA-DR/DQ or CTLA-4 polymorphisms, and the latter includes viral infection. Fulminant type 1 diabetes is the most severe form of diabetes because of the complete loss of pancreatic beta cells at disease onset, and it is also a high-risk subgroup for diabetic microangiopathy.

Key Words: Idiopathic, Epidemiology, HLA, CTLA-4, Virus, Complication

INTRODUCTION

In 2000, we reported on a series of 11 patients and proposed a novel clinical entity within diabetes mellitus known as "fulminant type 1 diabetes" (1, 2). The title of the first paper was "A novel subtype of type 1 diabetes mellitus characterized by a rapid onset and an absence of diabetes-related antibodies." A rapid onset and an absence of islet-related autoantibodies, such as islet cell antibodies (ICA), anti-glutamic acid decarboxyalse antibody (GADAb), insulin autoantibody (IAA), or anti-insulinoma-associated antigen 2 antibody (IA-2Ab), are still essential to this subtype of diabetes 8 yearslater, with a few exceptions. This subtype is tentatively classified as type 1B, an idiopathic form of the disease. This classification is appropriate because of the absence of islet-related autoantibodies, and it is consistent with the classification guidelines from the American Diabetes Association and the World Health Organization (3, 4). However, recent studies have revealed that an immune reaction is likely involved in the pathogenesis of this disease. If type 1A diabetes includes immune-mediated type 1 diabetes without autoantibodies, fulminant type 1 diabetes could also be classified as type 1A diabetes.

Like type 1A diabetes, fulminant type 1 diabetes also presents with high plasma glucose levels accompanied by ketosis or ketoacidosis; however, fulminant type 1 diabetes also exhibits nearly normal glycosylated hemoglobin levels, a high serum pancreatic enzyme concentration, and virtually no C-peptide secretion at the onset of the disease. This discrepancy comes from the rapid loss of pancreatic beta cells at the onset of fulminant type 1 diabetes. Sekine et al. reported a patient whose fasting blood glucose and serum C-peptide levels were monitored for a couple of weeks around the onset of fulminant type 1 diabetes. The blood glucose level was within the normal limit 1 day before the onset and suddenly increased at the onset with a fall in serum C-peptide levels (5).

To confirm our first report, a nationwide survey was performed, and 161 Japanese patients with fulminant type 1 diabetes were identified (6). Based on the clinical data of those 161 patients with fulminant type 1 diabetes and on the 137 patients with "classic" type 1A diabetes in this study, the Committee of Japan Diabetes Society of the Research of Fulminant Type 1 Diabetes Mellitus has set out the diagnostic criteria for definitively diagnosing the disease (Table 20.1) (7).

In this chapter, we compare fulminant type 1 diabetes with "classic" type 1A diabetes in epidemiology, in the mechanism of beta-cell destruction, and in prognosis. Classic type 1A diabetes is defined as a type 1 diabetes with acute onset (not latent onset) and islet autoantibodies.

Table 20.1

Fulminant type 1 diabetes mellitus is confirmed when the following three findings are satisfied
1. Occurrence of diabetic ketosis or ketoacidosis soon (around 7 days) after the onset of hyperglycemic symptoms (elevation of urinary and/or serum ketone bodies at first visit)
2. Plasma glucose level ≥16.0 mmol/l (288 mg/dl) and glycated hemoglobin level <8.5% at first visit
3. Urinary C-peptide level <10 μg/day or fasting plasma C-peptide level <0.3 and <0.5 ng/ml after intravenous glucagon (or after meal) load at onset
Related findings
(a) Islet-related autoantibodies such as antibodies to glutamic acid decarboxyalse, islet-associated antigen 2, and insulin are undetectable in general
(b) Duration of the disease before the start of insulin treatment can be 1–2 weeks
(c) Elevation of serum pancreatic enzyme levels (amylase, lipase, or elastase-1) is observed in 98% of the patients
(d) Flu-like symptoms (fever, upper respiratory symptoms, etc.) or gastrointestinal symptoms (upper abdominal pain, nausea and/or vomiting, etc.) precede the disease onset in 70% of the patients
(e) The disease can occur during the pregnancy or just after the delivery

EPIDEMIOLOGY

Fulminant type 1 diabetes has been mainly reported in East Asia, especially in Japan. The prevalence of fulminant type 1 diabetes among ketosis-onset type 1 diabetes was 19.4% (43 of 222 patients) in a Japanese nationwide survey (6). In this study, positivity for either GAD or IA-2 antibodies was present in 137 of 179 patients, indicating that at least 76.5% of acute-onset type 1 diabetic patients have classic type 1A diabetes. The prevalence of type 1A diabetes would increase if IAA and ZnT8 antibodies were measured (8). In the Ehime study, a regional hospital-based study for adult-onset diabetes, the prevalence of fulminant type 1 diabetes was 8.9% in all type 1 diabetic patients and 0.2% in 4,980 newly diagnosed patients with diabetes, including type 2, other types, and gestational diabetes (9). In this study, classic type 1A diabetes accounted for 62.3% of all type 1 diabetic patients and for 1.4% of all diabetic patients. Patients with fulminant type 1 diabetes were reported from all over Japan, and no significant seasonal or regional preference was observed. In addition, the number of newly diagnosed patients has not increased over the past 10 years, indicating that fulminant type 1 diabetes is not an emerging disease (7).

Recently, 7.1% of type 1 diabetic patients were classified as fulminant type 1 diabetic patients, and 68.7% were classified as autoimmune (type 1A) diabetic patients in Korea according to the Japanese criteria (10). Several cases have been reported in other Asian populations, such as Chinese or Filipino (11–14), and few cases have been reported outside of Asia.

In Caucasians, Pozzilli et al. reported no cases of fulminant type 1 diabetes, but they reported 59 cases of GAD-positive diabetes in 82 cases of newly diagnosed diabetes in Italy (15). Maldonado et al. also reported that no patients presented with fulminant type 1 diabetes in their study, but they reported 29 patients with islet autoantibodies in 103 consecutive ketosis-prone diabetic patients in Houston (16). Their patients were predominantly African-American, Hispanic-American, and Caucasian-American, with a few Asian-Americans. Balasubramanian et al. reported no patients susceptible to fulminant type 1 diabetes, and they found 54.5% of diabetic patients with islet autoantibodies in north Indian children (17). However, recently, Caucasian cases of fulminant type 1 diabetes were reported in France (18), suggesting that this clinical entity is observed beyond ethnicity.

Fulminant type 1 diabetes is equally observed in males and females. In a nationwide survey, 83 males and 78 females with fulminant type 1 diabetes were reported in Japan (5). On the other hand, 47 males and 90 females were reported to have classic type 1A diabetes, suggesting that females are predominant in this autoimmune disease. In an extended nationwide survey carried out until

30 June 2006, 3 patients under 4 years of age (one boy and two girls) suffered from fulminant type 1, and the other 12 of 250 patients under 20 years of age (three boys and nine girls) had fulminant type 1 diabetes (*19*). This finding suggests that fulminant type 1 diabetes occurs in children (*20*), but the number of patients is very small, which is clearly in contrast to the number of children with classic type 1A diabetes in Japan (*21*). In the extended nationwide survey, 24 patients over 65 years old (16 males and 8 females) suffered from fulminant type 1 diabetes, and the disease onset of the other 211 patients occurred between 20 and 64 years old (*20*).

Fulminant type 1 diabetes is not predominant in females, but pregnancy is sometimes associated with this disease (*5, 22, 23*). Almost all patients who suffered from type 1 diabetes in pregnancy showed characteristics similar to that of fulminant diabetes just after the delivery. Shimizu et al. reported the clinical characteristics of 22 patients with fulminant diabetes associated with pregnancy. In those 22 patients, 18 patients developed diabetes during pregnancy and 4 patients had diabetes immediately after the delivery. The disease onset of 13 patients occurred in the third trimester, and fetal demise occurred in 12 of 18 patients who developed fulminant diabetes during pregnancy. Five of six live fetal cases were rescued by Cesarean section (*23*). The patients with fulminant diabetes associated with pregnancy are presented with a more severe clinical form than those who are not associated with pregnancy at the onset of overt diabetes. In another nationwide survey in Japan, 9 of 12 patients with type 1 diabetes associated with pregnancy had fulminant type 1 diabetes (*24*).

MECHANISM OF BETA-CELL DESTRUCTION

Histological analysis has revealed that the area of pancreatic beta cells decreases to 1/255 of normal subjects and even to 1/37 of type 1A diabetes in fulminant type 1 diabetes (*25*), indicating that fulminant type 1 diabetes is a very severe form of type 1 diabetes. Several lines of evidence suggest that both genetic and environmental factors contribute to the beta-cell death in this disease (Fig. 20.1). As shown in the previous section, fulminant type 1 diabetes is rare in children, suggesting less contribution of genetic factors in this subtype than in classic type 1A diabetes. However, genetic factors such as *HLA-DR/DQ* and *CTLA-4*, both associated with immune reactions, have already been identified as factors in the development of fulminant type 1 diabetes. The genetic factors contributing to the development of fulminant and classic type 1A diabetes are listed in Table 20.2.

The prevalence of HLA-DR/DQ in fulminant type 1 diabetic patients was investigated in a nationwide survey (*26*). DR4–DQ4

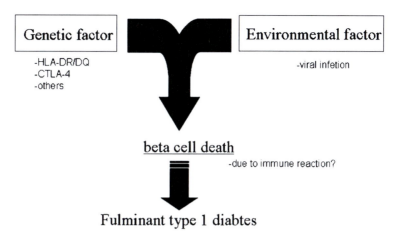

Fig. 20.1 Possible mechanism of beta-cell death in fulminant T1D.

Table 20.2

	Autoimmune	Fulminant
Susceptible HLA (Japanese)	DR9–DQ3	DR4–DQ4
(Caucasian)	DR3/DR4–DQ8	–
Resistance to DR2	Strong	Weak
INS VNTR	Class I	Unknown
CTLA-4	+49/G, CT60GG	CT60AA

(usually encoded by *DRB1*0405–DQB1*0401*) was observed in 41.8% of fulminant type 1 diabetic patients, which is significantly more frequent than its prevalence in the population as a whole. Both DR2–DQ1 (encoded by *DRB1*1501/*1502–DQB1*0602/*0601*) and DR8–DQ1 (encoded by *DRB1*0803–DQB1*0601*) were less frequently observed in fulminant type 1 diabetes. In type 1A diabetes, DR2–DQ1 was extremely rare, whereas DR9–DQ3 (encoded by *DRB1*0901–DQB1*0303*) was significantly more frequent. HLA-DR4–DQ1 (encoded by *DRB1*0401–DQB1*0302*) and DR3–DQ2 (encoded by *DRB1*0301–DQB1*0201*), which are susceptible haplotypes in Caucasian patients, were rare in fulminant, classic type 1A, and control subjects in Japanese populations (*27, 28*). In the combination analysis, the homozygote of DR4–DQ4 indicated a high odds ratio of 13.3 in fulminant type 1 diabetes. These results suggest that class II HLA contributes to the development of fulminant type 1 diabetes, but susceptibility and resistance of the class II HLA subtype to type 1 diabetes are distinct between fulminant and classic type 1A diabetes. The HLA-DR4–DQ4 haplotype is common in the Japanese population, but is rare in the Caucasian population, which might contribute to the different incidence of fulminant type 1 diabetes between Japanese and Caucasians. The role of class II HLA has been emphasized in the context of antigen-presenting processes in classic type 1A diabetes (*27*), but it remains to be elucidated in fulminant type 1 diabetes. Small pilot studies suggest that DR4–DQ4, which increases patient susceptibility to fulminant type 1 diabetes, is encoded by *DRB1*0405–DQB1*0401* (*29, 30*). On the other hand, no susceptibility or resistance to fulminant diabetes has been reported for HLA-A, a class I HLA.

Recently, differences in CTLA-4 gene polymorphisms were reported between fulminant type 1 diabetes and classic type 1A diabetes in Japan (*31*). Two polymorphisms had been reported in association with several autoimmune diseases, +49/G in the first exon, and CT60/G in the 3 untranslated region (*32, 33*). Fulminant type 1 diabetes was associated with the CT60AA subtype ($p = 0.021$, odd ratio 2.68) but not with the +49/G polymorphism. On the other hand, classical type 1A diabetes was associated with CT60GG ($p = 0.008$, odds ratio 1.89) and 49/GG ($p = 0.0005$, odds ratio 2.26) subtypes. Associations with these polymorphisms are also shown in Caucasian type 1 diabetes or autoimmune thyroid disease (*32, 33*). The mechanism regarding how CT60AA contributes to the development of fulminant type 1 diabetes is unknown; however, serum levels of soluble CTLA-4 were significantly lower in fulminant type 1 diabetes than those in classic type 1A diabetes and control subjects in this study.

These two genetic factors were found using the so-called candidate gene approach. Both HLA-DR/DQ and CTLA-4 were already known as genetic factors in Caucasian and Japanese type 1A diabetes. As an alternative approach, a genomewide association study would clarify the other genetic factors associated with fulminant type 1 diabetes.

As an environmental factor, viral infection could be involved in the pathogenesis of fulminant type 1 diabetes for the following reasons. First, a nationwide survey revealed that flu-like symptoms were observed in 71.2% of fulminant type 1 diabetic patients, whereas these symptoms were only observed in 26.9% of classic type 1A diabetic cases (*6*). Second, broad-reacting IgA antibody titers to enterovirus were significantly higher in fulminant type 1 diabetes than in either classic type 1A diabetes or controls, suggesting that fulminant type 1 diabetic patients are more susceptible to enterovirus infections than autoimmune diabetic patients and controls (*34*). Third, the encephalomyocarditis (EMC)-virus-induced diabetes model resembles fulminant type 1 diabetes in humans (*35*). Intraperitoneal injection of male DBA/2 mice with an EMC virus diabetic strain can induce a very rapid onset of diabetes with the involvement of exocrine tissue damage indicated by both histological findings and the high serum amylase level. In non-obese diabetic (NOD) mice, a model for classic type 1A diabetes, cellular infiltration is limited to the islet area (27). Fourth, several cases have been reported in which the onset of diabetes was accompanied by a reactivation of human herpesvirus (HHV)-6 (5, 12), the infection of herpes simplex virus (36), coxsackie B3 virus (37), influenza B virus (38), and mumps virus (39) in fulminant type 1 diabetes. Lastly, in a nationwide survey, the elevation of viral antibody was observed in 11 antibodies in 9 of 51 patients (i.e., cytomegalovirus Ig-M in three patients, rotavirus in two patients, and coxsackie virus type A4, A5, A6, and B1, Epstein–Barr virus Ig-M, HHV-6 Ig-M and Ig-G, HHV-7 Ig-G in one patient, respectively) (Table 20.3) (40). It is noteworthy that antibody titers to various viruses but not to a single virus was elevated around the disease onset in a subset of patients with fulminant type 1 diabetes. This finding suggests that immune reactions to virus might play more important roles in the development of fulminant diabetes than the virus itself, and pancreatic beta cells might be damaged in a by-stander manner, which has also been shown in the EMC-virus-induced diabetes model (41). Several case reports of various virus infections also support this hypothesis. Another hypothesis, that beta cells might be damaged by a single unknown virus, is also possible.

Viral infection is also emphasized in classic type 1A diabetes as a direct destroyer, a trigger of the immune reaction, or an additional destroyer of immunocytes. Detailed molecular mechanisms of diabetes involving viral infections should be clarified both in fulminant and in classic type 1A diabetes in the future.

Islet autoantibodies, a hallmark of type 1A diabetes, seldom appear in fulminant type 1 diabetes. In the extended nationwide survey, positivity for GAD antibodies was present only in 8.8% (16 of 182 patients) and IA-2 antibodies were not detected in fulminant diabetic patients at all (6). The contribution of GAD antibody positivity to the pathogenesis of fulminant type 1 diabetes is unknown. However, it might be produced in association with, and not be the cause of, beta-cell destruction in fulminant type 1 diabetes. These phenomena are also observed in subacute thyroiditis in which thyroid autoantibody is sometimes positive, but thyroid cells are damaged by a viral infection (42). Antibody to ZnT8, a novel autoantibody shown in 2007, was also negative in 34 patients with fulminant type 1 diabetes (43).

On the other hand, T-cell immunoreactivity to beta-cell antigens may be upregulated in fulminant type 1 diabetes after the onset of overt diabetes (44). The ELISPOT assay has revealed that GAD-reactive Th1 cells were identified in 69.2% of fulminant type 1 diabetes and in 46.9% of classic type 1A diabetes cases in peripheral blood mononuclear cells (45). The presence of these T cells does not necessarily mean that autoimmunity

Table 20.3

	Age	Sex	Associated symptoms	HLA-DR	Coxsackie virus	Rotavirus	CMV	EBV	HHV6	HHV7
1	77	F	Drowsiness, nausea, hypersensitivity syndrome	*1501/*1101	–	–	1.20 (IgM)	–	10 (IgM)	–
2	23	M	Drowsiness, nausea, upper abdominal pain, no diarrhea	*0405/–	–	x4/x16	–	–	–	–
3	45	F	Fever, nausea, upper abdominal pain	ND	–	–	–	–	–	x10/x80 (IgG)
4	57	M	Fever, nausea, upper abdominal pain, no diarrhea	*0405/–	–	<4/x8	–	3.2 (IgM)	x40/x160 (IgG)	–
5	38	M	Nausea, headache	ND	x16/x64 (A4) x16/x64 (B1)	–	–	–	–	–
6	34	M	ND	ND	x8/x32 (A6)	–	–	–	–	–
7	39	M	Fever, headache, upper abdominal pain	ND	x4/x16 (A5)	–	–	–	–	–
8	61	M	Fever, nausea, upper abdominal pain, diarrhea	ND	ND	ND	1.03 (IgM)	–	–	–
9	25	F	Fever, nausea, lower abdominal pain	ND	ND	ND	0.86 (IgM)	–	–	–

ND not determined, *CMV* cytomegalovirus, *EBV* Epstein–Barr virus, *HHV* human herpes virus plays a major role in the development of fulminant type 1 diabetes, but it is interesting that these T cells are present many years after the onset.

Of note, antibodies to exocrine pancreas were reported in patients with fulminant type 1 diabetes, although the number is small (*46*). Elevation of serum pancreatic amylase, lipase, elastase-1, or phospholipase level is usually observed around the onset of fulminant type 1 diabetes. Further examination would be necessary to clarify the contribution of abnormalities in the exocrine pancreas in the pathogenesis of fulminant type 1 diabetes.

Although the pathogenic role is unknown, hepatic dysfunction as defined by the elevated transaminase levels was common at the onset of fulminant type 1 diabetes (*1, 6*). Takaike et al. analyzed the data on liver transaminase from 108 patients with newly diagnosed type 1 diabetes complicated by ketosis, and 32 (60.4%) of 53 patients suffering from fulminant type 1 diabetes revealed a transient elevation of liver transaminase during the first month after starting insulin therapy. In the case of acute onset type 1 diabetes, this observation was noted in 16 (29.1%) of 55 patients. Fatty liver was found in 20% of the patients, and 65% of these patients exhibited transient elevation of liver transaminase (*47*).

THERAPY AND PROGNOSIS

Fulminant type 1 diabetes is usually accompanied by diabetic ketoacidosis as a result of acute insulin deficiency at the time of disease onset. Therefore, it is very important to diagnose fulminant type 1 diabetes without delay. After recovery from diabetic ketoacidosis, multiple insulin injection therapy is recommended. Owing to the complete loss of endogenous insulin secretion even at the onset of diabetes, some cases show brittleness in the blood glucose level. Nowadays, we are able to keep the hemoglobin A_{1c} level below 8%, even in patients with fulminant type 1 diabetes with intensive insulin therapy, by using ultra long-acting insulin analogs or continuous subcutaneous insulin injection (CSII) (Imagawa A et al., unpublished observation).

In a nationwide survey, insulin-secreting capacity did not recover in fulminant type 1 diabetic patients 5 years after its onset (*48*). No case of fulminant type 1 diabetes with a "honeymoon phase" was reported. Mean glycosylated hemoglobin levels were not significantly different between fulminant and classic type 1A diabetic patients (*6*).

Recently, we have shown that patients with fulminant type 1 diabetes are at a high-risk subgroup for diabetic microangiopathy (*49*). As part of a nationwide survey, 41 patients with fulminant type 1 diabetes and 76 age- and sex-matched patients with classic type 1A diabetes were followed. The 5-year cumulative incidence of microangiopathy was 24.4% in fulminant type 1 diabetes and 2.6% in type 1A diabetes (i.e., retinopathy was 9.8 vs. 0% ($p=0.014$), nephropathy 12.2 vs. 2.6% ($p=0.015$), and neuropathy 12.2 vs. 1.3% ($p=0.010$)). It is noteworthy that the mean HbA_{1c} levels were similar in the two groups during the follow-up periods (7.4 vs. 7.7%). However, the mean M value of 7 points blood glucose by self-monitoring, mean insulin dosages, and the frequency of severe hypoglycemic episodes were significantly higher, and the mean postprandial C-peptide level was significantly lower in the fulminant type 1 diabetes group. Irreversible loss of insulin production is associated with unstable blood glucose control and, therefore, there is a high incidence of diabetic complications in patients with low insulin production capacities. In addition, the lack of C-peptide itself might be also one of the causal factors in the development of microangiopathy in fulminant type 1 diabetic patients (*50*).

CONCLUSIONS

Fulminant type 1 diabetes mellitus was established in Japan by a hospital-based study in 2000 and by a nationwide survey in 2003. The accumulating evidence suggests that this subtype is the most severe subtype of diabetes, both from the pathological and the clinical points of view. Epidemiological data have increased in the past few years, but the pathogenesis of beta-cell death is still unknown. More studies are necessary to clarify the pathophysiology of fulminant type 1 diabetes.

ACKNOWLEDGMENT

We are indebted to the Osaka IDDM study group (shown in (*1*)) and the Committee of Japan Diabetes Society of the Research of Fulminant Type 1 Diabetes Mellitus [shown in (*6*)] for collaboration.

REFERENCES

1. Imagawa A, Hanafusa T, Miyagawa J, Matsuzawa Y, for the Osaka IDDM study group. A novel subtype of type 1 diabetes mellitus characterized by a rapid onset and an absence of diabetes-related antibodies. N Engl J Med 2000;342:301–307.
2. Imagawa A, Hanafusa T, Miyagawa J, Matsuzawa Y. A proposal of three distinct subtypes of type 1 diabetes mellitus based on clinical and pathological evidence. Ann Med 2000;32:539–543.
3. American Diabetes Association. Diagnosis and classification of diabetes mellitus. Diabetes Care 2008;31:S55–S60.
4. Alberti KG, Zimmet PZ. Definition, diagnosis classification of diabetes mellitus and its com-

plications. Part 1: diagnosis and classification of diabetes mellitus provisional report of a WHO consultation. Diabet Med 1998;15:539–553.
5. Sekine N, Motokura T, Oki T, et al. Rapid loss of insulin secretion in a patient with fulminant type 1 diabetes mellitus and carbamazepine hypersensitivity syndrome. JAMA 2001;285:1153–1154.
6. Imagawa A, Hanafusa T, Uchigata Y, et al. Fulminant type 1 diabetes: a nationwide survey in Japan. Diabetes Care 2003;26:2345–2352.
7. Hanafusa T, Imagawa A. Fulminant type 1 diabetes: a novel clinical entity requiring special attention by all medical practitioners. Nat Clin Pract Endocrinol Metab 2007;3:36–45.
8. Wenzlau JM, Juhl K, Yu L, et al. The cation efflux transporter ZnT8 (Slc30A8) is a major autoantigen in human type 1 diabetes. Proc Natl Acad Sci U S A 2007;104:17040–17045.
9. Takeda H, Kawasaki E, Shimizu I, et al. Clinical, autoimmune, and genetic characteristics of adult-onset diabetic patients with GAD autoantibodies in Japan (Ehime Study). Diabetes Care 2002;25:995–1001.
10. Cho YM, Kim JT, Ko KS, et al. Fulminant type 1 diabetes in Korea: high prevalence among patients with adult-onset type 1 diabetes. Diabetologia 2007;50:2276–2279.
11. Imagawa A, Hanafusa T. Fulminant type 1 diabetes-is it an Asian-oriented disease? Intern Med 2005;44:913–914.
12. Katsumata K, Katsumata K. A Chinese patient presenting with clinical signs of fulminant type 1 diabetes mellitus. Intern Med 2005;44:967–969.
13. Chiou CC, Chung WH, Hung SI, Yang LC, Hong HS. Fulminant type 1 diabetes mellitus caused by drug hypersensitivity syndrome with human herpesvirus 6 infection. J Am Acad Dermatol 2006;54:S14–S17.
14. Taniyama M, Katsumata R, Aoki K, Suzuki S. A Filipino patient with fulminant type 1 diabetes. Diabetes Care 2004;27:842–843.
15. Pozzilli P, Visalli N, Leslie D, IMDIAB Group. No evidence of rapid onset (Japanese) Type I diabetes in Caucasian patients. Diabetologia 2000;43:1332.
16. Maldonado M, Hampe CS, Gaur LK, et al. Ketosis-prone diabetes: dissection of a heterogeneous syndrome using an immunogenetic and β-cell functional classification, prospective analysis, and clinical outcomes. J Clin Endocrinol Metab 2003;88:5090–5098.
17. Balasubramanian K, Dabadghao P, Bhatia V, et al. High frequency of type 1B (idiopathic) diabetes in north Indian children with recent-onset diabetes. Diabetes Care 2003;26:2697–2697.
18. Moreau C, Drui D, Arnault-Ouary G, Charbonnel B, Chaillous L, Cariou B. Fulminant type 1 diabetes in Caucasians: a report of three cases. Diabetes Metab 2008;34:529–532.
19. Imagawa A, Hanafusa T, Iwahashi H, et al. Uniformity in clinical and HLA-DR status regardless of age and gender within fulminant type 1 diabetes. Diabetes Res Clin Pract 2008;82:233–237.
20. Urakami T, Nakagawa M, Morimoto S, Kubota S, Owada M, Harada K. A subtype of markedly abrupt onset with absolute insulin deficiency in idiopathic type 1 diabetes in Japanese children. Diabetes Care 2002;25:2353–2354.
21. Kida K, Mimura G, Kobayashi T, et al. ICA and organ-specific autoantibodies among Japanese patients with early-onset insulin-dependent diabetes mellitus – the JDS study. Diabetes Res Clin Pract 1994;23:187–193.
22. Otsubo M, Shiozawa T, Kimura K, Konishi I. Nonimmune "fulminant" type 1 diabetes presenting with diabetic ketoacidosis during pregnancy. Obstet Gynecol 2002;99:877–879.
23. Shimizu I, Makino H, Imagawa A, et al. Clinical and immunogenetic characteristics of fulminant type 1 diabetes associated with pregnancy. J Clin Endocrinol Metab 2006;91:471–476.
24. Kawasaki E, Shimizu I, Hanafusa T, et al. A nationwide survey of type 1 diabetes associated with pregnancy in Japan. Diabetes Pregnancy 2006;6:104–107 (in Japanese).
25. Sayama K, Imagawa A, Okita K, et al. Pancreatic beta and alpha cells are both decreased in patients with fulminant type 1 diabetes: a morphometrical assessment. Diabetologia 2005;48:1560–1564.
26. Imagawa A, Hanafusa T, Uchigata Y, et al. Different contribution of class II HLA in fulminant and typical autoimmune type 1 diabetes mellitus. Diabetologia 2005;48:294–300.
27. Eisenbarth GS, Polonsky KS, Buse JB. Type 1 diabetes mellitus. In: Reed Larsen P, et al., eds. Williams Textbook of Endocrinology. 11th ed. Philadelphia, PA: Saunders, 2008:1391–1416.
28. Ikegami H, Ogihara T. Genetics of insulin-dependent diabetes mellitus. Endocr J 1996;43:605–613.
29. Tanaka S, Kobayashi T, Nakanishi K, et al. Association of HLA-DQ genotype in autoantibody-negative and rapid-onset type 1 diabetes. Diabetes Care 2002;25:2302–2307.
30. Nakamura T, Nagasaka S, Kusaka I, Yatagai T, Yang J, Ishibashi S. HLA-DR-DQ haplotype in rapid-onset type 1 diabetes in Japanese. Diabetes Care 2003;6:1640–1641.
31. Kawasaki E, Imagawa A, et al. Differences in the contribution of CTLA4 gene to susceptibility

31. to fulminant and type 1A diabetes in Japanese patients. Diabetes Care 2008;31: 1608–1610.
32. Ueda H, Howson JM, Esposito L, et al. Association of the T-cell regulatory gene CTLA4 with susceptibility to autoimmune disease. Nature 2003;423:506–511.
33. Kavvoura FK, Akamizu T, Awata T, et al. Cytotoxic T-lymphocyte associated antigen 4 gene polymorphisms and autoimmune thyroid disease: a meta-analysis. J Clin Endocrinol Metab 2007;92:3162–3170.
34. Imagawa A, Hanafusa T, Makino H, Miyagawa JI, Juto P. High titres of IgA antibodies to enterovirus in fulminant type-1 diabetes. Diabetologia 2005;48:290–293.
35. Shimada A, Maruyama T. Encephalomyocarditis-virus-induced diabetes model resembles "fulminant" type 1 diabetes in humans. Diabetologia 2004;47:1854–1855.
36. Nagaoka T, Terada M, Miyakoshi H. Insulin-dependent diabetes mellitus following acute pancreatitis caused by herpes simplex virus; a case report. J Japan Diab Soc 2001;44: 335–340 (in Japanese).
37. Nishida W, Hasebe S, Kawamura R, Hashiramoto M, Onuma H, Osawa H, Makino H. A case of fulminant type 1 diabetes associated with high titer of coxsackie B3 virus antibody. J Japan Diab Soc 2005;48(Suppl 1):A23–A27 (in Japanese).
38. Sano H, Terasaki J, Tsutsumi C, Imagawa A, Hanafusa T. A case of fulminant type 1 diabetes mellitus after influenza B infection. Diabetes Res Clin Pract 2008;79:e8–e9.
39. Goto A, Takahashi Y, Kishimoto M, et al. A case of fulminant type 1 diabetes associated with significant elevation of mumps titers. Endocr J 2008;55:561–564.
40. Hanafusa T, Imagwa A, Iwahashi H, et al. Report of the committee of Japan Diabetes Society on the research of fulminant type 1 diabetes mellitus: analysis of anti-viral antibodies around the disease onset. J Japan Diab Soc 2008;51:531–536 (in Japanese).
41. Jun HS, Yoon JW. The role of viruses in type I diabetes: two distinct cellular and molecular pathogenic mechanisms of virus-induced diabetes in animals. Diabetologia 2001;44:271–285.
42. Pearce EN, Farwell AP, Braverman LE. Thyroiditis. N Engl J Med 2003;348: 2646–2655. Erratum in 349:620.
43. Kawasaki E, Nakamura H, et al. ZnT8 antibody in type 1 diabetes. Abstract book of the 6th meeting of the Japanese Study Group of Type 1 diabetes. 2008:31 (in Japanese).
44. Shimada A, Morimoto J, Kodama K, et al. T-cell-mediated autoimmunity may be involved in fulminant type 1 diabetes. Diabetes Care 2002;25:635–636.
45. Kotani R, Nagata M, Imagawa A, et al. T lymphocyte response against pancreatic beta cell antigens in fulminant Type 1 diabetes. Diabetologia 2004;47:1285–1291.
46. Taniguchi T, Okazaki K, Okamoto M, et al. Autoantibodies against the exocrine pancreas in fulminant type 1 diabetes. Pancreas 2005;30: 191–192.
47. Takaike H, Uchigata Y, Iwamoto Y, et al. Nationwide survey to compare the prevalence of transient elevation of liver transaminase during treatment of diabetic ketosis or ketoacidosis in new-onset acute and fulminant type 1 diabetes mellitus. Ann Med 2008;40:395–400.
48. Murase-Mishiba Y, Imagawa A, Hanafusa T. Fulminant type 1 diabetes as a model of nature to explore the role of C-peptide. Exp Diabetes Res 2008;8191:23.
49. Murase Y, Imagawa A, Hanafusa T, et al. Fulminant type 1 diabetes as a high risk group for diabetic microangiopathy – a nationwide 5-year-study in Japan. Diabetologia 2007;50: 531–537.
50. Wahren J, Ekberg K, Jörnvall H. C-peptide is a bioactive peptide. Diabetologia 2007;50: 503–509.

Chapter 21

Insulin Autoimmune Syndrome (Hirata Disease)

Yasuko Uchigata and Yukimasa Hirata

Summary

The insulin autoimmune syndrome (IAS), or Hirata's disease, is characterized by the combination of fasting hypoglycemia, high concentration of total immunoreactive insulin, and presence of autoantibodies to native human insulin in serum. Since Hirata et al. first described the disease in 1970, there have been 330 reported cases of IAS during the past 37 years in Japan. IAS is the third leading cause of spontaneous hypoglycemia in Japan while only 47 cases in Caucasians and 20 cases in East Asians excluding Japanese have been reported in the past 37 years. Insulin autoantibodies production is classified as monoclonal or polyclonal, with the majority of IAS cases classified as polyclonal. A striking association between human leukocyte antigen (HLA) class II alleles DRB1*0406/DQA1*0301/DQB1*0302 and Japanese IAS cases with polyclonal insulin autoantibodies, which we found in 1992, has been well confirmed. Glutamate at position 74 in the HLA-DR4β1-chain was shown to be essential to the production of polyclonal insulin autoantibodies in IAS, whereas alanine at the same position of the HLA-DRβ1-chain might be important in the production of monoclonal insulin autoantibodies. Another interesting finding is an exposure of reducing compounds with SH group ahead of development of IAS. After reducing human insulin, T-cell recognized fragmented human insulin molecule in the context of DRB1*0406 molecules. Although methimazole was a representative reducing compound for the development of IAS before 2003, an increasing number of alfa lipoic acid-induced IAS has been recently remarkable.

Key Words: Transglutaminase autoantibodies, HLA (human leukocyte antigen), HLA-DR3, gliadin, gluten-free diet genetics

INTRODUCTION

Although HLA and disease association has been studied for a tremendous number of diseases, only four diseases have been identified in which almost all patients have the same HLA antigen; B27 in 88% of ankylosing spondylitis (1), DR4 in 91% of patients with pemphigus vulgaris (2), DR2 in 100% of patients with narcolepsy (3), and DRw52a in 100% of patients with primary sclerosing cholangitis (4). When the first patient with spontaneous hypoglycemia associated with the production of insulin autoantibodies, so-called insulin autoimmune syndrome (IAS), was reported in Japan by Hirata et al. (5) in 1970, no one could forecast that IAS was the fifth disease with such a strong HLA association. Many questions were raised by the first case, including its differential diagnosis from factitious hypoglycemia, the causes of this syndrome, the mechanisms to produce hypoglycemia in this syndrome and so on, raised doubt whether IAS was a "disease." Immediately after the first patient was diagnosed with IAS, several other patients with the same symptoms and findings were reported over 5 years (6–9). The strong association of IAS with HLA-DR4 (10) gave IAS a citizenship of "disease," which was named Hirata's disease. One hundred and ninety-seven Japanese IAS patients have been registered from 1970 to 1992 (11), a total of 226 Japanese IAS patients have been registered until the end of 1996, and a total of 330 have been registered until the end of 2007 from the database of Japan Centra Revuo Medicina or personal communication. Besides the analysis of those reports, several studies concerning the cases of IAS and the hypoglycemia have been clarified by us.

INSULIN AUTOIMMUNE SYNDROME AS THE THIRD LEADING CAUSE OF SPONTANEOUS HYPOGLYCEMIA IN JAPAN

To determine the further characteristics of IAS in Japanese, we performed two nationwide surveys to identify the causes of cases with spontaneous hypoglycemia. Questionnaires were sent to 2,094 hospitals with more than 200 beds; the first, from 1979 to 1981, and the second, from 1985 to 1987. The first and the second surveys revealed the same results (12). Cases with hypoglycemia showed three main causes for the hypoglycemic attacks: insulinoma, extrapancreatic neoplasms, and IAS. IAS was found to be the third leading cause of spontaneous hypoglycemia in Japan. The third survey will be performed in 2009.

ONSET AGE AND SEX DISTRIBUTION, AND DURATION OF HYPOGLYCEMIA OF 330 JAPANESE IAS PATIENTS REGISTERED IN JAPAN FROM 1970 TO 2007

The records of 197 patients with IAS reported from 1970 to 1992 (11) and 133 patients from 1993 to 2007 were analyzed. The records of a total of 330 patients were obtained from the nationwide hypoglycemia surveys, abstracts in local or national medical congress, and personal communications to us.

Age of onset and sex distribution of the 330 patients are listed in Table 21.1. The age distribution was wide at the onset of IAS. The peak age of onset was 60–69 years for both sexes; there was no remarkable sex difference in the other age distribution except

Table 21.1
Age at Onset and Sex Distribution in Japanese IAS Patients, 1970–2007

IAS patient

Age at onset	Male (n)	Female (n)	Total
0–9	0	2	2
10–19	1	1	2
20–29	6	18	24
30–39	12	16	28
40–49	22	31	53
50–59	32	32	64
60–69	39	42	81
70–79	34	22	46
80–89	4	11	15
Total	155	175	330

20- to 29-year group, in which 75% were female IAS patients. It seems that the 20- to 29-year group had a larger number of female patients with Graves' disease. Such female dominancy has been confirmed from our previous report.

The duration of the transient and spontaneous hypoglycemia was shown to be less than 1 month in approximately 30% of the patients, more than 1 month and less than 3 months in 40% of the patients (11). A few of the patients have continued mild hypoglycemic attacks for more than 1 year.

The geographic distribution of IAS in Japan showed no characteristic pattern in the areas of residence of the patients.

DRUG EXPOSURE AHEAD OF DEVELOPMENT OF IAS AND ASSOCIATED DISEASES

As Hirata already noted in 1983, patients with Graves' disease who had received methimazole (MTZ) had a predisposition to develop IAS (13). In addition to methimazole (MTZ) for the treatment of Graves' disease, α-mercaptopropionyl glycine (MPG) for the treatment of chronic hepatitis, dermatitis, cataract and rheumatoid arthritis, and glutathione (GTT) for urticaria, which contained the sulfhydryl (SH) group, were proposed to be related to the development of IAS (11). Approximately 42% of Japanese IAS patients had received the drugs with SH group (Table 21.2).

Table 21.2
Drugs Exposure Ahead of the Development of Japanese IAS and Associated Diseases from 1970 to 2007, Total $n = 189$

Drugs	Diseases	n
Methimazole (MTZ)[a]	Graves' disease	64
α-Mercaptopropionyl glycine (MPG)[a]	Chronic liver dysfunction	33
α-Mercaptopropionyl glycine (MPG)[a]	Cataract	6
α-Mercaptopropionyl glycine (MPG)[a]	Dermatitis	5
α-Mercaptopropionyl glycine (MPG)[a]	Rheumatoid arthritis	2
Glutathione (GTT)[a]	Urticaria	8
Captopril[a]	Hypertension	1
Acegratone	Urinary bladder carcinoma	1
Steroid	Polymyositis	1
Interferon-α	Renal cell carcinoma	1
Loxoprofen sodium	Rheumatiod polymyositis/lumbar pain	1
Alfa lipoic acid[a]	Dieting/anti-aging supplement	17
S-Arylmercaptocysteine[a] in garlic	Tonic supplement	1
Miscellaneous		48

[a]Contains sulfhydryl compounds itself or after decomposition

After such drugs were discontinued, the hypoglycemic attacks subsided. We have four IAS patients who developed IAS at the second treatment after the interruption of MTZ therapy, one IAS patient who developed the disease after the third challenge (after two interruptions of MTZ therapy), and one IAS patient at both the first and the second MTZ treatment. Another three patients redeveloped IAS at MPG challenge (14). Such evidence may support the breakdown of T-cell immunotolerance in the circumstance described above.

We propose a new concept of disease entitled "drug-induced insulin autoimmune syndrome." Although MTZ had been a representative SH compound, as a drug exposed before the development of IAS as described above, an IAS patient induced by alfa lipoic acid was found in 2003 and an increasing number of alfa lipoic acid-induced IAS have been recently remarkable (15). Among 56 IAS patients from 2004 to 2007, MTZ for Graves' disease was prescribed for 11 IAS patients and alfa lipoic acid for dieting or anti-aging supplement for 17 IAS patients (15). By the end of 2007, there was another IAS patient with a history of taking alfa lipoic acid.

CLINICAL FEATURES OF IAS PATIENTS OUT OF JAPAN

Although there have been 330 IAS patients reported from 1970 to 2007 in Japan, 20 IAS patients have been reported in East Asians excluding Japanese patients (Table 21.3). Sixteen of 20 IAS patients have associated with Graves' disease with the treatment of MTZ or CMZ (Carbimazole), which is converted to MTZ in the body. Such patients were females and developed IAS at a younger age. HLA class II in three of them were analyzed, which was compatible with that in Japanese IAS patients and insulin autoantibodies were all polyclonal, as described later.

Table 21.3
Clinical Features in IAS Cases in East Asians Except Japanese

Patient	Age	Sex	Disease/drug	Race	Reference
1	5	M	Vasculitis?	Chinese	(31)
2	48	F	Graves'/MTZ*	Chinese	(31)
3	31	F	Graves'/MTZ*	Korean	(32)
4	18	F	Graves'/MTZ*	Chinese	(33)
5	67	F	–	Chinese	(34)
6	28	F	Graves'/MTZ*	Chinese	(34)
7	26	F	Graves'/MTZ*	Chinese	(34)
8	24	F	Graves'/MTZ*	Chinese	(34)
9	21	F	Graves'/MTZ*	Chinese	Unpublished[a]
10	11	F	Hashimoto/	Chinese	Unpublished[b]
11	34	M	Graves'/MTZ*	Chinese	(35)
12	26	F	Graves'/MTZ/CMZ*	Chinese	(36)
13	27	F	Graves'/MTZ/CMZ*	Chinese	(36)
14	27	M	Graves'/MTZ/CMZ*	Chinese	(36)
15	38	M	Graves'/MTZ/CMZ*	Chinese	(36)
16	31	F	Graves'/MTZ/CMZ*	Chinese	(36)
17	36	F	Graves'/MTZ/CMZ*	Chinese	(36)
18	27	F	Graves'/CMZ*	Chinese	(37)
19	44	F	Graves'/MTZ*	Chinese	(38)
20	00	–	Pulmonary TB/INH	Chinese	(39)

[a] Unpublished, kindly provided by Dr. Lin in Taiwan
[b] Unpublished, kindly provided by Dr. Wacharasindhu in Thailand

So far, 37 IAS patients in Caucasians have been reported in the past 37 years (Table 21.4). CMZ for the treatment of Graves' disease, penicillamine for the treatment of rheumatoid arthritis, pyritinol for the treatment of RA, and Penicillin G for tonsillitis were administered to six IAS patients, which all contained SH group. Insulin autoantibodies of nine IAS patients so far examined were monoclonal as described later.

Table 21.4
Clinical Features in IAS Cases Out of Asia

Patient	Age	Sex	Disease/drug	Race	Reference
1[a]	42	M	Pulmonary TB/INH	Norwegian	(7)
2	58	F	RA/?	White	(40)
3	43	F	–	Hispanic	(40)
4	3	M	–	?	(40)
5	26	F	–	White	(40)
6	48	F	Brain damage	White	(40)
7	5	M	–	Hispanic	(41)
8	82	F	Lupus/hydralazine	White	(42)
9	61	F	RA/asthma/penicillamine*	White	(43)
10[a]	55	F	Graves'/CMZ*	White	(43)
11	44	M	Pulmonary TB/INH	Morocco	(44)
12	84	F	RA/pyritinol*	White	(45)
13	74	M	Hypertension/hydralazine	Black	(46)
14	NS	NS	–	White	(47)
15	NS	NS	–	White	(47)
16	NS	NS	–	White	(47)
17	NS	NS	–	White	(47)
18	NS	NS	–	White	(48)
19	33	NS	RA/penicillamine*	White	(49)
20	NS	NS	RA/pyritinol*	White	(50)
21	NS	NS	–	White	(51)

(continued)

Table 21.4 (continued)

Patient	Age	Sex	Disease/drug	Race	Reference
22	63	M	–	White	(52)
23[a]	57	F	–	White	(53)
24[a]	5	M	–	White	(54)
25[a]	79	M	Malaria/?	White	Unpublished[b]
26	45	F	–	White	(22)
27	48	F	–	White	(55)
28	68	M	Urosepsis/imipenem	White	(56)
29	24	F	Tonsillitis/penicillin G*	White	(57)
30[a]	19	F	–	White	(57)
31	?	?	Systemic sclerosis/ penicillamine*	White	(58)
32	72	M	–	White	(59)
33[a]	45	F	–	White	(22)
34	–	–	Alcoholic cirrhosis	White	(60)
35	53	F	Rheumatoid disease/?	White	(61)
36	52	–	–	White	(62)
37	–	–	–	White	(63)
38	81	M	–	White	(64)
37	69	F	–	White	(65)
38	62	F	Hepatitis C/?	White	(66)
39	56	M	–	White	(67)
40[a]	73	F	SLE/?	White	(68)
41[a]	61	M	Ulcerative colitis	White	(68)
42	46	F	–	White	(68)
43	64	F	–	White	(68)
44	84	F	–	White	(68)
45	75	F	Graves?/PTU	White	(68)
46	72	F	–	White	(68)
47	55	M	–	White	(69)

RA rheumatoid arthritis, *INH* isoniatid, *TB* tuberculosis, – not stated, or no associated disease, *Imipenem* beta-lactam antibiotic, *PTU* propylthiouracil
[a]Monoclonal insulin autoantibody
[b]Unpublished by Dozio from Italy

INSULIN AND INSULIN AUTOANTIBODY IN THE SERA OF THE PATIENTS WITH IAS

The insulin in the sera of IAS patients was found to be native human insulin by HPLC analysis (*16*). The evidence that IAS patients after spontaneous remission had no hypoglycemia nor hyperglycemia may support that insulin in the sera of IAS patients is true human and not abnormal human insulin.

Figure 21.1 shows total extractable IRI (immunoreactive insulin) that consists of insulin free from insulin antibody and

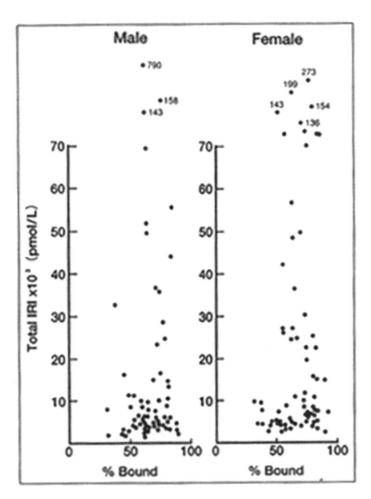

Fig. 21.1 Total extractable immunoreactive insulin (IRI), and ^{125}I-insulin binding percent of the sera of male and female patients, immediately after the diagnosis of insulin autoimmune syndrome (IAS). The methods for the IRI and ^{125}I-human insulin binding assay have been described elsewhere. At the diagnosis of IAS, the peak of the hypoglycemic attacks had been passed. The normal range of total IRI and ^{125}I-insulin binding was <71.8 pmol/L and <5%, respectively.

insulin bound to insulin antibody and ^{125}I-insulin binding of the sera of patients with IAS. The IRI levels during hypoglycemic attacks were quite enormous (8). A time course of total IRI and insulin autoantibody in the serum was clarified in a Japanese patient with IAS (17). When hypoglycemia was severe, Scatchard analysis of the insulin antibodies showed that a high-affinity (k1)/low-capacity (b1) population of the antibodies was changed to relatively low affinity with very high binding capacity compared with the same population of antibodies in insulin-treated diabetic patient (17). When the attacks were relieved, the total IRI was decreased, and the high-affinity (k1)/low-capacity (b1) population of antibodies showed a higher affinity constant and a lower binding capacity than those during the attacks (17).

A possible monoclonal insulin autoantibody in another Japanese patient with IAS which was of IgG1(γ) subclass and has a very low affinity constant and a large binding capacity against human insulin was found to be directed at a determinant at the asparagine site on insulin B-chain (18). One of idiotypic antibodies against the insulin autoantibody was found to express insulin action through the insulin receptor (19).

TWO GROUPS OF IAS DEFINED BY CLONALITY OF INSULIN AUTOANTIBODIES

The immunoglobulin class, the subclass, and the light chain types of insulin autoantibodies were examined (20). All insulin autoantibodies belonged to the IgG group with various ratios of κ:λ light chains.

Insulin autoantibodies from IAS patients were classified as polyclonal or monoclonal on the basis of affinity curves for binding to human insulin (Scatchard analysis) and presence of solitary light chain. So far, insulin autoantibodies in 2 among 330 Japanese IAS patients, 1 Norwegian, 1 Swiss, 3 Italian IAS patients (21), and 1 Netherlander IAS patient (22) were shown to have a single binding affinity to human insulin in Scatchard analysis, which means monoclonality (Table 21.4). In addition, three IAS patients out of Asia were found to have monoclonal insulin autoantibody from the literature (Table 21.4). On the other hand, Japanese IAS patients, in general, showed polyclonal autoantibodies to human insulin (Table 21.5) (21). Two Korean, one Chinese, and one Thai IAS patients were shown to possess a polyclonal insulin autoantibody. It is likely that the incidence of polyclonal IAS is relatively high among East Asians including Japan, whereas monoclonal IAS is more prevalent in Caucasians.

Table 21.5
Summary of Clinical Characteristics of IAS Polyclonal Responders at the Onset of IAS

Ethnic background	Patient no.	Age (years)	T-IRI sex	I-Insulin (pmol/1 × 10³)	Binding (%)	Drug	Associated disease	HLA-DR
Japanese	1	26	F	114.3	69	MTZ	Graves'	4, –
Japanese	2	52	F	54.1	73	GTG	Bronchial asthma	4, 13
Japanese	3	47	M	23.4	79	–	–	4, 9
Japanese	4	58	M	0.8	48	–	–	4, –
Japanese	5	54	F	60.0	70	MTZ	Graves'	4, –
Japanese	6	36	M	8.2	59	–	–	4, 9
Japanese	7	45	F	7.2	32	MTZ	Graves' Hashimot's IgA nephropathy	4, 8
Japanese	8	62	M	12.6	69	–	–	4, 9
Japanese	9	54	M	4.4	81	MPG	Liver dysfunction	2, 4
Japanese	10	61	F	5.1	72	MPG	Cataract	4, 9
Japanese	11	44	M	3.0	70	MPG	Dermatitis	2, 4
Japanese	12	39	F	2.7	69	MTZ	Graves'	4, –
Japanese	13	69	M	12.3	65	–	–	4, 6
Japanese	14	57	F	2.8	51	–	–	4, 9
Japanese	15	68	F	11.7	68	MPG	Liver dysfunction	4, 8

Insulin Autoimmune Syndrome (Hirata Disease)

Japanese	16	48	M	11.1	81	MTZ	Graves' Drug-induced arthritis	4, –
Japanese	17	64	M	4.6	82	MPG	Dermatitis	4, 13
Japanese	18	58	F	12.0	81	–	–	4, 12
Japanese	19	49	M	11.9	48	MPG	Liver dysfunction	4, 12
Japanese	20	69	F	167.2	67	TBM	NIDDM	4, –
Japanese	21	55	M	0.9	48	MPG	Liver dysfunction	4, 8
Japanese	22	53	F	35.0	55	–	–	4, 9
Japanese	23	69	M	47.0	65	MTZ	Graves'	4, 8
Japanese	24	36	F	192.5	79	MTZ	Graves'	2, 4
Japanese	25	43	F	23.0	57	MTZ	Graves'	4, –
Japanese	26	68	M	5.4	64	MPG	Liver dysfunction	4, 6
Japanese	27	66	F	21.0	57	MPG	Cataract	4, 9
Japanese	28	49	F	18.0	83	MTZ	Graves'	4, –
Japanese	29	54	M	3.4	67	MPG	Liver dysfunction	4, –
Japanese	30	70	F	46.8	94	MTZ	Graves'	4, –
Japanese	31	67	F	120.0	80	–	–	4, 8
Japanese	32	50	F	1.7	64	GTT	Urticaria	1, 4
Japanese	33	52	M	13.3	38	–	–	4, 6
Japanese	34	74	M	5.2	78	–	–	4, –
Japanese	35	54	M	3.0	76	–	–	4, 8

(continued)

Table 21.5 (continued)

Ethnic background	Patient no.	Age (years)	T-IRI sex	I-Insulin (pmol/1 × 10³)	Binding (%)	Drug	Associated disease	HLA-DR
Japanese	36	79	M	3.1	70	–	–	2, 4
Japanese	37	49	F	1.4	88	–	NIDDM	4, 9
Japanese	38	59	M	24.3	69	MPG	Liver dysfunction	4, 8
Japanese	39	66	M	6.2	91	–	Hypertension	4, –
Japanese	40	84	F	5.0	73	MPG	Liver dysfunction	4, 6
Japanese	41	42	F	2.5	24	MPG	Liver dysfunction	4, 6
Japanese	42	71	F	5.1	67	–	–	4, 15
Japanese	43	70	F	4.5	84	INF-α	Renal cell carcinoma	4, 8
Japanese	44	65	M	1.1	50	–	–	4, 8
Japanese	45	64	M	9.3	48	Steroid	Polymyositis	9, –
Japanese	46	49	F	5.4	75	–	–	2, 4
Japanese	47	71	M	3.0	68	MPG	Liver cirrhosis	4, 12
Japanese	48	81	M	1.4	92	–	–	4, 14
Japanese	49	77	M	0.7	64	Aceglatone	Urinary bladder carcinoma	9, –
Japanese	50	71	F	7.4	80	AHT drugs	Hypertension	4, 6
Korean	1	61	F	12.0	90	MTZ	Graves'	4, –

Korean	2	31	F	8.9	62	MTZ	Graves'	4, 9
Chinese	1	18	F	36.4	82	MTZ	Graves'	4, –
White American	1	61	F	4.8	1:64[a]	PNC	Rheumatoid arthritis	4, 5

Hypoglycemic attacks occurred 6 weeks after drug administration. All patients have remained healthy because of the resolution of hypoglycemic attacks. Abdominal computed tomography, abdominal ultrasound, abdominal angiography, and pancreatic cholangiography examinations performed in six patients failed to reveal the presence of pancreatic tumor. Total immunoreactive insulin (T-IRI) (normal range, <5 mU/ml) and I-labeled human insulin binding (normal range, <5%) were measured as previously described. Methimazole (MTZ) was administered orally for the treatment of Graves' disease. Gold thioglucose (GTG) was administered intramuscularly for the treatment of bronchial asthma. α-Mercaptopropionyl glycine (MPG) was administered orally for the treatment of liver dysfunction, cataracts, or dermatitis. Only one tablet (50 mg) of tolbutamide (TBM) was administered intravenously for the treatment of urticaria. Interferon-α (IFN-α) was administered intravenously for the treatment of renal cell carcinoma. The anti-cancer drug aceglatone was administered orally for the treatment of urinary bladder carcinoma. Japanese patient 50 was taking antihypertensive (AHT) drugs when IAS was developed. Penicillamine (PNC) was administered orally for the treatment of rheumatoid arthritis. Japanese patients 33, 36, 42, and 48 possessed the DRB1*0403 allele. Japanese patient 37 and the white American patient possessed the RB1*0407 allele. The remaining patients, with the exception of Japanese patients 45 and 49 (DR9 homozygotes), possessed the DRB1*0406 allele

[a]1:64 was expressed as positive

CRITICAL AMINO ACIDS FOR IAS POLYCLONAL RESPONDER AND IMPORTANCE OF DR GENE PRODUCTS IN THE PRESENTATION OF HUMAN INSULIN ANTIGEN

As reported in the study of serological typing of 27 Japanese IAS patients, Cw4/B62/DR4 was a highly prevalent allelic combination (*10*). Table 21.5 shows the summary of clinical characteristics of IAS polyclonal responders at the onset of IAS, which we examined. Japanese IAS polyclonal responders (except patients 45 and 49) possessed HLA-DR4/DQ3, whereas the remaining two (patients 45 and 49) possessed DR9/DQ3 and not DR4; the American white polyclonal responder possessed DR4/DQ3 (Table 21.5). Ninety-six percent (48/50) of Japanese IAS patients had DR4 (odds ratio, 39.9; $p < 10^{-4}$). DR9 was positive in 12 (24%) Japanese IAS patients, although this was not significant when compared with Japanese healthy controls (odds ratio, 0.8; $p > 0.65$).

The 48 DR4-positive Japanese IAS polyclonal responders consisted of 42 DRB1*0406-positive, 5 DRB1*0403-positive, and 1 DRB1*0407-positive patients (Table 21.6). All 48 DR4-positive Japanese IAS polyclonal responders possessed DQA1*0301/DQB1*0302 regardless of the differences in DR4 alleles. The two Korean and the Chinese IAS polyclonal responders were also positive for DRB1*0406/DQA1*0301/DQB1*0302. The phenotype of the American polyclonal responder was DRB1*0407/DQA1*0301/DQB1*0301. Thus, the DR4-positive IAS polyclonal responders possessed DRB1*0406, DRB1*0403, or DRB1*0407 for DR4 alleles, and DQA1*0301/DQB1*0302 or DQA1*0301/DQB1*0301 for DQ3 alleles.

For only DRB1*0406 individuals, incidence of B62/Cw4 was compared in Japanese IAS polyclonal responders and Japanese healthy controls. Sixty-seven percent (28/42) of Japanese IAS polyclonal responders had B62/Cw4, and 56% (5/9) of controls had B62/Cw4 (odds ratio, 1.6; 95% confidence interval, 0.37–6.91). It inculcates that the class I alleles are less important.

The differences in DQβ1 alleles encoding DQ3 among the IAS polyclonal responders suggest that DQ α- and DQ β-chains are not important in the development of IAS. We showed that T cells from polyclonal IAS patients with DRB1*0406/DQA1*0301/DQB1*0302 alleles proliferated in the presence of autologous antigen-presenting cells that had been exposed to 40 μM human insulin (*23*). The proliferative response of T cells was completely blocked by anti-HLA-DR but not by anti-HLA-DQ monoclonal antibodies (Fig. 21.2) (*24*). Moreover, experiments with DRB1*0406 transfectants supported the view that

Table 21.6
Incidence of DRB1 Alleles, Glu⁷⁴ in DRB1-chain, and DBQ1 Alleles in Japanese IAS Polyclonal Responders and Control Subjects

	IAS patients (n = 50)	Control (n = 106)	OR (95% confidence interval)	DRB1-chain amino acid residue 37	74	86
DRB1 allele						
DR4	48 (96)	40 (38)	39.6 (9.12–171)	–	–	–
DR9	12 (24)	29 (27)	0.8 (0.39–1.82)	Asn	Glu	Gly
DRB1*0406	42 (84)	9 (8)	56.6 (20.4–156)	Ser	Glu	Val
DRB1*0403	5 (10)	7 (7)	1.6 (0.47–5.22)	Tyr	Glu	Val
DRB1*0407	1 (2)	2 (2)	1.1 (0.09–12.0)	Tyr	Glu	Gly
Glu⁷⁴ in β-chain	50 (100)	70 (66)	52.3 (6.95–393)	–	–	–
DRQ1 allele						
DQA1*0301	50 (100)	74 (70)	44.1 (5.84–332)	–	–	–
DQB1*0302	48 (96)	26 (25)	73.8 (16.8–325)	–	–	–
DQA1*0301/ DQB1*0302	48 (96)	23 (22)	86.6 (18.8–380)	–	–	–

Data are n (%) or OR (95% confidence interval)

DR gene products participate in the presentation of human insulin antigens (24) (Table 21.7).

The HLA-DRβ1-chains encoded by DRB1*0406, DRB1*0403, and DRB1*0407 share a sequence motif (Leu-Leu-Glu-Gln-Arg-Arg-Ala-Glu) that spans the amino acid residues 67–74 of the third hypervariable region. The two DR9/DQ3 Japanese IAS polyclonal responders (patients 45 and 49) were DRB1*0901/DQA1*0301/DQB1*0303 homozygous. The products of DRB1*0406, DRB1*0403, and DRB1*0901 share the sequence motif Arg-Arg-Ala-Glu, corresponding to amino acid residues 71–74 of the DRβ1-chain. Comparison of this region of the DRβ1-chain and other DRB1 allele products reveals that Arg⁷¹ and especially Glu⁷⁴ may be important for polyclonal insulin autoantibody production in IAS, whereas residues 72 and 73 (Arg-Ala) are common in most of the DRB1 molecules (Table 21.5).

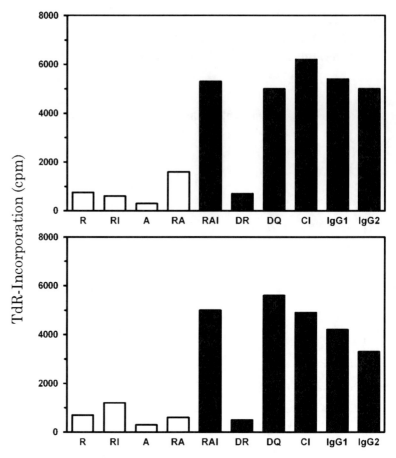

Fig. 21.2 T-cell responses (*top* from donor MI and *bottom* from donor SO) to human insulin blocked by anti-HLA-DR monoclonal antibody (mAb). Results represent the mean of triplicate (SD < 15% of the mean). *R* enriched T cells, *RI* R+ human insulin, *A* antigen-presenting cells, *DR* R+A+I+anti-HLA-DRmAb, *DQ* R+A+I+anti-HLA-DQmAB, *CI* R+A+I+anti-HLA class I mAb, *IgG1* R+A+I+mouse IgG1, *IgG2a* R+A+I+mouse IgG2a.

DIFFERENT AMINO ACIDS FOR IAS MONOCLONAL RESPONDER

The IAS monoclonal responder group consisted of six patients: one Japanese, one Norwegian, one Swiss, and three Italians (Table 21.8). Three of the six IAS monoclonal responders were DR4-positive, and their class II phenotypes were DRB1*0405/DQA1*0301/DQB1*0401, DRB1*0401/DQA1*0301/DQB1*0301, and DRB1*0402/DQA1*0301/DQB1*0301 (Table 21.8). The remaining three IAS monoclonal responders had non-DR4 and non-DR9 phenotypes. The IAS monoclonal responders, not Glu[74] but Ala,[74] as well as Asp[57] and Gly,[86] on the DRB1-chain were shared by the six monoclonal responders.

Table 21.7
HLA-DRB1*0406-Transfected L Cells Can Present Human Insulin to Enriched T Cell from a Healthy Donor or an IAS Patient with DRB1*0406 in the Presence of DTT[a]

	DRB1*	[3H]Thymidine incorporation (cpm)				
		R only	R+L	R+L+DTT	R+L+HI	R+L+HI+DTT
IAS patients						
IS	0406	1,834±23	905±79	1,554±138	16,267±306	12,692±374
SM	0406	2,396±199	5,167±263	6,104±413	ND	15,218±822
Healthy donors						
JJ	0406	247±141	3,711±465	3,493±572	7,280±1,874	11,854±538
KA	0406	208±25	1,618±465	1,518±391	5,727±607	7,492±248
NA	0405	328±25	457±4	ND	506±46	ND
ME	0405	1,563±416	2,819±251	1,309±15	572±32	630±59

[a] The 5×10^3 irradiated (80 Gy) L-cell transfectants (L) were incubated with or without 40 mM human insulin (HI) in a medium containing 2 mM DTT and cultured for 6 days with 5×10^4 enriched T cells (R, responder cells). [3H] Thymidine incorporation of L cells alone was 3,300±97 for DRB1*0406 transfectant and 1,586±94 for DRB1*0405 transfectant, respectively

One appropriate question that our data raise is whether antigen-presentation efficiency of insulin peptides in patients with Ala[74] in the DRβ1-chain is indeed reduced compared with that in Glu[74]-positive patients.

POSSIBLE ROLE OF THE SPECIFIC AMINO ACIDS ON THE DRβ-CHAIN IN IAS PATHOGENESIS

Based on the findings described above, we conclude that (1) DR4 is the dominant phenotype in terms of susceptibility to IAS, (2) DRB1*0406 is associated with the highest risk for the susceptibility to IAS, and (3) Glu[74] in the DR4β1-chain is essential for polyclonal IAA production in IAS. Ser[37] in the DR4β1-chain may have a significant additive effect on polyclonal autoantibody production (Table 21.6).

The three-dimensional structure of the HLA class II DR1 molecules determined by X-ray crystallography has shown an open-ended groove, in which the peptides processed by antigen-presenting cells are bound as straight extended chains (25) and an anchoring peptide side chain of the processed peptides was found to fit in a prominent non-polar pocket near one end of the binding groove (25). Matsushita et al. (26) reported that peptide of

Table 21.8
DRB1, DQA1, and DQB1 Alleles and Comparison of Amino Acid Residues in the DRB1-chain in IAS Monoclonal Responders

Ethnic background	Patient no.	DRB1	DQA1	DQB1	DRB1-chain amino acid residues				
					37	47	57	74	86
Japanese	51	0405/0803	0301/0103	0401/0601	Tyr	Tyr	Ser/Asp	Ala/Leu	Gly/Val
Norwegian	1	0401/–	0301/–	0301/–	Tyr	Tyr	Asp	Ala	Gly
Swiss	1	0101/0601	0101/0102	0501/0502	Ser	Tyr	Asp	Ala	Gly
Italian	1	1501/1502	0102/0103	0601/0602	Ser	Phe	Asp	Ala	Gly/Val
Italian	2	0701/1501	0201/0102	0201/0602	Ser/Phe	Phe/Tyr	Val/Asp	Ala/Gln	Gly/Val
Italian	3	0402/1101	0301/0501	0301/0302	Tyr	Phe/Tyr	Asp	Ala	Gly

human insulin α-chain (^{8}TSICSLYQLE^{17}) was shown to bind specifically to DRB1*0406 using its ^{10}IxxLxxQ^{15} motif. The second anchor residue was reported to exhibit allele specificity in binding, especially with the amino acid residue 74 of DRβ1-chain (26). However, the interaction of L (Leu) of insulin peptide with Glu^{74} in the DR4β1-chain has remained questionable because Leu was a hydrophobic residue and Glu was an acidic residue. Other portions of human insulin may be a candidate for presentation and recognition for T cells in IAS (in preparation).

Although there are controversial points in the antigen-HLA-DRB1*0406 molecule–T-cell receptor interaction, a reducing compound such as MTZ, MPG, or glutathione may cleave disulfide bonds in vivo and expose self-antigens such as insulin-derived peptides to DRB1*0406 molecules on antigen-presenting cells, resulting in insulin-specific proliferating T cells. As mentioned previously, T-cell recognition of human insulin in the context of DRB1*0406 molecules showed the highest risk for the susceptibility to IAS in the polyclonal IAS responders, whereas T-cell recognition in the context of DRB1*0403 or DRB1*0407 did not. When human insulin-derived peptides were tested (for example, amino acids 8–17 of α-chain), they were indeed recognized by T cells in the context of DRB1*0403 or DRB1*0407 (in preparation).

Because polyclonal IAS patients exhibit typical polyclonal immunoglobulin G response to human insulin, the response may be an antigen-driven immune one with the help of T cell. Accordingly, typical HLA- and peptide-restricted recognition may contribute to the initiating event in the pathogenesis of IAS, in which Glu^{74} may act as the primary residue in the peptide-binding interaction.

A CONCEPT OF DRUG-INDUCED INSULIN AUTOIMMUNE SYNDROME AND DRβ1-CHAIN

As shown in Table 21.2, patients with Graves' disease who developed IAS had received methimazole (MTZ). None of the Japanese IAS patients with Graves' disease had received propylthiouracil (PTU) before the onset of IAS. We examined differences in HLA class II genes between the patients with Graves' disease treated with MTZ who developed IAS and those who had received MTZ but did not develop IAS (27). All 13 patients with Graves' disease who developed IAS by MTZ therapy possessed a specific allelic combination, B62/Cw4/DR4 carrying DRB1*0406, whereas only 1 of 50 Graves' disease patients without IAS had B62/Cw4/DR4 and those 50 did not possess DRB1*0406 (odds ratio, 2,727; $p < 1 \times 10^{-10}$). It is highly likely that patients with Graves' disease develop IAS via treatment with MTZ when their B62/Cw4/DR4 carry DRB1*0406.

Since 2004, the number of alfa lipoic acid-induced IAS patient was increased. Generally, in Japan, alfa lipoic acid has gained popularity as a supplement for dieting and anti-aging since 2004, while it was formerly used as a remedy for diabetic neuropathy in the western countries. Alfa lipoic acid is a coenzyme of an enzyme that activates oxidative decarboxylation against pyruvic acid and alfa-keto acid in mitochondria. Among 56 IAS patients from 2004 to 2007, 17 IAS patients had a history of taking alfa lipoic acid for dieting or anti-aging supplement (*15*). The molecular typing of DRβ1-chain was done in 14 of them; DRB1*0406 in 12; and DRB1*0403 in 2 patients.

Although the development of IAS is clearly more frequent in Japanese than Caucasians with respect to the distribution of DBB1*0406 in the World (*28*), it is conceivable that those who carry DRB1*0403 or DRB1*0407, which are more frequent in Caucasians, could develop IAS when they take drugs such as alfa lipoic acid even though DRB1*0406 (odds ratio, 56.6) is stronger predisposition to risk of development of IAS than DRB1*0403 (odds ratio, 1.6) and DRB1*0407 (odds ratio, 1.7) (*10*).

POSTPRANDIAL HYPERGLYCEMIA IN IAS

To investigate the level of IRI in the sera, oral glucose tolerance test (GTT) has been often done when IAS was diagnosed. Table 21.9 is a summary of 143 reports that described the result of GTT from 1970 to 2003. Approximately 80% had diabetic pattern, and only 6% was of normal pattern. As shown in (*29*), blood glucose level before load was rather lower, but higher 2 h after

Table 21.9
Result of Oral Glucose Tolerance Test (GTT) in Japanese IAS from 1970 to 2003

Age at onset	IAS patient Male (*n*)	Female (*n*)	Total
GTT performed	71	72	143
Diabetic pattern	35	45	80 (59%)
Borderline pattern	31	23	54 (38%)
Normal pattern	5	4	7 (6%)

Allocated to the category of GTT by Diagnostic criteria of Japan Diabetes Society 1982; diabetic pattern, fasting glucose 140 mg/dl, and ≥200 mg/dl 2 h after glucose load; normal pattern, fasting glucose 100 mg/dl, and <120 mg/dl 2 h after glucose load; borderline pattern, neither diabetic nor normal pattern load. IAS is classified as a form of diabetes associated with other disease or conditions (the criteria of classification of diabetes by Japan Diabetes Society 1999).

A CONCEPT OF TYPE VII HYPERSENSITIVITY INTRODUCED BY INSULIN AUTOIMMUNE SYNDROME (HIRATA'S DISEASE)

Disorders resulting from aberrant, excessive, or uncontrolled immune responses are called hypersensitivity diseases. Hypersensitivity diseases that are supposed to be due to immune responses against self-antigens are called autoimmune diseases.

Based on the principal criterion of the type of immune responses that lead to tissue injury, the conventional classification consists of type I (immediate hypersensitivity), type II (antibody-mediated), type III (immune complex-mediated), and type IV (T-cell-mediated). Two new types V and VI have recently been derived from type II and proposed as "antibody-mediated hyperfunction of the target tissues" in which Graves' disease is representative and "antibody-dependent cell-mediated cytotoxicity (ADCC)," respectively. We propose a new concept of type VII hypersensitivity defined as immunologic diseases that are induced by the release of self-antigens from the bound autoantibodies in serum. The self-antigens in type VII hypersensitivity are supposed to be located in the liquid phase, different from the self-antigens on the cell membranes in types II and IV hypersensitivities. IAS is a representative disease in type VII hypersensitivity (*14*).

NATURAL HISTORY OF IAS

Table 21.10 shows the clinical course and IAS treatments. Approximately 80% of Japanese IAS patients had spontaneous remission/no statement. We can interpret "no statement" to spontaneous remission because there might be no special treatments except avoiding drug exposure for hypoglycemia of IAS. Spontaneous remission may have developed in less than 3 months (*30*).

Some patients needed medication to stop the persistent hypoglycemic attacks, steroids, azathioprine, or 6-mercaptopurine. In eight patients, plasmapheresis was performed to wash out insulin autoantibodies from sera. In the early 1970s, partial pancreas excision surgery was performed in six patients under misdiagnosis of insulinoma. Hyperplasia of the islet B cells in the excised part of the pancreas was reported in some IAS patients (*5, 6*).

The current treatment recommended is to take small meals divided into six or more and to avoid sweets except at the time of

Table 21.10
Disease Course and Treatment in Japanese IAS Patients from 1970 to 2007

	IAS patient Male n = 155	Female n = 175	Total n = 330
Spontaneous remission/no statement	121	139	260 (78.8%)
Treatment			
Steroids	10	20	30 (9.1%)
Pancreatic surgery	3	3	6 (1.8%)
Plasmapheresis	6	2	8 (2.4%)
Azathioprine	1	0	1 (0.3%)
6-Mercaptopurine	0	1	1 (0.3%)
Alfa glucosidase inhibitor	14	10	24 (7.3%)

hypoglycemic attacks. Alfa-glucosidase inhibitors may sometimes play a helpful role in decreasing immunoreactive insulin in the sera after taking a meal (*22*) (Table 21.10).

REFERENCES

1. Schlosstein L, Terasaki PI, Bluestone R, et al. High association of an HL-A antigen B27 with ankylosing spondylitis. N Engl J Med 1973;288:704–706.
2. Park MS, Terasaki PI, Ahmed AR, et al. HLA-DRw4 in 91% of Jewish pempemphigus vulgaris patients. Lancet 1979;2:441–443.
3. Juji T, Satake M, Honda Y, et al. HLA antigens in Japanese patients with narcolepsy. Tissue Antigens 1984;24:316–319.
4. Prochazka EJ, Terasaki PI, Park MS, et al. Association of primary sclerosing cholangitis with HLA-DRw52a. N Engl J Med 1990; 322:1842–1844.
5. Hirata Y, Ishizu H, Ouchi N, et al. Insulin autoimmunity in a case of spontaneous hypoglycemia. J Japan Diab Soc 1970; 13:312–320.
6. Hirata Y, Arimichi M. Insulin autoimmune syndrome – the second case. J Japan Diabetes Soc 1972;15:187–192.
7. Folling J, Norman N. Hyperglycemia, hypoglycemic attacks and production of anti-insulin autoantibodies without previous known immunization. Immunological and functional studies in a patient. Diabetes 1972;21:814–826.
8. Hirata Y, Tominaga M, Ito J, et al. Spontaneous hypoglycemia with insulin autoimmunity in Graves' disease. Ann Intern Med 1974;81:214–218.
9. Oneda A, Matsuda K, Sato M, et al. Hypoglycemia due to apparent autoantibodies to insulin. Characterization of insulin-binding protein. Diabetes 1974;23:41–50.
10. Uchigata Y, Kuwata S, Tokunaga K, et al. Strong association of insulin autoimmune syndrome with HLA-DR4. Lancet 1992;339:393–394.
11. Uchigata Y, Eguchi Y, Takayama-Hasumi S, et al. Insulin autoimmune syndrome (Hirata disease): clinical features and epidemiology in Japan. Diabetes Res Clin Pract 1994;22:89–94.
12. Takayama-Hasumi S, Eguchi Y, Sato A, et al. Insulin autoimmune syndrome is the third leading cause of spontaneous hypoglycemic attacks in Japan. Diabetes Res Clin Pract 1990;10:211–214.

13. Hirata Y. Methimazole and insulin autoimmune syndrome with hypoglycemia. Lancet 1983; 2:1037–1038.
14. Uchigata Y, Hirata Y, Omori Y. A nobel concept of type VII hypersensitivity induced by insulin autoimmune syndrome (Hirata's disease). Autoimmunity 1995;20:207–208.
15. Uchigata Y, Hirata Y, Iwamoto Y. Drug-induced insulin autoimmune syndrome. Diabetes Res Clin Pract 2009;89:e19–e20.
16. Wasada T, Eguchi Y, Takayama-Hasumi S, et al. Reverse phase high performance liquid chromatographic analysis of circulating insulin in the insulin autoimmune syndrome. J Clin Endocrinol Metab 1988;66:153–158.
17. Eguchi Y, Uchigata Y, Yao K, et al. Longitudinal changes of serum insulin concentration and insulin antibody features in persistent insulin autoimmune syndrome (Hirata's disease). Autoimmunity 1994;19:279–284.
18. Uchigata Y, Yao K, Takayama-Hasumi S, et al. Human monoclonal IgG1 insulin autoantibody from insulin autoimmune syndrome directed at determinant at asparagine site on insulin B-chain. Diabetes 1989;38:663–666.
19. Uchigata Y, Takayama-Hasumi S, Kawanishi K, et al. Inducement of antibody that mimics insulin action on insulin receptor by insulin autoantibody directed at determinant at asparagine site on human insulin B chain. Diabetes 1991;40:966–970.
20. Uchigata Y, Eguchi Y, Takayama-Hasumi S, et al. The immunoglobulin class, the subclass and the ratio of κ:λ light chain of autoantibodies to human insulin in insulin autoimmune syndrome. Autoimmunity 1983;3:289–297.
21. Uchigata Y, Tokunaga K, Nepom G, et al. Differential immunogenetic determinants of polyclonal insulin autoimmune syndrome (Hirata's disease) and monoclonal insulin autoimmune syndrome. Diabetes 1995;44:1227–1232.
22. Schlemper RJ, Uchigata Y, Frolich M, et al. Recurrent hypoglycemia caused by the insulin autoimmune syndrome: the first Dutch case. Neth J Med 1996;48:188–192.
23. Uchigata Y, Omori Y, Nieda M, et al. HLA-DR4 genotype and insulin-processing in insulin autoimmune syndrome. Lancet 1992;340:1467.
24. Ito Y, Nieda M, Uchigata Y, et al. Recognition of human insulin in the context of HLA-DRB1*0406 products by T cells of insulin autoimmune syndrome patients and healthy donors. J Immunol 1993;15:5770–5776.
25. Brown JHG, Jardetzky TS, Gorga JC, et al. Three-dimensional structure of the human class II histocompatibility antigen HLA-DR1. Nature 1993;364:33–39.
26. Matsushita S, Takahashi K, Motoki M, et al. Allele specificity of structural requirement for peptides bound to HLA-DRB1*0405 and DRB1*0406 complexes: implication for the HLA-associated susceptibility to methimazole-induced insulin autoimmune syndrome. J Exp Med 1994;180:873–883.
27. Uchigata Y, Kuwata S, Tsushima T, et al. Patients with Graves' disease who developed insulin autoimmune syndrome (Hirata disease) possess HLA-Bw62/Cw4/DR4 carrying DRB1*0406. J Clin Endocrinol Metab 1993;77:249–254.
28. Uchigata Y, Hirata Y, Omori Y, Iwamoto Y, Tokunaga K. Worldwide differences in incidence of insulin autoimmune syndrome (IAS, Hirata's disease) with respect to the evolution of HLA-DR4. Hum Genet 2000;61:154–157.
29. Yao K, Uchigata Y, Kyono H, Yokoyama H, Eguchi Y, Fukushima H, Yamauchi K, Hirata Y. Human insulin-specific IgG antibody and hypoglycemic attacks after the injection of gold thioglucose. J Endocrinol Invest 1992;15:43–47.
30. Hirata Y, Uchigata Y. Insulin autoimmune syndrome in Japan. Diabetes Res Clin Pract 1994;24(Suppl):S153–S157.
31. Benson EB, Ho P, Wang C, et al. Insulin autoimmunity as a cause of hypoglycemia. Arch Intern Med 1984;144:2351–2354.
32. Cho BY, Lee HK, Koh CS, et al. Spontaneous hypoglycemia and insulin autoantibodies in patients with Graves' disease. Diabetes Res Clin Pract 1987;3:119–124.
33. Lee Y-J, Shin S-J, Torng J-K, et al. Insulin autoimmune syndrome in a methimazole-treated Graves' disease with polyclonal anti-insulin autoantibodies. J Formos Med Assoc 1987;867:164–170.
34. Chen C-H, Huang M-J, Huang B-Y, et al. Insulin autoimmune syndrome as a cause of hypoglycemia – report of four cases. Chang Gung Med J 1990;13:134–142.
35. Lu CC, Lee JK, Yang CY, Han TM. Insulin autoimmune syndrome in a patient with methimazole and carbimazole-treated Graves' disease: a case report. Chin Med J 1994;54(5):353–358.
36. Lin H-D, Chen H-D, Chang R-Y, Lin C-Y, Ching K-N. Insulin autoimmune syndrome in methimazole or carbimazole treated Chinese patients of Graves' disease. Chin Med J 1988;42:163–168.

37. Wong ST, Ng WY, Thai AC. Case report: autoimmune insulin syndrome in a Chinese female with Graves' disease. Ann Acad Med Singapore 1996;25:882–885.
38. Masjhur JS. Insulin autoimmune syndrome (Hirata's disease): severe hypoglycemic episodes in Graves's hyperthyroidism patient treated with methimazole. Acta Med Indones 2005;37:214–216.
39. Wa WY, Won JG, Tang KT, Lin HD. Severe hypoglycemic coma due to insulin autoimmune syndrome. J Chin Med Assoc 2005;68:82–86.
40. Goldman J, Baldwin D, Rubenstein A, Klink DD. Characterization of circulating insulin and proinsulin-binding antibodies in autoimmune hypoglycemia. J Clin Invest 1979; 63(5):1050–1059.
41. Rovira A, Valverde I, Escorihuela R, et al. Autoimmunity to insulin in a child with hypoglycemia. Acta Paediatr Scand 1982;71:343–345.
42. Blackshear P, Rhil D, Roner HE, et al. Reactive hypoglycemia and insulin autoantibodies in drug-induced lupus erythematosus. Ann Intern Med 1983;99:182–184.
43. Sklenar I, Wilkin TJ, Diaz J-L, et al. Spontaneous hypoglycemia associated with autoimmunity specific to human insulin. Diabetes Care 1987;10:152–159.
44. Tenn G, Eryssenlein V, Mellinghoff HU, et al. Clinical and biochemical aspects of the insulin autoimmune syndrome (IAIS). Klin Wochenschr 1986;64:929–934.
45. Archambeaud-Mouveroux F, Canivet B, Fressinaud C, et al. Hypoglycemie autoimmune; responsabilite du pyritinol? Presse Med 1988;17:11733–11737.
46. Burch HB, Clement S, Sokol MS, et al. Reactive hypoglycemic coma due to insulin autoimmune syndrome: case report and literature review. Am J Med 1992;92:681–685.
47. Dozio N, Sodoyez-Goffaux F, Koch M. Are insulin autoantibodies different from exogenous insulin induced antibodies? Diabetologia 1987;30(Suppl):515A.
48. Anderson JH, Blackard WG, Goldman J, et al. Diabetes and hypoglycemia due to insulin antibodies. Am J Med 1978;64:8686–8873.
49. Benson EB, Healey LA, Barron EJ, et al. Insulin antibodies in patients receiving penicillamine. Am J Med 1985;78:857–861.
50. Faguer de Moustier B, Burgard M, Biotard C, et al. Syndrome hypoglycemique auto-immun iduit par le pyritinol. Diabete Metab 1988;14:423–429.

51. Discher T, Seipke G, Friedmann E, et al. Recurrent hypoglycemia in the insulin autoimmune syndrome. Dtsch Med Wochenschr 1990;115:1951–1955.
52. Sluiter WJ, Marrink J, Houwen B. Monoclonal gammopathy with an insulin binding IgG(κ) M-component, associated with severe hypoglycemia. Br J Haematol 1986;62:679–687.
53. Scavini M, Dozio N, Sartori S, et al. Effect of treatment on insulin bioavailability and ^{123}I insulin biodistribution in insulin immune hypoglycemia. Diabetologia 1992;35(Suppl):187A.
54. Meschi F, Dozio M, Bognetti E, et al. An unusual case of recurrent hypoglycemia; 10-year follow up of a child with insulin autoimmunity. Eur J Pediatr 1992;151:32–34.
55. Arnqvist H, Halban PA, Mathiesen UL, et al. Hypoglycemia caused by atypical insulin antibodies in a patient with benign monoclonal gammopathy. J Intern Med 1993; 234:421–427.
56. Lidar M, Rachmani R, Half E, Ravid M. Insulin autoimmune syndrome after therapy with imipramine Diabetes Care 1999;22:524–525.
57. Cavaco B, Uchigata Y, Porto T, Amparo-Santos M, Sobrinho L, Leite V. Hypoglycemia due to insulin autoimmune syndrome: report of two cases with characterization of HLA alleles and insulin autoantibodies. Eur J Endocrinol 2001;145:311–316.
58. Herranz L, Rovira A, Grande C, Suarez A, Artinez-Ara J, Pallardo LF, Gomez-Pan A. Autoimmune insulin syndrome in a patient with progressive systemic sclerosis receiving penicillamine. Horm Res 1992;37(1–2):78–80.
59. Discher T, Seipke G, Freidmann E, Velcovsky HG, Federlin K. Recurrent hypoglycemia in insulin autoimmune syndrome. Dtsch Med Wochenschr 1990;115(51–52):1950–1955.
60. Shah P, Mares D, Fineberg E, Pescovitz M, Filo R, Jindal R, Mahoney S, Lumeng L. Insulin autoimmune syndrome as a cause of spontaneous hypoglycemia in alcoholic cirrhosis. Gastroenterology 1995;109:1673–1676.
61. Gregersen G, Dinesen B, Pedersen OB. Autoimmune syndrome. The first Danish case report. Ugeskr Laeger 1998;160:4539–4540.
62. Casesnoves A, Mauri M, Dominguez JR, Alfayate R, Pico AM. Influence of anti-insulin antibodies on insulin immunoassays in the autoimmune insulin syndrome. Ann Clin Biochem 1998;35:768–774.
63. Virally ML, Timsit L, Chanson P, Warnet A, Guillausseau PJ. Insulin autoimmune syndrome; a rare cause of hypoglycemia not to be overlooked. Diabete Metab 1999;25:429–431.

64. Konijnendijk MA, Zandbergen AA, Verhaeul FE, Baggen MG. Insulin autoimmune syndrome: the second case. Neth J Med 2001;58:18–21.
65. Lohman T, Kratzsch J, Kellner K, Witzigmann H, Hauss J, Paschke R. Severe hypoglycemia due to insulin autoimmune syndrome with insulin autoantibodies crossreactive to proinsulin. Exp Clin Endocrinol Diabetes 2001;109:245–248.
66. Ruiz-Giardin JM, Cremades C, Romeo J, MArazuela M. Insulin autoimmune syndrome in a patient with viral hepatitis C. Clin Endocrinol 2002;57:411–412.
67. Moreira RO, Lima GA, Peixoto PC, Farias ML, Vaisman M. Insulin autoimmune syndrome: case report. Sao Paulo Med J 2004;122:178–180.
68. Basu A, Service FJ, Yu L, Heser D, Ferries LM, Eisenbarth G. Insulin autoimmunity and hypoglycemia in seven white patients. Endocr Pract 2005;11:97–103.
69. Paiva ES, Pereira AE, Lombardi MT, Nishida SK, Tachibana TT, Ferrer C, Hauache OM, Vieira JGH, Reis AF. Insulin autoimmune syndrome (Hirata disease) as differential diagnosis in patients with hyperinsulinemic hypoglycemia. Pancreas 2006;32:431–432.

Chapter 22

Lessons from Patients with Anti-Insulin Receptor Autoantibodies

Angeline Y. Chong and Phillip Gorden

Summary

Type B insulin resistance is a rare syndrome caused by autoantibodies to the insulin receptor. Patients typically present with severe insulin resistance and hyperglycemia, but some manifest hypoglycemia following a period of hyperglycemia or hypoglycemia alone. The syndrome is predominantly seen in middle-aged black women. Other clinical features of type B insulin resistance are acanthosis nigricans, hyperandrogenism in premenopausal women, autoimmune disorders, proteinuric renal disease, and hematologic abnormalities. In addition to dysglycemia, the metabolic characteristics of the syndrome include low serum triglyceride levels and high adiponectin levels. The autoantibody acts as an agonist at the insulin receptor at low titers, but functions as an antagonist at high titers. The partial agonist properties of the autoantibody are responsible for the spectrum of glycemic states observed in type B insulin resistance. The treatment of type B insulin resistance has been of limited success to date and protocols addressing multiple components of the underlying autoimmune process are being developed.

Key Words: Type B insulin resistance, Anti-insulin receptor autoantibody, Autoimmunity, Hyperglycemia, Hypoglycemia

INTRODUCTION

Type B insulin resistance is caused by autoantibodies against the insulin receptor. It belongs to a class of diseases characterized by autoantibodies against cell surface receptors (Table 22.1). The insulin receptor is a cell surface glycoprotein comprised of two external alpha subunits that form the binding component and two transmembrane beta subunits (Fig. 22.1). Each beta subunit contains an intracellular tyrosine phosphorylation site that is autophosphorylated following ligand binding and in turn transduces the insulin signal to downstream substrates. Other disorders in the same category as type B insulin resistance include

Table 22.1
Diseases Associated with Autoantibodies Against Cell Surface Receptors

Disease/dysfunction	Receptor
Hyperglycemia	Insulin
Hypoglycemia	Insulin
Hyperthyroidism (Graves' disease) (3)	Thyrotropin
Hypothyroidism (65)	Thyrotropin
Myasthenia gravis (1, 2)	Acetylcholine
Infertility, premature ovarian failure (66, 67)	Follicle-stimulating hormone Luteinizing hormone
Iron deficiency anemia (68)	Transferrin

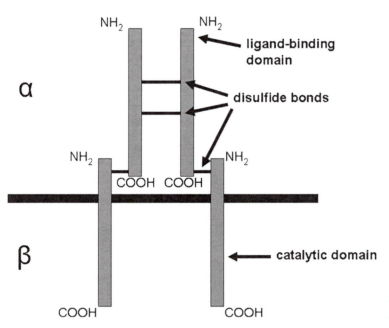

Fig. 22.1 Schematic diagram of the cell surface insulin receptor. In vivo, insulin or the autoantibody against the insulin receptor binds to the extracellular alpha subunit (although possibly at different sites). The binding event leads to autophosphorylation of the beta subunit, which in turn transduces the insulin signal to downstream substrates. It is of interest that the autoantibody can act as either an agonist or an antagonist for the insulin receptor while insulin acts only as an agonist.

Graves' disease and myasthenia gravis (Table 22.1). These diseases demonstrate that autoantibodies can form against diverse classes of cell surface receptors with a high degree of specificity for the individual receptors. Graves' disease is caused by autoantibodies against the thyroid stimulating hormone receptor, a G-protein coupled receptor, whereas myasthenia gravis is caused by autoantibodies against the acetylcholine receptor, a ligand-gated ion channel (1–3).

Type B insulin resistance is rare and its exact prevalence is unknown (4). It can result in a variety of glycemic abnormalities – extreme insulin resistance and hyperglycemia, hyperglycemia followed by hypoglycemia, or hypoglycemia alone. Type B insulin resistance is often associated with an underlying autoimmune disease, acanthosis nigricans, and hyperandrogenism in premenopausal women.

CLINICAL CHARACTERISTICS OF TYPE B INSULIN RESISTANCE

The typical patient with type B insulin resistance is a middle-aged black woman. To date, we have followed 34 patients with type B insulin resistance at the National Institutes of Health (NIH). Twenty-nine of 34 (85%) have been female and 29 of 34 (85%) have been black. We have evaluated five male patients (15%) and all of them have been black. In our series, the average age of affected women at presentation is 41 years and the average age of affected men is 57 years.

Acanthosis nigricans is a striking clinical feature of type B insulin resistance (4). Of our 34 patients, 31 (92%) have had acanthosis nigricans. The acanthosis nigricans most often affects the axillae, groin, and neck. A distinguishing feature of the acanthosis nigricans associated with type B insulin resistance is the involvement of the periocular, perioral, and labial regions (4). Because of this distinctive distribution of acanthosis nigricans, patients tend to have a characteristic facial appearance. In some patients, acanthosis nigricans can be found on the trunk, buttocks, lips, and vulva.

Ovarian enlargement and hyperandrogenism are also presenting characteristics in women with type B insulin resistance (4). In our NIH series, enlarged ovaries have been seen in most of the premenopausal female patients and are usually cystic. Arioglu et al. reported that 7 of 13 female patients who were between the ages of 14 and 50 had elevated testosterone levels (4). Since the publication of that paper, we have seen four additional women at the NIH with type B insulin resistance who have been under the age of 50 and three of them have manifested hypertestosteronemia. We observe a reduction in testosterone levels when a patient's autoantibody syndrome remits, suggesting that the hyperandrogenism is associated with the presence of the autoantibody or hyperinsulinemia (4).

Another common presenting feature of type B insulin resistance is autoimmune phenomena. The most common underlying autoimmune disorder is systemic lupus erythematosus (SLE) (*4*). Arioglu et al. noted that 11 of 24 (46%) NIH patients met the clinical criteria for SLE and 6 of 24 patients (25%) met three of four criteria for SLE (*4*). Of the ten additional patients we have seen since that 2002 paper, three patients have met the criteria for SLE. Two of our ten additional patients have met three of four criteria for SLE. One patient of the ten has mixed connective tissue disease. Twenty-nine (85%) of the 34 patients we have seen to date at the NIH have had positive antinuclear antibodies. Type B insulin resistance has also been associated with primary biliary cirrhosis, scleroderma, dermatomyositis, overlap syndrome, Sjögren syndrome, Hashimoto thyroiditis, autoimmune hepatitis, and autoimmune thrombocytopenia (*4*). Of note, the metabolic derangements caused by type B insulin resistance usually manifest after the onset of the systemic autoimmune disease.

Anti-insulin receptor autoantibodies may be related to a neoplasm rather than a systemic autoimmune disorder. At the NIH, we have seen type B insulin resistance associated with multiple myeloma in two cases. In addition, type B insulin resistance has been reported in patients with Hodgkin's disease and monoclonal gammopathy (*4–10*). In these instances, autoantibodies against the insulin receptor are a paraneoplastic manifestation.

Proteinuric renal disease can be associated with type B insulin resistance as well. Arioglu et al. reported that 13 of 24 (54%) NIH patients and 11 of 21 (52%) patients reported elsewhere in the literature had proteinuria (*4*). Although patients have uncontrolled hyperglycemia, they do not typically have diabetic nephropathy. Instead, different forms of lupus nephritis are seen on renal biopsy, such as mesangial lupus nephritis and proliferative lupus nephritis (*11, 12*). The co-occurrence of autoimmune disorders, especially SLE, may explain why lupus nephritis is so frequently observed.

Hematologic abnormalities are seen in type B insulin resistance and may also be related to underlying autoimmune diseases. Twenty-one (62%) of our 34 NIH patients have had leukopenia and 5 of 34 (15%) have had thrombocytopenia. Five of ten (50%) of our most recent type B patients have manifested anemia.

Type B insulin resistance is associated with high mortality. Fifteen of our 34 patients to date at the NIH have died. There is a relatively short interval between the time of presentation and the time of death. The average age at presentation of the 15 NIH patients who died was 49 years and the average age at death was 56 years. Four patients died from hypoglycemia; three of these initially presented with hyperglycemia and then later developed hypoglycemia. It appears then that the transition from a hyperglycemic to a hypoglycemic phase is a marker of poor outcome. The other causes of death were SLE (five patients), cardiovascular or cerebrovascular disease (three cases), and malignancy (two patients).

In other case reports in the literature, patients have died of hypoglycemia, bronchopneumonia and gastrointestinal bleeding (4, 5, 13, 14).

METABOLIC CHARACTERISTICS OF TYPE B INSULIN RESISTANCE

Most patients with type B insulin resistance present with moderate to severe hyperglycemia that is usually associated with profound glucosuria and polyuria. The onset of hyperglycemia is relatively acute and patients generally have dramatic weight loss. Arioglu et al. reported that the average blood glucose at presentation was 371 mg/dL and the average weight loss was 43 lb in 24 NIH patients (4). Endogenous serum insulin levels are high (over 200 mUnits/mL) prior to exogenous insulin therapy (Figs. 22.2 and 22.3). The hyperglycemia of type B insulin resistance can resolve with spontaneous disappearance of the insulin receptor antibody. In the 2002 NIH series, six patients who presented with hyperglycemia had spontaneous remission of their disease with disappearance of the autoantibody over a course of 11–48 months (4).

Other patients with type B insulin resistance can develop hypoglycemia after a period of hyperglycemia (Figs. 22.2 and 22.3). The hypoglycemia may occur in the fasting or the postprandial state. Instead of having a preceding period of hyperglycemia, some patients can initially present with spontaneous hypoglycemia and never manifest hyperglycemia. In our experience at the NIH, 24% of patients (8 of 34) have manifested some form of hypoglycemia during the course of their illness.

Importantly, insulin binding in type B insulin resistance does not change with fasting. In the typical obese patient with insulin resistance, fasting results in increased binding of ^{125}I-labeled insulin because of an increase in the number of insulin receptors at the

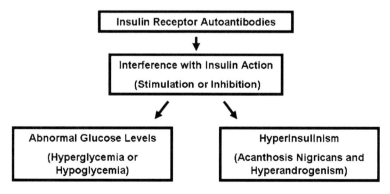

Fig. 22.2 Scheme by which binding of an autoantibody to the insulin receptor may produce diverse metabolic and clinical effects.

Determinants of Glycemic Status in Type B Insulin Resistance

- **Autoantibody titer**
    - Higher titer – inhibition of insulin action
        - Hyperglycemia
    - Lower titer – stimulation of insulin action
        - Hypoglycemia

- **Internal factors specific to the patient**
    - Insulin receptor number
    - Other hormonal or immunological factors

- **Change in the biological properties of the autoantibody**
    - Has not been seen in the NIH series

Fig. 22.3

cell surface (*15*). Therefore, with fasting, obese patients become more sensitive to insulin. On the other hand, fasting in the type B insulin-resistant patient does not change the amount of insulin bound to the cell surface (*16*).

Type B insulin resistance has other metabolic features. Unlike other syndromes of insulin resistance, fasting serum triglyceride levels are low. In the NIH series of 24 patients published in 2002, the average fasting triglyceride level was 54 mg/dL (*4*). Among our ten additional patients since 2002, fasting serum triglycerides at presentation have ranged from 25 to 68 mg/dL with an average of 49 mg/dL. Low fasting triglyceride levels are also seen in patients with mutations in the insulin receptor and appear to be a unique feature of insulin receptor dysfunction as opposed to non-receptor-mediated insulin resistance.

Another characteristic of type B insulin resistance is hyperadiponectinemia. Semple et al. have reported paradoxically high plasma adiponectin levels in patients with type B insulin resistance (*17*). Adiponectin is produced by adipose tissue and levels are typically low in insulin-resistant patients. In type B insulin resistance, adiponectin levels normalize as the titers of insulin receptor autoantibodies fall and insulin resistance resolves. High adiponectin levels, like low fasting triglyceride levels, are also observed in patients with insulin receptor mutations (*18*). Therefore, hyperadiponectinemia is another marker of insulin receptor pathology.

CHARACTERISTICS OF THE ANTI-INSULIN RECEPTOR AUTOANTIBODY

Autoantibodies against the insulin receptor are primarily polyclonal IgGs (*19*). While type B insulin resistance is often associated with hypergammaglobulinemia and some cases have occurred in the setting of multiple myeloma, there have been no reports of patients with monoclonal antibodies to the insulin receptor. Most autoantibodies can be detected by their ability to inhibit insulin binding. A series of experiments demonstrated that when circulating monocytes were exposed to the serum of patients with type B insulin resistance, there was markedly reduced binding of ^{125}I-labeled insulin to the cell surface (*16, 20*). Furthermore, the antibodies bound to the insulin receptor with high avidity. After the monocytes were incubated with patients' serum, they were washed prior to assaying ^{125}I-labeled insulin binding. The inhibition of insulin binding persisted despite this extensive washing (*20, 21*).

There has been discussion about whether some antireceptor autoantibodies can bind to the insulin receptor, but not inhibit insulin binding. For example, Bloise et al. described one patient with type B insulin resistance in whom antireceptor antibodies could not be detected by a binding inhibition assay (*22*). Bloise et al. then covalently cross-linked ^{125}I-labeled insulin to insulin receptors and found that this patient's antireceptor antibodies did immunoprecipitate labeled receptors. Similarly, Boden et al. reported several patients with diabetes whose anti-insulin receptor antibodies immunoprecipitated radiolabeled insulin receptors, but did not inhibit insulin binding to cultured rat hepatocytes (*23*). However, the finding of antibodies that immunoprecipitate insulin receptors but do not inhibit insulin binding may be explained by differences in the sensitivity of the two assays. Rodriguez et al. showed a tight coupling between the ability of antireceptor autoantibodies to immunoprecipitate receptors and their ability to block insulin binding (*24*). They studied the same patient as Bloise et al. (*22*) and demonstrated that the patient's purified immunoglobulins both inhibited insulin binding and immunoprecipitated the insulin receptor. They proposed that variations in technique were responsible for the different results.

Antireceptor autoantibodies tend to be specific for the insulin receptor, but some demonstrate low affinity binding to type 1 insulin-like growth factor (IGF) receptors. Kasuga et al. observed that sera from some patients with type B insulin resistance immunoprecipitated both human placental insulin receptors and type I IGF receptors (*25*). Antireceptor autoantibodies also appear to be specific for the insulin receptor in its native conformation as binding is lost when receptors are denatured. Zhang and Roth identified a region of the insulin receptor to which autoantibodies bind, residues 450–601 of the carboxy terminal half of the alpha subunit (*26*). This region is distinct from the domain of the receptor that contains the binding site for insulin, which is located primarily in the amino terminus of the alpha subunit (Fig. 22.1). Therefore, antireceptor antibodies can inhibit the binding of insulin without binding to the same site as insulin. It has been proposed that the antibodies may cause allosteric inhibition, steric hindrance, or misalignment of the insulin-binding site (*4, 26*).

Of note, the endogenous insulin receptor is normal in patients with type B resistance (*27*). Muggeo et al. exposed peripheral monocytes from patients with type B insulin resistance to an acid wash, a procedure that removed cell-bound antibodies. After the acid wash, they found an increase in insulin binding and insulin receptor affinity. In one patient whose type B insulin resistance spontaneously remitted and whose antireceptor antibody titers fell, the insulin receptors on monocytes had normal binding in equilibrium binding, kinetic, and specificity studies.

In addition to inhibiting insulin binding, another mechanism by which antireceptor antibodies may cause insulin resistance is by accelerating insulin receptor degradation. When human lymphoblastoid cells are incubated with antibodies from type B patients, washing the cells to dissociate the antibodies only partially reverses inhibition of ^{125}I-insulin binding (*28*). This observation suggests that the antibodies cause a decrease in the number of insulin receptors at the cell surface. It has been demonstrated that antibodies decrease the number of cell surface receptors by accelerating receptor turnover. When cells are incubated with antireceptor antibodies, there is an increased rate of degradation of ^{125}I-labeled cell surface insulin receptors (*28*). Down-regulation of insulin receptors has also been observed when a rabbit antibody against the insulin receptor is incubated with murine fibroblasts (*29*). The down-regulation of insulin receptors appears to be dependent on protein synthesis. Shimoyama et al. demonstrated that cycloheximide, a protein synthesis inhibitor, prevented down-regulation of insulin receptors on rat hepatocytes in response to human antireceptor antibodies (*30*).

Three different assays exist for detecting anti-insulin receptor autoantibodies. The first is binding inhibition. Cells are incubated with a patient's serum and washed. Then, the amount of ^{125}I-labeled insulin that can bind to the cells is ascertained (*21, 31*). The second assay is immunoprecipitation, which is currently the most sensitive and specific method for detecting receptor antibodies. A patient's serum is incubated with solubilized insulin receptors and antibody-bound receptors are precipitated with antihuman IgG (Fc specific) antibody (*4, 17, 21, 32*). Western blotting is then performed by transferring the immune complexes to membranes and probing with an antibody directed against the insulin receptor. Unfortunately, immunoprecipitation is not a commercially available assay. Therefore, before requesting that a specialized laboratory test a patient's serum, it is important to have a high index of suspicion for type B insulin resistance based on the patient's clinical and metabolic features. Finally, the third assay involves measuring the biological activity of the anti-insulin receptor antibody. The ability of a patient's serum or immunoglobulin fraction to stimulate glucose oxidation or lipogenesis in animal cells is determined (21, 31). However, since cells from different animal species are used, the bioactivity of a patient's antibody might not be detected because of its specificity to the human insulin receptor.

THE PARADOX OF HYPERGLYCEMIA AND HYPOGLYCEMIA

It seems paradoxical that antireceptor antibodies can cause either insulin resistance or hypoglycemia. An explanation for these dual effects is that the autoantibodies act as partial agonists for the insulin receptor. Antireceptor antibodies have been shown to stimulate autophosphorylation of the insulin receptor (33, 34). When autoantibodies to the insulin receptor are injected into fasting rats, severe and persistent hypoglycemia is induced in a dose-dependent manner (35). The hypoglycemic effect occurs within 2–4 h of injection and lasts 8–24 h. In vitro, antireceptor antibodies stimulate 2-deoxyglucose uptake and glucose oxidation in murine fatty fibroblasts and rat adipocytes (34–37). Human adipocytes incubated with antireceptor antibodies also show increased glucose oxidation (38). The insulinomimetic effect of antireceptor antibodies requires bivalency. Bivalent Fab_2 fragments can be prepared from IgG receptor antibodies by pepsin digestion. A bivalent Fab_2 retains the ability to stimulate glucose oxidation in adipocytes (39, 40). Monovalent Fab fragments, however, have little ability to stimulate glucose oxidation and act as competitive antagonists to insulin at its receptor (39, 40). Insulinomimetic properties can be restored by adding antihuman antibodies directed against the Fab portion (41). An anti-Fab antibody crosslinks two monovalent Fab fragments, effectively recreating a bivalent Fab_2.

On the other hand, when antibodies are administered at high doses for several days to fed rats, hyperglycemia is observed instead (35). Similar results have been seen in cultured murine fatty fibroblasts. Autoantibodies acutely stimulate deoxyglucose uptake and glucose oxidation in these cells, but with extended exposure, the insulinomimetic effect is lost and the cells become resistant to insulin (41, 42). Thus, autoantibodies to the insulin receptor can mimic the effects of insulin when given acutely; however, with chronic administration, they induce persistent hyperglycemia and insulin resistance.

The partial agonist activity of antireceptor antibodies is related to the observation that, in general, low antibody titers are associated with hypoglycemia and high antibody titers are associated with hyperglycemia (31, 43). At low titers, the insulin-like activity of the antibody is seen whereas at high titers, the antagonist effect predominates. In some patients, the transition from severe insulin resistance to hypoglycemia is heralded by a fall in antibody titer (31, 43). The onset of hypoglycemia, however, does not always correlate with titers of the antireceptor antibody. Arioglu et al. reported one NIH patient who had no change in antibody titer or characteristics when she transitioned from hyperglycemia to hypoglycemia (4). Two other patients in that series had episodes of hypoglycemia associated with significant drops in antibody titer.

The shift between hypoglycemic and insulin-resistant states could also be due to a change in the qualitative characteristics of the antireceptor antibody from agonist to antagonist. De Pirro et al. described a patient with hypoglycemia who had several distinct populations of IgG antireceptor antibodies (44). These populations differed in their ability to inhibit insulin binding and stimulate deoxyglucose transport. The investigators suggested that the manifestation of hyperglycemia or hypoglycemia depended on the relative concentrations of these different IgG antibodies. Tsushima et al. used isoelectric focusing to demonstrate heterogeneous populations of antireceptor antibodies in patients with type B insulin resistance (45). Different fractions of antibodies from the same patient exhibited varying abilities to inhibit insulin binding and increase glucose incorporation into lipids.

Finally, hypoglycemia might be caused by an increase in the number of insulin receptors at the cell surface. During the hypoglycemic phase of NIH patient B2, ^{125}I-insulin binding to the patient's monocytes increased (46). The increased binding was attributed to a proliferation of insulin receptors at the cell surface.

TREATMENT OF TYPE B INSULIN RESISTANCE

The goal of definitive therapy for type B insulin resistance is to eliminate the autoantibodies to the insulin receptor. In our experience, this goal has been difficult to achieve. A variety of immunosuppressive treatments have been used by different groups. Glucocorticoids, plasmapheresis, cyclophosphamide, azathioprine, intravenous immunoglobulin, cyclosporine, and mycophenolate mofetil have all been tried (5, 12, 13, 32, 47–63). The decision to target the production of autoantibodies is complicated by the fact that many patients undergo spontaneous remission without any immunomodulatory therapy (4). Therefore, debate exists as to whether immunosuppression affects remission rates or alters the natural history of the disease.

At times, the patient's underlying autoimmune or neoplastic illness requires immunosuppression in its own right. For example, treatment of a patient's associated lupus nephritis may be accompanied by remission of the type B insulin resistance (64). In the past, we have used the patient's underlying autoimmune disease to guide us in our choice of immunosuppressant's (4).

More recently, we have attempted to develop a rational approach to immunosuppressive therapy for type B insulin resistance. Since antibodies are produced by B cells, we have used rituximab to effect B-cell depletion. Rituximab is an antibody against CD20, a cell surface molecule expressed widely by B cells. Rituximab, however, does not affect plasma cells, which can survive for months to years. To target plasma cells, we have used pulses of high-dose glucocorticoids. Rituximab and glucocorticoids have been combined with classic immunosuppressive agents, such as cyclophosphamide, in an ongoing clinical trial. However, developing a treatment protocol with these agents is a work in progress and our experience is limited thus far.

The hypercatabolism and hyperglycemia of type B insulin resistance can be controlled with high doses of insulin regardless of whether the patient receives immunosuppression (Fig. 22.4). Given the massive amounts of insulin that are usually required, we typically use concentrated insulin U-500. The dose of insulin required to ameliorate the severe catabolic and hyperglycemic state may range from several hundred to several thousand units a day.

Therapy for Glycemic Control in Type B Insulin Resistance

Hyperglycemia
Goal is to reverse the catabolic state and reduce glucosuria
- High-dose insulin (e.g., over 1000 units/day). U-500 insulin is preferred.
- Oral antidiabetic agents are of little use.

Hypoglycemia
Goal is to avoid dangerously low blood glucose levels
- Steroids (effect occurs within 12-24 hours, prior to immunomodulatory action)

Fig. 22.4

CONCLUSIONS

Type B insulin resistance belongs to a class of diseases in which antibodies are directed against cell surface receptors. These receptors are of widely varying types and serve diverse functions, from metabolic control to neuromuscular signaling. It appears that the receptor antibody itself is the fundamental pathologic component in this class of disease. The inherent pathogenicity of the receptor antibody makes these diseases different from other autoimmune disorders that are caused by T-cell-mediated injury.

REFERENCES

1. Lindstrom JM. Acetylcholine receptors and myasthenia. Muscle Nerve 2000;23(4): 453–477.
2. Toyka KV, Drachman DB, Griffin DE, et al. Myasthenia gravis. Study of humoral immune mechanisms by passive transfer to mice. N Engl J Med 1977;296(3):125–131.
3. Zakarija M, Garcia A, McKenzie JM. Studies on multiple thyroid cell membrane-directed antibodies in Graves' disease. J Clin Invest 1985;76(5):1885–1891.
4. Arioglu E, Andewelt A, Diabo C, Bell M, Taylor SI, Gorden P. Clinical course of the syndrome of autoantibodies to the insulin receptor (type B insulin resistance): a 28-year perspective. Medicine 2002;81(2):87–100.
5. Braund WJ, Naylor BA, Williamson DH, et al. Autoimmunity to insulin receptor and hypoglycaemia in patient with Hodgkin's disease. Lancet 1987;1(8527):237–240.
6. Chan JC, Zhu SQ, Ho SK, Cockram CS. Hypoglycaemia and Hodgkin's disease. Br J Haematol 1990;76(3):434–436.
7. Khokher MA, Avasthy N, Taylor AM, Fonseca VA, Dandona P. Insulin-receptor antibody and hypoglycaemia associated with Hodgkin's disease. Lancet 1987;1(8534):693–694.
8. Walters EG, Tavare JM, Denton RM, Walters G. Hypoglycaemia due to an insulin-receptor antibody in Hodgkin's disease. Lancet 1987;1(8527):241–243.
9. Sluiter WJ, Marrink J, Houwen B. Monoclonal gammopathy with an insulin binding IgG(K) M-component, associated with severe hypoglycaemia. Br J Haematol 1986;62(4): 679–687.
10. Wasada T, Eguchi Y, Takayama S, Yao K, Hirata Y, Ishii S. Insulin autoimmune syndrome associated with benign monoclonal gammopathy. Evidence for monoclonal insulin autoantibodies. Diabetes Care 1989;12(2):147–150.
11. Musso C, Javor E, Cochran E, Balow JE, Gorden P. Spectrum of renal diseases associated with extreme forms of insulin resistance. Clin J Am Soc Nephrol 2006;1(4):616–622.
12. Tsokos GC, Gorden P, Antonovych T, Wilson CB, Balow JE. Lupus nephritis and other autoimmune features in patients with diabetes mellitus due to autoantibody to insulin receptors. Ann Intern Med 1985;102(2):176–181.
13. Varga J, Lopatin M, Boden G. Hypoglycemia due to antiinsulin receptor antibodies in systemic lupus erythematosus. J Rheumatol 1990;17(9):1226–1229.
14. O'Brien TD, Rizza RA, Carney JA, Butler PC. Islet amyloidosis in a patient with chronic massive insulin resistance due to antiinsulin receptor antibodies. J Clin Endocrinol Metab 1994;79(1):290–292.
15. Archer JA, Gorden P, Roth J. Defect in insulin binding to receptors in obese man. Amelioration with calorie restriction. J Clin Invest 1975;55(1):166–174.
16. Kahn CR, Flier JS, Bar RS, et al. The syndromes of insulin resistance and acanthosis nigricans. Insulin-receptor disorders in man. N Engl J Med 1976;294(14):739–745.
17. Semple RK, Halberg NH, Burling K, et al. Paradoxical elevation of high-molecular weight adiponectin in acquired extreme insulin resistance due to insulin receptor antibodies. Diabetes 2007;56(6):1712–1717.
18. Semple RK, Soos MA, Luan J, et al. Elevated plasma adiponectin in humans with genetically defective insulin receptors. J Clin Endocrinol Metab 2006;91(8):3219–3223.
19. Flier JS, Kahn CR, Jarrett DB, Roth J. Characterization of antibodies to the insulin

receptor: a cause of insulin-resistant diabetes in man. J Clin Invest 1976;58(6):1442–1449.
20. Flier JS, Kahn CR, Roth J, Bar RS. Antibodies that impair insulin receptor binding in an unusual diabetic syndrome with severe insulin resistance. Science 1975;190(4209):63–65.
21. Taylor SI, Underhill LH, Marcus-Samuels B. Assay of antibodies directed against cell surface receptors. Methods Enzymol 1985;109:656–667.
22. Bloise W, Wajchenberg BL, Moncada VY, Marcus-Samuels B, Taylor SI. Atypical antiinsulin receptor antibodies in a patient with type B insulin resistance and scleroderma. J Clin Endocrinol Metab 1989;68(1):227–231.
23. Boden G, Fujita-Yamaguchi Y, Shimoyama R, et al. Nonbinding inhibitory antiinsulin receptor antibodies. A new type of autoantibodies in human diabetes. J Clin Invest 1988;81(6):1971–1978.
24. Rodriguez O, Collier E, Arakaki R, Gorden P. Characterization of purified autoantibodies to the insulin receptor from six patients with type B insulin resistance. Metabolism 1992;41(3):325–331.
25. Kasuga M, Sasaki N, Kahn CR, Nissley SP, Rechler MM. Antireceptor antibodies as probes of insulinlike growth factor receptor structure. J Clin Invest 1983;72(4):1459–1469.
26. Zhang B, Roth RA. A region of the insulin receptor important for ligand binding (residues 450–601) is recognized by patients' autoimmune antibodies and inhibitory monoclonal antibodies. Proc Natl Acad Sci U S A 1991;88(21):9858–9862.
27. Muggeo M, Kahn CR, Bar RS, Rechler M, Flier JS, Roth J. The underlying insulin receptor in patients with antireceptor autoantibodies: demonstration of normal binding and immunological properties. J Clin Endocrinol Metab 1979;49(1):110–119.
28. Taylor SI, Marcus-Samuels B. Anti-receptor antibodies mimic the effect of insulin to down-regulate insulin receptors in cultured human lymphoblastoid (IM-9) cells. J Clin Endocrinol Metab 1984;58(1):182–186.
29. Grunfeld C. Antibody against the insulin receptor causes disappearance of insulin receptors in 3T3-L1 cells: a possible explanation of antibody-induced insulin resistance. Proc Natl Acad Sci U S A 1984;81(8):2508–2511.
30. Shimoyama R, Shelmet JJ, Savage CR Jr, Boden G. Effects of anti-insulin receptor antibodies (AIRA) on downregulation and turnover of insulin receptors on cultured hepatocytes. Diabetes 1986;35(1):28–32.
31. Gorden P, Collier E, Roach P. Autoimmune mechanisms of insulin resistance and hypoglycemia. In: Moller DE, ed. Insulin Resistance. Chichester: John Wiley & Sons Ltd, 1993:123–142.
32. Coll AP, Morganstein D, Jayne D, Soos MA, O'Rahilly S, Burke J. Successful treatment of type B insulin resistance in a patient with otherwise quiescent systemic lupus erythematosus. Diabet Med 2005;22(6):814–815.
33. Zick Y, Rees-Jones RW, Taylor SI, Gorden P, Roth J. The role of antireceptor antibodies in stimulating phosphorylation of the insulin receptor. J Biol Chem 1984;259(7):4396–4400.
34. Takayama-Hasumi S, Tobe K, Momomura K, et al. Autoantibodies to the insulin receptor (B-10) can stimulate tyrosine phosphorylation of the beta-subunit of the insulin receptor and a 185,000 molecular weight protein in rat hepatoma cells. J Clin Endocrinol Metab 1989;68(4):787–795.
35. Dons RF, Havlik R, Taylor SI, Baird KL, Chernick SS, Gorden P. Clinical disorders associated with autoantibodies to the insulin receptor. Simulation by passive transfer of immunoglobulins to rats. J Clin Invest 1983;72(3):1072–1080.
36. Kasuga M, Akanuma Y, Tsushima T, Suzuki K, Kosaka K, Kibata M. Effects of antiinsulin receptor autoantibody on the metabolism of rat adipocytes. J Clin Endocrinol Metab 1978;47(1):66–77.
37. Van Obberghen E, Spooner PM, Kahn CR, et al. Insulin-receptor antibodies mimic a late insulin effect. Nature 1979;280(5722):500–502.
38. Kasuga M, Akanuma Y, Tsushima T, et al. Effects of anti-insulin receptor autoantibodies on the metabolism of human adipocytes. Diabetes 1978;27(9):938–945.
39. Kahn CR, Baird KL, Flier JS, Jarrett DB. Effects of autoantibodies to the insulin receptor on isolated adipocytes. J Clin Invest 1977;60:1094–1106.
40. Kahn CR, Baird KL, Jarrett DB, Flier JS. Direct demonstration that receptor crosslinking or aggregation is important in insulin action. Proc Natl Acad Sci U S A 1978;75(9):4209–4213.
41. Grunfeld C, Jones DS, Shigenaga JK. Autoantibodies against the insulin receptor. Dissociation of the acute effects of the antibodies from the desensitization seen with prolonged exposure. Diabetes 1985;34(3):205–211.
42. Grunfeld C, Van Obberghen E, Karlsson FA, Kahn CR. Antibody-induced desensitization of the insulin receptor. Studies of the mechanism of desensitization in 3T3-L1 fatty fibroblasts. J Clin Invest 1980;66(5):1124–1134.

43. Taylor SI, Grunberger G, Marcus-Samuels B, et al. Hypoglycemia associated with antibodies to the insulin receptor. N Engl J Med 1982;307(23):1422–1426.
44. De Pirro R, Roth RA, Rossetti L, Goldfine ID. Characterization of the serum from a patient with insulin resistance and hypoglycemia. Evidence for multiple populations of insulin receptor antibodies with different receptor binding and insulin-mimicking activities. Diabetes 1984;33(3):301–304.
45. Tsushima T, Omori Y, Murakami H, Hirata Y, Shizume K. Demonstration of heterogeneity of autoantibodies to insulin receptors in type B insulin resistance by isoelectric focusing. Diabetes 1989;38(9):1090–1096.
46. Flier JS, Bar RS, Muggeo M, Kahn CR, Roth J, Gorden P. The evolving clinical course of patients with insulin receptor autoantibodies: spontaneous remission or receptor proliferation with hypoglycemia. J Clin Endocrinol Metab 1978;47(5):985–995.
47. Bao S, Root C, Jagasia S. Type B insulin resistance syndrome associated with systemic lupus erythematosus. Endocr Pract 2007;13(1):51–55.
48. Eriksson JW, Bremell T, Eliasson B, Fowelin J, Fredriksson L, Yu ZW. Successful treatment with plasmapheresis, cyclophosphamide, and cyclosporin A in type B syndrome of insulin resistance. Case report. Diabetes Care 1998;21(8):1217–1220.
49. Fareau GG, Maldonado M, Oral E, Balasubramanyam A. Regression of acanthosis nigricans correlates with disappearance of anti-insulin receptor autoantibodies and achievement of euglycemia in type B insulin resistance syndrome. Metabolism 2007;56(5):670–675.
50. Freeland BS, Paglia RE, Seal DL. Clinical challenges of type B insulin resistance: a case study. Diabetes Educ 1998;24(6):728–733.
51. Gehi A, Webb A, Nolte M, Davis J Jr. Treatment of systemic lupus erythematosus-associated type B insulin resistance syndrome with cyclophosphamide and mycophenolate mofetil. Arthritis Rheum 2003;48(4):1067–1070.
52. Kato Y, Ichiki Y, Kitajima Y. A case of systemic lupus erythematosus presenting as hypoglycemia due to anti-insulin receptor antibodies. Rheumatol Int 2008;29(1):103–105.
53. Kawanishi K, Kawamura K, Nishina Y, Goto A, Okada S. Successful immunosuppressive therapy in insulin resistant diabetes caused by anti-insulin receptor autoantibodies. J Clin Endocrinol Metab 1977;44(1):15–21.
54. Kramer N, Rosenstein ED, Schneider G. Refractory hyperglycemia complicating an evolving connective tissue disease: response to cyclosporine. J Rheumatol 1998;25(4):816–818.
55. Moller DE, Ratner RE, Borenstein DG, Taylor SI. Autoantibodies to the insulin receptor as a cause of autoimmune hypoglycemia in systemic lupus erythematosus. Am J Med 1988;84(2):334–338.
56. Muggeo M, Flier JS, Abrams RA, Harrison LC, Deisserroth AB, Kahn CR. Treatment by plasma exchange of a patient with autoantibodies to the insulin receptor. N Engl J Med 1979;300(9):477–480.
57. Nagayama Y, Morita H, Komukai D, Watanabe S, Yoshimura A. Type B insulin resistance syndrome induced by increased activity of systemic lupus erythematosus in a hemodialysis patient. Clin Nephrol 2008;69(2):130–134.
58. Page KA, Dejardin S, Kahn CR, Kulkarni RN, Herold KC, Inzucchi SE. A patient with type B insulin resistance syndrome, responsive to immune therapy. Nat Clin Pract Endocrinol Metab 2007;3(12):835–840.
59. Rochet N, Blanche S, Carel JC, et al. Hypoglycaemia induced by antibodies to insulin receptor following a bone marrow transplantation in an immunodeficient child. Diabetologia 1989;32(3):167–172.
60. Selinger S, Tsai J, Pulini M, Saperstein A, Taylor S. Autoimmune thrombocytopenia and primary biliary cirrhosis with hypoglycemia and insulin receptor autoantibodies. A case report. Ann Intern Med 1987;107(5):686–688.
61. Tardella L, Rossetti L, De Pirro R, et al. Circulating anti-insulin receptor antibodies in a patient suffering from lupus nephritis and hypoinsulinemic hypoglycaemia. J Clin Lab Immunol 1983;12(3):159–165.
62. Toyota T, Suzuki H, Sugawara H, et al. Remission of insulin resistant diabetes in two patients with anti-insulin receptor antibodies. Tohoku J Exp Med 1982;138(2):187–197.
63. Vesely DL, Coleman MJ, Kohler PO, Jordan RM, Stanley S. Hyperalimentation as cause of markedly worsened metabolic control in a patient with autoantibodies to the insulin receptor. Am J Med 1985;79(4):504–508.
64. Sims RE, Rushford FE, Huston DP, Cunningham GR. Successful immunosuppressive therapy in a patient with autoantibodies to insulin receptors and immune complex glomerulonephritis. South Med J 1987;80(7):903–906.

65. Sato K, Okamura K, Yoshinari M, et al. Goitrous hypothyroidism with blocking or stimulating thyrotropin binding inhibitor immunoglobulins. J Clin Endocrinol Metab 1990;71(4):855–860.
66. Moncayo H, Moncayo R, Benz R, Wolf A, Lauritzen C. Ovarian failure and autoimmunity. Detection of autoantibodies directed against both the unoccupied luteinizing hormone/human chorionic gonadotropin receptor and the hormone-receptor complex of bovine corpus luteum. J Clin Invest 1989;84(6):1857–1865.
67. Sluss PM, Schneyer AL. Low molecular weight follicle-stimulating hormone receptor binding inhibitor in sera from premature ovarian failure patients. J Clin Endocrinol Metab 1992;74(6):1242–1246.
68. Larrick JW, Hyman ES. Acquired iron-deficiency anemia caused by an antibody against the transferrin receptor. N Engl J Med 1984;311(4):214–218.

Chapter 23

Islet and Pancreas Transplantation

Gaetano Ciancio, Alberto Pugliese, George W. Burke, and Camillo Ricordi

Summary

Transplantation of whole pancreas or of purified pancreatic islets can restore insulin secretion in patients with insulin-dependent, type 1 diabetes (T1D). Both procedures reverse diabetes in most patients, improving chronic complications and quality of life, but require chronic, systemic immunosuppression. Given the side effects and health risks associated with immunosuppression, exogenous insulin therapy remains the mainstay of treatment for most patients with T1D, unless patients cannot adequately control their metabolism with exogenous insulin or develop life-threatening complications (such as severe hypoglycemia and kidney failure) that can be corrected by transplantation. While pancreas transplantation is presently associated with longer graft survival and function than islet transplantation, it requires invasive surgery compared to the less invasive islet infusion procedure and has a higher risk of perioperative mortality and morbidity. Thus, clinical indications and patient selection criteria for the two procedures are different. Islet transplants are mostly performed in patients with brittle diabetes and severe hypoglycemia. Patients with end stage renal disease are candidates for simultaneous-kidney pancreas transplantation, which accounts for the majority of pancreas transplants. This chapter will review the current status of both islet and pancreas transplantation and discuss major challenges and future directions.

Key Words: Islet transplantation, Pancreas transplantation, Immunosuppression, Type 1 diabetes, Tolerance, Rejection, Autoimmunity

ISLET TRANSPLANTATION

The goal of islet transplantation (ITX) is to provide a platform technology for the development of a cell-based treatment for type 1 diabetes (T1D). For ITX to be considered a cure, it has to be a part of a combination strategy that will also allow for the restoration of self-tolerance to correct the autoimmune condition that was at the base of T1D onset and prevention of rejection of the transplanted insulin-producing cells, without the use of life-long recipient immunosuppression. ITX is considered the first step of cell-based approaches for diabetes treatment that eventually requires the development of an unlimited source of insulin-producing cells (e.g., expansion of adult islet cells, stem cell-derived insulin-producing cells, tissue reprograming, or xenogeneic sources) to really become a treatment option that could be offered to most of the patients with diabetes who could benefit from this procedure.

At present, the requirement for systemic immunosuppression limits the indications of ITX to the most severe cases of T1D, where the main goal of the procedure is the normalization of glucose metabolism and the prevention of severe hypoglycemic episodes to improve the quality of life. Insulin independence, although often obtained, is not an absolute requirement to achieve these goals (1, 2). Thus, candidates for islet transplantation alone are patients with frequent life-threatening hypoglycemic episodes, severe hyperglycemia or recurrent ketoacidosis, or suffer from incapacitating physical and emotional problems with insulin therapy (1). Patients with imminent or current end-stage renal disease (ESRD) may receive a simultaneous islet–kidney (SIK) transplant from the same donor and those who already had a kidney transplant may receive an islet after kidney (IAK) transplant from a different donor.

Islet Isolation Procedures

Pancreatic islets are purified using a semi-automated method of enzymatic dissociation in a digestion-dissociation chamber (Ricordi chamber) (3). Both choice of enzyme blend and variability among lots are critical to the outcome of islet isolations (4). Digestion is followed by centrifugation on density gradients to separate endocrine from exocrine cells. Once islets are purified, they are cultured for 2 days prior to the transplant to allow beta cells to recover from the isolation process, increasing the islet viability while preserving the islet mass. The cell culture medium is enriched with trophic and antioxidants to prevent oxidative stress, apoptosis, and promote beta-cell function and survival (5). This time window also allows starting induction therapies early, to reduce the risk of acute rejection. Another advantage is that islets can be shipped to remote clinical sites for transplantation (6). Preparations are routinely assessed for islet purity, survival, insulin content, and function to ensure product clinical suitability using FDA-approved tests (7). The islet mass is estimated as the number of islet equivalents (IEQ) based on a standard islet diameter of 150 μm. A transplant is generally considered possible when a minimum of 350,000 IEQ or 5,000 IEQ/kg of recipient body weight is available.

Islet Infusion Procedure

The islet transplant is performed by gravity infusion from a closed-bag system containing the heparinized-islet product. This is infused in the main portal vein through percutaneous transhepatic catheterization, under fluoroscopic and ultrasound guidance, with close monitoring of portal pressure, using local anesthesia (*8*). The procedure results in the microembolization of the islets into the hepatic portal venous system, which is followed by engraftment and revascularization. This minimally invasive, interventional radiology procedure lasts for approximately 1 h, and patients are usually discharged within 24–48 h. In SIK, or if contraindications to this approach exist (e.g., risk of hemorrhage, anatomical anomalies), cannulation of a tributary of the portal vein, such as the mesenteric or umbilical vein, is performed by laparotomy or laparoscopy (*9*).

ITX Outcomes

ITX has been improving over time in parallel with methodological advances in procurement, isolation procedures, and the availability of more effective immunosuppressive regimens. During the first decade of trials, mostly based on the use of steroids and calcineurin inhibitors, islet graft survival was limited, with high rates of primary nonfunction. Only about 10% of islet recipients maintained insulin independence at 1 year (*10*). In the late 1990s, the introduction of mTOR inhibitors (Sirolimus and Everolimus) and TNFα blockers (Infliximab and Etanercept) allowed using steroid-free regimens and a significant reduction in the Tacrolimus doses (*11*). In 2000, the Edmonton group reported remarkable results from a steroid-free protocol, based on induction with daclizumab, high-dose Sirolimus (trough levels of 12–15 ng/ml during the first 3 months and then 10–12 ng/ml) plus low-dose Tacrolimus as maintenance immunosuppression. Insulin independence was obtained infusing more than 10,000 IEQ/kg or >700,000 IEQ total, thus infusing essentially a full islet mass. Achieving this mass required multiple infusions from two or more donors in most patients (*12, 13*). Virtually all recipients were insulin-free at 1 year, had normalized HbA1c, and no longer suffered from severe hypoglycemia (*12*). The initial success of the Edmonton protocol was a major turning point in the field. Since then, about 400 patients have been transplanted (receiving about 700 islet transplants) with Edmonton-like protocols in approximately 50 centers worldwide, as reported by the Clinical Islet Transplant Registry (CITR) (*14*). Insulin independence at 1 year was reported in 70–80% of the patients transplanted at the most experienced centers (*14, 15*). With longer follow-up, insulin independence using the Edmonton protocol declines to 50% at 2 years, 30% at 3 years, and 10% at 5 years. This progressive loss of function seems mainly due to chronic alloimmunity and autoimmunity, and there are concerns that FK506 and rapamycin (but not MMF) are permissive for the homeostatic proliferation of autoreactive memory T cells (*16*). Moreover, several of the immunosuppressive drugs used have deleterious effects on islet cell function, survival, and replication (*17*).

Overall, the Edmonton protocol showed that restoring a sufficient islet mass with islet infusions from multiple donors could restore insulin independence in most patients, albeit its duration was limited. Yet, significant metabolic improvements are maintained even with only partial islet graft function, such as stability of glucose control with normalized HbA1c, amelioration of insulin sensitivity with reduced insulin requirements, lack of severe hypoglycemia with restored hypoglycemia awareness, and improved quality of life (*18, 19*). Glucagon responses to hypo- and hyperglycemia are improved, with recovery of sympathoadrenal responses and reduced hepatic glucose output (*20–24*).

Exenatide in ITX

Recent studies have shown that islet graft function can be aided by islet supportive therapy. The incretin-mimetic Exenatide might also aid in protecting the beta cells from the immunosuppression-related toxicity. In recent studies, Exenatide has been given from the time of the first islet infusion (University of Illinois), or after islet graft dysfunction (Miami and Vancouver). Our group also used Exenatide in patients receiving islet retransplants, beginning treatment prior to the supplemental islet infusion. Exenatide seems to improve islet engraftment as well as islet graft function and survival, normalizing glucose control, and favoring insulin independence (*25–27*). Exenatide has manageable side effects (e.g., vomit, nausea) but there is a small risk of pancreatitis and of possible worsening of preexistent diabetic gastroparesis (*28*).

Challenges and Future Perspectives in ITX

While significant advances have been made during the last decade, several hurdles limit the success and widespread applicability of ITX. At present, suboptimal pancreases are generally available for ITX, since the best organs (nonobese and donors of less than age 50) are first offered to whole organ, pancreas transplant programs. As a consequence, <50% of pancreata processed with intent to transplant yield a sufficient islet number. Twenty to more than 50% of the pancreatic islet content can be lost during the isolation process due to donor braindeath-related events, suboptimal organ preservation, deficient isolation process, and inadequate beta cell cytoprotection. Overall, these events limit the chances of a satisfactory islet yield from a single pancreas, such that more than one donor is often required to achieve insulin independence (*29*). Given the limited supply of organ donors for ITX, however, the use of multiple donors would not be sustainable on a large scale. Moreover, allosensitization has been observed in recipients of multiple islet donors after graft failure and the discontinuation of immunosuppression (*30, 31*). To avoid this potential risk, trials in the post-Edmonton protocol era are focusing on single-donor protocols. Access to better quality donor pancreases, further improvements in islet procurement strategies, isolation methods, and cytoprotective treatments are required to improve the yield and the overall final quality of islet cell products, which in turn will provide better short- and long-term outcomes.

The lengthened islet allograft survival observed in recent years has meant prolonged exposure to immunosuppression, and similar to organ transplantation, this has paralleled immunosuppression-related side effects that have been observed in several recipients, such as those with common or opportunistic infections (skin, respiratory, and urinary tract). Serious adverse events requiring hospitalization have also been observed (e.g., profound neutropenia, pneumonia, and ovarian cysts). Reactivation of latent viral infections (e.g., EBV and CMV) and de novo malignancies have been rare, with only 13 neoplasms reported by the CITR in 400 IT recipients (14). Some reports noted declining kidney function on follow-up (32–34), likely explained by accelerated diabetic nephropathy from the renal toxicity of immunosuppressive drugs. Antihypertensive and nephroprotective therapy, together with selection criteria that focus on patients with virtually normal renal function, could help limiting posttransplant kidney toxicity (35), which will be likely completely avoided only by the development of immunomodulatory strategies that will not include nephrotoxic immunosuppressive agents. The Edmonton protocol has also been tested in several IAK and SIK trials, with rates of insulin independence varying between 30 and 70% at 1 year. However, long-term stabilization of glucose control and sustained C-peptide secretion were achieved. In these settings, kidney graft function and survival appeared to be improved (36–39). IAK transplantation can induce sustained improvements in cardiovascular and endothelial function, reduce the atherothrombotic profile, and is associated with fewer cardiovascular events and improved survival. Thus, ITX per se might protect kidney graft function and could increase its longevity. Even partial C-peptide secretion may reduce nerve dysfunction and increase blood flow in cardiac and renal districts, with myocardial and glomerular vasodilatation, improving cardiovascular and kidney function, and slowing the progression of diabetic macro- and microangiopathy, including retinopathy (40–48).

Trials are now testing new immunosuppressive regimens aiming at reduced toxicity toward the islet grafts and importantly the native kidneys. Considering that a much longer function is reported in patients receiving islet autografts after chronic pancreatitis (49), it is clear that ITX could become a more successful and safer therapeutic option if we could more effectively control the immune system and fully prevent chronic allo- and autoimmune responses. The Minneapolis group has been using rabbit ATG (rATG) or a modified humanized OKT3 (hOKT3γ Ala-Ala), together with Etanercept, achieving insulin independence from a single donor with less than 10,000 IEQ/kg, which is considered a marginal islet mass. Sirolimus plus low-dose Tacrolimus or MMF was used for maintenance immunosuppression (50, 51). The same group has reported 60% insulin independence rates for over 3 years posttransplant, using rATG and Etanercept as induction together with mTOR inhibitors and CNI/MMF as maintenance (52). More recently, the Miami and Edmonton centers have been using Alemtuzumab, an antiCD52 lymphodepleting monoclonal antibody, as an induction agent, and replaced Tacrolimus or Sirolimus with MMF. These studies show significant improvements in islet function and survival (53, 54). Induction with rATG and Etanercept followed by maintenance with Sirolimus, Efalizumab, an antiLFA1/CD11a monoclonal antibody is also being tested (55).

New regimens and hopefully more tolerogenic strategies, including more selective lymphodepleting drugs, costimulatory blockade, and antiinflammatory agents, will be tested in future trials. The Clinical Islet Transplant Consortium, including centers in North America and Europe, is starting several phase II–III trials using combinations of several agents, including antiCD20 (Rituximab) for B-cell depletion, antiCD80/86 (Belatacept) for costimulatory blockade, Deoxyspergualin for immunomodulation, Lysofilline as antiinflammatory, and low-molecular weight dextran to block instant blood-mediated inflammatory reaction. Conceptually, these regimens remain based on chronic, systemic immunosuppression. Our group is conducting experimental studies in animal models to explore the concept of localized immunosuppression, based on the use of an implantation device engineered to deliver immunosuppression only within the graft microenvironment and at the same time to create a graft site that is supportive of islet function and survival (56). Major innovations in strategies to induce transplantation tolerance and restore self-tolerance will be required to bring ITX to the next level. For example, employing short courses of immunomodulatory therapy associated with the administration of tolerogenic cells may allow for more effective and long-lasting effects on the immune system with much reduced toxicity.

PANCREAS TRANSPLANTATION

The goal of pancreas transplantation (PT) is to restore euglycemia providing long-term insulin independence, increase patient survival, stabilize or improve diabetic retinopathy and neuropathy, and, in combination with kidney transplantation, eliminate the need for dialysis. Simultaneous kidney–pancreas (SPK) transplant results have improved consistently over the past decade (57, 58) as a consequence of advances in immunosuppressive strategies (59, 60), improvements in surgical technique, and better understanding of intra and postoperative care (*61*). At the University of Miami (UM), PT has been performed since 1990. Most (>95%) have been SPK transplants. SPK transplantation is considered the best treatment option for patients with T1D and ESRD (*57, 58, 62*).

Hypercoagulable State in T1D/ESRD

The pancreas transplant portion of SPK has historically been more prone to thrombosis than other solid organ transplants, accounting for up to 15–20% of pancreas graft loss. When viewed in the context of Virchow's triad (hypercoagulability, endothelial cell damage, and venous stasis), thrombosis may in fact be predicted, since all three criteria are met: (a) hypercoagulability is clearly defined by the thromboelastogram (TEG, vide infra) (*63*); (b) endothelial cell damage, which results from an ischemia/reperfusion injury and mediated by cytokines, O_2 radicals, nitric oxide, etc. Furthermore, immunosuppression, particularly calcineurin inhibitors (Tacrolimus, cyclosporine A), can induce endothelial cell damage by eliciting procoagulants (*64*); (c) venous stasis occurs when the spleen is removed from the tail of the pancreas, as the major source of blood return through the splenic vein is lost. The pancreas portion of the splenic vein remains with its high capacitance, but there is only limited flow from the pancreas. The superior mesenteric vein similarly no longer receives venous return from the small bowel, but is limited to small pancreatic venous radicals. Thus, the pancreas transplant fulfills Virchow's triad for propensity to venous thrombosis.

Indeed, at UM, we perform a TEG at the time of SPK transplant surgery, which consistently demonstrates a hypercoagulable pattern (*63*). Generally, rheologic assessment including the combination of (a) shortened prothrombin time, INR, and partial thromboplastin time and (b) elevated platelet count, fibrinogen, and hematocrit along with hyperlipidemia, which are all features associated with hypercoagulability, are conceptually integrated into the TEG. Since each of these factors may vary over time, the performance of the intraoperative TEG allows a "real time" evaluation of the degree of hypercoagulability at the time of transplantation. Although the uremic effect on platelets could offset the hypercoagulability associated with T1D, our experience suggests that it does not. This has led us to use heparin intraoperatively, when the degree of hypercoagulability is matched with the degree of operative field hemostasis. The PT loss rate of 1% from thrombosis shows that this has been an effective strategy, while reoperating from bleeding is also low (2%) (*63*).

When seen in the context of other risk factors for atherosclerosis – e.g., hypertension, obesity, diabetes mellitus, insulin resistance, dyslipidemia (components of the metabolic syndrome) – the greatest benefit of the demonstration of the hypercoagulable state may lie in its long-term therapy. While SPK transplant prolongs patient survival (*62, 65*), recognition and treatment of the hypercoagulable state along with new approaches to inflammation and atherosclerosis may allow further improvement.

Pancreas Transplant, Technical Aspects: Exocrine Drainage

Pancreas transplantation is performed primarily for its endocrine function, based on the vascularized islet cell, with the exocrine function, i.e., digestive enzymes including amylase and lipase, etc., nearly irrelevant in most cases. Drainage of the pancreas/duodenum graft has evolved over time. It is performed either into the bladder or the small bowel. Bladder drainage is used in our center foremost for safety reasons, since it avoids intraabdominal enteric spill. Bladder drainage also allows monitoring of urine amylase, which provides an insight into pancreatic graft function, typically useful in diagnosing acute rejection. After the administration of antirejection therapy, the need for repeat pancreatic biopsy can also be avoided if urine amylase returns to baseline levels. However, bladder-drained pancreas transplants are associated with multiple urological and metabolic complications, requiring enteric conversion in 14–50% of most reported series, although only 8% in our 390 consecutive SPK transplants (*58*). When exocrine pancreas secretions are enterically drained, metabolic acidosis and dehydration are avoided. However, rejection episodes may progress undiagnosed before treatment is started, and this delay increases the likelihood of allograft loss. The most serious complication of the enteric-drained pancreas transplant is a leak from the anastomotic site with the resultant intraabdominal sepsis.

Pancreas Transplant, Technical Aspects: Venous Drainage

Venous effluent from the portal vein of the pancreas transplant is usually through the systemic circulation (external iliac vein), which results in loss of first-pass insulin through the liver, and typically hyper-c-peptidemia. Alternatively, the pancreas transplant portal vein can be anastomosed to a mesenteric venous radical leading to the liver, a more physiologic placement, avoiding hyper-c-peptidemia. The combination of exocrine enteric drainage and venous portal drainage was attempted to achieve a more physiologic transplant but has not gained wide acceptance (*66*).

Immunosuppression in Pancreas Transplantation

Recent protocols in pancreas transplantation include attempts to: (a) reduce calcineurin inhibitor short- and long-term nephrotoxicity, (b) reduce or avoid corticosteroids, (c) use adjunctive maintenance antiproliferative agents or mTOR inhibitors, and (d) utilize new induction antibodies. These include nondepleting monoclonals (daclizumab or basiliximab), or depleting monoclonals (alemtuzumab) and polyclonal antibodies (Thymoglobulin). The goal is to reduce the incidence and severity of acute rejection (AR) as well as to prevent long-term chronic allograft dysfunction (*59*).

Induction with Daclizumab

The results of a multicenter survey from 2001 using daclizumab (antiCD25 antibody) as induction therapy revealed a low incidence of acute rejection in combination with Tacrolimus, MMF, and steroids in SPK recipients (*67*). MMF as primary immunosuppression was later investigated in a multicenter, open label, comparative trial (*68*). SPK recipients were randomized to one of the three groups. The rate of renal allograft AR was similar in the two daclizumab arms, however significantly higher in the no antibody arm. Although the follow-up was short, this study emphasized the important role of induction antibody in reducing AR (*69*).

Induction with Daclizumab in Combination with Thymoglobulin

In our center, SPK recipients were randomized prospectively to MMF or rapamycin, starting in September 2000. Patients received daclizumab and Thymoglobulin as induction immunosuppression as well as tapering steroids and Tacrolimus. Patient, kidney, and pancreas survival rates were similar in the two arms. However, kidney-specific (biopsy proven) AR occurred more often in the MMF vs. the rapamycin arm. Similarly, pancreas-specific AR (biopsy proven or clinically suspected) occurred more often in the MMF vs. rapamycin arm. GI symptoms led to dose reductions or withholding MMF in the first year, significantly more often than in the rapamycin group. Excellent kidney and pancreas graft survival was achieved using MMF or rapamycin-based immunosuppression in this long-term study. Rates of AR for pancreas and biopsy-proven kidney transplantation were statistically significantly better with rapamycin than MMF. It appears that rapamycin is better tolerated than MMF from the GI standpoint in this patient population with T1D, in whom 60% have gastroparesis (*70*).

Induction with Alemtuzumab

A nonrandomized study of 75 SPK and pancreas recipients who received alemtuzumab (antiCD52) (four doses for induction and up to 12 doses within the first year) and MMF (2 g/day) monotherapy was reported from Minnesota in 2005 (*71*). Patient and pancreas survival rates were not compared to an historical group of 266 consecutive pancreas recipients on Thymoglobulin (induction) and Tacrolimus (maintenance). The interim conclusion was that the combination of alemtuzumab and MMF was associated with an acceptable rejection rate (albeit higher than expected for SPK transplantation), and good (graft and native) kidney function; however, it eliminated the undesired calcineurin inhibitor and steroid-related side effects. Longer follow-up appears warranted. Kaufman et al. (*72*) compared the effects of alemtuzumab to those of Thymoglobulin as induction agents, given a steroid-free regimen in combination with Tacrolimus/Sirolimus-based maintenance therapy. The 1-year actual patient survival rates and AR were not statistically different (*72*). Viral infectious complications were statistically significantly lower in the alemtuzumab group. Although steroid-free protocols for pancreas transplantation are effective, questions remain regarding optimal patient selection and long-term outcome (*11*).

Pancreas Transplantation Outcomes

Pancreas transplantation restores euglycemia and provides long-term insulin independence in most patients. In our experience, 10-year survival rates for patients and pancreas are 84 and 76%, respectively, among patients with T1D and ESRD (*65*). Similar rates are reported by other centers while 15-year actuarial patient survival was recently reported to be 56% for SPK, 42% for PAK, and 59% for pancreas transplantation alone (PTA) with pancreas survival rates of 36, 18 and 16%, respectively (*62*). PT also ameliorates some diabetic complications. It can reverse preexisting histological lesions of diabetic nephropathy in the native kidneys, but reversal requires more than 5 years of normoglycemia (*73*). There is also evidence for improvement of renal function after pancreas transplantation, documented by the reduction of proteinuria and stable creatinine clearance (*74*). The majority of patients who undergo SPK transplant have already developed some degree of retinopathy and most have received laser therapy. For those patients without ESRD, the percentage of patients with improved or stabilized retinopathy was significantly higher among those receiving PTA than those treated with intensive insulin (*75*). For SPK recipients with longer duration of T1D (mean 24.6 years) and ESRD, more than 90% of patients have stable diabetic retinopathy, following transplantation (*76*). Some improvement in gastroparesis, as well as postural hypotension, generally occurs after PT (*77*). Sensory and motor neuropathy, as shown by nerve conduction studies, have also improved after SPK (*78*).

Challenges and Future Perspectives in Pancreas Transplantation

The present challenge is finding the balance between benefit (protection from rejection and resultant long-term graft function) and risk (side effects, infection, cancers) for patients with T1D and ESRD. Advances in immunosuppression protocol based on novel induction antibodies and effective maintenance agents have resulted in low rates of AR and excellent graft survival. Some centers, including our own, have also witnessed a low rate of viral sequelae and lymphoproliferative disorders. Similar to ITX, the major hurdle is the requirement for chronic immunosuppression and the inability of current regimens to achieve transplantation tolerance and prevent recurrent autoimmunity. At our center, we are intensively monitoring our patients for the possible recurrence of autoimmune diabetes, and have identified several who have developed T1D in the transplanted pancreas, in the absence of rejection (*79, 80*). Improved immune monitoring for both rejection and autoimmunity will also be required to develop tolerogenic protocols that would ideally provide freedom from chronic immunosuppression.

REFERENCES

1. Ryan EA, Bigam D, Shapiro AM. Current indications for pancreas or islet transplant. Diabetes Obes Metab 2006;8(1):1–7.
2. Leitao CB, Cure P, Tharavanij T, Baidal DA, Alejandro R. Current challenges in islet transplantation. Curr Diab Rep 2008;8(4):324–331.
3. Ricordi C, Lacy PE, Finke EH. Automated method for isolation of human pancreatic islets. Diabetes 1988;37:413–420.
4. Antonioli B, Fermo I, Cainarca S, et al. Characterization of collagenase blend enzymes for human islet transplantation. Transplantation 2007;84(12):1568–1575.
5. Ichii H, Wang X, Messinger S, et al. Improved human islet isolation using nicotinamide. Am J Transplant 2006;6(9):2060–2068.
6. Ichii H, Sakuma Y, Pileggi A, et al. Shipment of human islets for transplantation. Am J Transplant 2007;7(4):1010–1020.
7. Ichii H, Inverardi L, Pileggi A, et al. A novel method for the assessment of cellular composition and beta-cell viability in human islet preparations. Am J Transplant 2005;5(7):1635–1645.
8. Baidal DA, Froud T, Ferreira JV, Khan A, Alejandro R, Ricordi C. The bag method for islet cell infusion. Cell Transplant 2003;12(7):809–813.
9. Goss JA, Soltes G, Goodpastor SE, et al. Pancreatic islet transplantation: the radiographic approach. Transplantation 2003;76(1):199–203.
10. Bretzel RG, Brandhorst D, Brandhorst H, et al. Improved survival of intraportal pancreatic islet cell allografts in patients with type-1 diabetes mellitus by refined peritransplant management. J Mol Med 1999;77(1):140–143.
11. Mineo D, Sageshima J, Burke GW, Ricordi C. Minimization and withdrawal of steroids in pancreas and islet transplantation. Transpl Int 2009;22(1):20–37.
12. Shapiro AM, Lakey JR, Ryan EA, et al. Islet transplantation in seven patients with type 1 diabetes mellitus using a glucocorticoid-free immunosuppressive regimen. N Engl J Med 2000;343(4):230–238.
13. Ryan EA, Lakey JR, Paty BW, et al. Successful islet transplantation: continued insulin reserve provides long-term glycemic control. Diabetes 2002;51(7):2148–2157.
14. Alejandro R, Barton FB, Hering BJ, Wease S. 2008 Update from the Collaborative Islet Transplant Registry. Transplantation 2008;86(12):1783–1788.
15. Shapiro AM, Ricordi C, Hering BJ, et al. International trial of the Edmonton protocol for islet transplantation. N Engl J Med 2006;355(13):1318–1330.
16. Monti P, Scirpoli M, Maffi P, et al. Islet transplantation in patients with autoimmune diabetes induces homeostatic cytokines that expand autoreactive memory T cells. J Clin Invest 2008;118(5):1806–1814.
17. Nir T, Melton DA, Dor Y. Recovery from diabetes in mice by beta cell regeneration. J Clin Invest 2007;117(9):2553–2561.
18. Leitao CB, Tharavanij T, Cure P, et al. Restoration of hypoglycemia awareness after islet transplantation. Diabetes Care 2008;31(11):2113–2115.
19. Tharavanij T, Betancourt A, Messinger S, et al. Improved long-term health-related quality of life after islet transplantation. Transplantation 2008;86(9):1161–1167.
20. Luzi L, Perseghin G, Brendel MD, et al. Metabolic effects of restoring partial beta-cell function after islet allotransplantation in type 1 diabetic patients. Diabetes 2001;50(2):277–282.
21. Paty BW, Ryan EA, Shapiro AM, Lakey JR, Robertson RP. Intrahepatic islet transplantation in type 1 diabetic patients does not restore hypoglycemic hormonal counterregulation or symptom recognition after insulin independence. Diabetes 2002;51(12):3428–3434.
22. Rickels MR, Schutta MH, Mueller R, et al. Glycemic thresholds for activation of counterregulatory hormone and symptom responses in islet transplant recipients. J Clin Endocrinol Metab 2007;92(3):873–879.
23. Rickels MR, Schutta MH, Markmann JF, Barker CF, Naji A, Teff KL. {beta}-Cell function following human islet transplantation for type 1 diabetes. Diabetes 2005;54(1):100–106.
24. Rickels MR, Schutta MH, Mueller R, et al. Islet cell hormonal responses to hypoglycemia after human islet transplantation for type 1 diabetes. Diabetes 2005;54(11):3205–3211.
25. Ghofaili KA, Fung M, Ao Z, et al. Effect of exenatide on beta cell function after islet transplantation in type 1 diabetes. Transplantation 2007;83(1):24–28.
26. Froud T, Faradji RN, Pileggi A, et al. The use of exenatide in islet transplant recipients with chronic allograft dysfunction: safety, efficacy, and metabolic effects. Transplantation 2008;86(1):36–45.
27. Gangemi A, Salehi P, Hatipoglu B, et al. Islet transplantation for brittle type 1 diabetes: the

28. Cure P, Pileggi A, Alejandro R. Exenatide and rare adverse events. N Engl J Med 2008;358(18):1969–1970.
29. Ponte GM, Pileggi A, Messinger S, et al. Toward maximizing the success rates of human islet isolation: influence of donor and isolation factors. Cell Transplant 2007;16(6):595–607.
30. Campbell PM, Senior PA, Salam A, et al. High risk of sensitization after failed islet transplantation. Am J Transplant 2007;7(10): 2311–2317.
31. Cardani R, Pileggi A, Ricordi C, et al. Allosensitization of islet allograft recipients. Transplantation 2007;84(11):1413–1427.
32. Fung MA, Warnock GL, Ao Z, et al. The effect of medical therapy and islet cell transplantation on diabetic nephropathy: an interim report. Transplantation 2007;84(1):17–22.
33. Maffi P, Bertuzzi F, De TF, et al. Kidney function after islet transplant alone in type 1 diabetes: impact of immunosuppressive therapy on progression of diabetic nephropathy. Diabetes Care 2007;30(5):1150–1155.
34. Senior PA, Zeman M, Paty BW, Ryan EA, Shapiro AM. Changes in renal function after clinical islet transplantation: four-year observational study. Am J Transplant 2007;7(1): 91–98.
35. Leitao CB, Cure P, Messinger S, et al. Stable renal function after islet transplantation: importance of patient selection and aggressive clinical management. Transplantation 2009;87(5):681–688.
36. Toso C, Baertschiger R, Morel P, et al. Sequential kidney/islet transplantation: efficacy and safety assessment of a steroid-free immunosuppression protocol. Am J Transplant 2006;6(5 Pt 1):1049–1058.
37. Cure P, Pileggi A, Froud T, et al. Improved metabolic control and quality of life in seven patients with type 1 diabetes following islet after kidney transplantation. Transplantation 2008;85(6):801–812.
38. Tan J, Yang S, Cai J, et al. Simultaneous islet and kidney transplantation in seven patients with type 1 diabetes and end-stage renal disease using a glucocorticoid-free immunosuppressive regimen with alemtuzumab induction. Diabetes 2008;57(10):2666–2671.
39. Gerber PA, Pavlicek V, Demartines N, et al. Simultaneous islet-kidney vs pancreas-kidney transplantation in type 1 diabetes mellitus: a 5 year single centre follow-up. Diabetologia 2008;51(1):110–119.
40. Johansson BL, Borg K, Fernqvist-Forbes E, Kernell A, Odergren T, Wahren J. Beneficial effects of C-peptide on incipient nephropathy and neuropathy in patients with Type 1 diabetes mellitus. Diabet Med 2000;17(3): 181–189.
41. Hansen A, Johansson BL, Wahren J, von Bibra H. C-peptide exerts beneficial effects on myocardial blood flow and function in patients with type 1 diabetes. Diabetes 2002;51(10): 3077–3082.
42. Del CU, Fiorina P, Amadio S, et al. Evaluation of polyneuropathy markers in type 1 diabetic kidney transplant patients and effects of islet transplantation: neurophysiological and skin biopsy longitudinal analysis. Diabetes Care 2007;30(12):3063–3069.
43. Fiorina P, Gremizzi C, Maffi P, et al. Islet transplantation is associated with an improvement of cardiovascular function in type 1 diabetic kidney transplant patients. Diabetes Care 2005;28(6):1358–1365.
44. Fiorina P, Venturini M, Folli F, et al. Natural history of kidney graft survival, hypertrophy, and vascular function in end-stage renal disease type 1 diabetic kidney-transplanted patients: beneficial impact of pancreas and successful islet cotransplantation. Diabetes Care 2005;28(6):1303–1310.
45. Fiorina P, Folli F, Maffi P, et al. Islet transplantation improves vascular diabetic complications in patients with diabetes who underwent kidney transplantation: a comparison between kidney-pancreas and kidney-alone transplantation. Transplantation 2003;75(8):1296–1301.
46. Fiorina P, Folli F, Bertuzzi F, et al. Long-term beneficial effect of islet transplantation on diabetic macro-/microangiopathy in type 1 diabetic kidney-transplanted patients. Diabetes Care 2003;26(4):1129–1136.
47. Thompson DM, Begg IS, Harris C, et al. Reduced progression of diabetic retinopathy after islet cell transplantation compared with intensive medical therapy. Transplantation 2008;85(10):1400–1405.
48. Warnock GL, Thompson DM, Meloche RM, et al. A multi-year analysis of islet transplantation compared with intensive medical therapy on progression of complications in type 1 diabetes. Transplantation 2008;86(12):1762–1766.
49. Sutherland DE, Gruessner AC, Carlson AM, et al. Islet autotransplant outcomes after total pancreatectomy: a contrast to islet allograft outcomes. Transplantation 2008;86(12): 1799–1802.
50. Hering BJ, Kandaswamy R, Harmon JV, et al. Transplantation of cultured islets from two-layer preserved pancreases in type 1 diabetes with anti-CD3 antibody. Am J Transplant 2004;4(3):390–401.

51. Hering BJ, Kandaswamy R, Ansite JD, et al. Single-donor, marginal-dose islet transplantation in patients with type 1 diabetes. JAMA 2005;293(7):830–835.
52. Bellin MD, Kandaswamy R, Parkey J, et al. Prolonged insulin independence after islet allotransplants in recipients with type 1 diabetes. Am J Transplant 2008;8(11):2463–2470.
53. Froud T, Baidal DA, Faradji R, et al. Islet transplantation with alemtuzumab induction and calcineurin-free maintenance immunosuppression results in improved short- and long-term outcomes. Transplantation 2008;86(12):1695–1701.
54. Shapiro AMJ, Koh A, Kin T, et al. Outcomes following Alemtuzumab induction in clinical islet transplantation. Am J Transplant 2008;8(Suppl 2):S213.
55. Posselt A, Szot G, Frasssseto L, et al. Ilset allograft survival in type 1 diabetics using a calcineurin-free based on Efalizumab and Sirolimus. Am J Transplant 2008;8(Suppl 2):S253.
56. Pileggi A, Molano RD, Ricordi C, et al. Reversal of diabetes by pancreatic islet transplantation into a subcutaneous, neovascularized device. Transplantation 2006;81(9):1318–1324.
57. Leichtman AB, Cohen D, Keith D, et al. Kidney and pancreas transplantation in the United States, 1997–2006: the HRSA Breakthrough Collaboratives and the 58 DSA Challenge. Am J Transplant 2008;8(4 Pt 2):946–957.
58. Burke GW, Ciancio G, Sollinger HW. Advances in pancreas transplantation. Transplantation 2004;77(9 Suppl):S62–S67.
59. Ciancio G, Burke GW, Miller J. Current treatment practices in immunosuppression. Expert Opin Pharmacother 2000;1:1307–1330.
60. Ciancio G, Mattiazzi A, Roth D, Kupin W, Miller J, Burke GW. The use of daclizumab as induction therapy in combination with tacrolimus and mycophenolate mofetil in recipients with previous transplants. Clin Transplant 2003;17(5):428–432.
61. Burke GW, Ciancio G. Critical care issues in the renal and pancreatic allograft recipient. In: Civetta JM, Taylor RW, Kirby RR, eds. Critical Care. 3rd ed. Philadelphia: J.B. Lippincott Company, 1997:1311–1315.
62. White SA, Shaw JA, Sutherland DE. Pancreas transplantation. Lancet 2009;373(9677):1808–1817.
63. Burke GW, III, Ciancio G, Figueiro J, et al. Hypercoagulable state associated with kidney-pancreas transplantation. Thromboelastogram-directed anti-coagulation and implications for future therapy. Clin Transplant 2004;18(4):423–428.
64. Burke GW, Ciancio G, Cirocco R, et al. Microangiopathy in kidney and simultaneous pancreas/kidney recipients treated with tacrolimus: evidence of endothelin and cytokine involvement. Transplantation 1999;68(9):1336–1342.
65. Burke GW, Ciancio G, Olson L, Roth D, Miller J. Ten-year survival after simultaneous pancreas/kidney transplantation with bladder drainage and tacrolimus-based immunosuppression. Transplant Proc 2001;33(1–2):1681–1683.
66. Stratta RJ, Shokouh-Amiri MH, Egidi MF, et al. Long-term experience with simultaneous kidney-pancreas transplantation with portal-enteric drainage and tacrolimus/mycophenolate mofetil-based immunosuppression. Clin Transplant 2003;17 Suppl 9:69–77.
67. Bruce DS, Sollinger HW, Humar A, et al. Multicenter survey of daclizumab induction in simultaneous kidney-pancreas transplant recipients. Transplantation 2001;72(10):1637–1643.
68. Stratta RJ, Alloway RR, Hodge E, Lo A. A multicenter, open-label, comparative trial of two daclizumab dosing strategies vs. no antibody induction in combination with tacrolimus, mycophenolate mofetil, and steroids for the prevention of acute rejection in simultaneous kidney-pancreas transplant recipients: interim analysis. Clin Transplant 2002;16(1):60–68.
69. Stratta RJ, Alloway RR, Hodge E, Lo A. A multicenter, open-label, comparative trial of two daclizumab dosing strategies versus no antibody induction in simultaneous kidney-pancreas transplantation: 6-month interim analysis. Transplant Proc 2002;34(5):1903–1905.
70. Burke GW, Ciancio G, Gaynor JJ, et al. Lower rate of acute rejection with rapamycin versus mycophenolate mofetil in simultaneous kidney transplant recipients: eight year follow-up. Am J Transplant 2009;9(Suppl 2):216.
71. Gruessner RW, Kandaswamy R, Humar A, Gruessner AC, Sutherland DE. Calcineurin inhibitor- and steroid-free immunosuppression in pancreas-kidney and solitary pancreas transplantation. Transplantation 2005;79(9):1184–1189.
72. Kaufman DB, Leventhal JR, Gallon LG, Parker MA. Alemtuzumab induction and prednisone-free maintenance immunotherapy in simultaneous pancreas-kidney transplantation comparison with rabbit antithymocyte globulin induction - long-term results. Am J Transplant 2006;6(2):331–339.

73. Fioretto P, Sutherland DE, Najafian B, Mauer M. Remodeling of renal interstitial and tubular lesions in pancreas transplant recipients. Kidney Int 2006;69(5):907–912.
74. Coppelli A, Giannarelli R, Vistoli F, et al. The beneficial effects of pancreas transplant alone on diabetic nephropathy. Diabetes Care 2005;28(6):1366–1370.
75. Giannarelli R, Coppelli A, Sartini MS, et al. Pancreas transplant alone has beneficial effects on retinopathy in type 1 diabetic patients. Diabetologia 2006;49(12):2977–2982.
76. Pearce IA, Ilango B, Sells RA, Wong D. Stabilisation of diabetic retinopathy following simultaneous pancreas and kidney transplant. Br J Ophthalmol 2000;84(7):736–740.
77. Hathaway DK, Hartwig MS, Milstead J, Elmer D, Evans S, Gaber AO. Improvement in quality of life reported by diabetic recipients of kidney-only and pancreas-kidney allografts. Transplant Proc 1994;26(2):512–514.
78. Navarro X, Sutherland DE, Kennedy WR. Long-term effects of pancreatic transplantation on diabetic neuropathy. Ann Neurol 1997;42(5):727–736.
79. Laughlin E, Burke G, Pugliese A, Falk B, Nepom G. Recurrence of autoreactive antigen-specific CD4+ T cells in autoimmune diabetes after pancreas transplantation. Clin Immunol 2008;128(1):23–30.
80. Diamantopoulos S, Allende G, Martin-Pagola A, et al. Recurrence of type 1 diabetes (T1DR) after simultaneous pancreas-kidney (SPK) transplantation is associated with islet cell autoantibody conversion. Acta Diabetol 2007;44(S1):S13.

Chapter 24

Addison's Disease

Alberto Falorni

Summary

Autoimmune Addison's disease (AAD) represents 70–90% of all cases of primary adrenal insufficiency (PAI) in western countries and Japan. The adrenal autoimmune process is made evident by the appearance of autoantibodies, directed against steroid-21-hydroxylase (21OHAb), the gold marker to identify AAD in patients with clinical and biochemical signs of adrenal insufficiency. 21OHAb have no major pathogenic role, and the disease is thought to be caused by a cell-mediated immune process. In 21OHAb-negative patients, adrenal imaging and very long-chain fatty acids determination should be performed to exclude other causes of PAI such as posttuberculosis Addison's disease or X-linked adrenoleukodystrophy. AAD is a major component of autoimmune polyendocrine syndrome (APS) type 1 and type 2. Isolated AAD and APS2-related AAD are strongly associated with HLA-DRB1*0301–DQA1*0501–DQB1*0201 (DR3–DQ2) and DRB1*04–DQA1*0301–DQB1*0302 (DR4–DQ8). HLA-DRB1*0403 is strongly protective for the development of AAD. Other genetic factors that contribute to the risk of AAD include MICA5.1, and the polymorphisms of the CTLA-4, PTPN22, and MHC2TA genes. Around two-thirds of AAD subjects show clinical or biochemical signs of other autoimmune diseases, the most common being thyroid autoimmune diseases, type 1 diabetes mellitus, and primary ovarian insufficiency. Presence of 21OHAb in subjects with no clinical signs of adrenal insufficiency and with normal basal cortisol levels identifies the so-called subclinical AAD. In subjects with subclinical AAD, a stimulation test with 1 μg of synthetic ACTH should be performed to discriminate between an early and potentially reversible adrenal dysfunction and a progressive form of the disease.

Key Words: ACTH, Adrenal insufficiency, Autoantibodies, Cortisol, HLA, 21-hydroxylase, MICA, prediction

INTRODUCTION

Primary adrenal insufficiency (PAI) is a clinical condition due to the destruction or impaired function of adrenocortical cells (1). The reduction of adrenocortical cell mass is responsible for a deficiency of glucocorticoids and, in some cases, of mineralocorticoids and androgens.

The disease is also known as Addison's disease, after the name of the English hematologist who described it in 1855. It must, however, be noted that of the 11 cases initially described by Thomas Addison, ten were caused by tuberculosis infection or metastatic localization of nonadrenal tumors, with only one case being clinically idiopathic (possibly of autoimmune origin). Accordingly, the definition of Addison's disease can be applied to posttuberculosis adrenal insufficiency (posttuberculosis Addison's disease) and to autoimmune adrenal insufficiency (autoimmune Addison's disease, AAD), but not to other etiological agents today known to cause PAI.

The clinical spectrum of adrenal insufficiency has indeed considerably expanded in the last decades to include rare genetic diseases such as X-linked adrenoleukodystrophy (present in approximately 10% of males with PAI), adrenal hypoplasia congenita, triple A syndrome, familiar glucocorticoid deficiency, Smith–Lemli–Opitz syndrome, or Kearns–Sayre syndrome (*2–8*). Other causes of PAI include: sarcoidosis, amyloidosis, mycosis (paracoccidiomycosis, coccidiomycosis, histoplasmosis, blastomycosis, cryptococcosis), infection by cytomegalovirus or atypical mycobacteria in AIDS patients, adrenal hemorrhages, the antiphospholipid syndrome, drugs (such as ketoconazole, rifampicin, barbiturates, mitotane, metyrapone, and aminoglutethimide), or toxics (paraquat).

The disease was considered rare in the past, but recent epidemiological studies have shown that it occurs in approximately one individual of every 7,000–7,500 people in European countries (*9, 10*) (prevalence of 120–150 cases per million inhabitants), with a higher prevalence among females than males. It is still unclear if this increased prevalence, as compared to the initial data from the 1970s, is the consequence of a more accurate diagnosis or if it reflects a higher frequency of PAI.

DIAGNOSIS AND CLINICAL MANAGEMENT OF PAI

From a clinical standpoint, PAI often has a progressive evolution that can even last for years. In the early phases, clinical signs are evident only in stressful conditions. With the progression of the glandular damage, an increased hypophyseal release of ACTH and POMC-derived peptides is associated with reduced glucocorticoid secretion. In parallel, the insufficient production of mineraloactive steroids implies an increased plasmatic renin activity (PRA) with an excessive generation of angiotensin II (*11*). The clinical signs and symptoms of PAI are nonspecific and correct diagnosis may be dangerously delayed. Melanodermia is the major and most characteristic clinical sign of PAI. The most intensely colored areas are those exposed to light (face, neck, back of the hand), those already normally hyperpigmented (areola of the nipple, scrotum, labia), those that undergo friction or microtraumas, the linea alba, and the palmar folds. A conspicuous increase in cutaneous nevi can also be evident. Scars acquired after the development of PAI tend to darken. The pigmentation of the mucosae has important diagnostic significance: small brownish patches appear on the lips, the palate, the tongue, and the gingivae at the dental neck. Although melanodermia is often considered an inevitable sign of PAI, a few cases of the so-called "White Addison's disease," associated with a high degree of melanosome degradation in secondary lysosomes at skin biopsy, have been reported. Other clinical signs and symptoms include profound asthenia, weight loss in adults, slowed weight growth in children, hypotension, nausea, vomiting, abdominal pain, anemia, oligo-amenhorrea, reduction in the amount of axillary and pubic hair, muscular pain and neurological disturbances, with depression, irritability and inability to concentrate, hypersensitivity to tastes and smells, and headache.

The electrolytic picture is characterized by hyponatremia, hyperkaliemia, hyperchloremic acidosis, and hypercalcemia. When all are present, these alterations are highly suggestive of adrenal insufficiency. Dehydration is a frequent condition and is consequent to the complex hydroelectrolytic equilibrium disorder.

Once suspected on clinical ground, diagnosis is made according to low levels of basal cortisol (<3 µg/dl) and increased basal ACTH levels (>100 pg/ml). Low aldosterone and high PRA are typically present in AAD, but can be absent in other forms of PAI. In stressful conditions, such as septic shock, the cutoff level for diagnosis of adrenal insufficiency is higher, at around 15 µg/dl (12).

Treatment of PAI is based on substitutive therapy with oral hydrocortisone or cortisone acetate, and, in case of mineralocorticoid deficiency, with fluorohydrocortisone. New strategies for physiological glucocorticoid replacement have been recently suggested, including a modified release hydrocortisone preparation (13) that may become a clinical routine in the future.

The aim of the therapy is to revert the symptoms, improve quality of life, and prevent the occurrence of an Addisonian crisis. Addisonian crisis is a serious medical emergency that can manifest in subjects with no previous diagnosis of PAI or in diagnosed patients as a consequence of an intercurrent illness or major stressful event. If adequate parenteral therapy with high-dose hydrocortisone is not carried out, death ensues within 12–48 h of hypovolemic shock.

ADRENAL AUTOANTIBODIES AND DIAGNOSIS OF AAD

Until 25–30 years ago, the most frequent cause of PAI was tubercular adrenal infiltration (posttuberculosis Addison's disease) and this is still the case in developing countries. Autoimmune destructive adrenalitis has become the most common cause of PAI in western countries and Japan, representing 68–94% of cases in different studies (14, 15). The adrenal autoimmune process is made evident by the appearance of adrenocortical autoantibodies (ACA), detected in about two-thirds of PAI patients using indirect immunofluorescence techniques on cryostatic sections of adrenal gland tissue (14, 15).

ACA has been the gold marker for identification of AAD until the demonstration that the enzyme steroid 21 hydroxylase (21OH) is the major adrenocortical autoantigen, target of adrenal autoantibodies (16, 17). Sensitive immunoprecipitation assays with recombinant human 21OH, radiolabeled with either ^{35}S (18, 19) or ^{125}I (20), have been used to demonstrate that 21OH autoantibodies (21OHAb) have a high diagnostic sensitivity and specificity for AAD (13, 14). 21OHAb can be detected in approximately 70–90% of patients with PAI, representing over 95% of cases with clinically idiopathic adrenal insufficiency. 21OHAb are directed mostly to epitopes located in the central and COOH-terminal domains of the enzyme, and naturally occurring mutations, associated with the development of congenital adrenal hyperplasia, inhibit the binding of human autoantibodies to recombinant 21OH (21, 22). In vitro studies have shown that 21OHAb inhibit the enzymatic activity of the autoantigen (23), but no 21OH inhibition can be observed in vivo in 21OHAb-positive individuals, during the natural history of the disease (24, 25). Accordingly, 21OHAb do not appear to have a major pathogenic role in the development of adrenal insufficiency. They can be detected in approximately 0.5% of healthy subjects who do not necessarily progress toward clinical adrenal insufficiency.

Furthermore, 21OHAb cross the placental barrier and can be detected in the newborn of 21OHAb-positive women, without being associated with any sign of clinical or preclinical adrenal insufficiency (26). Hence, 21OHAb are an immunological marker of the ongoing adrenal autoimmune process, rather than an effector of the destructive autoimmune process, as it is the case for many other organ-specific autoantibodies. The presence of circulating 21OHAb identifies the autoimmune origin of PAI. However, it must be noted that the presence of low-titer adrenal autoantibodies does not enable the unequivocal diagnosis of AAD in all cases, as ACA and 21OHAb have sporadically been found also in patients with posttuberculosis Addison's disease (27, 28). A comprehensive flowchart for the etiological classification of

PAI, that takes into consideration immunological, biochemical, and imaging data, has been developed (29). According to this flowchart, adrenal autoantibodies should be the first marker to be analyzed. In the case of a simultaneous presence of both ACA and 21OHAb, the probability of an accurate diagnosis of AAD is higher than 99%, and no further tests, such as adrenal imaging or determination of plasmatic very long-chain fatty acids (VLCFA), are needed (29). All patients with AAD should undergo additional autoantibody analyses, as approximately two-thirds of AAD patients show clinical or preclinical signs of another autoimmune disease. Autoimmune AAD can be diagnosed also in the presence of medium–high levels of either 21OHAb or ACA. At present, no clear and standardized cutoff is available to discriminate between low and medium–high-level autoantibody titers, and workshops for the standardization of adrenal autoantibody assays are strongly needed. However, published data indicate that the accuracy of the 21OHAb immunoradiometric assay is higher than that of the ACA immunofluorescence assay, for the accurate identification of AAD (29), and 21OHAb must be considered the gold standard for the detection of adrenal autoantibodies. In the case of patients positive only for 21OHAb or ACA at low levels, as well as in autoantibody-negative subjects, adrenal imaging should be performed to exclude an infiltrative form of adrenal insufficiency (such as posttuberculosis, sarcoidosis, mycosis, or metastatic localization of nonadrenal tumors) (29). In male patients negative for both adrenal autoantibody measurement and adrenal imaging analysis, determination of plasmatic VLCFA must be performed to exclude X-linked ALD. Only after having performed adrenal imaging and VLCFA analysis, to reduce the risk of false positivity for adrenal autoantibodies, a low positivity for 21OHAb or ACA can be considered sufficient to formulate an accurate diagnosis of AAD. Etiological classification in 345 Italian patients with PAI is shown in Table 24.1.

Table 24.1
Etiological Classification of Primary Adrenal Insufficiency in 345 Patients from Italy

Disease	Frequency
AAD (including APS 1)	77% in males, 85% in females
Posttuberculosis Addison's disease	13%
X-linked adrenoleukodystrophy	8% of male patients
Other causes (such as postsepsis, adrenal hypoplasia congenita, or sarcoidosis)	2%

The coexistence of AAD with clinical or preclinical signs of other autoimmune diseases configures the so-called autoimmune polyendocrine syndromes (APS). APS1 is a genetic disease caused by mutations of the Autoimmune Regulator gene on chromosome 21. Clinical diagnosis of APS1 is formulated on the existence of at least two of three major disease components: chronic candidiasis, AAD, and hypoparathyroidism. APS2 represents the association of AAD with other endocrine autoimmune diseases, more often thyroid autoimmune diseases, and/or type 1 diabetes mellitus (T1DM). Thyroid autoantibodies are detected in over 50% of AAD patients, with clinical signs of a thyroid disease reported in 4–32% of cases in different studies (15). T1DM is present in approximately 5–20% of cases (15). Autoimmune primary ovarian insufficiency affects 10–20% of AAD women (15). Other autoimmune diseases associated with AAD include: vitiligo (2–16% of cases), atrophic gastritis (3–20% of cases), celiac disease (1–8% of cases), alopecia (1–12% of cases), multiple sclerosis (2–3% of cases), Sjögren's syndrome (1–2% of cases), and lymphocytic hypophysitis (<1% of cases) (15).

Although 21OHAb represent the major immune marker of AAD, other adrenal autoantibodies are also found in the sera collected from patients with PAI. They include 17α-hydroxylase autoantibodies (17OHAb) and P450 side-chain cleavage autoantibodies (P450sccAb). These autoantibodies can be detected in approximately 15–20% of sera from AAD patients (15, 30). It must be noted that 21OH is selectively expressed in the adrenal cortex, while 17OH and P450scc are expressed not only in the adrenal gland, but also in other organs such as the ovary, the testis, and the placenta. 17OH and P450scc represent the major autoantigenic targets of steroid cell autoantibodies (StCA), detected by indirect immunofluorescence on cryostatic sections of adrenal, ovary, and testis. StCA can be detected in approximately 20% of patients with AAD and in over 90% of women with both AAD and autoimmune primary ovarian insufficiency (also known as premature ovarian failure, POF) (15, 30). 17OHAb and P450sccAb are each detected in 50–70% of women with autoimmune POF (15, 30). The presence of StCA, 17OHAb, and P450sccAb in women with AAD identifies subjects at high risk to develop primary ovarian insufficiency within a few years. Positivity for steroidogenic enzyme autoantibodies identifies autoimmune POF that represents a subgroup of 4–5% of women with primary ovarian insufficiency. Autoimmune POF is constantly associated with positivity for 21OHAb and with clinical or subclinical signs of autoimmune adrenal insufficiency. Interestingly, StCA react specifically with androgen-producing cells in both the ovary (theca cells) and the testis (Leydig cells). Immunohistochemistry studies have demonstrated that oophoritis can be detected only in the presence of steroidogenic autoantibodies and is mainly located around the antral follicles. Thus, a diagnosis of autoimmune POF can be formulated only in the presence of 21OHAb and steroidogenic autoantibodies. Recent studies have demonstrated that the ovarian autoimmune process causes the selective destruction of theca cells, with lack of substrates for the production of estradiol by viable and functioning granulosa cells that react to the increase levels of gonadotropins, with an increase in production of inhibin A and inhibin B (*31, 32*).

Other autoantibodies, such as those directed against cytochrome P450 1A2, aromatic l-amino acid decarboxylase, tryptophan hydroxylase, or histidine decarboxylase, can also be detected in AAD patients, but they are typically associated with APS1 and are only sporadically found in patients with isolated or APS2-associated AAD.

GENETICS OF ISOLATED AND APS-2 ASSOCIATED AAD

The accurate identification of patients with AAD is critical for the identification of genetic factors associated with disease risk. The major genetic markers associated with AAD are located in the HLA region on chromosome 6. More specifically, the disease is strongly and positively associated with both HLA-DRB1*0301–DQA1*0501–DQB1*0201 (DR3–DQ2) and DRB1*04–DQA1*0301–DQB1*0302 (DR4–DQ8) (*33*). The odds ratio of these associations ranged from 3.0 to 8.5 for DR3–DQ2 and from 2.5 to 4.5 for DR4–DQ8, in different studies, respectively. The HLA-DRB1*01–DQA1*01–DQB1*0501 and DRB1*13–DQA1*0103–DQB1*0603 haplotypes are negatively associated with genetic risk for AAD, with odds ratio of 0.1–0.2. It is noteworthy that the HLA predisposing haplotypes are shared with a long series of other endocrine and nonendocrine autoimmune diseases, along with T1DM.

In several studies, it has been shown that the association of HLA class II haplotypes is still highly significant in patients with isolated AAD and does not depend on the coexistence of other autoimmune disorders in the same patient. In the attempt to dissect the genetic predisposition to different endocrine autoimmune diseases, some studies have focused their attention on the frequency of HLA-DRB1*04 subtypes in different populations of AAD and T1DM patients and healthy control subjects. It was observed that DRB1*0404 was more frequent among DRB1*04-positive AAD patients from USA (*34*) and Norway (*35*), as compared to both DRB1*04-positive healthy control subjects and DRB1*04-positive T1DM patients. The DRB1*0401 subtype was strongly and positively associated with T1DM, but not with AAD (*34, 35*). These results were interpreted to indicate that two different genetic markers (namely DRB1*0401 and DRB1*0404) conferred a differential risk for T1DM or AAD. However, a more recent study from Italy (36) did not confirm this hypothesis. In that study (36), it was observed that no statistically different distribution of DRB1*0401 and DRB1*0404 was detectable among T1DM patients and AAD patients. On the other hand, it was observed that the DRB1*0403 subtype, which was already known to confer strong protection for T1DM, was absent among 56 DRB1*04-positive AAD patients, but present in 27% DRB1*04-positive healthy control subjects, thus conferring protection also for the development of AAD. Furthermore, the endogenous LTR13 retrovirus-like element, which is located 1.3 kb upstream of the DQB1 gene and had previously been found to be positively associated with both T1DM (37) and AAD (38), was virtually absent among DRB1*0403-positive individuals (36), thus providing a potential explanation for DRB1*0403-mediated protection. However, multivariate logistic regression analysis demonstrated that DRB1*0403 is primarily and negatively associated with disease risk, while LTR13 is associated with human endocrine autoimmune disorders only because of a positive linkage disequilibrium with DQB1*0302 and a negative linkage disequilibrium with DRB1*0403 (36).

So far, it is not possible to clearly discriminate the HLA-related genetic background associated with AAD from that associated with other endocrine autoimmune diseases such as T1DM. The frequency of "at risk" HLA haplotypes and genotypes in the general population from different countries correlates positively with the incidence rate of T1DM (39), thus suggesting that genetic factors are a major determinant of the risk for T1DM. Although the frequency of the "high-risk" HLA markers is approximately threefold higher in Scandinavia than in the Mediterranean countries, the prevalence rate of AAD is only slightly higher in Norway (10) than in Italy (9), and the relative contribution of genetic factors and environmental agents for the development of clinical AAD remains to be elucidated. More specifically, the frequency of DRB1*0401 in Caucasian populations is not significantly different from that of DRB1*0404 and cannot alone explain the 10- to 20-fold higher prevalence of T1DM, as compared to AAD.

Several lines of evidence support the hypothesis that other HLA and nonHLA genes contribute to the risk for AAD, including the observation that the frequency of at-risk HLA haplotypes in the general population is several fold higher than that of the disease. Among the disease-associated gene marker is the MHC class I chain-related A (MICA) gene polymorphism. The MICA gene is located within the HLA class III region, though it encodes for a membrane-bound polypeptide, whose predicted domain structure is considered to be similar to that of the classical HLA class I chains. However, MICA, which is a ligand for an activating receptor (NKG2D) present on γδ T cells, CD8+CD28− αβ T cells, natural killer cells, and CD4+CD28− αβ cells, has no role in antigen presentation, and the significance of MICA gene polymorphism has not yet been clarified, even though there are speculations that might influence the affinity for the NKG2D receptor. AAD is strongly associated with the transmembrane MICA 5.1 allele, with odds ratio similar to that observed for HLA class II haplotypes (*40, 41*). MICA6 appears to be negatively associated with the disease risk for AAD (OR = 0.13) (*40*).

Although the association of MICA with AAD appears to be independent from that with HLA class II haplotypes, the strong linkage disequilibrium existing within the DRB1*03–DQA1*0501–DQB1*0201–MICA5.1-HLA-B extended haplotype has so far limited the possibility to discriminate the relative contribution of each gene marker, and further studies on large populations are needed to provide an answer to this specific question.

Similar to T1DM and other autoimmune diseases, the genetic background for AAD also includes other genes believed to modulate the function of the immune system. Accordingly, the CTLA-4 gene polymorphism and the PTPN22 gene polymorphism have been found to modulate the genetic risk for AAD (*33*). Recently, two independent European studies have shown the association of the class II transactivator (CIITA) (also denominated MHC2TA) gene with AAD (*42, 43*). The class II expression on antigen presenting cells is under the control of CIITA that exhibits cell-specific, cytokine-inducible, and differentiation-specific expression and is expressed in the same cells that express class II molecules such as B cells, monocytes, dendritic cells, and activated T cells. The association of CIITA with AAD appears to be independent from that with HLA gene markers. Other reported AAD genetic associations include the vitamin D receptor and the CYP27B1 (25-hydroxyvitamin D3-1a-hydroxylase) gene (*33*).

CELLULAR AUTOIMMUNITY AND AAD

The unavailability of spontaneous animal models of autoimmune adrenal insufficiency has so far limited the studies of the pathogenetic mechanisms responsible for the immune-mediated destruction of adrenocortical cells. The effector cells of the autoimmune-mediated destruction of adrenocortical cells are thought to be T lymphocytes (*44, 45*). Patients with autoimmune adrenal insufficiency have T cells that are reactive against fetal adrenal extracts or adrenal mitochondrial fraction (*46, 47*) and have an increased expression of circulating Ia-positive T cells, when compared to healthy control subjects (*48*). T cell proliferation in response to stimulation with adrenal proteins fractionated according to molecular weight was also demonstrated. Patients with APS type II, but not individuals with isolated Addison's disease, seem to have CD4+CD25+regulatory T cells with defective suppressive capacity (*49*). According to these studies, and to information derived from other organ-specific endocrine autoimmune diseases, a major role of cellular immunity in the autoimmune destruction of the adrenocortical cells in Addison's disease can be speculated, with a predominance of Th1 type of immune responses. However, it is still unclear why the prevalence of AAD is so dramatically lower than that of other endocrine autoimmune diseases such as Hashimoto's thyroiditis, Graves' disease, or T1DM. Studies of chemokine expression have shown that patients with AAD have increased circulating levels of CXCL10, a Th1 autoimmune-associated chemokine (*50*). In addition, CXCL10 secretion by cells from the fasciculata zona of the adrenal cortex is strongly induced by IFN-γ and by TNF-α, while hydrocortisone inhibits cytokine-induced CXCL10 secretion, in vitro (*50*). Accordingly, it can be speculated that the adrenal cortex cells participate in the maintenance of the autoimmune-mediated inflammatory process by producing chemokines, such as CXCL10, and that the endogenous production of cortisol acts as a modulator of this process, determining an autocrine and paracrine anti-inflammatory effect in the adrenal cortex.

SUBCLINICAL AAD

The presence of adrenal autoantibodies in patients with normal basal cortisol concentration and no clinical signs of adrenal insufficiency identifies the so-called subclinical AAD. 21OHAb can be found in around 0.5–1.5% T1DM patients, 0.5–1.5% patients with autoimmune thyroid diseases, and 4–6% women with primary ovarian insufficiency (*14, 15*). Subjects with subclinical AAD exhibit a variable degree of adrenal dysfunction that can be classified into four different stages (*51*). In stage 0, a normal ACTH–cortisol and PRA–aldosterone axis activity is present; stage 1 is characterized by an initial increase of PRA, with normal ACTH–cortisol axis response; in stage 2, an impaired response to the ACTH stimulation test is documented. Finally, stage 3 represents the preclinical stage characterized by increased basal ACTH levels, along with the dysfunctions observed in stages 1 and 2. A substitutive therapy is recommended in stage 3, because patients are at high risk to develop an Addisonian crisis, as a consequence of a stressful event. Substitutive therapy is not recommended in the other stages, but patients with an impaired response to the ACTH stimulation test need a strict follow-up, with hormonal and clinical evaluation every 6–9 months.

Several studies have attempted to identify the factors associated with progression toward clinical adrenal insufficiency, characterized by low-basal cortisol levels (stage 4) (52–56). It was shown that adrenal autoantibody levels increase during the progression of the adrenal dysfunction (54), especially at stages 2 and 3, when a destructive autoimmune attack of the adrenocortical cells is believed to take place. It was also shown that the response to the ACTH stimulation test discriminates between early potentially reversible stages (stage 0 and stage 1) and a more advanced and irreversible dysfunction (stage 2 and stage 3) (52–56). Indeed, approximately 80% of patients with stage 0 and stage 1 do not progress to clinical AAD and may show a spontaneous remission of the preclinical dysfunction, with possible disappearance of circulating autoantibodies (Table 24.2). On the other hand, no such spontaneous remission can occur in patients with stage 2 and stage 3, in whom progression to clinical AAD is observed in over 95% of cases (Table 24.2). Accordingly, in subjects positive for 21OHAb and/or ACA, an ACTH stimulation test is mandatory.

Typically, the ACTH stimulation test is performed with a highdose of 250 µg of synthetic ACTH. It has, however, been shown that such a dose is supra-maximal and that as little as 1 µg of synthetic ACTH can determine a maximal stimulation of the adrenocortical cells (57). It has also been shown that the low-dose test (LDT) with 1 µg of ACTH has a high-diagnostic sensitivity and specificity for preclinical adrenal dysfunction and can substitute the classical high-dose test (HDT) (25, 58).

Table 24.2
Estimated Risk of Progression Toward AAD in Patients Positive for 21OHAb

Response to the ACTH stimulation test	Outcome at 10-year follow-up (%)
Normal (stages 0–1)	
Progression to clinical AAD	25
No progression	50
Regression from stage 1 to stage 0	25
Subnormal (stages 2–3)	
Adrenal insufficiency stages 3–4	95
Pre-clinical AAD stage 2	5
Regression to stages 0–1	0

Factors increasing significantly the risk of progression toward clinical adrenal insufficiency, in subjects with subclinical AAD, include: male gender, presence of other concomitant autoimmune diseases, impaired response to the LDT, and a high 21OHAb titer (56). Among genetic factors, HLA-DR3-DQ2, DR4-DQ8, and CTLA-4 gene polymorphisms are significantly associated with the appearance of 21OHAb, but do not influence the natural history of the disease and do not predict future clinical adrenal insufficiency [(56) and Falorni et al., unpublished data]. Homozygosis for MICA5.1 was found to increase significantly the risk of progression toward clinical adrenal insufficiency (55), but larger, prospective studies are needed to confirm this finding. The high-predictive value of 21OHAb for future AAD, which is higher than 30% at 10 years of follow-up, warrants the use of this marker in patients with endocrine autoimmune diseases to identify subjects with subclinical adrenal insufficiency.

REFERENCES

1. Oelkers W. Adrenal insufficiency. N Engl J Med 1996;335:1206–1212.
2. Aubourg P. On the front of X-linked adrenoleukodystrophy. Neurochem Res 1999;24:515–520.
3. McCabe ER. DAX1: increasing complexity in the roles of this novel nuclear receptor. Mol Cell Endocrinol 2007;265–266:179–182.
4. Achermann JC, Ito M, Ito M, Hindmarsh PC, Jameson JL. A mutation in the gene encoding steroidogenic factor-1 causes XY sex reversal and adrenal failure in humans. Nat Genet 1999;22:125–126.
5. Clark AJ, McLoughlin L, Grossman A. Familial glucocorticoid deficiency associated with point mutation in the adrenocorticotropin receptor. Lancet 1993;341:461–462.
6. Weber A, Wienker TF, Jung M, Easton D, Dean HJ, Heinrichs C, Reis A, Clark A. Linkage of the gene for the triple A syndrome to chromosome 12q13 near the type II keratin gene cluster. Hum Mol Genet 1996;5:2061–2066.
7. North K, Korson MS, Krawiecki N, Shoffner JM, Holm IA. Oxidative phosphorylation defect associated with primary adrenal insufficiency. J Pediatr 1996;128:688–692.
8. Andersson HC, Frentz J, Martínez JE, Tuck-Muller CM, Bellizaire J. Adrenal insufficiency in Smith–Lemli–Opitz syndrome. Am J Med Genet 1999;82:382–384.
9. Laureti S, Vecchi L, Santeusanio F, Falorni A. Is the prevalence of Addison's disease underestimated? J Clin Endocrinol Metab 1999;84:1762.
10. Lovas K, Husebye ES. High prevalence and increasing incidence of Addison's disease in Western Norway. Clin Endocrinol 2002;56:787–791.
11. Laureti S, Santeusanio F, Falorni A. Recent advances in the diagnosis and therapy of primary adrenal insufficiency. Curr Med Chem Immunol Endocr Metab Agents 2002;2:251–272.
12. Cooper MS, Stewart PM. Corticosteroid insufficiency in acutely ill patients. N Engl J Med 2003;348:727–734.
13. Newell-Price J, Whiteman M, Rostami-Hodjegan A, Darzy K, Shalet S, Tucker GT, Ross RJM. Modified-release hydrocortisone for circadian therapy: a proof-of-principle study in dexamethasone-suppressed normal volunteers. Clin Endocrinol 2008;68:130–135.
14. Falorni A, Laureti S, Santeusanio F. Autoantibodies in polyendocrine syndrome type II. Endocrinol Metab Clin North Am 2002;31:369–389.
15. Betterle C, Dal Pra C, Mantero F, Zanchetta R. Autoimmune adrenal insufficiency and autoimmune polyendocrine syndromes: autoantibodies, autoantigens, and their applicability in diagnosis and disease prediction. Endocr Rev 2002;23:327–364.
16. Winqvist O, Karlsson FA, Kämpe O. 21-Hydroxylase, a major autoantigen in idiopathic Addison's disease. Lancet 1992;339:1559–1562.
17. Bednarek J, Furmaniak J, Wedlock N, Kiso Y, Baumann-Antczak A, Fowler SSS, Krishnan H,

Craft JA, Rees Smith B. Steroid 21-hydroxylase is a major autoantigen involved in adult onset autoimmune Addison's disease. FEBS Lett 1992;309:51–55.
18. Falorni A, Nikoshkov A, Laureti S, Grenbäck E, Hulting AL, Casucci G, Santeusanio F, Brunetti P, Luthman H, Lernmark Å. High diagnostic accuracy for idiopathic Addison's disease with a sensitive radiobinding assay for autoantibodies against recombinat human 21-hydroxylase. J Clin Endocrinol Metab 1995;80:2752–2755.
19. Colls J, Betterle C, Volpato M, Prentice L, Smith BR, Furmaniak J. Immunoprecipitation assay for autoantibodies to steroid 21-hydroxylase in autoimmune adrenal diseases. Clin Chem 1995;41:375–380.
20. Tanaka H, Perez MS, Powell M, Sanders JF, Sawicka J, Chen S, Prentice L, Asawa T, Betterle C, Volpato M, Rees Smith B, Furmaniak J. Steroid 21-hydroxylase autoantibodies: measurements with a new immunoprecipitation assay. J Clin Endocrinol Metab 1997;82:1440–1446.
21. Chen S, Sawicka J, Prentice L, Sanders J, Tanaka H, Petersen V, Betterle C, Volpato M, Roberts S, Powell M, Rees Smith B, Furmaniak J. Analysis of autoantibody epitopes on steroid 21-hydroxylase (21-OH) using a panel of monoclonal antibodies. J Clin Endocrinol Metab 1998;83:2977–2986.
22. Nikoshkov A, Falorni A, Lajic S, Laureti S, Wedell A, Lernmark Å, Luthman H. A conformation-dependent epitope in Addison's disease and other endocrinological autoimmune diseases maps to a carboxyl-terminal functional domain of human steroid 21-hydroxylase. J Immunol 1999;162:2422–2426.
23. Furmaniak J, Kominami S, Asawa T, Wedlock N, Colls J, Rees-Smith B. Autoimmune Addison's disease. Evidence for a role of steroid 21-hydroxylase autoantibodies in adrenal insufficiency. J Clin Endocrinol Metab 1994;79:1517–1521.
24. Boscaro M, Betterle C, Volpato M, Fallo F, Furmaniak J, Rees-Smith B, Sonino N. Hormonal responses during various phases of autoimmune adrenal failure: no evidence for 21-hydroxylase enzyme activity block in vivo. J Clin Endocrinol Metab 1996;81:2801–2804.
25. Laureti S, Candeloro P, Aglietti MC, Giordano R, Arvat E, Ghigo E, Santeusanio F, Falorni A. Dehydroepiandrosterone, 17α-hydroxyprogesterone and aldosterone responses to the low-dose (1 mg) ACTH test in subjects with preclinical adrenal autoimmunity. Clin Endocrinol 2002;57:677–683.

26. Betterle C, Pra CD, Pedini B, Zanchetta R, Albergoni MP, Chen S, Furmaniak J, Smith BR. Assessment of adrenocortical function and autoantibodies in a baby born to a mother with autoimmune polyglandular syndrome Type 2. J Endocrinol Invest 2004;27:618–621.
27. Nomura K, Depura H, Saruta T. Addison's disease in Japan: characteristics and changes revealed in a nationwide survey. Intern Med 1994;33:602–604.
28. de Carmo Silva R, Kater CE, Dib SA, Laureti S, Forini F, Casentino A, Falorni A. Autoantibodies against recombinant human steroidogenic enzyme 21-hydroxylase, side-chain cleavage and 17 α-hydroxylase in Addison's disease and autoimmune polyendocrine syndrome type III. Eur J Endocrinol 2000;142:187–194.
29. Falorni A, Laureti S, De Bellis A, Zanchetta R, Tiberti C, Arnaldi G, Bini V, Bizzarro A, Dotta F, Mantero F, Bellastella A, Betterle C, Santeusanio F. Italian Addison Network Study: update of diagnostic criteria for the etiological classification of primary adrenal insufficiency. J Clin Endocrinol Metab 2004;89:1598–1604.
30. Falorni, A, Laureti S, Candeloro P, Perrino S, Coronella C, Bizzarro A, Bellastella A, Santeusanio F, De Bellis A. Steroid-cell autoantibodies are preferentially expressed in women with premature ovarian failure who have adrenal autoimmunity. Fertil Steril 2002;78:270–279.
31. Welt CK, Falorni A, Taylor AE, Martin KA, Hall JE. Selective theca cell destruction accounts for the multifollicular development, decreased estradiol and elevated inhibin B levels in autoimmune premature ovarian failure. J Clin Endocrinol Metab 2005;90:3069–3076.
32. Tsigkou A, Marzotti S, Borges L, Brozzetti A, Candeloro P, Bacosi ML, Bini V, Petraglia F, Falorni A. High serum inhibin concentration discriminates autoimmune oophoritis from other forms of primary ovarian insufficiency. J Clin Endocrinol Metab 2008;93:1263–1269.
33. Falorni A, Brozzetti A, La Torre D, Tortoioli C, Gambelunghe G. The association of genetic polymorphisms and autoimmune Addison's disease. Exp Rev Clin Immunol 2008;4:441–456.
34. Yu L, Brewer KW, Gates S, Wu A, Wang T, Babu SR, Gottlieb PA, Freed BM, Noble J, Erlich HA, Rewers MJ, Eisenbarth GS. DRB1*04 and DQ alleles: expression of 21-hydroxylase autoantibodies and risk of

progression to Addison's disease. J Clin Endocrinol Metab 1999;84:328–335.
35. Myhre AG, Undlien DE, Løvås K, Uhlving S, Nedrebø BG, Fougner KJ, Trovik T, Sørheim JI, Husebye E. Autoimmune adrenocortical failure in Norway autoantibodies and human leukocyte antigen class II associations related to clinical features. J Clin Endocrinol Metab 2002;87:618–623.
36. Gambelunghe G, Kockum I, Bini V, De Giorgi G, Celi F, Betterle C, Giordano R, Libè R, Falorni A. Retrovirus-like long terminal repeat DQ-LTR13 and genetic susceptibility to type 1 diabetes mellitus and autoimmune Addison's disease. Diabetes 2005;54:900–905.
37. Bieda K, Pani MA, Van der Auwera B, Seidl C, Tönjes RR, Gorus F, Usadel KH, Badenhoop K. A retroviral long terminal repeat adjacent to the HLA DQB1 gene (DQ-LTR13) modifies Type I diabetes susceptibility on high risk DQ haplotypes. Diabetologia 2002;45:443–447.
38. Pani MA, Seidl C, Bieda K, Seissler J, Krause M, Seifried E, Usadel KH, Badenhoop K. Preliminary evidence that an endogenous retroviral long-terminal repeat (LTR13) at the HLA-DQB1 gene locus confers susceptibility to Addison's disease. Clin Endocrinol 2002;56:773–777.
39. Rønningen KS, Keiding N, Green A, EURODIAB ACE Study Group. Correlations between the incidence of childhood-onset type I diabetes in Europe and HLA genotypes. Diabetologia 2001;44(Suppl 3):B51–B59.
40. Gambelunghe G, Falorni A, Ghaderi M, Laureti S, Tortoioli C, Santeusanio F, Brunetti P, Sanjeevi CB. Microsatellite polymorphism of the MHC class I chain-related (MIC-A and MIC-B) genes marks the risk for autoimmune Addison's disease. J Clin Endocrinol Metab 1999;84:3701–3707.
41. Park YS, Sanjeevi CB, Robles D, Yu L, Rewers M, Gottlieb PA, Fain P, Eisenbarth GS. Additional association of intra-MHC genes, MICA and D6S273, with Addison's disease. Tissue Antigens 2002;60:155–163.
42. Ghaderi M, Gambelunghe G, Tortoioli C, Brozzetti A, Jatta K, Gharizadeh B, De Bellis A, Pecori Giraldi F, Terzolo M, Betterle C, Falorni A. MHC2TA single nucleotide polymorphism and genetic risk for autoimmune adrenal insufficiency. J Clin Endocrinol Metab 2006;91:4107–4111.
43. Skinningsrud B, Husebye E, Pearce SH, McDonald DO, Brandal K, Bøe Wolff A, Løvas K, Egeland T, Undlien DE. Polymorphisms in CLEC16A and CIITA at 16p13 are associated with primary adrenal insufficiency. J Clin Endocrinol Metab 2008;93:3310–3317.
44. Freeman M, Weetman AP. T and B cell reactivity to adrenal antigens in autoimmune Addison's disease. Clin Exp Immunol 1992;88:275–279.
45. Hayashi Y, Hiyoshi T, Takemura T, Kurashima C, Hirokawa K. Focal lymphocytic infiltration in the adrenal cortex of the elderly: immunohistological analysis of infiltrating lymphocytes. Clin Exp Immunol 1989;77:101–105.
46. Nerup J, Andersen V, Bendixen G. Anti-adrenal, cellular hypersensitivity in Addison's disease. Clin Exp Immunol 1969;4:355–363.
47. Nerup J, Andersen V, Bendixen G. Anti-adrenal, cellular hypersensitivity in Addison's disease. IV. In vivo and in vitro investigations on the mitochondrial fraction. Clin Exp Immunol 1970;6:733–739.
48. Rabinowe SL, Jackson RA, Dluhy RG, Williams GH. Ia-positive T lymphocytes in recently diagnosed idiopathic Addison's disease. Am J Med 1984;77:597–601.
49. Kriegel MA, Lohmann T, Gabler C, Blank N, Kalden JR, Lorenz HM. Defective suppressor function of human $CD4^+CD25^+$ regulatory T cells in autoimmune polyglandular syndrome type II. J Exp Med 2004;199:1285–1291.
50. Rotondi M, Falorni A, De Bellis A, Laureti S, Ferruzzi P, Romagnani P, Buonamano A, Mannelli M, Santeusanio F, Bellastella A, Serio M. Elevated serum interferon-g inducible chemokine IP-10/CXCL10 in autoimmune primary adrenal insufficiency and in vitro expression in human adrenal cells primary cultures after stimulation with proinflammatory cytokines. J Clin Endocrinol Metab 2005;90:2357–2363.
51. Betterle C, Scalici C, Presotto F, Pedini B, Moro L, Rigon F, Mantero F. The natural history of adrenal function in autoimmune patients with adrenal autoantibodies. J Endocrinol 1988;117:467–475.
52. De Bellis A, Bizzarro A, Rossi R, Paglionico VA, Criscuolo T, Lombardi G, Bellastella A. Remission of subclinical adrenocortical failure in subjects with adrenal autoantibodies. J Clin Endocrinol Metab 1993;76:1002–1007.
53. Betterle C, Volpato M, Rees-Smith B, Furmaniak J, Chen S, Greggio NA, Sanzari M, Tedesco F, Pedini B, Boscaro M, Presotto F. I. Adrenal cortex and steroid 21-hydroxylase autoantibodies in adult patients with organ-specific autoimmune diseases: markers of low progression to clinical Addison's disease. J Clin Endocrinol Metab 1997;82:932–938.

54. Laureti S, De Bellis A, Muccitelli VI, Calcinaro F, Bizzarro A, Rossi R, Bellastella A, Santeusanio F, Falorni A. Levels of adrenocortical autoantibodies correlate with the degree of adrenal dysfunction in subjects with preclinical Addison's disease. J Clin Endocrinol Metab 1998;83:3507–3511.
55. Barker JM, Ide A, Hostetler C, Yu L, Miao D, Fain PR, Eisenbarth GS, Gottlieb PA. Endocrine and immunogenetic testing in individuals with type 1 diabetes and 21-hydroxylase autoantibodies: Addison's disease in a high-risk population. J Clin Endocrinol Metab 2005;90:128–134.
56. Coco G, Dal Pra C, Presotto F, Albergoni MP, Canova C, Pedini B, Zanchetta R, Chen S, Furmaniak J, Rees Smith B, Mantero F, Betterle C. Estimated risk for developing autoimmune Addison's disease in patients with adrenal cortex autoantibodies. J Clin Endocrinol Metab 2006;91:1637–1645.
57. Arvat E, Di Vito L, Laffranco F, Maccario M, Baffoni C, Rossetto R, Aimaretti G, Camanni F, Ghigo E. Stimulatory effect of adrenocorticotropin on cortisol, aldosterone, and dehydroepiandrosterone secretion in normal humans: dose–response study. J Clin Endocrinol Metab 2000;88:3141–3146.
58. Laureti S, Arvat E, Candeloro P, Di Vito L, Ghigo E, Santeusanio F, Falorni A. Low dose (1 mg) ACTH test in the evaluation of adrenal dysfunction in pre-clinical Addison's disease. Clin Endocrinol 2000;53:107–115.

Chapter 25

Animal Models of Autoimmune Thyroid Disease

Yuji Nagayama and Norio Abiru

Summary

Autoimmune thyroid disease includes Graves' disease and Hashimoto's thyroiditis; the former is characterized by hyperthyroidism induced by agonistic antithyrotropin receptor (TSHR), whereas the latter by hypothyroidism mediated by cytotoxic T lymphocytes against thyroglobulin and/or thyroid peroxidase and cytokine-induced thyroid cell apoptosis. Animal models of autoimmune thyroid diseases, including spontaneous and inducible models of Hashimoto's thyroiditis and inducible models of Graves' hyperthyroidism, have an approximately 50-year history. Extensive studies with these models have provided us insights into the numerous aspects of the pathogenesis of autoimmune thyroid diseases, for example, (1) the genetic and environmental factors affecting disease development, (2) characterization of lymphocyte subsets involved in the disease pathogenesis, and (3) significance of peripheral and central tolerance to thyroid autoimmunity. Thus, animal models have substantially contributed to accumulating numerous novel findings on the pathogenesis of autoimmune thyroid diseases and to updating of our current understanding of the etiology of these diseases.

Key Words: Graves' hyperthyroidism, Hashimoto's thyroiditis, Thyrotropin receptor, Thyroglobulin, Thyroid peroxidase, Effector T cells, Regulatory T cells

INTRODUCTION

Autoimmune thyroid disease consists of Graves' disease and Hashimoto's thyroiditis, which stand at opposite ends of a continuum of this disease entity. Although both diseases are literally of autoimmune nature, each disease is mediated by different immune responses with different consequences. Thus, the former is caused by abnormal humoral immune response that elicits agonistic antithyrotropin receptor (TSHR) autoantibody (called thyroid stimulating antibody, TSAb) and leads to diffuse enlargement of the thyroid gland and hyperthyroidism (hyperfunction of the target organ), whereas the latter by abnormal cellular immune response that induces cytotoxic T lymphocytes and cytokine-induced thyroid cell apoptosis, and results in thyroid destruction and hypothyroidism (hypofunction of the target organ) (1).

Animal models of human autoimmune diseases provide an invaluable means for delineating the pathogenesis of these conditions because studies with human materials have nonnegligible limitations. Thus, numerous animal models of autoimmune thyroid diseases have been generated for the last five decades and are currently being used widely. In this review, animal models of Hashimoto's thyroiditis and Graves' hyperthyroidism so far reported are first briefly introduced, and then how these models contribute to clarification of the pathogenesis of these diseases is discussed.

HISTORY OF ANIMAL MODELS OF AUTOIMMUNE THYROID DISEASES

Experimental autoimmune thyroiditis induced by immunizing rabbits with thyroid extracts together with complete Freund's adjuvant reported in 1956 by Rose et al. (2) is the first animal model of autoimmune thyroid disease. Thyroglobulin (Tg) and thyroid peroxidase (TPO) were subsequently identified as specific autoantigens in thyroid extracts (3–5). Thus immunization of susceptible mice (see below) with these antigen proteins emulsified with classic adjuvants (3, 4) or professional antigen-presenting dendritic cells (DC) pulsed with Tg efficiently induced autoimmune thyroiditis (6). Animals that spontaneously develop autoimmune thyroiditis have also been established such as Obese Strain (OS) chicken, BioBreeding (BB) rats, nonobese diabetic (NOD) mice, and NOD-H2^{h4} mice (7, 8). Recently, transgenic mice expressing the T cell receptor gene of a TPO-specific human T-cell clone have also been generated that spontaneously develop severe thyroiditis and hypothyroidism (9).

In contrast, spontaneous animal model of Graves' hyperthyroidism has never been established, and generation of the authentic inducible mouse Graves' model had been awaited until 1996 (10), although anti-TSHR autoantibody was identified to be responsible for hyperthyroidism in 1970s (11). In 1996, Shimojo et al. have demonstrated induction of Graves' hyperthyroidism by repetitive immunization of mice with syngeneic fibroblasts stably expressing recombinant MHC class II and the TSHR (10). They expected that the fibroblasts expressing both the autoantigen TSHR and MHC class II would work as antigen-presenting cells (12). A similar approach was later reported using a B cell line that constitutively expressed endogenous MHC class II and exogenous recombinant TSHR (13). B cells are also professional antigen-presenting cells. Subsequently, genetic immunization with the eukaryotic expression plasmid (*14*) or recombinant adenoviral vector (*15, 16*) has been reported to be effective at inducing Graves' hyperthyroidism. Particularly, repeated intramuscular immunization with adenovirus coding the TSHR (Ad-TSHR) efficiently induced hyperthyroidism in mice (*15*). As for experimental autoimmune thyroiditis, immunization with DC expressing the TSHR also worked well (*16*). These immunization approaches were later improved by using the TSHR A-subunit, instead of the full-length receptor cDNA (see below for a detail) (*17, 18*) and/or combined with in vivo electroporation in the case of plasmid (*19*), with the incidence of disease being increased up to 60–80%. As easily understood, all the models mentioned above use the TSHR cDNA. Thus, establishment of these models is largely attributed to the cloning of the TSHR cDNA during 1989–1990 (*20*). It should be, however, noted here that it is reported that immunization with the TSHR extracellular domain protein can also induce hyperthyroidism (*13*), but purification of large amounts of native TSHR protein is a daunting task.

GENETIC FACTORS

It is well known that both genetic and environmental factors contribute to development of autoimmune thyroid disease. In Tg-induced mouse autoimmune thyroiditis models, studies with different mouse strains including mice congenic for different MHC haplotypes revealed that disease susceptibility is closely linked to this genetic locus; thus, mice with $H\text{-}2^{k,\,q,\,\text{and}\,s}$ (CBA/J, DBA/1J, SJL/J, etc.) are good responders, and those with $H\text{-}2^{b\,\text{and}\,d}$ (C57BL/6, BALB/c, etc.) respond poorly (*21*) (Table 25.1).

Susceptibility of each inbred mouse strain to TPO immunization is quite different from those to Tg. For example, C57BL/6 ($H\text{-}2^b$) are susceptible, and BALB/c ($H\text{-}2^d$), CBA/J ($H\text{-}2^k$) and SJL/J ($H\text{-}2^s$) are resistant (*4, 5*). Of interest, the existence of at least one non-H-2-linked susceptible gene is also suggested.

Regarding the susceptibility to the TSHR autoimmunity, the data are not identical among different models (*7*). At least in the Ad-TSHR model, BALB/c mice ($H\text{-}2^d$) are a good responder, C57BL/6 ($H\text{-}2^b$) a poor responder, and CBA/J ($H\text{-}2^k$) and DBA/1J ($H\text{-}2^q$) nonresponders (*15*). SJL/J ($H\text{-}2^s$) mice are a good responder in terms of (nonstimulating) antibody production, but resistant to development of hyperthyroidism. Studies with mice congenic for different MHC haplotypes revealed that non-MHC genes are the major determinants for development of Graves' hyperthyroidism (*22*). However, studies with transgenic mice expressing human DR3 (*23*) and also linkage studies

Table 25.1
Susceptibility of Different Mouse Strains in Different Mouse Models of Experimental Autoimmune Thyroid Diseases

Mouse strains (H-2)	Tg-induced thyroiditis Incidence of thyroiditis	Tg-induced thyroiditis Antibody titers	TPO-induced thyroiditis Incidence of thyroiditis	TPO-induced thyroiditis Antibody titers	Ad-TSHR-induced Graves' disease Incidence of hyperthyroidism	Ad-TSHR-induced Graves' disease Antibody titers
AJ (a)	+	+	+	++	n.d.[a]	n.d.
C57BL/6 (b)	–	±	++	+	±	++
BALB/c (d)	–	±	–	±	++	++
CBA/1J (k)	++	++	–	±	–	–
DBA/1J (q)	++	++	n.d.	n.d.	–	–
SJL/J (s)	++	++	–	±	–	++

*, –, ±, +, and ++ means no, poor, moderate, and good, respectively, responders
[a] Not examined

performed with recombinant inbred BALB/c × C57BL/6 and × C3H/He strains (24, 25) show the contribution of both MHC and non-MHC genes for susceptibility to hyperthyroidism. It was shown that susceptibility rather than resistance to hyperthyroidism is dominant while using BALB/c × C57BL/6 hybrid mice (26).

ENVIRONMENTAL FACTORS

One of the most critical environmental factors for autoimmune thyroiditis is, no doubt, iodine. Indeed, NOD-H2^{h4} mice develop autoimmune thyroiditis after provision of iodine in the drinking water (27). It is now recognized that exacerbation of thyroiditis by excessive iodine is related to higher immunogenecity in iodinated Tg (28).

Infectious agents have long been suspected to induce autoimmune diseases. The discovery of the Toll-like receptors (TLRs), the receptors recognizing pathogen-specific molecular patterns in infectious agents, contributed to recent progress in understanding this concept (29). For example, TLR3, the receptor for double-stranded RNA and synthetic poly I:C (a viral mimic), has recently been reported to be expressed on a normal differentiated Fisher rat thyroid cell line FRTL5 and Hashimoto's thyrocytes, which are assumed to induce the innate immune response in the thyroid and subsequently thyroiditis (*30*). Administration of poly I:C (high doses for a short period or low doses for a longer period) had, however, no effect on development of anti-Tg antibodies and autoimmune thyroiditis in NOD-H2^{h4} mice (our unpublished data).

In Graves' model with Ad-TSHR, maintaining mice in a conventional housing or administration of microbial components such as *Escherichia coli* lipopolysaccharide or *Saccharomyces cerevisiae* zymosan A (the ligands for TLR 4 and 2, respectively) (*22*) did not show a significant impact on incidence of Graves' disease. However, infection with live microorganisms such as *Schistosoma mansoni* and *Mycobacterium bovis* Bacillus Calmette–Guerin significantly suppressed disease development (*31, 32*). Since these microorganisms polarized TSHR-specific immune response toward T helper type 2 (Th2; see below) and Th1, respectively, the suppressive effect cannot be explained by altered Th1/Th2 balance. Instead, these data fits well the hygiene hypothesis, a concept that reduced exposure to microorganisms during childhood impairs the development of an appropriately educated immune system, and leads to development of not only Th1-type autoimmune disease but also Th2-type allergic disease. Collectively, the development of Graves' disease may be affected by certain infectious pathogens.

CHARACTERIZATION OF IMMUNE RESPONSES

It should be, at first, noted here that due to some differences in the features of immune responses elicited in distinct models (*7, 33*) and also due to space limitation, the main focus is put on the Graves' model with Ad-TSHR and the Hashimoto's model with NOD-H2^{h4} mice in the following sections.

Briefly, acquired immune response is initiated with phagocytosis of an antigen by professional antigen-presenting cells such as DC, macrophages, and B cells, followed by the presentation of the antigenic peptides by antigen-presenting cells to naïve CD4$^+$ helper T cells. CD4$^+$ T cells can largely be divided into two different subsets; effector (pathogenic) T cells (T$_{eff}$) and regulatory T cells (T$_{reg}$), which positively and negatively regulate immune responses, respectively. Dependent on cytokine environments, activated CD4$^+$ T$_{eff}$ cells differentiate into either Th1 cells or Th2 cells (*34*). Th1 cells are largely induced by interferon (IFN)-g and interleukin (IL)-12 and represents cell-mediated immune response, while Th2 cells involve antibody-mediated immune response regulated by IL-4.

In addition, Th17 cells have recently been identified as an additional new helper T$_{eff}$ cell lineage (*35, 36*). Th17 cells (T cells producing a strong proinflammatory IL-17) can be derived from naïve CD4⁺ T cells by IL-6 and transforming growth factor-b in mice (*37*). It has recently been shown that Th17 cells play a critical role in arthritis and experimental autoimmune encephalomyelitis, both of which had previously been thought to be the Th1-dominant diseases.

It has long been believed, as I mentioned in the "Introduction," that Hashimoto's thyroiditis is cellular immune response-mediated, while Graves' disease is humoral immune response-mediated. This concept was readily confirmed by antibody-mediated depletion of T cell subsets. Thus, in Graves' model, depletion of CD4⁺, but not CD8⁺, T cells completely suppressed disease development (our unpublished data), while depletion of either CD4⁺ or CD8⁺ T cells both inhibited induction of autoimmune thyroiditis in NOD-H2^{h4} mice (*38, 39*).

Although cellular and humoral immune responses in general correspond to Th1 and Th2, respectively, understanding of Th1/Th2 (or Th1/Th2/Th17) balance in experimental Graves' disease is challenging. In Graves' model with Ad-TSHR, both Th1 and Th2 IgG subclass anti-TSHR antibodies are elicited against the TSHR (Th1-type being dominant), and the Th1 cytokine IFN-g, not the Th2 cytokine IL-4, is secreted by splenocytes in in vitro recall assay, suggesting the elicitation of both Th2 and particularly Th1 immune responses against the TSHR (*40*). Exogenous IL-4 indeed suppresses development of Graves' hyperthyroidism (*40*). In the studies with knockout (KO) mice, disease induction is severely impaired in both IFN-g and IL-4 KO mice (*41*). However, of interest, IL-17 defect has little effect on disease development (our unpublished data). Thus, although Graves' disease is clearly humoral immune-mediated, Th2 and particularly Th1, but not Th17, immune responses appear to play a crucial role in developing Graves' hyperthyroidism.

However, these data are considerably different from those in NOD-H2^{h4} mice in which disease development was significantly suppressed in IFN-g KO (*42*) and IL-17 KO mice (our unpublished data), but not in IL-4 KO mice (*42*). Thus, Th1 and Th17, not Th2, immune responses are crucial for developing autoimmune thyroiditis in NOD-H2^{h4} mice. Of interest, the ability of thyrocytes to respond to IFN-g is somehow essential for development of autoimmune thyroiditis in these mice (*43*).

Although B cells have been long recognized to contribute to the pathogenesis of autoimmune disease as antibody-producing cells, recent studies revealed B cells have numerous functions besides antibody production (*44*). For example, in B cell-deficient mice, T cell response in recall assay is abolished in Graves' model (*45*), and disease development is suppressed in NOD-H2^{h4} mice (*46*). Similar results were also observed in anti-CD20 antibody-mediated B cell depletion studies in both models (our unpublished data, and (*47*)). These data support positive regulation of immune response by antigen-presentation function of B cells (*44*). Actually, anti-CD20 monoclonal antibody (rituximab) was used for treatment of Graves' disease in a clinical trial (*48*), showing a potential of this agent for treatment of the patients with mild Graves' hyperthyroidism.

However, B cells are also reported to exert their negative regulatory function on immune response as regulatory cells (*49*). The aforementioned studies with anti-CD20 antibody suggest regulatory B cell-mediated suppression of T_{reg} (*50*).

PERIPHERAL TOLERANCE

As mentioned earlier, CD4⁺ T cells include not only T_{eff} but also T_{reg} that negatively regulate immune response (*51*). It is now well known that some autoreactive T_{eff} escape central tolerance in the thymus and migrate to the periphery in all individuals (see below) but are kept in an anergic state by T_{reg}. Thus, T_{reg} play a central role in peripheral tolerance of autoreactive T_{eff}.

T_{reg} can be divided into two subpopulations; naturally occurring versus inducible. Naturally occurring CD4⁺CD25⁺ T_{reg} (*52*), CD8⁺CD122⁺ T_{reg} (*53*), and natural killer T (NKT) cells (*31*) are so far identified as the subsets of T_{reg} participating in the pathogenesis of Graves' disease. Thus, depletion of either CD4⁺CD25⁺ T cells or CD8⁺CD122⁺ T cells by anti-CD25 or CD122 enhances disease development/severity, respectively (*52, 53*). Repetitive stimulation of NKT cells with its synthetic agonistic ligand a-galactosylceramide polarize anti-TSHR immune response toward a Th2 phenotype and suppress disease induction in the Graves' model with Ad-TSHR (*31*). An important role for CD4⁺CD25⁺ T_{reg} in the development of Hashimoto's thyroiditis has also been demonstrated recently by antibody-mediated depletion (*54–56*).

Of interest, it has been previously shown that CD4⁺CD45RC⁻ suppressor T cells from athyroitic rats adoptively transferred to recipient rats having thyroids are unable to prevent thyroiditis, but able to prevent diabetes (*57*). These data, together with studies on other autoimmune diseases (*58, 59*), indicate that the presence of the self-antigen in the peripheral tissue is a requisite for maintenance of effective numbers of autoantigen-specific T_{reg}.

CENTRAL TOLERANCE

It is generally believed that tolerance to "self" antigens is mediated by two steps: the thymus and the periphery (central and peripheral tolerance, respectively). As mentioned above, T_{reg} are one of the critical factors for peripheral tolerance. Central tolerance is established (but not completely) in the thymus by deletion of T cells that bind with high affinity to peptides derived from self proteins. The *auto*i*m*mune *r*egulator (Aire)-positive thymic medullary epithelial cells play a crucial role in this process. The Aire is a transcriptional factor involved in promiscuous expression of various tissue-specific autoantigens in these cells (*60*). Indeed, inactivation of the Aire gene causes a rare recessive disorder, autoimmune polyendocrine syndrome 1 (APS1) in humans (*61*).

Therefore, central tolerance can generally be abolished by genetic disruption of the Aire gene. Thus, Aire KO mice spontaneously develop lymphocyte infiltration into numerous organs including the thyroid glands (*62–64*). In addition, Goodnow and his colleagues generated transgenic mice expressing hen egg lysosome (HEL) exclusively in the thyroid gland using the Tg promoter, and crossed them with HEL-specific TCR transgenic mice (*65*). The double transgenic mice shows partial reduction in numbers of CD4+CD8+ thymocytes and peripheral CD4+ T and CD8+ T cells. In addition, peripheral CD4+ T cells displayed reduced proliferative ability in response to HEL. However, high local concentrations of HEL in the thyroid gland reactivated partially tolerized autoreactive T cells, leading to intrathyroidal lymphocyte infiltration. To elucidate whether this partial tolerance is attributed to the promiscuous expression of HEL in the thymus by Aire, the double transgenic mice mentioned above were further crossed with Aire KO mice (*66*). Loss of Aire expression abolished thymic expression of HEL, and concomitantly, restored the partial reduction of autoreactive T cells mentioned above. Thus, at least in the studies with the Tg promoter, thymic Aire expression plays a crucial role in central tolerance to the thyroid specific autoantigens.

Regarding the TSHR, thyroid-specific TSHR A-subunit transgenic mice, generated by using the Tg promoter, were found to be tolerant to low-dose Ad-TSHR A-subunit immunization (*67*). The authors speculate that higher thymic expression of the TSHR A-subunit by the Tg promoter in transgenic mice is responsible for the enhanced central tolerance. Supporting these assumptions, anti-TSHR immune response was enhanced in the Aire KO BALB/c mice (*68*). However, such an enhanced immune response was not observed in the TSHR KO mice immunized with TSHR-plasmid (*69*), which must lack central (and also peripheral) tolerance.

Of interest, it has recently been demonstrated the induction of extensive intrathyroidal lymphocyte infiltration and in some cases hypothyroidism by antibody-mediated depletion of CD4+CD25+ or CD8+CD122+ T_{reg} in the A-subunit transgenic mice (*70*). This observation is particularly interesting in that, in most thyroiditis models, the animals are euthyroid. The similar, albeit weaker, intrathyroidal lymphocyte infiltration was also observed in wt C57BL/6 mice depleted of T_{reg} with anti-CD25 or anti-CD122 antibodies (52, 53). The mechanisms responsible for lymphocytic infiltration and thyroid destruction are yet to be elucidated. Nevertheless, these observations suggest that immune response to the TSHR can trigger thyroid gland destruction. It remains to be clarified why intrathyroidal lymphocytic infiltration is only induced in resistant mice (wt C57BL/6 and A-subunit transgenic BALB/c), but not susceptible mice (wt BALB/c).

CONCLUSIONS

Animal models have contributed to accumulating numerous new findings on the pathogenesis of autoimmune thyroid diseases and improved enormously our current understanding of the etiology of these diseases. For example, the results obtained suggest the major importance of MHC locus in Hashimoto's models and non-MHC genes in Graves' model. Possible involvement of microbial infection in the disease pathogenesis (via innate immunity or hygiene hypothesis) is also indicated. The immune responses elicited appear mainly to be of Th1 and to a lesser degree Th2 types in Graves' disease, and Th1 and Th17 types in Hashimoto's thyroiditis. B cells likely function not only as antibody-producing cells but also as antigen-presenting cells. In addition, naturally occurring regulatory T cells (CD4+CD25+ and CD8+CD122+ T cells) and thymic expression of autoantigens play a role in peripheral and central tolerance, respectively.

Although numerous questions remain unanswered, continuation of studies with these mouse models will make further progress in understanding the pathogenesis of autoimmune thyroid diseases and enable development of novel therapeutic interventions, although attempts in developing novel therapeutic approaches are not discussed in this review. For example, it will hopefully become possible to manipulate antigen-presenting cells (DC and B cells) or T_{reg}, to provide new avenues for immunotherapy of autoimmune thyroid diseases in the near future.

REFERENCES

1. Braverman LE, Utiger RD, eds. Werner & Ingbar's the Thyroid. Eighth Edition. Tokyo: Lippincott Williams & Wilkins, 2000.
2. Rose NR, Witebsky E. Studies on organ specificity. V. Changes in the thyroid glands of rabbits following active immunization with rabbit thyroid extracts. J Immunol 1956;76:417–427.
3. Rose NR, Kite Jr, JH, Doebbler TK, Spier R, Skelton FR, Witebsky E. Studies on experimental thyroiditis. Ann N Y Acad Sci 1965;124:201–230.
4. Kotani T, Ueki K, Hirai K, Ohtaki S. Experimental murine thyroiditis induced by porcine thyroid peroxidase and its transfer by the antigen-specific T cell line. Clin Exp Immunol 1990;80:11–18.
5. McLachlan SM, Atherton MC, Nakajima Y, Napier J, Jordan RK, Clark F, Rees Smith B.

Thyroid peroxidase and the induction of autoimmune thyroid disease. Clin Exp Immunol 1990;79:182–188.
6. Knight AC, Farrant J, Chan J, Bryant A, Bedford PA, Bateman C. Induction of autoimmunity with dendritic cells: studies on thyroiditis in mice. Clin Immunol Immunopathol 1988;48:277–289.
7. McLachlan SM, Nagayama Y, Rapoport B. Insight into Graves' hyperthyroidism from animal models. Endocr Rev 2005;26: 800–832.
8. Podolin PL, Pressey A, DeLarato NH, Fischer PA, Peterson LB, Wicker LS. I-E$^+$ nonobese diabetic mice develop insulitis and diabetes. J Exp Med 1993;178:793–803.
9. Quaratino S, Badami E, Pang YY, Bartok I, Dyson J, Kioussis D, Londei M, Maiuri L. Degenerate self-reactive human T-cell receptor causes spontaneous autoimmune disease in mice. Nat Med 2004;10:920–926.
10. Shimojo N, Kohno Y, Yamaguchi K, Kikuoka S, Hoshioka A, Niimi H, Hirai A, Tamura Y, Saito Y, Kohn LD, Tahara K. Induction of Graves-like disease in mice by immunization with fibroblasts transfected with the thyrotropin receptor and a class II molecule. Proc Natl Acad Sci U S A 1996;93:11074–11079.
11. Rees Smith B, Hall R. Thyroid-stimulating immunoglobulins in Graves' disease. Lancet 1974;2:427–431.
12. Bottazzo GF, Pujol-Borrell R, Hanafusa T, Feldmann M. Role of aberrant HLA-DR expression and antigen presentation in induction of endocrine autoimmunity. Lancet 1983;2:1115–1118.
13. Kaithamana S, Fan J, Osuga Y, Liang S-G, Prabhakar BS. Induction of experimental autoimmune Graves' disease in BALB/c mice. J Immunol 1999;163:5157–5164.
14. Costagliola S, Many M-C, Dehef J-F, Pohlenz J, Refetoff S, Vassart G. Genetic immunization of outbred mice with thyrotropin receptor cDNA provides a model of Graves' disease. J Clin Invest 2000;105:803–811.
15. Nagayama Y, Kita-Furuyama M, Nakao K, Ando T, Mizuguchi H, Hayakawa T, Eguchi K, Niwa M. A novel murine model of Graves' hyperthyroidism with intramuscular injection of adenovirus expressing thyrotropin receptor. J Immunol 2002;168:2789–2794.
16. Kita-Furuyama M, Nagayama Y, Pichurin P, McLachlan SM, Rapoport B, and Eguchi K. Dendritic cells infected with adenovirus expressing the thyrotropin receptor induce Graves' hyperthyroidism in BALB/c mice. Clin Exp Immunol 2003;131:234–240.
17. Chen C-R, Pichurin P, Nagayama Y, Latrofa F, Rapoport B, McLachlan SM. The thyrotropin receptor autoantigen in Graves' disease is the culprit as well as the victim. J Clin Invest 2003;111:1897–1904.
18. Mizutori Y, Saitoh O, Eguchi K, Nagayama Y. Adenovirus coding the thyrotropin receptor A-subunit improves the efficacy of dendritic cell-based mouse model of Graves' hyperthyroidism. J Autoimmun 2006;26:32–36.
19. Kaneda T, Honda A, Hakozaki A, Fuse T, Muto A, Yoshida T. An improved Graves' disease model established by using in vivo electroporation exhibited long-term immunity to hyperthyroidism in BALB/c mice. Endocrinology 2007;148:2335–2344.
20. Rapoport B, Chazenbalk GD, Jaume JC, McLachlan SM. The thyrotropin (TSH) receptor: interaction with TSH and autoantibodies. Endocr Rev 1998;19:673–616.
21. Vladutiu AO, Rose NR. Autommune murine thyroiditis relation to histocompatibility (H-2) type. Science 1971;174:1137–1139.
22. Nagayama Y, McLachlan SM, Rapoport B, Niwa M. A major role for non-major histocompatibility complex genes but not for microorganisms in a novel murine model of Graves' hyperthyroidism. Thyroid 2003;13: 235–240.
23. Pichurin P, Chen C-R, Pichurin O, David C, Rapoport B, McLachlan SM. Thyrotropin receptor-DNA vaccination of transgenic mice expressing HLA-DR3 or HLA-DQ6b. Thyroid 2003;13:911–917.
24. Aliesky HA, Pichurin PN, Chen C-R, Williams RW, Rapoport B, McLachlan SM. Probing the genetic basis for thyrotropin receptor antibodies and hyperthyroidism in immunized CXB recombinant inbred mice. Endocrinology 2006;147:2789–2800.
25. McLachlan SM, Aliesky HA, Pichurin PN, Chen C-R, Williams RW, Rapoport B. Shared and unique susceptibility genes in a mouse model of Graves' disease determined in BXH and CXB recombinant inbred mice. Endocrinology 2008;149:2001–2009.
26. Chen C-R, Aliesky H, Pichurin PN, Nagayama Y, McLachlan SM, Rapoport B. Susceptibility rather than resistance to hyperthyroidism is dominant in a thyrotropin receptor adenovirus-induced animal model of Graves' disease as revealed by BALB/c–C57BL/6 hybrid mice. Endocrinology 2004;145:4927–4933.
27. Rassoly L, Burek CL, Rose NR. Iodine-induced autoimmune thyroiditis in NOD-H-2^{h4} mice. Clin Immunol Immunopathol 1996;81:287–292.

28. Barin JG, Talor MV, Sharma RB, Rose NR. Iodination of murine thyroglobulin enhances autoimmune activity in the NOD.H-2^{h4} mice. Clin Exp Immunol 2005;142:251–259.
29. Kaisho T, Akira S. Toll-like receptors as adjuvant receptors. Biochim Biophys Acta 2002; 1589:1–13.
30. Harii N, Lewis CJ, Vasko V, McCall K, Benavides-Peralta U, Sun X, Ringel MD, Saji M, Giuliani C, Napolitano G, Goetz DJ, Kohn LD. Thyrocytes express a functional toll-like receptor 3: overexpression can be induced by viral infection and reversed by phenylmethimazole and is associated with Hashimoto's autoimmune thyroiditis. Mol Endocrinol 2005;19:1231–1250.
31. Nagayama Y, Niwa M, McLachlan SM, Rapoport B. *Schistosoma mansoni* and α-galactosylceramide: prophylactic effect of Th1 immune suppression in a mouse model of Graves' hyperthyroidism. J Immunol 2004;173:2167–2173.
32. Nagayama Y, McLachlan SM, Rapoport B, Oishi K. Graves' hyperthyroidism and the hygiene hypothesis in a mouse model. Endocrinology 2004;145:5075–5079.
33. Fang Y, Yu S, Braley-Mullen H. Contrasting roles of IFN-g in murine models of autoimmune thyroid diseases. Thyroid 2007;17:989–994.
34. Mosmann TR, Coffman RL. Th1 and Th2 cells: different patterns of lymphokine secretion lead to different functional properties. Annu Rev Immunol 1989;7:145–173.
35. Weaver CT, Harrington LE, Mangan PR, Gavrieli M, Murphy KM. Th17: an effector CD4 T cell lineage with regulatory T cell ties. Immunity 2006;24:677–688.
36. Steinman L. A brief history of T$_H$17, the first major revision in the T$_H$1/T$_H$2 hypothesis of T cell-mediated tissue damage. Nat Med 2007;13:139–145.
37. Veldhoen M, Hocking RJ, Atkins CJ, Locksley RM, Stockinger B. TGFb in the context of an inflammatory cytokine milieu supports de novo differentiation of IL-17 producing T cells. Immunity 2006;24:179–189.
38. Hutchings PR, Verma S, Phillips JM, Harach SZ, Howlett S, Cooke A. Both CD4$^+$ and CD8$^+$ T cells are required for iodine accelerated thyroiditis in NOD mice. Cell Immunol 1999;192:113–121.
39. Braley-Mullen H, Sharp GC, Medling B, Tang H. Spontaneous autoimmune thyroiditis in NOD.H-2^{h4} mice. J Autoimmun 1999;12:157–165.
40. Nagayama Y, Mizuguchi H, Hayakawa T, Niwa M, McLachlan SM, Rapoport B. Prevention of autoantibody-mediated Graves'-like hyperthyroidism in mice by IL-4, a Th2 cytokine. J Immunol 2003;170:3522–3527.
41. Nagayama Y, Saitoh O, McLachlan SM, Rapoport B, Kano H, Kumazawa Y. TSH receptor-adenovirus-induced Graves' disease is attenuated in both interferon-g and interleukin-4 knockout mice; implications for the Th1/Th2 paradigm. Clin Exp Immunol 2004;138:417–422.
42. Yu S, Sharp GC, Braley-Mullen H. Dual role for IFN-g, but not for IL-4, in spontaneous autoimmune thyroiditis in NOD.H-2^{h4} mice. J Immunol 2002;169:3999–4007.
43. Yu S, Sharp G, Braley-Mullen H. Thyrocytes responding to IFN-g are essential for development of lymphocytic spontaneous autoimmune thyroiditis and inhibition of thyrocyte hyperplasia. J Immunol 2006;176:1259–1265.
44. Yanaba K, Bouaziz J-D, Matsushita T, Margo CM, St. Clair EW, Tedder TF. B-lymphocyte contributions to human autoimmune disease. Immunol Rev 2008;223:284–299.
45. Pichurin P, Aliesky H, Chen, C-R, Nagayama Y, Rapoport B, McLachlan SM. Thyrotropin receptor-specific memory T cell responses require normal B cells in a murine model of Graves' disease. Clin Exp Immunol 2003;134:396–402.
46. Braley-Mullen H, Yu S. Early requirement of B cells for development of spontaneous autoimmune thyroiditis in NOD.H-2^{h4} mice. J Immunol 2000;165:7262–7269.
47. Yu S, Dunn R, Kehry MR, Braley-Mullen H. B cell depletion inhibits spontaneous autoimmune thyroiditis in NOD.H-2h4 mice. J Immunol 2008;180:7706–7713.
48. Fassi DE, Nielasen CH, Bonnema SJ, Hasselbach HC, Hegedus LB. Lymphocyte depletion with the monoclonal antibody rituximab in Graves' disease: a control pilot study. J Clin Endocrinol Metab 2007;92:1769–1772.
49. Jamin C, Morva A, Lemoine S, Daridon C, de Mendoza AR, Youinou P. Regulatory B lymphocytes in humans. Arthritis Rheum 2008;58:1900–1906.
50. Yu S, Maiti PK, Dyson M, Jain R, Braley-Mullen H. B cell-deficient NOD.H-2^{h4} mice have CD4$^+$CD25$^+$ T regulatory cells that inhibit the development of spontaneous autoimmune thyroiditis. J Exp Med 2006;203:349–358.
51. Sakaguchi S. Naturally arising Foxp3-expressing CD4$^+$CD25$^+$ regulatory T cells in immunological tolerance to self and non-self. Nat Immunol 2005;6:345–352.

52. Saitoh O, Nagayama Y. Regulation of Graves' hyperthyroidism with naturally occurring CD4+CD25+ regulatory T cells in a mouse model. Endocrinology 2006;147: 2417–2422.
53. Saitoh O, Abiru N, Nakahara M, Nagayama Y. CD8+CD122+ T cells, a newly identified regulatory T subset, negatively regulate Graves' hyperthyroidism in a murine model. Endocrinology 2007;148:6040–6048.
54. Wei WZ, Jacob JB, Zielinski JF, Flynn JC, Shim KD, Alsharabi G, Girado AA, Kong YM. Concurrent induction of antitumor immunity and autoimmune thyroiditis in CD4+CD25+ regulatory T cell-depleted mice. Cancer Res 2005;65:8471–8478.
55. Wei WZ, Morris GP, Kong YM. Anti-tumor immunity and autoimmunity: a balancing act of regulatory T cells. Cancer Immunol Immunother 2004;53:73–78.
56. Nagayama Y, Horie I, Saitoh O, Nakahara M, Abiru N. CD4+CD25+ naturally occurring regulatory T cells and not lymphopenia play a role in the pathogenesis of iodine-induced autoimmune thyroiditis in NOD-H2h4 mice. J Autoimmun 2007;29:195–202.
57. Seddon B, Mason D. Peripheral autoantigen induces regulatory T cells that prevent autoimmunity. J Exp Med 1999;189:877–882.
58. Samy ET, Setiady YY, Ohno K, Pramoonjago P, Sharp C, Tung KS. The role of physiological self-antigen in the acquisition of and maintenance of regulatory T-cell function. Immunol Rev 2006;212:170–184.
59. Suri-Payer E, Fritzsching B. Regulatory T cells in experimental autoimmune disease. Springer Semin Immunopathol 2006;28: 3–16.
60. Su MA, Anderson MS. Aire: an update. Curr Opin Immunol 2004;16:746–752.
61. Nagamine K, Peterson P, Scott HS, Kudoh J, Minoshita S, Heino M, Krohn KJ, Lalioti MD, Mullis PE, Antonarakis SE, et al. Positional cloning of the APECED gene. Nat Genet 1997;17:393–398.
62. Ramsy C, Winqvist O, Puhakka L, Halonen M, Moro A, Kämpe O, Eskelin P, Pelto-Huikko M, Peltonen L. Aire deficient mice develop multiple features of APECED phenotype and show altered immune response. Hum Mol Genet 2002;11:397–409.
63. Anderson MS, Venanzi ES, Klein L, Chen Z, Berzins SP, Turley SJ, von Boehmer H, Bronson R, Dierich A, Benoist C, Mathis D. Projection of an immunological self shadow within the thymus by the aire protein. Science 2002;298:1395–1401.
64. Kuroda N, Mitani T, Takeda N, Ishimaru N, Arakaki R, Hayashi Y, Bando Y, Izumi K, Takahashi T, Nomura T, Sakaguchi S, Ueno T, Takahama Y, Uchida D, Sun S, Kajiura F, Mouri Y, Han H, Matsushima A, Yamada G, Matsumoto M. Development of autoimmunity against transcriptionally unrepressed target antigen in the thymus of aire-deficient mice. J Immunol 2005;174:1862–1870.
65. Akkaraju S, Ho WY, Leoong D, Canaan K, Davis MM, Goodnow CC. A range of CD4 T cell tolerance: partial inactivation to organ-specific antigen allows nondestructive thyroiditis or insulitis. Immunity 1997;7: 255–271.
66. Liston A, Gray DHD, Lesage S, Fletcher AL, Wilson J, Webster KE, Scott HS, Boyd RL, Peltonen L, Goodnow CC. Gene dosage-limiting role of aire in thymic expression, clonal deletion and organ-specific autoimmunity. J Exp Med 2004;200:1015–1026.
67. Pichurin PN, Chen C-R, Chazenbalk GD, Aliesky H, Pham N, Rapoport B, McLachlan SM. Targeted expression of the human thyrotropin receptor A-subunit to the mouse thyroid: insight into overcoming the lack of response to A-subunit adenovirus immunization. J Immunol 2006;176:668–676.
68. Misharin A, Aliesky H, Nagayama Y, Rapoport B, McLachlan SM. Aire-deficiency modulates induction of TSHR antibodies and hyperthyroidism in a mouse model of Graves' disease. The Abstract in the 90th Annual Meeting of Endocrine Society. 2008:R50–R52.
69. Pichurin P, Pichurina O, Marians RC, Chen C-R, Davies TF, Rapoport B, McLachlan SM. Thyrotropin receptor knockout mice: studies on immunological tolerance to a major thyroid autoantigen. Endocrinology 2004;14: 1294–1301.
70. McLachlan SM, Nagayama Y, Pichurin PN, Mizutori Y, Chen C-R, Misharin A, Aliesky HA, Rapoport B. The link between Graves' disease and Hashimoto's thyroiditis: a role for regulatory T cells. Endocrinology 2007;148: 5724–5733.

Chapter 26

Genetics of Thyroid Autoimmunity

Yaron Tomer

Summary

Autoimmune thyroid diseases (AITD) including Graves' disease (GD) and Hashimoto's thyroiditis (HT) are the commonest autoimmune endocrine diseases, affecting up to 5% of the general population. Genetic factors play a major role in the etiology of AITD as evidenced by the strong familial aggregation of the AITD and the high concordance rates in monozygotic twins. The past decade has witnessed significant progress in our understanding of the genetic contribution to the etiology of AITD, and several major AITD susceptibility genes have been identified and characterized. Some susceptibility genes are specific to either Graves' disease or Hashimoto's thyroiditis, while others are common to both conditions. The first AITD susceptibility gene locus identified was the HLA-DR gene locus. Subsequently, five major non-HLA genes, including the CTLA-4, CD40, PTPN22, thyroglobulin, and TSH receptor (TSHR) gene, have been shown to contribute to the susceptibility to AITD; other putative genes are still being tested and confirmed. Excitingly, we are now beginning to unravel the mechanisms by which these AITD susceptibility genes confer risk for disease.

Key Words: Thyroid, Genes, Association, Linkage, Graves' disease, Hashimoto's thyroiditis, Autoimmune thyroiditis, HLA

INTRODUCTION

The major autoimmune thyroid diseases (AITD) include Graves' disease (GD) and Hashimoto's thyroiditis (HT), both of which are characterized pathologically by infiltration of the thyroid by T and B cells, reactive to thyroid antigens, resulting in the production of thyroid autoantibodies. Clinically, HT manifests by hypothyroidism often with goiter, while GD manifests by hyperthyroidism, goiter, and in some patients ophthalmopathy (1, 2). Additional forms of AITD include post-partum thyroiditis (3–5), drug-induced thyroiditis, such as interferon-induced thyroiditis (IIT) (6), thyroiditis associated with polyglandular autoimmune syndromes (reviewed in ref. (*7*)), and the presence of thyroid antibodies (TAbs) with no apparent clinical disease (*8*). The etiology of AITD involves a complex interplay between genetic factors and environmental triggers. Indeed, there now exist solid evidence for a major genetic influence on the development of AITD (*9*). In this chapter, we discuss recent exciting advances in our understanding of the genetic basis of AITD.

EPIDEMIOLOGICAL OBSERVATIONS

The familial occurrence of AITD has been noted for many years. Early studies, by Hall and colleagues, have shown that 33% of siblings of patients with GD or HT developed AITD themselves and 56% of siblings had thyroid antibodies (TAbs) without clinical disease (*10*). More recently, we have shown that 36% of GD patients with ophthalmopathy had a family history of AITD and 23% had a first degree relative with AITD (*11*).

However, the fact that a disease cluster in families does not necessarily mean that it is genetic since family members share many environmental exposures such as diet and infections. One way to estimate the genetic contribution to familial aggregation of a disease is by computing the sibling risk ratio (λs). The sibling risk ratio is the ratio of the prevalence of the disease in siblings of affected individuals, compared to the prevalence of the disease in the general population (*12*). In a recent study, we computed the λs for AITD to be 16.9, a very high value, supporting a strong genetic influence on the development of AITD (*13*).

Twin studies also lend strong support to a genetic susceptibility to AITD. Several large twin studies have been performed in AITD, all showing significantly higher concordance rates in monozygotic (MZ) twins than in dizygotic (DZ) twins. In Graves' disease, the concordance was 35% in MZ twins and 3% in DZ twins (*14–16*). For Hashimoto's thyroiditis, the concordance rates were 55% and 0% for MZ and DZ twins, respectively (*17*), and for TAbs MZ twins had 80% concordance and DZ twins had 40% concordance (*17*). Thus, the sibling risk ratio and twin data support a significant inherited risk for AITD.

IMMUNE REGULATOR GENES AND SUSCEPTIBILITY TO AITD

AITD are characterized by breakdown of tolerance to self-antigens. Therefore, immune regulatory genes are likely to play a role in the genetic susceptibility to AITD. Moreover, one would expect immune regulatory genes to confer risk for several autoimmune

HLA-DR

diseases with similar pathogenesis (e.g., HT and type 1 diabetes (T1D), both T-cell mediated diseases, which affect one target organ).

The major histocompatibility complex (MHC) region, encoding the HLA glycoproteins, consists of a complex of genes located on chromosome 6p21 (*18*). HLA class II genes were the first genes to be tested in AITD. While initial studies analyzed different HLA-DR and DQ alleles in AITD (*19*), more recent studies focused on specific peptide binding pocket sequences and 3-D structures that predispose to disease (*20, 21*). GD is strongly associated with HLA-DR3 (*9*). The frequency of DR3 in GD patients was generally 40–50% and in the general population ~15–30%, resulting in an odds ratio (OR) for people with HLA-DR3 of up to 4.0 (*22*). Among Caucasians, HLA-DQA1*0501 was also shown to be associated with GD (*23, 24*), but it appears that the primary susceptibility allele in GD is indeed HLA-DR3 (HLA-DRB1*03) (*25*). However, the exact amino acid sequence in the DRb1 chain conferring susceptibility to GD was until recently unknown. In other autoimmune diseases including T1D (*26*), there is convincing evidence that the disease is associated with specific amino acid sequences of the DRB1 and DQ genes. We recently identified arginine at position 74 of the HLA-DRb1 chain (DRb-Arg-74) as the critical DR amino acid conferring susceptibility to GD (*20*). In contrast, the presence of glutamine at position 74 of the DRβ1 chain was protective from disease. These data were replicated in an independent dataset (*27*). Moreover, structural modeling analysis demonstrated that the change at position 74 from glutamine to arginine significantly modified the 3-D structure of the P4 peptide-binding pocket, potentially modifying the interaction of the DR peptide binding pocket with antigenic peptides during presentation to T cells.

Data on HLA alleles in HT have been less definitive than in GD. Earlier studies showed an association of goitrous HT with HLA-DR5 (RR = 3.1) (*28*) and of atrophic HT with DR3 (RR = 5.1) in Caucasians (*29*). Later studies in Caucasians reported weak associations of HT with HLA-DR3 (*30, 31*) and HLA-DR4 (*32*). Recently, we have identified a pocket HLA-DR amino acid signature, consisting of tyrosine at position 26 (Tyrosine-26), Tyrosine-30, Glutamine-70, Lysine-71, and Arginine-74, that conferred strong risk for HT resulting in an OD of 3.7 (*21*). This pocket amino acid signature resulted in a unique pocket structure that is likely to influence pathogenic peptide binding and presentation to T cells (*21*).

CTLA-4

The cytotoxic T lymphocyte-associated factor 4 (CTLA-4) gene is a major negative regulator of T-cell activation (*33*). Indeed, CTLA-4 knockout mice succumb early in life due to high levels of activation of T cells that infiltrate and destroy multiple organs (*34*). CTLA-4 may play a role in autoimmunity as CTLA-4 activation has been shown to suppress several experimental autoimmune diseases including murine lupus (*35*), collagen-induced arthritis (*36*), experimental autoimmune glomerulonephritis (*37*), and diabetes in NOD mice (*38*).

Since the original publication by DeGroot and colleagues of an association between a CTLA-4 polymorphism and GD (*39*), CTLA-4 was shown in numerous studies to be linked and associated with all AITD phenotypes including GD, HT, and Tab (*40–45*). Several CTLA-4 polymorphisms have been investigated, and the most consistent associations were found with three variants: an AT-repeat microsatellite at the 3′ untranslated region (3′UTR) of the CTLA-4 gene [(AT)n] (*39, 42*), an A/G SNP at position 49 in the signal peptide resulting in an alanine/threonine substitution (A/G49) (*11, 41, 46–48*), and an A/G SNP located downstream and outside of the 3′UTR of the CTLA-4 gene (designated CT60) (*44*). The association between GD and CTL-4 has been consistent across different ethnic groups, pointing to the importance of CTLA-4 as an AITD susceptibility gene (*39, 49–51*). Hashimoto's thyroiditis (HT) was also associated with CTLA-4 across populations of different ethnicities and geographic locations including Caucasians (*42, 46, 52*) and Japanese (*50, 53*). Moreover, CTLA-4 was shown to confer susceptibility to the production of TAbs alone without clinical disease. Our group has shown strong evidence for linkage between the CTLA-4 gene region and the production of TAbs (*54*). Another study has reported an association between the G allele of the CTLA-4 A/G49 SNP and the thyroid autoantibody diathesis (*55, 56*). Further analysis by our group showed that the involvement of CTLA-4 in the genetic architecture of AITD is more complex than originally thought. While the main contribution of CTLA-4 is to the propensity to develop TAbs, CTLA-4 also influences the risk to develop high-level TAb and clinical AITD when interacting with other loci (*57*). Moreover, both the G allele (previously reported to be associated with AITD) and the A allele (reported to be protective) of the A/G49 SNP may predispose to disease when interacting with different loci (*57*).

It is still not known which CTLA-4 variant is the causative variant and by what mechanism it confers susceptibility to autoimmunity. To identify the causative variant, functional studies are needed as all associated variants are in tight linkage disequilibrium. Mechanistically, a polymorphism that reduced CTLA-4 expression/function would be expected to augment T-cell activation, and potentially, lead to autoimmunity. The A/G49 SNP causing a Thr > Ala substitution in the signal peptide was reported to cause misprocessing of CTLA-4 in the ER resulting in less efficient glycosylation and diminished surface expression of

CTLA-4 protein (*58*). However, these data need to be confirmed. Kouki et al. (*59*) have shown an association between the G allele of the A/G49 SNP and reduced inhibition of T-cell proliferation, results which were later replicated by us (*45*). However, this association could be due to a direct effect of the A/G49 SNP on CTLA-4 expression/function or due to the effects of another variant in linkage disequilibrium with the A/G49 SNP. Further direct functional studies demonstrated that when a T-cell line, devoid of endogenous CTLA-4 expression, was transiently transfected with a CTLA-4 construct harboring either the G or the A allele of the A/G49 SNP, there was no difference in CTLA-4 expression/function (*60*). These data suggest that A/G49 is not the causative SNP but rather is in linkage disequilibrium with the causative variant. Functional analysis of the CT60 SNP in a small number of patients suggested that the GG (disease susceptible) genotype was associated with reduced mRNA expression of the soluble form of CTLA-4 (*44*). However, a recent large study could not replicate these results (*61*). Another CTLA-4 variant that could affect CTLA-4 functionality is the 3 UTR (AT)n. Indeed, carriage of the longer repeats (associated with disease) was associated with reduced CTLA-4 inhibitory function (*62*), and the long repeats were associated with significantly shorter half-life of CTLA-4 mRNA compared with the short repeats (*63*). Moreover, the region of the CTLA-4 3 UTR in which the AT-repeat is located contains three AUUUA motifs, which may affect mRNA stability (*64*). This could provide an attractive mechanism for the association between the short alleles of (AT)n and AITD as well as other autoimmune diseases. Alternatively, it is possible that no one CTLA-4 variant is causative and that a haplotype consisting of several variants is responsible for the association with autoimmunity. Indeed, recent data points to the existence of signatures of extended haplotypes across the CTLA-4 gene that is preferentially preserved in certain populations (*65*).

CD40

CD40 is a member of the TNF-R receptor (TNFR) family of molecules, which is expressed primarily but not exclusively on B-cells and other antigen-presenting cells (APCs) (*66*). CD40 plays a fundamental role in B-cell activation inducing, upon ligation, B-cell proliferation, immunoglobulin class switching, antibody secretion, and generation of memory cells (*67, 68*). Other professional APCs, such as macrophages and dendritic cells, also require CD40 signaling for their activation (*69*). CD40 signaling cascade has been shown to play a role in a number of autoimmune conditions. For example, the introduction of antibodies against CD154 (CD40 ligand) suppressed several experimental autoimmune diseases, with a strong humoral component, such as experimental autoimmune myasthenia gravis (*70*) and experimental Graves' disease (*71*). Additionally, when Graves' thyroid tissue was xenografted into severe combined immunodeficient (SCID) mice, its humoral response was inhibited by blocking CD40 activation (72).

Recently, using a combination of linkage and association studies, we and others have identified CD40 as a novel susceptibility gene for GD (73–77). A C/T single-nucleotide polymorphism (SNP) at the 5′UTR of CD40 was associated with GD, with the CC genotype of this SNP conferring risk for disease (74). With the exception of a sole report (78), the association between the CC genotype and GD has been replicated in several studies performed in Caucasians (79, 80), Koreans (76), and Japanese (77, 81). Moreover, a metaanalysis showed a highly significant association between the CC genotype and GD (79). We have recently shown that the association of the CC genotype was stronger in the subset of GD patients that had persistently high levels of TAbs after treatment (82).

How can the CC genotype predispose to GD? Functional studies demonstrated that the CD40 Kozak SNP influences CD40 translational efficiency. The C allele of the polymorphism increases the translation of CD40 mRNA transcripts by 20–30% compared to the T allele (83, 84). Therefore, it is possible that increased CD40 expression driven by the C allele contributes to disease etiology by lowering the threshold of autoreactive B cells for activation to thyroidal antigens (83). Another possibility is that the C allele enhances CD40 expression on thyrocytes (85, 86). CD40 signaling in thyrocytes can result in cytokine secretion (e.g., IL-6 (85)) and activation of resident T cells in the thyroid by bystander mechanisms (82).

Since CD40 is a major APC and B-cell costimulatory molecule, the question arises whether the CD40 Kozak SNP could play a role in other autoimmune conditions? Association studies in Hashimoto's thyroiditis (74) and T1D (87), both cell-mediated autoimmune diseases with strong Th1 component showed no association. However, a recent study has shown that the C allele of the CD40 Kozak SNP was strongly associated with high IgE levels in asthma (84).

The Protein Tyrosine Phosphatase-22 Gene

The lymphoid tyrosine phosphatase (LYP), encoded by the protein tyrosine phosphatase-22 (PTPN22) gene, is a 110-kDa protein tyrosine phosphatase that, like CTLA-4, is a powerful inhibitor of T-cell activation (88). A tryptophan/arginine substitution at codon 620 (R620W) of PTPN22 was found to be associated with AITD including Graves' disease (89) and Hashimoto's thyroiditis (90) as well as with other autoimmune diseases (91–94).

Mechanistically, the disease-associated tryptophan variant makes the protein an even stronger inhibitor of T cells, as it is a gain-of-function variant (95). One possible explanation for this surprising finding is that a lower T-cell receptor signaling would lead to a tendency for self-reactive T cells to escape thymic deletion and thus remain in the periphery.

THYROID-SPECIFIC GENES IN AITD

While immune regulatory genes are critical for the genetic susceptibility to AITD, thyroid-specific genes could explain the targeting of the immune response to the thyroid. Of the four main thyroid antigens, thyroglobulin (Tg), TSHR, thyroid peroxidase (TPO), and sodium-iodide symporter (NIS) only Tg and TSHR were shown to play a key role in the genetic susceptibility to AITD.

Thyroglobulin

Tg is a 660-kDa homodimeric protein that serves as a precursor and storehouse for thyroid hormones (96). Tg is one of the main targets of the immune response in AITD, and all AITD phenotypes are characterized by the development of Tg antibodies. Mouse models have provided additional evidence for the importance of Tg in the development of thyroid autoimmunity. The mouse model for Hashimoto's thyroiditis, murine experimental autoimmune thyroiditis (EkAT), can be induced, in genetically susceptible mice, by immunization with thyroglobulin (97). EAT, like its human disease counterpart, is characterized by a cellular infiltrate of the thyroid, anti-Tg T-cell responses, as well as high titers of anti-Tg autoantibodies (96). Thus, Tg is a critical thyroid-specific protein for the development of AITD in humans and EAT in mice.

Tg undergoes several important posttranslational modifications, the most important of which is iodination (98). Iodination is believed to be a contributor to disease (reviewed in ref. (99)). However, reports showing that the immunogencity of peptides, containing potential sites of iodination, is a function of amino acid sequence rather than iodination (100, 101), may suggest that iodinated thyroglobulin is not a prerequisite for the initiation of thyroiditis but may exert an effect on disease maintenance and/ or severity.

Recently, the Tg gene was established as a major AITD susceptibility gene (102–104). Linkage studies mapped an AITD locus to the Tg gene region on chromosome 8q24 (102, 105, 106). Further detailed sequencing analysis of the Tg gene identified three amino acid substitutions that were significantly associated with AITD, A734S, V1027M, and W1999R (107).

What is the mechanism by which amino acid variants in Tg could predispose to GD and HT? One potential mechanism is by altering Tg peptide presentation by APCs to T cells within HLA class II molecules. Such a mechanism would imply that there exist an interaction between Tg variants and HLA-DR variants predisposing to AITD. Indeed, we have shown that the W1999R variant had a statistical interaction with the Arg74 polymorphism of HLA-DR, resulting in a high odds ratio of 15 for GD (*108*). This statistical interaction may imply a biological interaction between Tg and HLA-DR. For example, the Tg peptide repertoire generated in individuals with the R allele of W1999R (associated with AITD) could be pathogenic, while DRβ-Arg74 could optimally present these pathogenic Tg peptides to T cells.

TSH Receptor

The hallmark of Graves' disease is the presence of stimulating TSHR antibodies (*1*), and therefore, the TSHR was an attractive candidate gene for GD. Prior to the completion of the human genome project and the availability of detailed SNP maps, three missense SNPs of the TSHR have been examined for association with GD (*109*), an aspartic acid to histidine substitution at position 36 (D36H), a proline to threonine substitution at position 52 (P52T), and a glutamic acid to aspartic acid substitution at position 727 (D727E). Studies of these SNPs gave inconsistent results with some showing associations (*110, 111*) and others not (*112–115*). However, one group in Japan consistently reported associations of the TSHR with GD in the Japanese (*50, 53*). More recently, it was found that noncoding SNPs of the TSHR are associated with GD (*116, 117*). The most consistent association has been with an intron 1 SNP (*118, 119*). It is still not known how the intron 1 SNP of the TSHR could predispose to GD, but it could theoretically influence TSHR gene expression and/or splicing (*120*).

CONCLUSIONS: FROM GENE MAPPING TO MECHANISMS

Genetic studies have revolutionized our understanding of complex diseases. As new genes and loci are being identified, novel mechanisms are being unraveled. For example, the identification of NOD2 as a major Crohn's disease gene revealed the importance of innate immune responses in the etiology of inflammatory bowel disease (*121*). In another example, genetic studies demonstrating an association of variants of complement factors with age related macular degeneration, for the first time, shed light on the pathogenesis of this disease (*122*). Similarly, with the identification of novel AITD susceptibility genes significant progress has been made in our understanding of the pathogenesis of AITD. What has become apparent is that most of the AITD susceptibility identified participates in the immunological synapse (Fig. 26.1). The immunological synapse is the interface formed between APCs and T cells during antigen presentation (*123, 124*). Among the

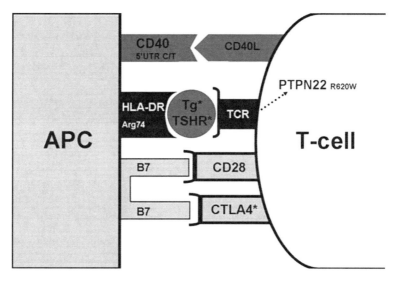

Fig. 26.1

components of the immunological synapse involve in the genetic susceptibility to AITD are the target antigens presented to T cells (Tg and TSHR), the HLA-DR molecules presenting peptide antigens to T cells, costimulatory molecules (CTLA-4, CD40), and genes regulating TCR signaling pathways (PTPN22). Another mechanism for regulating the activation of T cells is through regulatory T cells (Treg) (*125*). Recently, we have shown that variants in the FOXP3 gene, which is the master regulator of Treg differentiation, were associated with AITD (*126*). Thus, it is likely that the genetic risk factors for AITD influence disease by enabling presentation of pathogenic Tg and TSHR peptides to T cells and augmenting their responses to the presented peptides.

The next step in understanding the role of the AITD susceptibility genes in the etiology of AITD is to investigate the functional consequences of these gene variants and to analyze for gene–gene and genetic–epigenetic interactions. Gene–gene interaction studies have already demonstrated significant interaction between HLA-DR and Tg conferring a high risk for GD (*108*). It is clear that other interactions exist and their identification will be crucial to dissecting the mechanisms of thyroid autoimmunity. Progress is rapidly being made in our understanding of the genetic etiology of AITD, and it is hoped that this progress will lead to a better understanding of the molecular mechanisms causing AITD and other autoimmune disease.

ACKNOWLEDGMENTS

This work was supported in part by grants DK061659 and DK067555 from NIDDK.

REFERENCES

1. Menconi F, Oppenheim YL, Tomer Y. Graves' disease. In: Shoenfeld Y, Cervera R, Gershwin ME, eds. Diagnostic Criteria in Autoimmune Diseases. Totowa, NJ: Humana, 2008:231–235.
2. Weetman AP. Chronic autoimmune thyroiditis. In: Braverman LE, Utiger RD, eds. Werner and Ingbar's the Thyroid. Philadelphia, PA: Lippincott Williams and Wilkins, 2000:721–732.
3. Stagnaro-Green A. Clinical review 152: postpartum thyroiditis. J Clin Endocrinol Metab 2002;87:4042–4047.
4. Roti E, Uberti E. Post-partum thyroiditis – a clinical update. Eur J Endocrinol 2002;146: 275–279.
5. Muller AF, Drexhage HA, Berghout A. Postpartum thyroiditis and autoimmune thyroiditis in women of childbearing age: recent insights and consequences for antenatal and postnatal care. Endocr Rev 2001;22: 605–630.
6. Mandac JC, Chaudhry S, Sherman KE, Tomer Y. The clinical and physiological spectrum of interferon-alpha induced thyroiditis: toward a new classification. Hepatology 2006;43:661–672.
7. Huber A, Menconi F, Corathers S, Jacobson EM, Tomer Y. Joint genetic susceptibility to type 1 diabetes and autoimmune thyroiditis: from epidemiology to mechanisms. Endocr Rev 2008;29(6):697–725.
8. Hall R, Dingle PR, Roberts DF. Thyroid antibodies: a study of first degree relatives. Clin Genet 1972;3:319–324.
9. Tomer Y, Davies TF. Searching for the autoimmune thyroid disease susceptibility genes: from gene mapping to gene function. Endocr Rev 2003;24:694–717.
10. Hall R, Stanbury JB. Familial studies of autoimmune thyroiditis. Clin Exp Immunol 1967;2:719–725.
11. Villanueva RB, Inzerillo AM, Tomer Y, Barbesino G, Meltzer M, Concepcion ES, Greenberg DA, Maclaren N, Sun ZS, Zhang DM, Tucci S, Davies TF. Limited genetic susceptibility to severe Graves' ophthalmopathy: no role for ctla-4 and evidence for an environmental etiology. Thyroid 2000; 10:791–798.
12. Risch N. Linkage strategies for genetically complex traits. II. The power of affected relative pairs. Am J Hum Genet 1990;46:229–241.
13. Villanueva R, Greenberg DA, Davies TF, Tomer Y. Sibling recurrence risk in autoimmune thyroid disease. Thyroid 2003;13:761–764.
14. Brix TH, Christensen K, Holm NV, Harvald B, Hegedus L. A population-based study of Graves' diseases in Danish twins. Clin Endocrinol 1998;48:397–400.
15. Brix TH, Kyvik KO, Christensen K, Hegedus L. Evidence for a major role of heredity in Graves' disease: a population-based study of two Danish twin cohorts. J Clin Endocrinol Metab 2001;86:930–934.
16. Ringold DA, Nicoloff JT, Kesler M, Davis H, Hamilton A, Mack T. Further evidence for a strong genetic influence on the development of autoimmune thyroid disease: The California twin study. Thyroid 2002;12: 647–653.
17. Brix TH, Kyvik KO, Hegedus L. A population-based study of chronic autoimmune hypothyroidism in Danish twins. J Clin Endocrinol Metab 2000;85:536–539.
18. Todd JA, Acha-Orbea H, Bell JI, Chao N, Fronek Z, Jacob CO, McDermott M, Sinha AA, Timmerman L, Steinman L. A molecular basis for MHC class II – associated autoimmunity. Science 1988;240:1003–1009.
19. Jacobson EM, Huber A, Tomer Y. The HLA gene complex in thyroid autoimmunity: from epidemiology to etiology. J Autoimmun 2008;30:58–62.
20. Ban Y, Davies TF, Greenberg DA, Concepcion ES, Osman R, Oashi T, Tomer Y. Arginine at position 74 of the HLA-DRb1 chain is associated with Graves' disease. Genes Immun 2004;5:203–208.
21. Menconi F, Monti MC, Greenberg DA, Oashi T, Osman R, Davies TF, Ban Y, Jacobson EM, Concepcion ES, Li CW,

Tomer Y. Molecular amino acid signatures in the MHC class II peptide-binding pocket predispose to autoimmune thyroiditis in humans and in mice. Proc Natl Acad Sci USA 2008;105:14034–14039.
22. Farid NR. Graves' disease. In: Farid NR, ed. HLA in Endocrine and Metabolic Disorders. London: Academic, 1981:85–143.
23. Barlow ABT, Wheatcroft N, Watson P, Weetman AP. Association of HLA-DQA1*0501 with Graves' disease in English caucasian men and women. Clin Endocrinol 1996;44:73–77.
24. Yanagawa T, Mangklabruks A, Chang YB, Okamoto Y, Fisfalen M-E, Curran PG, DeGroot LJ. Human histocompatibility leukocyte antigen-DQA1*0501 allele associated with genetic susceptibility to Graves' disease in a caucasian population. J Clin Endocrinol Metab 1993;76:1569–1574.
25. Zamani M, Spaepen M, Bex M, Bouillon R, Cassiman JJ. Primary role of the HLA class II DRB1*0301 allele in Graves disease. Am J Med Genet 2000;95:432–437.
26. Todd JA, Bell JI, McDevitt HO. HLA-DQbeta gene contributes to susceptibility and resistance to insulin-dependent diabetes mellitus. Nature 1987;329:599–604.
27. Simmonds MJ, Howson JM, Heward JM, Cordell HJ, Foxall H, Carr-Smith J, Gibson SM, Walker N, Tomer Y, Franklyn JA, Todd JA, Gough SC. Regression mapping of association between the human leukocyte antigen region and Graves disease. Am J Hum Genet 2005;76:157–163.
28. Farid NR, Sampson L, Moens H, Barnard JM. The association of goitrous autoimmune thyroiditis with HLA-DR5. Tissue Antigens 1981;17:265–268.
29. Moens H, Farid NR, Sampson L, Noel EP, Barnard JM. Hashimoto's thyroiditis is associated with HLA-DRw3. N Engl J Med 1978;299:133–134.
30. Tandon N, Zhang L, Weetman AP. HLA associations with Hashimoto's thyroiditis. Clin Endocrinol (Oxf) 1991;34:383–386.
31. Ban Y, Davies TF, Greenberg DA, Concepcion ES, Tomer Y. The influence of human leucocyte antigen (HLA) genes on autoimmune thyroid disease (AITD): results of studies in HLA-DR3 positive AITD families. Clin Endocrinol (Oxf) 2002;57:81–88.
32. Petrone A, Giorgi G, Mesturino CA, Capizzi M, Cascino I, Nistico L, Osborn J, Di Mario U, Buzzetti R. Association of DRB1*04-DQB1*0301 haplotype and lack of association of two polymorphic sites at CTLA-4 gene with Hashimoto's thyroiditis in an Italian population. Thyroid 2001;11:171–175.
33. Teft WA, Kirchhof MG, Madrenas J. A molecular perspective of CTLA-4 function. Annu Rev Immunol 2006;24:65–97.
34. Tivol EA, Borriello F, Schweitzer AN, Lynch WP, Bluestone JA, Sharpe AH. Loss of CTLA-4 leads to massive lymphoproliferation and fatal multiorgan tissue destruction, revealing a critical negative regulatory role of CTLA-4. Immunity 1995;3:541–547.
35. Finck BK, Linsley PS, Wofsy D. Treatment of murine lupus with CTLA4Ig. Science 1994;265:1225–1227.
36. Knoerzer DB, Karr RW, Schwartz BD, Mengle-Gaw LJ. Collagen-induced arthritis in the BB rat. Prevention of disease by treatment with CTLA-4-Ig. J Clin Invest 1995;96:987–993.
37. Nishikawa K, Linsley PS, Collins AB, Stamenkovic I, McCluskey RT, Andres G. Effect of CTLA-4 chimeric protein on rat autoimmune anti-glomerular basement membrane glomerulonephritis. Eur J Immunol 1994;24:1249–1254.
38. Lenschow DJ, Herold KC, Rhee L, Patel B, Koons A, Qin HY, Fuchs E, Singh B, Thompson CB, Bluestone JA. CD28/B7 regulation of Th1 and Th2 subsets in the development of autoimmune diabetes. Immunity 1996;5:285–293.
39. Yanagawa T, Hidaka Y, Guimaraes V, Soliman M, DeGroot LJ. CTLA-4 gene polymorphism associated with Graves' disease in a caucasian population. J Clin Endocrinol Metab 1995;80:41–45.
40. Nistico L, Buzzetti R, Pritchard LE, Van der Auwera B, Giovannini C, Bosi E, Larrad MT, Rios MS, Chow CC, Cockram CS, Jacobs K, Mijovic C, Bain SC, Barnett AH, Vandewalle CL, Schuit F, Gorus FK, Tosi R, Pozzilli P, Todd JA. The CTLA-4 gene region of chromosome 2q33 is linked to, and associated with, type 1 diabetes. Begian Diabetes Registry. Hum Mol Genet 1996;5:1075–1080.
41. Donner H, Rau H, Walfish PG, Braun J, Siegmund T, Finke R, Herwig J, Usadel KH, Badenhoop K. CTLA4 alanine-17 confers genetic susceptibility to Graves' disease and to type 1 diabetes mellitus. J Clin Endocrinol Metab 1997;82:143–146.
42. Kotsa K, Watson PF, Weetman AP. A CTLA-4 gene polymorphism is associated with both Graves' disease and autoimmune hypothyroidism. Clin Endocrinol 1997;46:551–554.
43. Kouki T, Gardine CA, Yanagawa T, DeGroot LJ. Relation of three polymorphisms of the

44. Ueda H, Howson JM, Esposito L, Heward J, Snook H, Chamberlain G, Rainbow DB, Hunter KM, Smith AN, Di Genova G, Herr MH, Dahlman I, Payne F, Smyth D, Lowe C, Twells RC, Howlett S, Healy B, Nutland S, Rance HE, Everett V, Smink LJ, Lam AC, Cordell HJ, Walker NM, Bordin C, Hulme J, Motzo C, Cucca F, Hess JF, Metzker ML, Rogers J, Gregory S, Allahabadia A, Nithiyananthan R, Tuomilehto-Wolf E, Tuomilehto J, Bingley P, Gillespie KM, Undlien DE, Ronningen KS, Guja C, Ionescu-Tirgoviste C, Savage DA, Maxwell AP, Carson DJ, Patterson CC, Franklyn JA, Clayton DG, Peterson LB, Wicker LS, Todd JA, Gough SC. Association of the T-cell regulatory gene CTLA4 with susceptibility to autoimmune disease. Nature 2003;423:506–511.

45. Ban Y, Davies TF, Greenberg DA, Kissin A, Marder B, Murphy B, Concepcion ES, Villanueva RB, Barbesino G, Ling V, Tomer Y. Analysis of the CTLA-4, CD28 and inducible co-stimulator (ICOS) genes in autoimmune thyroid disease. Genes Immun 2003;4:586–593.

46. Nithiyananthan R, Heward JM, Allahabadia A, Franklyn JA, Gough SC. Polymorphism of the CTLA-4 gene is associated with autoimmune hypothyroidism in the United Kingdom. Thyroid 2002;12:3–6.

47. Braun J, Donner H, Siegmund T, Walfish PG, Usadel KH, Badenhoop K. CTLA-4 promoter variants in patients with Graves' disease and Hashimoto's thyroiditis. Tissue Antigens 1998;51:563–566.

48. Yanagawa T, Taniyama M, Enomoto S, Gomi K, Maruyama H, Ban Y, Saruta T. CTLA4 gene polymorphism confers susceptibility to Graves' disease in Japanese. Thyroid 1997;7:843–846.

49. Heward JM, Allahabadia A, Armitage M, Hattersley A, Dodson PM, Macleod K, Carr-Smith J, Daykin J, Daly A, Sheppard MC, Holder RL, Barnett AH, Franklyn JA, Gough SC. The development of Graves' disease and the CTLA-4 gene on chromosome 2q33. J Clin Endocrinol Metab 1999;84:2398–2401.

50. Akamizu T, Sale MM, Rich SS, Hiratani H, Noh JY, Kanamoto N, Saijo M, Miyamoto Y, Saito Y, Nakao K, Bowden DW. Association of autoimmune thyroid disease with microsatellite markers for the thyrotropin receptor gene and CTLA-4 in Japanese patients. Thyroid 2000;10:851–858.

51. Park YJ, Chung HK, Park DJ, Kim WB, Kim SW, Koh JJ, Cho BY. Polymorphism in the promoter and exon 1 of the cytotoxic T lymphocyte antigen-4 gene associated with autoimmune thyroid disease in Koreans. Thyroid 2000;10:453–459.

52. Donner H, Braun J, Seidl C, Rau H, Finke R, Ventz M, Walfish PG, Usadel KH, Badenhoop K. Codon 17 polymorphism of the cytotoxic T lymphocyte antigen 4 gene in Hashimoto's thyroiditis and Addison's disease. J Clin Endocrinol Metab 1997;82:4130–4132.

53. Sale MM, Akamizu T, Howard TD, Yokota T, Nakao K, Mori T, Iwasaki H, Rich SS, Jennings-Gee JE, Yamada M, Bowden DW. Association of autoimmune thyroid disease with a microsatellite marker for the thyrotropin receptor gene and CTLA-4 in a Japanese population. Proc Assoc Am Physicians 1997;109:453–461.

54. Tomer Y, Greenberg DA, Barbesino G, Concepcion ES, Davies TF. CTLA-4 and not CD28 is a susceptibility gene for thyroid autoantibody production. J Clin Endocrinol Metab 2001;86:1687–1693.

55. Zaletel K, Krhin B, Gaberscek S, Pirnat E, Hojker S. The influence of the exon 1 polymorphism of the cytotoxic T lymphocyte antigen 4 gene on thyroid antibody production in patients with newly diagnosed Graves' disease. Thyroid 2002;12:373–376.

56. Zaletel K, Krhin B, Gaberscek S, Hojker S. Thyroid autoantibody production is influenced by exon 1 and promoter CTLA-4 polymorphisms in patients with Hashimoto's thyroiditis. Int J Immunogenet 2006;33:87–91.

57. Vieland VJ, Huang Y, Bartlett C, Davies TF, Tomer Y. A multilocus model of the genetic architecture of autoimmune thyroid disorder, with clinical implications. Am J Hum Genet 2008;82:1349–1356.

58. Anjos S, Nguyen A, Ounissi-Benkalha H, Tessier MC, Polychronakos C. A common autoimmunity predisposing signal peptide variant of the cytotoxic T-lymphocyte antigen 4 results in inefficient glycosylation of the susceptibility allele. J Biol Chem 2002;277:46478–46486.

59. Kouki T, Sawai Y, Gardine CA, Fisfalen ME, Alegre ML, DeGroot LJ. CTLA-4 gene polymorphism at position 49 in exon 1 reduces the inhibitory function of CTLA-4 and contributes to the pathogenesis of Graves' disease. J Immunol 2000;165:6606–6611.

60. Xu Y, Graves P, Tomer Y, Davies T. CTLA-4 and autoimmune thyroid disease: lack of influence of the A49G signal peptide polymorphism on functional recombinant human

CTLA-4. Cell Immunol 2002;215: 133–140.
61. Mayans S, Lackovic K, Nyholm C, Lindgren P, Ruikka K, Eliasson M, Cilio CM, Holmberg D. CT60 genotype does not affect CTLA-4 isoform expression despite association to T1D and AITD in northern Sweden. BMC Med Genet 2007;8:3.
62. Takara M, Kouki T, DeGroot LJ. CTLA-4 AT-repeat polymorphism reduces the inhibitory function of CTLA-4 in Graves' disease. Thyroid 2003;13:1083–1089.
63. Wang XB, Kakoulidou M, Giscombe R, Qiu Q, Huang D, Pirskanen R, Lefvert AK. Abnormal expression of CTLA-4 by T cells from patients with myasthenia gravis: effect of an AT-rich gene sequence. J Neuroimmunol 2002;130:224–232.
64. Shaw G, Kamen R. A conserved AU sequence from the 3 untranslated region of GM-CSF mRNA mediates selective mRNA degradation. Cell 1986;46:659–667.
65. Butty V, Roy M, Sabeti P, Besse W, Benoist C, Mathis D. Signatures of strong population differentiation shape extended haplotypes across the human CD28, CTLA4, and ICOS costimulatory genes. Proc Natl Acad Sci USA 2007;104:570–575.
66. Banchereau J, Bazan F, Blanchard D, Briere F, Galizzi JP, van Kooten C, Liu YJ, Rousset F, Saeland S. The CD40 antigen and its ligand. Annu Rev Immunol 1994;12: 881–922.
67. Armitage RJ, Macduff BM, Spriggs MK, Fanslow WC. Human B cell proliferation and Ig secretion induced by recombinant CD40 ligand are modulated by soluble cytokines. J Immunol 1993;150:3671–3680.
68. Arpin C, Dechanet J, van Kooten C, Merville P, Grouard G, Briere F, Banchereau J, Liu YJ. Generation of memory B cells and plasma cells in vitro. Science 1995;268:720–722.
69. van Kooten C, Banchereau J. Functions of CD40 on B cells, dendritic cells and other cells. Curr Opin Immunol 1997;9:330–337.
70. Im SH, Barchan D, Maiti PK, Fuchs S, Souroujon MC. Blockade of CD40 ligand suppresses chronic experimental myasthenia gravis by down-regulation of Th1 differentiation and up-regulation of CTLA-4. J Immunol 2001;166:6893–6898.
71. Chen CR, Aliesky HA, Guo J, Rapoport B, McLachlan SM. Blockade of costimulation between T cells and antigen-presenting cells: an approach to suppress murine Graves' disease induced using thyrotropin receptor-expressing adenovirus. Thyroid 2006;16: 427–434.
72. Resetkova E, Kawai K, Enomoto T, Arreaza G, Togun R, Foy TM, Noelle RJ, Volpe R. Antibody to gp39, the ligand for CD40 significantly inhibits the humoral response from Graves' thyroid tissues xenografted into severe combined immunodeficient (SCID) mice. Thyroid 1996;6:267–273.
73. Tomer Y, Barbesino G, Greenberg DA, Concepcion ES, Davies TF. A new Graves disease-susceptibility locus maps to chromosome 20q11.2. Am J Hum Genet 1998;63:1749–1756.
74. Tomer Y, Concepcion E, Greenberg DA. A C/T single nucleotide polymorphism in the region of the CD40 gene is associated with Graves' disease. Thyroid 2002;12: 1129–1135.
75. Pearce SH, Vaidya B, Imrie H, Perros P, Kelly WF, Toft AD, McCarthy MI, Young ET, Kendall-Taylor P. Further evidence for a susceptibility locus on chromosome 20q13.11 in families with dominant transmission of Graves disease. Am J Hum Genet 1999;65: 1462–1465.
76. Kim TY, Park YJ, Hwang JK, Song JY, Park KS, Cho BY, Park DJ. A C/T polymorphism in the 5'-untranslated region of the CD40 gene is associated with Graves' disease in Koreans. Thyroid 2003;13:919–926.
77. Ban Y, Tozaki T, Taniyama M, Tomita M, Ban Y. Association of a C/T single-nucleotide polymorphism in the 5' untranslated region of the CD40 gene with Graves' disease in Japanese. Thyroid 2006;16: 443–446.
78. Houston FA, Wilson V, Jennings CE, Owen CJ, Donaldson P, Perros P, Pearce SH. Role of the CD40 locus in Graves' disease. Thyroid 2004;14:506–509.
79. Kurylowicz A, Kula D, Ploski R, Skorka A, Jurecka-Lubieniecka B, Zebracka J, Steinhof-Radwanska K, Hasse-Lazar K, Hiromatsu Y, Jarzab B, Bednarczuk T. Association of CD40 gene polymorphism (C-1T) with susceptibility and phenotype of Graves' disease. Thyroid 2005;15:1119–1124.
80. Tomer Y, Davies TF, Greenberg DA. What is the contribution of a Kozak SNP in the CD40 gene to Graves' disease? Clin Endocrinol 2005;62:258.
81. Mukai T, Hiromatsu Y, Fukutani T, Ichimura M, Kaku H, Miyake I, Yamada K. A C/T polymorphism in the 5' untranslated region of the CD40 gene is associated with later onset of Graves' disease in Japanese. Endocr J 2005;52:471–477.
82. Jacobson EM, Huber AK, Akeno N, Sivak M, Li CW, Concepcion E, Ho K, Tomer Y. A

CD40 Kozak sequence polymorphism and susceptibility to antibody-mediated autoimmune conditions: the role of CD40 tissue-specific expression. Genes Immun 2007;8: 205–214.
83. Jacobson EM, Concepcion E, Oashi T, Tomer Y. A Graves' disease-associated Kozak sequence single-nucleotide polymorphism enhances the efficiency of CD40 gene translation: a case for translational pathophysiology. Endocrinology 2005;146:2684–2691.
84. Park JH, Chang HS, Park CS, Jang AS, Park BL, Rhim TY, Uh ST, Kim YH, Chung IY, Shin HD. Association analysis of CD40 polymorphisms with asthma and the level of serum total IgE. Am J Respir Crit Care Med 2007;175:775–782.
85. Metcalfe RA, McIntosh RS, Marelli-Berg F, Lombardi G, Lechler R, Weetman AP. Detection of CD40 on human thyroid follicular cells: analysis of expression and function. J Clin Endocrinol Metab 1998;83: 1268–1274.
86. Smith TJ, Sciaky D, Phipps RP, Jennings TA. CD40 expression in human thyroid tissue: evidence for involvement of multiple cell types in autoimmune and neoplastic diseases. Thyroid 1999;9:749–755.
87. Cooper JD, Smyth DJ, Bailey R, Payne F, Downes K, Godfrey LM, Masters J, Zeitels LR, Vella A, Walker NM, Todd JA. The candidate genes TAF5L, TCF7, PDCD1, IL6 and ICAM1 cannot be excluded from having effects in type 1 diabetes. BMC Med Genet 2007;8:71.
88. Cloutier JF, Veillette A. Cooperative inhibition of T-cell antigen receptor signaling by a complex between a kinase and a phosphatase. J Exp Med 1999;189:111–121.
89. Velaga MR, Wilson V, Jennings CE, Owen CJ, Herington S, Donaldson PT, Ball SG, James RA, Quinton R, Perros P, Pearce SH. The codon 620 tryptophan allele of the lymphoid tyrosine phosphatase (LYP) gene is a major determinant of Graves' disease. J Clin Endocrinol Metab 2004;89:5862–5865.
90. Criswell LA, Pfeiffer KA, Lum RF, Gonzales B, Novitzke J, Kern M, Moser KL, Begovich AB, Carlton VE, Li W, Lee AT, Ortmann W, Behrens TW, Gregersen PK. Analysis of families in the multiple autoimmune disease genetics consortium (MADGC) collection: the PTPN22 620W allele associates with multiple autoimmune phenotypes. Am J Hum Genet 2005;76:561–571.
91. Begovich AB, Carlton VE, Honigberg LA, Schrodi SJ, Chokkalingam AP, Alexander HC, Ardlie KG, Huang Q, Smith AM, Spoerke JM, Conn MT, Chang M, Chang SY, Saiki RK, Catanese JJ, Leong DU, Garcia VE, McAllister LB, Jeffery DA, Lee AT, Batliwalla F, Remmers E, Criswell LA, Seldin MF, Kastner DL, Amos CI, Sninsky JJ, Gregersen PK. A missense single-nucleotide polymorphism in a gene encoding a protein tyrosine phosphatase (PTPN22) is associated with rheumatoid arthritis. Am J Hum Genet 2004;75:330–337.
92. Kyogoku C, Langefeld CD, Ortmann WA, Lee A, Selby S, Carlton VE, Chang M, Ramos P, Baechler EC, Batliwalla FM, Novitzke J, Williams AH, Gillett C, Rodine P, Graham RR, Ardlie KG, Gaffney PM, Mose KL, Petri M, Begovich AB, Gregersen PK, Behrens TW. Genetic association of the R620W polymorphism of protein tyrosine phosphatase PTPN22 with human SLE. Am J Hum Genet 2004;75:504–507.
93. Bottini N, Musumeci L, Alonso A, Rahmouni S, Nika K, Rostamkhani M, MacMurray J, Meloni GF, Lucarelli P, Pellecchia M, Eisenbarth GS, Comings D, Mustelin T. A functional variant of lymphoid tyrosine phosphatase is associated with type I diabetes. Nat Genet 2004;36:337–338.
94. Smyth D, Cooper JD, Collins JE, Heward JM, Franklyn JA, Howson JM, Vella A, Nutland S, Rance HE, Maier L, Barratt BJ, Guja C, Ionescu-Tirgoviste C, Savage DA, Dunger DB, Widmer B, Strachan DP, Ring SM, Walker N, Clayton DG, Twells RC, Gough SC, Todd JA. Replication of an association between the lymphoid tyrosine phosphatase locus (LYP/PTPN22) with type 1 diabetes, and evidence for its role as a general autoimmunity locus. Diabetes 2004;53:3020–3023.
95. Vang T, Congia M, Macis MD, Musumeci L, Orru V, Zavattari P, Nika K, Tautz L, Tasken K, Cucca F, Mustelin T, Bottini N. Autoimmune-associated lymphoid tyrosine phosphatase is a gain-of-function variant. Nat Genet 2005;37:1317–1319.
96. Charreire J. Immune mechanisms in autoimmune thyroiditis. Adv Immunol 1989;46:263–334.
97. Stafford EA, Rose NR. Newer insights into the pathogenesis of experimental autoimmune thyroiditis. Int Rev Immunol 2000;19:501–533.
98. Kondo Y, Ui N. Iodination of thyroglobulin by thyroid cellular fractions and the role of thyrotropic hormone. Biochim Biophys Acta 1961;48:415–416.
99. Rose NR, Bonita R, Burek CL. Iodine: an environmental trigger of thyroiditis. Autoimmun Rev 2002;1:97–103.

100. Kong YC, McCormick DJ, Wan Q, Motte RW, Fuller BE, Giraldo AA, David CS. Primary hormonogenic sites as conserved autoepitopes on thyroglobulin in murine autoimmune thyroiditis. Secondary role of iodination. J Immunol 1995;155: 5847–5854.
101. Wan Q, Motte RW, McCormick DJ, Fuller BE, Giraldo AA, David CS, Kong YM. Primary hormonogenic sites as conserved autoepitopes on thyroglobulin in murine autoimmune thyroiditis: role of MHC class II. Clin Immunol Immunopathol 1997;85: 187–194.
102. Tomer Y, Greenberg DA, Concepcion E, Ban Y, Davies TF. Thyroglobulin is a thyroid specific gene for the familial autoimmune thyroid diseases. J Clin Endocrinol Metab 2002;87:404–407.
103. Collins JE, Heward JM, Carr-Smith J, Daykin J, Franklyn JA, Gough SCL. Association of a rare thyroglobulin gene microsatellite variant with autoimmune thyroid disease. J Clin Endocrinol Metab 2003;88:5039–5042.
104. Tomer Y, Greenberg D. The thyroglobulin gene as the first thyroid-specific susceptibility gene for autoimmune thyroid disease. Trends Mol Med 2004;10:306–308.
105. Sakai K, Shirasawa S, Ishikawa N, Ito K, Tamai H, Kuma K, Akamizu T, Tanimura M, Furugaki K, Yamamoto K, Sasazuki T. Identification of susceptibility loci for autoimmune thyroid disease to 5q31-q33 and Hashimoto's thyroiditis to 8q23-q24 by multipoint affected sib-pair linkage analysis in Japanese. Hum Mol Genet 2001;10:1379–1386.
106. Tomer Y, Ban Y, Concepcion E, Barbesino G, Villanueva R, Greenberg DA, Davies TF. Common and unique susceptibility loci in Graves and Hashimoto diseases: results of whole-genome screening in a data set of 102 multiplex families. Am J Hum Genet 2003;73:736–747.
107. Ban Y, Greenberg DA, Concepcion E, Skrabanek L, Villanueva R, Tomer Y. Amino acid substitutions in the thyroglobulin gene are associated with susceptibility to human and murine autoimmune thyroid disease. Proc Natl Acad Sci USA 2003;100: 15119–15124.
108. Hodge SE, Ban Y, Strug LJ, Greenberg DA, Davies TF, Concepcion ES, Villanueva R, Tomer Y. Possible interaction between HLA-DRbeta1 and thyroglobulin variants in Graves' disease. Thyroid 2006;16:351–355.
109. Tonacchera M, Pinchera A. Thyrotropin receptor polymorphisms and thyroid diseases. J Clin Endocrinol Metab 2000;85: 2637–2639.
110. Cuddihy RM, Dutton CM, Bahn RS. A polymorphism in the extracellular domain of the thyrotropin receptor is highly associated with autoimmune thyroid disease in females. Thyroid 1995;5:89–95.
111. Chistyakov DA, Savost'anov KV, Turakulov RI, Petunina NA, Trukhina LV, Kudinova AV, Balabolkin MI, Nosikov VV. Complex association analysis of Graves disease using a set of polymorphic markers. Mol Genet Metab 2000;70:214–218.
112. Allahabadia A, Heward JM, Mijovic C, Carr-Smith J, Daykin J, Cockram C, Barnett AH, Sheppard MC, Franklyn JA, Gough SC. Lack of association between polymorphism of the thyrotropin receptor gene and Graves' disease in United Kingdom and Hong Kong Chinese patients: case control and family-based studies. Thyroid 1998;8:777–780.
113. Kotsa KD, Watson PF, Weetman AP. No association between a thyrotropin receptor gene polymorphism and Graves' disease in the female population. Thyroid 1997;7:31–33.
114. Simanainen J, Kinch A, Westermark K, Winsa B, Bengtsson M, Schuppert F, Westermark B, Heldin NE. Analysis of mutations in exon 1 of the human thyrotropin receptor gene: high frequency of the D36H and P52T polymorphic variants. Thyroid 1999;9:7–11.
115. Kaczur V, Takacs M, Szalai C, Falus A, Nagy Z, Berencsi G, Balazs C. Analysis of the genetic variability of the 1st (CCC/ACC, P52T) and the 10th exons (bp 1012–1704) of the TSH receptor gene in Graves' disease. Eur J Immunogenet 2000;27:17–23.
116. Hiratani H, Bowden DW, Ikegami S, Shirasawa S, Shimizu A, Iwatani Y, Akamizu T. Multiple SNPs in intron 7 of thyrotropin receptor are associated with Graves' disease. J Clin Endocrinol Metab 2005;90: 2898–2903.
117. Ho SC, Goh SS, Khoo DH. Association of Graves' disease with intragenic polymorphism of the thyrotropin receptor gene in a cohort of Singapore patients of multi-ethnic origins. Thyroid 2003;13:523–528.
118. Dechairo BM, Zabaneh D, Collins J, Brand O, Dawson GJ, Green AP, Mackay I, Franklyn JA, Connell JM, Wass JA, Wiersinga WM, Hegedus L, Brix T, Robinson BG, Hunt PJ, Weetman AP, Carey AH, Gough SC. Association of the TSHR gene with Graves' disease: the first disease specific locus. Eur J Hum Genet 2005;13: 1223–1230.

119. Yin X, Latif R, Bahn R, Tomer Y, Davies TF. Influence of the TSH receptor gene on susceptibility to Graves' disease and Graves' ophthalmopathy. Thyroid 2008;18:1201–1206.
120. Graves PN, Tomer Y, Davies TF. Cloning and sequencing of a 1.3 kb variant of human thyrotropin receptor mRNA lacking the transmembrane domain. Biochem Biophys Res Commun 1992;187:1135–1143.
121. Van Limbergen J, Russell RK, Nimmo ER, Ho GT, Arnott ID, Wilson DC, Satsangi J. Genetics of the innate immune response in inflammatory bowel disease. Inflamm Bowel Dis 2007;13(3):338–355.
122. Yates JR, Sepp T, Matharu BK, Khan JC, Thurlby DA, Shahid H, Clayton DG, Hayward C, Morgan J, Wright AF, Armbrecht AM, Dhillon B, Deary IJ, Redmond E, Bird AC, Moore AT. Complement C3 variant and the risk of age-related macular degeneration. N Engl J Med 2007;357:553–561.
123. Grakoui A, Bromley SK, Sumen C, Davis MM, Shaw AS, Allen PM, Dustin ML. The immunological synapse: a molecular machine controlling T cell activation. Science 1999;285:221–227.
124. Dustin ML. T-cell activation through immunological synapses and kinapses. Immunol Rev 2008;221:77–89.
125. Abbas AK, Lohr J, Knoechel B. Balancing autoaggressive and protective T cell responses. J Autoimmun 2007;28:59–61.
126. Ban Y, Tozaki T, Tobe T, Ban Y, Jacobson EM, Concepcion ES, Tomer Y. The regulatory T cell gene FOXP3 and genetic susceptibility to thyroid autoimmunity: An association analysis in Caucasian and Japanese cohorts. J Autoimmun 2007;28:201–207.

Chapter 27

Immunopathogenesis of Thyroiditis

Su He Wang and James R. Baker

Summary

Thyroiditis consists of a number of different inflammatory processes in thyroid and is caused by a variety of factors. Among the various inflammatory thyroid lesions, Hashimoto's thyroiditis is the most common, and we will focus on the mechanisms involved in this disease. While extensive studies have been performed to elucidate the immunopathogenesis of Hashimoto's thyroiditis, the processes underlying this disease are still not fully understood. However, significant progress has been made in areas related to the roles that iodine, $CD4^+CD25^+$ regulatory T cells, and apoptosis play in autoimmune-mediated thyroid damage, the defining feature of Hashimoto's thyroiditis.

Key Words Hashimoto's thyroiditis, Iodine, T and B cells, Regulatory T cells, Apoptosis

INTRODUCTION

Thyroiditis is an inflammatory process in the thyroid gland that can be classified into one of several subtypes depending on the eliciting factor and thyroid pathology. The subtypes include subacute (granulomatous) thyroiditis, postpartum thyroiditis, drug-induced thyroiditis, radiation-induced thyroiditis, acute (suppurative) thyroiditis, and Hashimoto's thyroiditis (HT), also known as chronic lymphocytic thyroiditis or autoimmune thyroiditis. HT represents the most common form of thyroiditis and is the most frequent cause of hypothyroidism in adults [1]. It ranks third among autoimmune diseases in the United States [2], and its incidence in women is five to tenfold higher than that observed in men [2]. Since most of the advances in understanding thyroiditis have occurred in Hashimoto's disease, this chapter will focus on the immunopathogenesis of HT.

HT is characterized by lymphocytic infiltration of the thyroid parenchyma, causing a dense accumulation of lymphocytes, plasma

George S. Eisenbarth (ed.), *Immunoendocrinology: Scientific and Clinical Aspects,* Contemporary Endocrinology,
DOI 10.1007/978-1-60327-478-4_27, © Springer Science+Business Media, LLC 2011

cells, and macrophages. The lymphoid architecture is very organized, producing structures such as germinal centers that are normally only seen in lymph nodes. The inflammation is intense and leads, at least initially, to thyroid enlargement that can be confused with a goiter. The hallmark of HT is the presence of thyroid autoantibodies to thyroglobulin (Tg) and thyroid peroxidase (TPO) in the serum of patients with this disease. It is thought that all patients with HT have antibodies to these autoantigens, and patients lacking these antibodies on normal immunoassays using porcine antigens often have human Tg-specific antibodies (3). Despite this, there is no specific immune response to thyroid autoantigens that is known to cause clinical expression of HT (4). As with all autoimmune diseases, it is thought that HT is the result of interplay of genetic, environmental, and endogenous factors. Although the relative contribution of each factor is not clearly defined, it is clear that all are involved in the dysregulation of the immune system. This results in the activation of immune cells and increased apoptosis in thyrocytes, leading to the destruction of the thyroid.

MAJOR HISTOCOMPATIBILITY COMPLEX ANTIGENS AND HT

Major histocompatibility complex (MHC) class II antigens appear to have several roles in thyroid autoimmunity. The aberrant expression of HLA-DR by the thyrocytes and/or intrathyroidal T cells has been reported in HT, potentially augmenting the immunogenicity of thyrocytes (Table 27.1) (1, 12, 13). It is unclear whether the expression of HLA-DR molecules on thyrocytes is involved

Table 27.1
Association of HLA Molecules with Hashimoto's Thyroiditis

Population studied	HLA associated	Reference
Caucasian (Canada)	DR4, DR5	(5)
Caucasian (Canada + UK)	DR4, DR5	(6)
Caucasian (Denmark)	Dw5	(7)
Caucasian (Hungary)	DR3	(8)
Caucasian (UK)	DR3	(9)
Oriental (China)	DR9, Bw46	(10)
Oriental (Japan)	DRB4*0101, A2	(4)
Oriental (Japan)	DR53	(6)
Oriental (Korea)	DR8, DQB1*0302	(11)

with initiating autoimmunity. Initiation of autoimmunity would require this expression to occur before the immune infiltration of the thyroid; it is a sign that autoimmunity has already been initiated. The doubt that autoimmunity initiation results from MHC class II expression in thyrocytes was initially raised by the fact that MHC class II expression can be induced by gamma interferon from infiltrating inflammatory cells. An in vivo animal study also demonstrated that thyrocytes did not express MHC class II molecules prior to lymphocytic infiltration (*14*). Therefore, the expression of MHC class II molecules on thyroid cells is not responsible for initiating the immunologic attack on the thyroid, but may be important to facilitate or perpetuate the autoimmune response (*15*).

It is possible that other MHC class II positive cells, such as tissue macrophages and dendritic cells, present in the thyroid prior to the lymphocytic infiltration activate autoreactive T cells and are responsible for the initiation of the autoimmune response against the thyroid. A recent study found that there is a quantitative increase in CD4$^+$CD25^{high}HLA-DR$^+$ cells in newly diagnosed HT patients. This may represent a compensatory expansion of CD4$^+$CD25$^+$ T cells in an attempt to suppress an autoimmune response to thyrocytes (*16*). It would be interesting to probe the function of this subset of T cells and track how their population changes over the course of the disease, as these early events in the thyroid are crucial to disease pathogenesis.

The phenomenon of aberrant MHC expression is coupled with the finding that MHC genes may be one of the major genetic factors predisposing an individual to autoimmunity. In this regard, it has been shown that there is an increased frequency of specific MHC class II molecules such as HLA-DQw3.1 and DQA2 in patients with HT (*5*). The DRw52 allele has been found to be present in 80% of HT patients compared with 50% in normal individuals (*12*). The pathogenic role of these molecules has been proven in animal studies; the NOD H2^{h4} mouse with a MHC class II haplotype is prone to suffering spontaneous thyroiditis, which closely resembles human HT (*17*). In class II-knockout mice on the NOD background, DR3 transgenic mice are susceptible to experimental autoimmune thyroiditis (EAT) induction by mouse thyroglobulin (mTg) and human (h) Tg, but DQ8 transgenic mice are weakly susceptible only to hTg (*18*). This reinforces the central role of MHC susceptibility to the development of HT.

IODINE AND THYROID AUTOIMMUNITY

Iodine is necessary for normal thyroid hormonogenesis and is required for the synthesis of the thyroid hormones T3 and T4. However, there also is strong evidence indicating that iodine is one of the major environmental agents responsible for increased risk of thyroid autoimmunity. Epidemiological studies have shown there is a high prevalence of

HT in adolescents and schoolchildren who have received treatment for iodine deficiency (*19, 20*). These epidemiological observations are further supported by a study in which the levels of Tg autoantibodies are increased in patients receiving the iodine-rich, antiarrhythmic drug, amiodarone (*15*). Furthermore, animal studies have confirmed that high iodine intake accelerates autoimmune thyroiditis in autoimmune-prone animal models (*21–23*).

Several mechanisms have been suggested for the induction of thyroid autoimmunity by excess iodine. *First*, iodine may stimulate macrophage myeloperoxidase activity, initiating local inflammation. This can promote the maturation of dendritic cells, increase the number of circulating T cells, and stimulate B-cell immunoglobulin production (*24*). *Second*, iodination of Tg may lead to the production of novel iodine-containing antigenic determinants, which may trigger an autoimmune response (*25, 26*). *Third*, iodine may enhance the uptake, processing, and presentation of Tg by antigen-presenting cells (APCs) such as dendritic cells, macrophages, and B cells (*26*). *Fourth*, iodined Tg may promote the affinity of critical peptides to MHC class II molecules, activating Tg-specific T cells and B cells, and inhibiting suppressor T cells (*27, 28*). Peripheral blood lymphocytes from HT patients and normal controls are able to proliferate in response to normal Tg or highly iodinated Tg, but they do not respond to nontoxic goiter Tg that lacks iodine (*25*). In vitro and in vivo studies have shown that iodine treatment inhibits the number of suppressor T cells and increases B cell activity (*29*). *Fifth*, if iodine increases the affinity of the TcR for the MHC class II peptide complex to a threshold level sufficient for T cell and B cell activation, the effector function of autoreactive T-cell clones can be switched on or off by the neoantigenic determinant of iodinated Tg peptides (*30*). It was found that iodotyrosyl formation can enhance (p179, a.a. 179–194), suppress (p2540, a.a. 2,540–2,554), or not alter (p2529, a.a. 2,529–2,545) the immunogenic profiles of the Tg peptides at the T-cell level (*31*). On the other hand, iodination neither altered the MHC-restriction profile of p2529 and p2540 [A(k)-binders] or p179 [A(k)- and E(k)-binder] nor significantly influenced the pathogenicity of these determinants. At the B-cell level, addition of an iodine atom on Y192 in p179 generated a neoantigenic determinant, but analogous effects were not discernible in p2529 or p2540. Therefore, the variations in the iodine content of Tg may significantly alter the hierarchy of antigenic determinants to which the immune system may or may not be tolerant. *Sixth*, high doses of iodine are shown to damage human thyrocytes via the production of reactive oxygen species, resulting in the release of thyroid autoantigens and the activation of autoreactive T cells (*15, 32*). *Finally*, iodine may induce the expression of MHC class I molecules on thyroid follicular cells and the infiltrated CD4(+) and CD8(+) T cells (*32, 33*). However, depletion of CD8(+) T cells at early stages of disease induction not only inhibited lymphocytic infiltration in the thyroid and autoantibody production but also reduced the levels of MHC expression in thyroid, suggesting that the increased MHC expression requires the presence of CD8(+) T cells that are affected by iodine. From this list, it is clear how central iodine may be to the induction of thyroiditis.

T AND B CELLS IN THYROID AUTOIMMUNITY

In the early phase of thyroid autoimmunity leading to HT, two separate immune processes may take place. In the first stage, an increased number of intrathyroidal APCs is a primary indication of the initiation of an autoimmune reaction. The presentation of antigen by APCs can be facilitated by iodine through one or more mechanisms described above. Presentation of antigen may also be promoted by other factors such as toxins, and a localized viral or bacterial infection. In the second stage, lymphocytes interact with the presented autoantigens, immune tolerance is broken, and antigen-specific T and B cells are activated. It is reported that both CD4(+) and CD8(+) T cells are required for the initiation of autoimmune thyroiditis (34, 35). However, CD8(+) T cells may not be critical in maintaining thyroiditis after the thyroid lesions have developed, since the depletion of CD4(+), but not CD8(+) T cells, markedly reduced the severity of the disease (36). The infiltrating CD4(+) T cells may play a number of roles in the development of autoimmune thyroiditis. For example, CD4(+) T cells can produce cytokines such as IFNγ which may damage thyrocytes, as well as up-regulate MHC class II molecules on thyrocytes and adhesion molecules involved in the recruitment of mononuclear cells into the thyroid (34). CD4(+) T cells also promote B cell activation to facilitate cellular immune responses against the thyroid. CD8(+) T cells may damage thyrocytes by releasing perforin/granzymes or by producing TNFα. The importance of CD8(+) T cells in the initiation of HT is highlighted in an animal study in which depletion of CD8(+) T cells before the development of thyroid lesions was shown to reduce the severity of lymphocytic infiltration of the thyroid (36).

B cells appear to be as important as T cells in the initiation of HT. Experiments have demonstrated that NOD H2^{h4} mice depleted of B cells develop minimal autoimmune thyroiditis (37), indicating that B cells are necessary for initiation as well as progression and maintenance of autoimmune thyroiditis (38). CD4$^+$CD25$^+$ T regulatory cells can be increased in B cell-deficient NOD H2^{h4} mice to inhibit the development of autoimmune thyroiditis (39). In addition, B cells are required for the activation or selection of autoreactive T cells. This is evidence that the autoreactive T cells are apparently unable to respond to autoantigens if B cells are absent (*37*). ,Owing to this B-cell depletion has been used as a protocol against autoimmune thyroiditis (*40*). Thus, all immune cells are important in the pathogenesis of HT.

CD4+CD25+ T REGULATORY CELLS AND THYROID AUTOIMMUNITY

From the aforementioned discussion, it is clear that the immune systems in individuals susceptible to HT are sensitive to changes in the microenvironment and endogenous elements. One immune component these alterations can suppress is the activity of T regulatory (Treg) cells (*41–44*), which plays an important role in the maintenance of self-tolerance. It has been shown that the removal of CD4+CD25+ Treg cells from mice that do not normally develop autoimmune disease can result in autoimmune thyroiditis (*41*), while EAT is prevented in mice given Treg cells (*18, 42–44*). The explanation for why fewer and/or dysfunctional Treg cells are present in mice with autoimmune disease remains unclear. However, in several autoimmune disease models, a mutation of the forkhead box protein P3 (Foxp3) gene, which is a characteristic and functional marker of Treg cells, has been observed (*45*). Mutations such as these may be responsible for the autoimmune response by either inducing autoreactive T cells to break self-tolerance or reducing the number of functional Treg cells that suppress autoimmunity (*46*). Nevertheless, depletion of Treg cells in normal hosts can result in defects in the immune surveillance system, leading to an "unchecked" status with a decrease, or defect, in the inhibitory function of CD4[(+)] and CD8[(+)] T cells and their cytokine production. In this situation, the host permits the defective immunological tolerance and eventually develops autoimmune diseases (*47, 48*). Experiments have demonstrated that TRAIL is able to regulate the immune system by promoting Treg cells (*49, 50*). In fact, treatment of EAT with TRAIL inhibits the development of the disease (*51*). Recent studies have shown that this effect occurs via the promotion of Treg cells in EAT or autoimmune thyroiditis in NOD H2^{h4} mice (*52, 53*).

It is not known how the thyroid microenvironment leads to a defect in the CD4+CD25+ Treg cells in the thyroid. The Treg cells appear to be abundant in inflamed thyroid tissues; however, they are apparently dysfunctional and unable to downregulate the autoimmune response (*18, 41–44*). The expression of Fas in CD4+CD25+ Treg cells is greater in patients with severe HT than in those with mild HT (*54*), and this is consistent with reports of high numbers of apoptotic CD4+CD25+ Treg cells when compared with CD4+CD25− T cells in the thyroid of AITD. In addition to the high expression of Fas in CD4+CD25+ Treg cells of thyroid, these cells strongly express other proapoptotic genes such as TRAIL and TNFα, but weakly express antiapoptotic genes such as Bcl-2, making the Treg cells susceptible to Fas-ligand mediated apoptosis (*55,*

56). Therefore, it has been proposed that the defect or reduction of CD4⁺CD25⁺ Treg cells results from the increased apoptosis of CD4⁺CD25⁺ Treg cells in inflamed thyroid (57).

Despite intense recent investigations (*18, 41–48*), the molecular mechanisms by which Treg cells exert their immunosuppressive activity remains undiscovered. Changes in the cytokine microenvironment in the thyroid correlate with the induction of autoimmunity. One of the important functions of Treg cells is to inhibit Th1-driven autoimmune and inflammatory responses (*58, 59*). Defective Treg cells are unable to inhibit Th1 cell function, resulting in the overproduction of Th1 cytokines including IL-1β, IFNγ, and TNFα (Fig. 27.1). The Th1 cytokine production pattern occurs not only in intrathyroidal but also in peripheral CD4$^{(+)}$ and CD8$^{(+)}$ T lymphocytes in HT patients (*60*), which suggests that the cytokine predisposition to HT is related to defective Treg activity (*61, 62*).

While the defect in the CD4⁺CD25⁺ Treg results in the activation of Th1 cells and the overproduction of Th1 cytokines, it may also promote autoimmune response by the downregulation of a number of molecules that are known to have immunosuppressive effects. These molecules include CD25, IL-2, CTLA-4, IL-10, GITR, LAG-3, Foxp3, and TGFβ (Fig. 27.1). Although the regulation of these molecules is not singly responsible for autoimmune pathogenesis, it is possible that the reduction of several of these molecules may enhance the activity of autoreactive B cells, produce anti-TPO and anti-Tg antibodies, the clinical hallmarks of HT (*63, 64*).

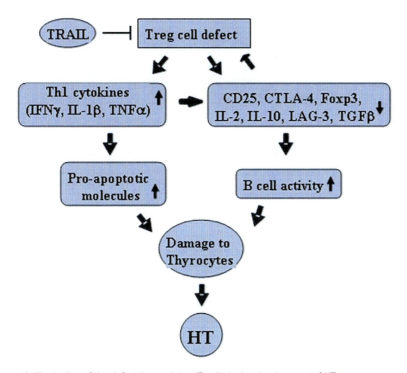

Fig. 27.1 Schematic illustration of the defect in regulatory T cells in the development of HT.

APOPTOSIS AND THYROID AUTOIMMUNITY

As discussed above, the defect in Treg cells may enhance the production of the Th1 cytokines in the thyroid, resulting in a change in the microenvironment. Such a change can facilitate the induction of apoptosis in thyroid cells (65, 66), and evidence indicates that the destruction of thyroid follicles in HT occurs through apoptosis rather than by necrosis or autophagy (65, 67). Thyroid cells are known to express apoptotic molecules, such as TNFα, Fas, and TRAIL (68). However, under normal physiological conditions, only limited apoptosis occurs, since the apoptotic pathways remain inactivated. In their native, controlled environment, thyrocytes constitutively express Fas and do not undergo apoptosis even in the presence of excess anti-Fas antibodies (69). Therefore, under normal conditions, thyrocytes are protected from indiscriminant apoptosis. In contrast, apoptosis appears to regulate the low-level lymphocytic infiltration in the thyroid by inducing autologous lymphocyte apoptosis through Fas ligand expression on these lymphocytes (70). Thus, it is crucial that the thyrocytes are normally resistant to Fas–FasL apoptosis to protect them from normal trafficking lymphocytes.

The exact molecules responsible for the regulation of apoptosis in thyrocytes remain unknown. However, apoptosis inhibition can be reversed by the administration of cycloheximide, an inhibitor of protein translation, suggesting that the inhibitor(s) is a labile protein(s) (69). Interestingly, the Fas pathway in thyrocytes can be activated by Fas ligand in the presence of combinations of proinflammatory cytokines such as IL-1β, IFNγ, and TNFα, although not by any single one of these cytokines (66–68, 71). The induction of apoptosis in thyrocytes has been correlated with an increase of caspases 8, 10, and 7, Bid and Bak levels, but a decrease of p44/42 mitogen-activated protein kinase activity (65, 66, 71). Therefore, it appears that Fas apoptotic pathway activity is further amplified by the bridge proapoptotic molecule Bid, leading to the release of Bak from the mitochondria and activation of caspases. These observations suggest that apoptosis of thyrocytes in HT is dependent on both cell-death receptors and mitochondrial elements. In contrast to most apoptotic activity, apoptotic cell death in HT is not antiinflammatory. Instead, apoptotic thyroid cells and secondary necrotic cells induce a proinflammatory environment (72), which may provide sufficient levels of self-antigens to intensify a dysregulated immune response. Therefore, the apoptosis of thyrocytes in HT may not just be the end result of defective immunological tolerance, but may also serve as a positive feedback loop to exacerbate damage to the thyroid.

CONCLUSIONS

HT is a multifactor autoimmune disorder (Fig. 27.2). There are various factors involved in the dysregulation of immune system at many levels that combine to lead to the development of HT. The expression of particular MHC class II molecules may determine

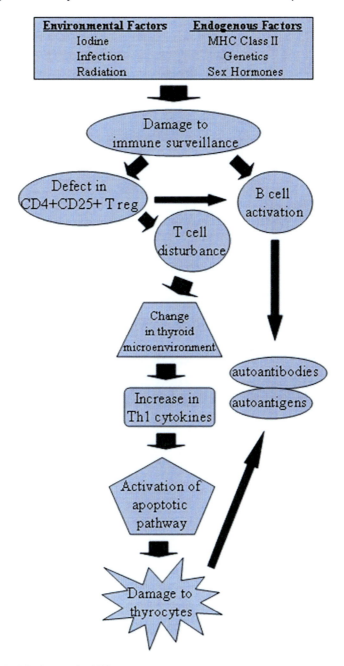

Fig. 27.2 Pathogenesis of HT.

the susceptibility of individuals to the development of HT. In the presence of environmental factors, such as iodine, the autoantigens of the thyroid are altered, and the tolerance to the immune surveillance is broken. This can lead to the activation of T and B cells, especially in individuals with defective Treg cells. These changes in the immunoregulatory cells can result in increased production of Th1 cytokines, which changes the microenvironment of the thyroid and releases the inhibitory mechanisms that inactivate thyroid apoptotic pathways. Eventually, the thyrocytes are damaged via apoptosis and the disease develops. Unchecked, this process is self-reinforcing and self-fulfilling and eventually results in the complete destruction of the thyroid gland.

REFERENCES

1. Weetman AP. Autoimmune thyroid disease. Autoimmunity 2004;37:337–340.
2. Jacobson DL, Gange SJ, Rose NR, Graham NM. Epidemiology and estimated population burden of selected autoimmune diseases in the United States. Clin Immunol Immunopathol 1997;84:223–243.
3. Baker JR Jr, Saunders NB, Wartofsky L, Tseng YC, Burman KD. Seronegative Hashimoto thyroiditis with thyroid autoantibody production localized to the thyroid. Ann Intern Med 1988;108:26–30.
4. Vargas MT, Bropnes-Urbina R, Gladman D, Papsin FR, Walfish PG. Antithyroid microsomal autoantibodies and HLA-DR5 are associated with postpartum thyroid dysfunction: evidence supporting an endocrine pathogenesis. J Clin Endocrinol Metab 1988;67:327–333.
5. Badenhoop K, Schwarz G, Walfish PG, Drummond V, Usadel KH, Bottazzo GF. Susceptibility to thyroid autoimmune disease: molecular analysis of HLA-D region genes identifies new markers for goitrous Hashimoto's thyroiditis. J Clin Endocrinol Metab 1990;71:1131–1137.
6. Wan XL, Kimura A, Dong RP, Honda K, Tamai H, Sasazuki T. HLA-A and DRB4 genes in controlling the susceptibility to Hashimoto's thyroiditis. Hum Immunol 1995;42:131–136.
7. Thomsen M, Ryder LP, Bech K, Bliddal H, Feldt-Rasmussen U, Molholm J, Kappelgaard E, Nielsen H, Svejgaard A. HLA-D in Hashimoto's thyroiditis. Tissue Antigens 1983;21:173–175.
8. Weetman AP. Autoimmune thyroiditis: predisposition and pathogenesis. Clin Endocrinol 1992;36:307–323.
9. Onuma H, Ota M, Sugenoya A, et al. Association between HLA and Hashimoto thyroiditis in Japanese. In: Nagataki S, Mori T, Torizuka K, eds. 80 Years of Hashimoto Disease. Amsterdam: Elsevier, 1993:65–68.
10. Cho BY, Chung JH, Lee HK, Koh C-S. Immunogenetic heterogeneity of atrophic antoimmune thyroiditis according to thyrotropin receptor blocking antibody. In: Nagataki S, Mori T, Torizuka K, eds. 80 Years of Hashimoto Disease. Amsterdam: Elsevier, 1993:45–50.
11. Cho BY, Chung JH, Shong YK, et al. A strong association between thyrotropin receptor-blocking antibody-positive atrophic autoimmune thyroiditis and HLA-DR8 and HLA-DQB1*0302 in Koreans. J Clin Endocrinol Metab 1993;77:611–615.
12. Ayadi H, Hadj Kacem H, Rebai A, Farid NR. The genetics of autoimmune thyroid disease. Trends Endocrinol Metab 2004;15:234–239.
13. Pujol-Borrell R, Todd I, Londei M, Foulis A, Feldmann M, Bottazzo GF. Inappropriate major histocompatibility complex class II expression by thyroid follicular cells in thyroid autoimmune disease and by pancreatic beta cells in type I diabetes. Mol Biol Med 1986;3:159–165.
14. Bonita RE, Rose NR, Rasooly L, Caturegli P, Burek CL. Kinetics of mononuclear cell infiltration and cytokine expression in iodine-induced thyroiditis in the NOD-H2^{h4} mouse. Exp Mol Pathol 2003;74:1–12.
15. Rose NR, Bonita R, Burek CL. Iodine: an environmental trigger of thyroiditis. Autoimmun Rev 2002;1:97–103.
16. Fountoulakis S, Vartholomatos G, Kolaitis N, Frillingos S, Philippou G, Tsatsoulis A. HLA-DR expressing peripheral T regulatory cells in newly diagnosed patients with different forms of autoimmune thyroid disease. Thyroid 2008;18:1195–2000.
17. Caturegli P, Kimura H, Rocchi R, Rose NR. Autoimmune thyroid diseases. Curr Opin Rheumatol 2007;19:44–48.

18. Flynn JC, Meroueh C, Snower DP, David CS, Kong YM. Depletion of CD4+CD25+ regulatory T cells exacerbates sodium iodide-induced experimental autoimmune thyroiditis in human leucocyte antigen DR3 (DRB1*0301) transgenic class II-knock-out non-obese diabetic mice. Clin Exp Immunol 2007;147:547–554.
19. Zois C, Stavrou I, Kalogera C. High prevalence of autoimmune thyroiditis in schoolchildren after elimination of iodine deficiency in northwestern Greece. Thyroid 2003;13:485–489.
20. Bastemir M, Emral R, Erdogan G, Gullu S. High prevalence of thyroid dysfunction and autoimmune thyroiditis in adolescents after elimination of iodine deficiency in the Eastern Black Sea Region of Turkey. Thyroid 2006;16:1265–1271.
21. Rasooly L, Burek CL, Rose NR. Iodine-induced autoimmune thyroiditis in NOD-H-2^{h4} mice. Clin Immunol Immunopathol 1996;81:287–292.
22. Bagchi N, Brown TR, Sundick RS. Thyroid cell injury is an initial event in the induction of autoimmune thyroiditis by iodine in obese strain chickens. Endocrinology 1995;136:5054–5060.
23. Mooij P, de Wit HJ, Drexhage HA. An excess of dietary iodine accelerates the development of a thyroid-associated lymphoid tissue in autoimmune prone BB rats. Clin Immunol Immunopathol 1993;69:189–198.
24. Allen EM, Appel MC, Braverman LE. Iodine-induced thyroiditis and hypothyroidism in the hemithyroidectomized BB/W rat. Endocrinology 1987;121:481–485.
25. Rasooly L, Rose NR, Saboori AM, Ladenson PW, Burek CL. Iodine is essential for human T cell recognition of human thyroglobulin. Autoimmunity 1998;27:213–219.
26. Saboori AM, Rose NR, Bresler HS, Vladut-Talor M, Burek CL. Iodination of human thyroglobulin (Tg) alters its immunoreactivity. I. Iodination alters multiple epitopes of human Tg. Clin Exp Immunol 1998;113:297–302.
27. Rayner DC, Champion BR, Cooke A. Thyroglobulin as autoantigen and tolerogen. Immunol Ser 1993;59:359–376.
28. Sundick RS, Bagchi N, Brown TR. The role of iodine in thyroid autoimmunity: from chickens to humans: a review. Autoimmunity 1992;13:61–68.
29. Wilson R, McKillop JH, Jenkins C, Thomson JA. In vivo and in vitro studies into the immunological changes following iodine 131 therapy for Graves' disease. Eur J Nucl Med 1991;18:265–268.
30. Jiang HY, Li HS, Carayanniotis K, Carayanniotis G. Variable influences of iodine on the T-cell recognition of a single thyroglobulin epitope. Immunology 2007;121:370–376.
31. Li HS, Jiang HY, Carayanniotis G. Modifying effects of iodine on the immunogenicity of thyroglobulin peptides. J Autoimmun 2007;28:171–176.
32. Burek CL, Rose NR. Autoimmune thyroiditis and ROS. Autoimmun Rev 2008;7:530–537.
33. Verma S, Hutchings P, Guo J, McLachlan S, Rapoport B, Cooke A. Role of MHC class I expression and CD8(+) T cells in the evolution of iodine-induced thyroiditis in NOD-H2(h4) and NOD mice. Eur J Immunol 2000;30:1191–1202.
34. Hutchings PR, Verma S, Phillips JM, Harach SZ, Howlett S, Cooke A. Both CD4(+) T cells and CD8(+) T cells are required for iodine accelerated thyroiditis in NOD mice. Cell Immunol 1999;192:113–121.
35. Fuller BE, Giraldo AA, Waldmann H, Cobbold SP, Kong YC. Depletion of CD4+ and CD8+ cells eliminates immunologic memory of thyroiditogenicity in murine experimental autoimmune thyroiditis. Autoimmunity 1994;19:161–168.
36. Braley-Mullen H, Sharp GC, Medling B, Tang H. Spontaneous autoimmune thyroiditis in NOD.H-2^{h4} mice. J Autoimmun 1999;12:157–165.
37. Braley-Mullen H, Yu S. Early requirement for B cells for development of spontaneous autoimmune thyroiditis in NOD.H-2^{h4} mice. J Immunol 2000;165:7262–7269.
38. Yu S, Dunn R, Kehry MR, Braley-Mullen H. B cell depletion inhibits spontaneous autoimmune thyroiditis in NOD.H-2h4 mice. J Immunol 2008;180:7706–7713.
39. Yu S, Maiti PK, Dyson M, Jain R, Braley-Mullen H. B cell-deficient NOD.H-2h4 mice have CD4+CD25+ T regulatory cells that inhibit the development of spontaneous autoimmune thyroiditis. J Exp Med 2006;203:349–358.
40. Hasselbalch HC. B-cell depletion with rituximab – a targeted therapy for Graves' disease and autoimmune thyroiditis. Immunol Lett 2003;88:85–86.
41. Wei WZ, Jacob JB, Zielinski JF, et al. Concurrent induction of antitumor immunity and autoimmune thyroiditis in CD4+ CD25+ regulatory T cell-depleted mice. Cancer Res 2005;65:8471–8478.
42. Verginis P, Li HS, Carayanniotis G. Tolerogenic semimature dendritic cells suppress experimental autoimmune thyroiditis by activation of thyroglobulin-specific CD4+CD25+ T cells. J Immunol 2005;174:7433–7439.
43. Gangi E, Vasu C, Cheatem D, Prabhakar BS. IL-10-producing CD4+CD25+ regulatory

T cells play a critical role in granulocyte-macrophage colony-stimulating factor-induced suppression of experimental autoimmune thyroiditis. J Immunol 2005;174:7006–7013.
44. Nagayama Y, Horie I, Saitoh O, Nakahara M, Abiru N. CD4+CD25+ naturally occurring regulatory T cells and not lymphopenia play a role in the pathogenesis of iodide-induced autoimmune thyroiditis in NOD-H2^{h4} mice. J Autoimmun 2007;29:195–202.
45. Hori S, Nomura T, Sakaguchi S. Control of regulatory T cell development by the transcription factor Foxp3. Science 2003;299:1057–1061.
46. Chen Y, Cuda C, Morel L. Genetic determination of T cell help in loss of tolerance to nuclear antigens. J Immunol 2005;174:7692–7702.
47. Lan RY, Ansari AA, Lian ZX, Gershwin ME. Regulatory T cells: development, function and role in autoimmunity. Autoimmun Rev 2005;4:351–363.
48. Torgerson TR. Regulatory T cells in human autoimmune diseases. Springer Semin Immunopathol 2006;28:63–76.
49. Ren X, Ye F, Jiang Z, Chu Y, Xiong S, Wang Y. Involvement of cellular death in TRAIL/DR5-dependent suppression induced by CD4(+)CD25(+) regulatory T cells. Cell Death Differ 2007;14:2076–2084.
50. Hirata S, Matsuyoshi H, Fukuma D, et al. Involvement of regulatory T cells in the experimental autoimmune encephalomyelitis-preventive effect of dendritic cells expressing myelin oligodendrocyte glycoprotein plus TRAIL. J Immunol 2007;178:918–925.
51. Wang SH, Cao Z, Wolf JM, Van Antwerp M, Baker JR Jr. Death ligand tumor necrosis factor-related apoptosis-inducing ligand inhibits experimental autoimmune thyroiditis. Endocrinology 2005;146:4721–4726.
52. Nakahara M, Nagayama Y, Saitoh O, Sogawa R, Tone S, Abiru N. Expression of immunoregulatory molecules by thyrocytes protects NOD-H2^{h4} mice from developing autoimmune thyroiditis. Endocrinology 2008;150(3):1545–1551.
53. Wang SH, Chen GH, Fan Y, Van Antwerp M, Baker JR Jr. TRAIL inhibits experimental autoimmune thyroiditis by the expansion of CD4+CD25+ regulatory T cells. Endocrinology 2009;150(4):2000–2007.
54. Marazuela M, Garcia-Lopez MA, Figueroa-Vega N, et al. Regulatory T cells in human autoimmune thyroid disease. J Clin Endocrinol Metab 2006;91:3639–3646.
55. Maruoka H, Watanabe M, Matsuzuka F, Takimoto T, Miyauchi A, Iwatani Y. Increased intensities of fas expression on peripheral T-cell subsets in severe autoimmune thyroid disease. Thyroid 2004;14:417–423.
56. Kasprowicz DJ, Droin N, Soper DM, Ramsdell F, Green DR, Ziegler SF. Dynamic regulation of FoxP3 expression controls the balance between CD4+ T cell activation and cell death. Eur J Immunol 2005;35:3424–3432.
57. Taams LS, Smith J, Rustin MH, Salmon M, Poulter LW, Akbar AN. Human anergic/suppressive CD4(+)CD25(+) T cells: a highly differentiated and apoptosis-prone population. Eur J Immunol 2001;31:1122–1131.
58. Baecher-Allan C, Hafler DA. Human regulatory T cells and their role in autoimmune disease. Immunol Rev 2006;212:203–216.
59. Daniel C, Sartory N, Zahn N, Geisslinger G, Radeke HH, Stein JM. FTY720 ameliorates Th1-mediated colitis in mice by directly affecting the functional activity of CD4+CD25+ regulatory T cells. J Immunol 2007;178:2458–2468.
60. Mazziotti G, Sorvillo F, Naclerio C, et al. Type-1 response in peripheral CD4+ and CD8+ T cells from patients with Hashimoto's thyroiditis. Eur J Endocrinol 2003;148:383–388.
61. Colin IM, Isaac J, Dupret P, Ledant T, D'Hautcourt JL. Functional lymphocyte subset assessment of the Th1/Th2 profile in patients with autoimmune thyroiditis by flow-cytometric analysis of peripheral lymphocytes. J Biol Regul Homeost Agents 2004;18:72–76.
62. Phenekos C, Vryonidou A, Gritzapis AD, Baxevanis CN, Goula M, Papamichail M. Th1 and Th2 serum cytokine profiles characterize patients with Hashimoto's thyroiditis (Th1) and Graves' disease (Th2). Neuroimmunomodulation 2004;11:209–213.
63. Baker JR Jr. Immunologic aspects of endocrine diseases. Ann Intern Med 1988;108:26–30.
64. Bonger U, Finke R, Hegedus L, Hanseb JM, Schleusener H. Cytotoxicity and antithyroid peroxidase antibodies in patients with autoimmune thyroiditis. In: Nagataki S, Mori T, Torizuka K, eds. 80 Years of Hashimoto Disease. Amsterdam: Elsevier, 1993:383–388.
65. Wang SH, Mezosi E, Wolf JM, et al. IFNgamma sensitization to TRAIL-induced apoptosis in human thyroid carcinoma cells by upregulating Bak expression. Oncogene 2004;23:928–935.
66. Mezosi E, Wang SH, Utsugi S, et al. Interleukin-1beta and tumor necrosis factor (TNF)-alpha sensitize human thyroid epithelial cells to TNF-related apoptosis-inducing ligand-induced apoptosis through increases in procaspase-7 and bid, and the down-regulation of p44/42 mitogen-activated protein kinase activity. J Clin Endocrinol Metab 2004;89:250–257.

67. Baker JR Jr. Dying (apoptosing?) for a consensus on the Fas death pathway in the thyroid. J Clin Endocrinol Metab 1999;84:2593–2595.
68. Arscott PL, Baker JR Jr. Apoptosis and thyroiditis. Clin Immunol Immunopathol 1998;87:207–217.
69. Arscott PL, Knapp J, Rymaszewski M, et al. Fas (APO-1, CD95)-mediated apoptosis in thyroid cells is regulated by a labile protein inhibitor. Endocrinology 1997;138:5019–5027.
70. Batteux F, Tourneur L, Trebeden H, Charreire J, Chiocchia G. Gene therapy of experimental autoimmune thyroiditis by in vivo administration of plasmid DNA coding Fas ligand. J Immunol 1999;162:603–608.
71. Mezosi E, Wang SH, Utsugi S, et al. Induction and regulation of Fas-mediated apoptosis in human thyroid epithelial cells. Mol Endocrinol 2005;19:804–811.
72. Ren Y, Tang J, Mok MY, Chan AW, Wu A, Lau CS. Increased apoptotic neutrophils and macrophages and impaired macrophage phagocytic clearance of apoptotic neutrophils in systemic lupus erythematosus. Arthritis Rheum 2003;48:2888–2897.

Chapter 28

Immunopathogenesis of Graves' Disease

Syed A. Morshed, Rauf Latif, and Terry F. Davies

Key Words: Graves' disease, autoimmune thyroid disease, TSH receptor antibodies, Thyroid-specific T cells, Genetic susceptibility, Environmental influences

INTRODUCTION

Graves' disease (GD) was one of the first human autoimmune diseases to be characterized following the discovery of thyroid-stimulating antibodies in hyperthyroid patients in 1956 (*1*). GD is now known to be the most common cause of hyperthyroidism between the ages of 20 and 50 years. In females, the annual incidence ranges from 15 to 200 per 100,000 per year (*2*). The rates observed in males are about one tenth of those in females, and the disease is more common in iodine-sufficient regions (*3*). The hyperactivity of the thyroid gland is due to the presence of thyroid stimulating antibodies, and these are now known to recognize and activate the thyroid-stimulating hormone receptor (TSHR). These TSHR stimulating antibodies increase the growth and the function of the thyroid follicular cells, leading to the excessive production of thyroid hormones (both T3 and T4) and symptoms of tachycardia, anxiety, and weight loss among others. Pathologically, the disease is characterized by a heterogeneous lymphocytic infiltration of the thyroid parenchyma as well as infiltration of retroorbital and dermal tissues (*4–6*) (see Chap. 31). Transplacental antibody transferred to the infants of affected mothers during pregnancy can induce symptoms similar to the mother by causing neonatal Graves' disease (*7, 8*). Similarly, antibodies from patients with GD when injected into experimental animals and even humans can induce thyroid activation (*9*).

AUTOIMMUNITY AND GRAVES' DISEASE

The pathologic processes involved in GD are similar to that of other autoimmune diseases, with the emphasis on the antibodies as the most unique aspect. These characteristics include a lymphocytic infiltrate at the target organs, the presence of antigen-reactive T and B cells and antibodies, and the establishment of animal models of GD by antibody transfer or immunization with antigen. Similar to other autoimmune diseases, risk factors for Graves' disease include the presence of multiple susceptibility genes, including certain human leukocyte antigen (HLA) alleles, and the TSHR gene itself, which are discussed in Chap. 28. In addition, a variety of known risk factors and precipitators have been characterized including the influence of sex and sex hormones, pregnancy, stress, infection, iodine, and other potential environmental factors (*10*).

THE TSH RECEPTOR ANTIGEN OF GRAVES' DISEASE

In GD, the main autoantigen is the TSHR, which is expressed primarily in the thyroid and also in adipocytes, bone cells, and a variety of additional sites including the heart (*11*) (Fig. 28.1). We have reviewed this antigen in detail elsewhere (*12, 13*). The TSHR is a G-protein-coupled receptor with seven transmembrane-spanning domains. TSH, acting via the TSHR, regulates thyroid growth and thyroid hormone production and secretion. The TSHR undergoes complex posttranslational processing involving dimerization and intramolecular cleavage; the latter modification leaves a two-subunit structural form of the receptor (*14*). Data suggest that there is eventual shedding or degradation of the TSHR ectodomain (*15–17*), although this has not been confirmed in vivo. Each of these posttranslational events may influence the antigenicity of the receptor, and furthermore, this complex processing may contribute to the break in TSHR self-tolerance. For example, the affinity of TSHR antibodies for the TSHR ectodomain is greater than for the holoreceptor itself (*15*). However, factors that contribute to TSHR presentation as a target for the immune system when expressed at different sites are not well understood.

HUMORAL IMMUNITY TO THE TSHR

One of the unique characteristics of GD, not found in normals nor the entire animal kingdom, is the presence of TSHR antibodies (TSHR-Ab), easily detectable in the vast majority of patients (*18*).

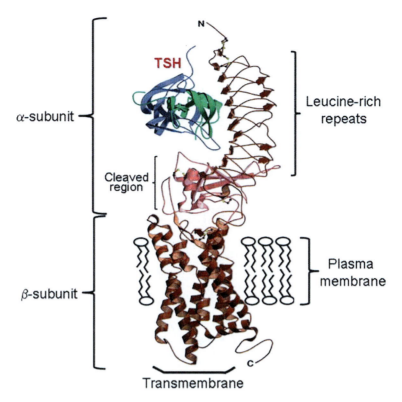

Fig. 28.1 A computer model of the TSH receptor based on the crystal structure of the receptor ectodomain and seven transmembrane domains derived from the rhodopsin receptor structure. The large ectodomain is made of ten leucine-rich repeats (LRRs), which form the characteristic "horseshoe-" shaped structure with a concave inner surface, which harbors the major ligand and autoantibody binding regions. The unique 50aa cleaved region in the ectodomain is shown in gray is characteristic only of the TSHR among the glycoprotein hormone receptor family (*13*).

B cells in lymph node germinal centers undergo somatic hypermutation that can produce self-specific B cells. Normally, such cells are removed by apoptosis when exposed to soluble self-antigen. In patients with GD, as for other antigens in other autoimmune diseases, TSHR-reactive B cells survive and secrete autoantibodies to the TSHR. Furthermore, such B cells can potentially present thyroid autoantigen to T cells and can also produce proinflammatory cytokines as seen in other autoimmune diseases (*19*). These findings suggest, therefore, that B cells play a central role in mediating chronic inflammatory thyroid disease. Whether it is the B cells or the T cells that play a primary role in GD is controversial but most likely both are intimately involved (*20*).

Many self-specific B cells escape destruction but are prevented from responding to self-antigen by several additional mechanisms such as clonal anergy, clonal deletion, or peripheral or central suppression. B cells recognizing specific self-antigen in the secondary lymphoid organs are trapped in the T cell areas; if not activated by T cells available to provide help, the B cells will die by apoptosis (*21*), while B cells which bind soluble self-antigen will undergo anergy, downregulate membrane IgM expression, and survive for only a short time. The mechanisms of B-cell self-tolerance also include receptor editing and autoreactive B-cell receptor (BCRs) allelic exclusion, as well as clonal ignorance (lack of recognition) (*21*).

TYPES OF TSHR ANTIBODIES

The TSHR is the likely cause of, as well as the target of, various types of TSHR antibodies recognized in the serum of patients with GD. Clear delineation of the characteristics of these antibody types has resulted from the analysis of monoclonal antibodies to the TSHR (TSHR-mAbs) raised in animal models of GD (*22–24*). Three varieties of TSHR-Ab are common in GD: stimulating, blocking, and neutral antibodies (Fig. 28.2). Stimulating antibodies, which bind only to the naturally conformed TSHR, not only induce cAMP generation but also block TSH-mediated activation of thyroid function. The first stimulating mAb called MS-1 is illustrated in Fig. 28.3. The activity of such antibodies is similar to that of TSH ligand itself. In addition, TSHR blocking antibodies, whose primary biological action is to prevent TSH

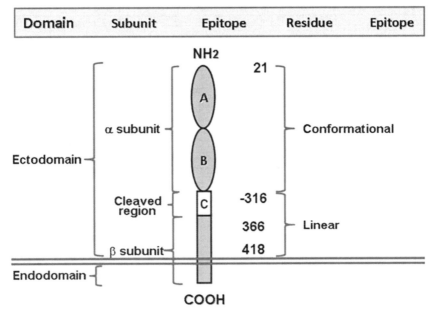

Fig. 28.2 A cartoon depicting the epitope geography of the TSHR. The capital letters A–C indicate the three major epitopes recognized by the antibodies. The epitopes shown as *oval* indicate conformational recognition and *squares* indicate linear recognition regions. The ~50aa region removed by TSHR cleavage is shown in *white* (*24*).

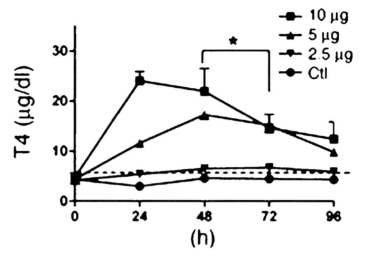

Fig. 28.3 CBA/J mice were injected with the indicated doses of a thyroid-stimulating monoclonal antibody (MS-1) or control antibody (Ctl), and serum T4 levels were measured every 24 h. The *broken line* in the graph indicates the upper level of control mouse serum T4 (*38*).

binding to the receptor to such an extent that alone they may induce hypothyroidism, may also act as weak TSH agonists (*25*). Some such blocking antibodies are conformationally dependent, while others have a high affinity for reduced TSHR antigen and/or linear peptides. On the other hand, neutral TSHR antibodies neither block TSH binding or action nor do they induce cAMP production. These neutral TSHR-Abs bind exclusively with linear epitopes. The presence of differing proportions of high-affinity TSHR-Abs with different biological activity in autoimmune thyroid disease patients determines the disease phenotypes, varying from hyperthyroidism to hypothyroidism.

In the last 5 years, insight into the contribution of autoreactive B cells to the normal human B-cell repertoire and their regulation at self-tolerance checkpoints has come from the analysis of monoclonal antibodies cloned from single purified B cells at different stages during their development (*21*). Since diversity by V(D)J recombination and somatic hypermutation provides protective humoral immunity and also generates potentially harmful autoreactive B cell clones, attempts to thwart autoimmunity are ensured by several checkpoints at which developing autoreactive B cells are counterselected. Thus, defects in central and peripheral checkpoints for B cell tolerance may also be involved in the autoimmunity of GD. Indeed, B cell survival factors such as B-cell-activating factor (BAFF) and proliferation-inducing ligand (APRIL) have been shown to be important in a Graves' animal model (*26*). Both BAFF-Fc and BCMA-Fc treatments lead to amelioration of hyperthyroid GD induced by TSHR immunization in mice, indicating that such treatment may lead to better targeted therapies for GD. Therefore, the concept that B cells may play a central role in balancing autoimmune thyroid reactivity is clinically important. Indeed, recent studies using gene silencing, targeting BAFF, inhibited proinflammatory cytokine expression, suppressed plasma cell generation and Th17 cells, and caused marked amelioration in autoimmune arthritis (27). Similar early clinical studies using B cell suppression in Graves' ophthalmopathy with Rituximab add further support to this concept (28). These findings clearly indicate that targeting B cells and factors that regulate B cell function may be highly applicable to the modulation of clinical GD.

TSH RECEPTOR ANTIBODY EPITOPES

Monoclonal Antibodies to the TSHR

Monoclonal antibodies to the TSHR raised against a variety of antigen preparations, including recombinant proteins and synthesized peptides, proved to be all of the blocking variety. Only when intact natural TSH receptors or genetic immunization was used was it possible to induce an animal model of hyperthyroidism (29) and subsequently isolate relatively rare B cells secreting TSHR antibodies with stimulating activity (22). The most well-defined stimulating monoclonal TSHR-Abs include MS-1 raised in hamsters (22) and M-22 obtained from a patient with hyperthyroid GD (30). In addition, blocking and neutral mAbs have been well characterized by a number of groups (25, 31, 32).

Epitopes of Stimulating TSHR-Abs

The TSHR ectodomain has been recently crystallized with a stimulating monoclonal Fab fragment bound to the TSHR in situ (33). Several amino acids distributed along an extensive part of the concave surface of the leucine-rich repeat region (LRR) of the TSHR ectodomain were found to be important for antibody binding, but the same region did not appear to be important for TSH binding and stimulation (Fig. 28.4) (33). Most of the amino acids important for antibody interactions were common for six stimulating monoclonals, suggesting that different TSHR stimulating antibodies interact with the same region of the TSHR, although there were subtle differences in the actual amino acids that make contact with the different stimulating antibodies (34). However, from several studies of TSHR antibodies (30, 35–37), it has also been concluded that epitope differences are probably responsible for their different biological activities. Our recent study of three stimulating TSHR-mAbs showed variation in their patterns of signal transduction and is consistent with this conclusion (25). Further studies are needed to relate epitope binding to signal transduction patterns (see below).

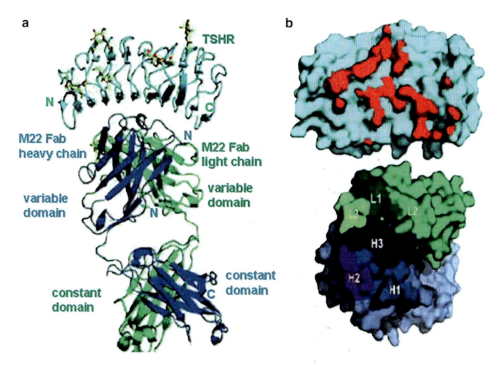

Fig. 28.4 Two views of the complex of the thyroid-stimulating hormone leucine-rich domain (LRD) and Fab fragment of a human TSH receptor-stimulating antibody M22 obtained by analysis of crystal structure of TSHR260-M22 Fab complex at 2.55 Å resolution. (a) In the structure the TSHR LRD is in cyan, the M22 Fab light chain (LC) is in *green*, the M22 heavy chain (HC) is in *blue*, and N-linked carbohydrates are in *yellow*. (b) An open view of the interface. TSHR LRD residues are shown in *red* if within 4.0 Å from M22 Fab residues. The hypervariable regions of M22 are highlighted in different colors and labeled as heavy (H) and light (L).

Epitopes of Blocking TSHR-Abs

Epitopes for TSHR blocking antibodies appear to be more widely distributed than for stimulating antibodies. These can be both conformational and nonconformational. Experimentally produced blocking TSHR-mAbs have been shown to bind to independent linear or conformational epitopes (*38*) on the α subunit, although at least one linear epitope on the α/β subunit has been described (*39*). TSHR autoantibodies from patients with Graves' and autoimmune (Hashimoto's) thyroiditis have been shown to compete with a blocking TSHR-mAb to the N-terminus of the β TSHR α subunit (amino acids 382–415) (*40*). Hence, blocking antibodies that cause hypothyroidism are heterogeneous and their epitopes may lie broadly upstream of the α subunit or downstream of the β subunit (*41*). Clearly, there appear to be multiple epitopes involved in this repertoire of antibodies.

Epitopes for Neutral TSHR-Abs

Neutral TSHR antibodies were thought to have no influence on thyroid cell function (see below). In animal models of Graves' disease (*42, 43*), the major linear epitopes recognized are mainly N-terminus peptides (~20 amino acids) and those in the TSHR cleavage region (Fig. 28.1) (*13*). Neither of these epitopes is involved in the TSH binding pocket (*44*) and thus neutral TSHR-mAbs fail to block TSH binding to the receptor.

THYROCYTE SIGNAL TRANSDUCTION BY TSHR ANTIBODIES

To help determine the functional consequences of TSHR-Abs, we have recently characterized the signaling pathways on rat thyroid cells (*25*). Our studies on the characterization of TSHR antibody-mediated signaling demonstrated that stimulating TSH receptor antibodies used signaling pathways similar to TSH for cell activation and growth (Fig. 28.5). However, some TSHR blocking and neutral TSHR mAbs also resulted in signal responses demonstrating that such TSHR-mAbs may be weak agonists or

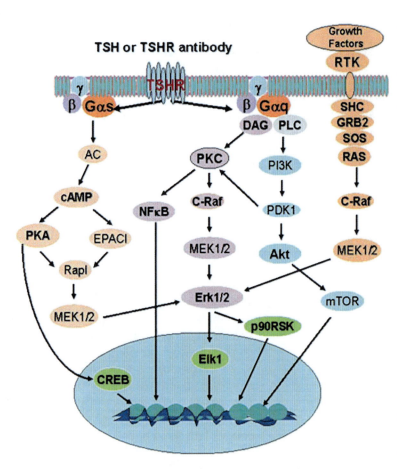

Fig. 28.5 Simplified diagrammatic illustration of the major signaling pathways stimulated by TSH receptor antibodies. Note the five pathways from *left* to *right*: cAMP/PKA/ERK or PKA/CREB, PI3/Akt/mTOR, PKC/NFkB, PKC/c-raf/ERK/p90RSK, and Ras/c-Raf/ERK (*25*).

inverse agonists (*25*). These observations help explain how TSHR-Abs may contribute to different clinical phenotypes in autoimmune thyroid disease. Most striking was that two of the blocking antibodies we examined, resulted not only in signal initiation, but they also showed different pathway dominance (*25*). More study is necessary to correlate the effector mechanisms used by the TSHR-Abs with their different epitopes.

Of general interest was our characterization of two neutral TSHR-Abs on signaling cascades and downstream effectors, which identified two separate mechanisms working in the rat thyroid cells. For example, one antibody showed suppression of signaling activity, including cell proliferation, whereas the other neutral antibody activated cell signaling and induced cell proliferation. Both failed to inhibit TSH binding (by definition) and activate cAMP generation. The amino acid sequences for these neutral antibody binding sites (*38*) showed an overlap of 5 amino acids (337–341 residues), and we deduced that the last 16 amino acids (341–356) may, therefore, be critical to signal-activating events. A conformational monoclonal antibody with a possible binding site at the LRR domain (residues 260–289) has also been described as an inverse agonist that suppressed TSHR constitutive activity (*45*) as assessed by cAMP generation. These findings raise the possibility that multiple domains in the ectodomain of the TSHR that suppress or stimulate the TSHR may exist.

HUMORAL IMMUNITY TO OTHER ANTIGENS IN GRAVES' DISEASE

It would be an omission to ignore the fact that the vast majority of patients with GD also express significant titers of antibodies to thyroperoxidase and thyroglobulin (*46*). However, animal models of TSHR immunization do not express an intrathyroidal infiltrate unless outbred animals are used. This may be telling us that autoimmune thyroiditis is a complex genetic disorder on top of which GD develops. Factors in favor of this explanation include the finding that such antibodies do not transfer thyroid disease and are polyclonal in character (*46*). Recent reports of antibodies to pendrin and the sodium iodide symporter indicate that such antibodies are also not confined to GD but are more common in autoimmune thyroiditis but are of uncertain importance (*47, 48*).

Recent work has also suggested that antibodies to the IGF-1 receptor are present in the serum of patients with GD, especially those with Graves' ophthalmopathy (*49, 50*). The IGF-1 receptor is widely expressed but may be overexpressed in B cells and fibroblasts from such patients (*51*). Synergism between antibodies to the TSHR and the IGF-1 receptor may be an important concept in activating the thyrocyte.

T CELLS AND GRAVES' DISEASE

Antigen-Specific T Cells

T cells play a central role in the pathogenesis of GD (*52–56*) as reflected by their presence in the intrathyroidal infiltrate, both Th1 and Th2 (*52, 53*), and their reactivity to TSHR antigen and TSHR peptides (*52–57*) (Fig. 28.6). Oligoclonal use of T-cell receptor (TCR) genes has been identified in the T cells infiltrating the thyroid gland (and retroorbital tissues) from patients with GD (*52, 53*), indicative of clonal expansion and suggesting the primary nature of the T-cell responses. However, variations in actual TCR usage is seen among different patients (*54, 58*) as would be expected, since T cells recognize the TSHR only in the context of MHC (major histocompatibility complex) molecules. Studies with TSHR peptides in patients with GD have shown a variety of T cell epitopes with none dominant (*58*). However, some restriction related to HLA types has been reported (*57*).

Regulatory T Cells

Recently, much attention has been focused on regulatory CD4+ T cells (Tregs). These cells express CD25 (α chain of the IL-2 receptor) on their cell surface and also express FoxP3 (*59*), a critically

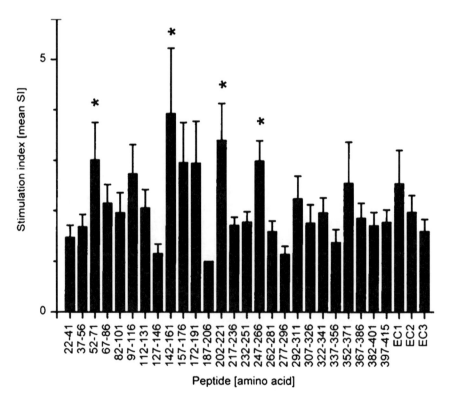

Fig. 28.6 T-cell reactivity to TSHR peptides. Proliferative responses of PBMC obtained from thyroid patients to different TSHR peptides. The results are expressed as stimulation indices (Mean SI). As baseline, the peptide with the lowest median response (187–206) was used (*57*).

important transcription factor of the forkhead family which is necessary for development and maintenance of Treg function. Tregs have suppressive functions on effector T cells, and the lack of these cells induces autoimmunity (60). Treg function in animal models of autoimmune thyroid disease has been extensively explored, and recent data suggests similar suppressive effects (61–63). The relevance of such immunization-induced models to immune regulation in human disease is questionable. However, increased numbers of Tregs within the thyroid, as well as in peripheral blood, have been reported in patients with GD, but they had defective suppressive immune function, (64) indicating that Tregs may be deficient in their downregulatory effects in GD. Of note, however, taking 633 unrelated GD patients, Owen et al. (65) genotyped the *FOXP3* locus and identified no association with the disease, suggesting that any defect may be secondary to the immune response.

Th17 Cells

Recent evidence indicates that naïve CD4+ T cells can be differentiated into Th1, Th2, Th17, and Tregs depending on the local cytokine milieu. Both in vitro and in vivo murine and human CD4+ T cells document polarization of certain cytokines toward Th17 cells (66–68) that produce IL-17 cytokine. In these studies, IL-12 skews toward Th1, IL-4 toward Th2, TGF-β toward Tregs, and IL-6 plus TGF-β toward Th17 (69). It has been proposed that Th17 or Th1 responses rather than Treg differentiation may be responsible for the development and/or progression of autoimmune disease (69). Recently, the role Th17 cells in GD has been described in a patient who underwent CD34+-selected autologous stem-cell transplantation (70). The same group identified an additional two out of 25 cases that underwent autologous hematopoietic stem-cell transplantation (71). Increases in IL-6 and TGF-β cytokines preceded the increased Th17 levels in this patient indicating that priming of these cells by both IL-6 and TGF-β was required to induce pathogenic Th17 cells and subsequent development of TSHR-specific autoreactive B cells.

INTRATHYROIDAL ANTIGEN-PRESENTATION IN GRAVES' DISEASE

There are at least three clear routes for TSHR antigen to be presented to thyroid-specific T cells: by the thyroid cells themselves, via intrathyroidal or extrathyroidal dendritic cells, and by using B cells directly. Patients with GD demonstrate increases in anti-apoptotic Bcl-2 expression and a reduced apoptotic Fas expression on thyrocytes while exhibiting opposite effects on the infiltrating lymphocytes (72–74). These findings suggest that the induction of lymphocyte death ensures thyrocyte survival possibly by downmodulating inflammatory cytokines. However, there remains an element of ongoing apoptosis of thyroid cells in GD glands (*73*), providing ample thyroid antigen for presentation in addition to the hypothetical shedding of the TSHR ectodomain (*72, 74*). Clearly these observations highlight the important role of regulating apoptosis in thyroid autoimmunity.

Thyrocytes as Antigen Presenting Cells

It has been known for some time now that thyroid epithelial cells can express MHC class I and class 2 antigens in autoimmune thyroid disease (*75*). MHC class I antigen expression endows the ability to present viral antigen to T cells (*76*) and thyroid antigen to thyroid-specific T cells (*77, 78*) (Fig. 28.7). What remains unclear is how important this mechanism is in the context of thyroid autoimmunity.

Intrathyroidal Dendritic Cells

Dendritic cells within the thyroid gland itself have been implicated in autoimmune thyroid disease, in thyroiditis more than Graves' disease, but there have been surprisingly limited numbers of studies. For example, necrotic thyrocytes facilitated maturation of dendritic cells in a mouse model of thyroiditis (*79*), and T cell interactions with dendritic cells have been implicated in intrathyroidal lymphoid hyperplasia (*80*). It is therefore to be assumed that such cells have a major role in thyroid antigen presentation in GD, and that immunization of mice with TSHR-loaded dendritic cells has been successful in inducing hyperthyroidism (*81*). Furthermore, characterization of thyroidal dendritic cells in GD has shown their adherence to thyrocytes (*82, 83*) indicative of a major role in the disease.

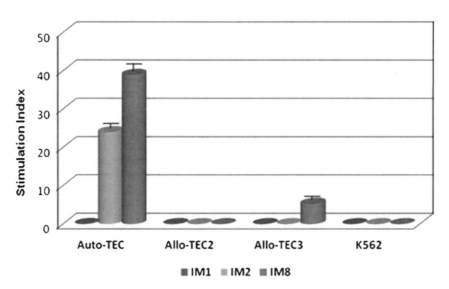

Fig. 28.7 Thyroid-specific T-cell reactivity: cytotoxicity assay was measured using ^{51}Cr release with autologous thyroid epithelial cells (TEC), allogeneic TEC and K562 cell line. Significant increases in cytotoxicity by IM8 and IM2 T cell clones were noted with autologous TEC. TECs were treated for 5 days with bovine TSH (10 mU/ml), and Thytroper (1 U/mg) to induce human Tg secretion, and M-Ag expression. Recombinant human γ-interferon (100 U/ml) was used to induce HLA-DR antigen expression. Cytotoxicity is expressed as % ^{51}Cr release (Mean ± SEM) (*78*).

The CD1 molecule, which resembles MHC I, is a family of four cell surface proteins (CD1 a, b, c, and d) (*84*). Both dendritic and B cells express CD1 molecules and present lipid antigens to T cells to regulate antimicrobial and antitumor responses and to balance between tolerance and autoimmunity (*84*). To determine whether CD1 played a role in the generation of thyroid autoimmunity, Roura-Mir et al. (*85*) studied CD1⁺ APCs (antigen presenting cells) and CD1-restricted T cells within the thyroid glands of affected GD and autoimmune thyroiditis patients. CD1-expressing APCs infiltrated the thyroid gland in large numbers during the acute and chronic stages of both patient groups. Fresh thyroid-derived lymphocytes and short-term T cell lines isolated from the glands were able to lyse target cells that expressed CD1 proteins. These findings indicate that CD1-restricted intrathyroidal T cells may play a critical role in orchestrating inflammasomes, which include both innate and adaptive immunity (*86*) during human autoimmune thyroid disease.

Antigen Presentation by B Cells

Thyroglobulin antigen has been shown to be presented by B cells in animal models (*87*), but to date, there are no data on TSHR presentation. However, as with all antigens, B cells are powerful antigen presenters and are able by their antibody specificity to capture specific antigens, even those in sparse supply such as the TSHR.

PRECIPITATING GRAVES' DISEASE: THE ENVIRONMENT VERSUS GENETIC SUSCEPTIBILITY

Epidemiological data indicate that genetics cannot account for all susceptibility to complex autoimmune diseases such as GD. One of the commonest claims for evidence that the environment is important in the precipitation of AITD is the fact that identical twins are not always in synchrony. While nonidentical twins have an expected low concordance for AITD of ~2%, identical twins have a concordance of only ~20–40% rather than 100% (*88*), although it is likely that the older such twins become the greater the concordance (reaching, for example, 60% by 60 years in Type 1 diabetes) (*89*). These types of data, seen in many autoimmune diseases, suggest that genes are not the only causative factor. But the immune systems of identical, monozygous twins are far from identical. The variable (V) genes of T-cell receptors and immunoglobulins undergo random rearrangements throughout life and so identical twins become less similar as time goes by, and different environmental stimuli are experienced (*58*). Hence, it is significant that the concordance rate for AITD remains so high in identical twins, and this provides evidence for the powerful effects of non-V genes, such as the MHC genes, CTLA-4, PTPN22, etc. discussed in Chap. 28 (*90*). However, such observations also leave room for the possibility that the environment is an important component in the etiology of autoimmune disease. Indeed, exploring a unique 756 twin pair data set, Hansen et al. in 2006, using thyroid autoantibodies as a marker for AITD, determined, via structural equation modeling, that only 60–70% of the risk for such markers was genetic (*91*).

ENVIRONMENTAL PRECIPITATORS

Several factors may be involved in the initiation of GD, and many of these factors are similar to other autoimmune disorders. While some have long been implicated, there are remarkably few data in this area (Table 28.1) (*92*). These factors include irradiation, as with the children of Chernobyl who developed increased thyroid autoantibodies, (*93*) and radioiodine treatment, which may pre-

Table 28.1
Environmental Influences on AITD

Fetal size
Iodine intake
Selenium intake
Hormones – female sex   Oral contraceptives
Pregnancy and Parity
Fetal microchimerism
Stress and direct trauma
Seasonal variation
Allergy
Smoking
Drugs – amiodarone, antiretrovirals, campath anti-CD52, interferon alpha, IL-2, GM-CSF

Irradiation – external
    RAI
    Nuclear fall out

Viral infections
Bacterial infections
Lack of infections – the hygiene hypothesis

cipitate Graves' disease, (*94*) and iodine – itself or within amiodarone, which can precipitate thyroiditis or Graves' disease (*95, 96*). Smoking has also been shown to be an important factor, especially in Graves' ophthalmopathy (see Chap. 31) (*97*), and stress, though less well documented, is widely considered a precipitator by its effects on immune reactivity (*98*). However, these additive causes can only account for a small fraction of patients developing these disorders, leaving more environmental and stochastic causes to be determined. This is why infections have been so widely implicated, and the lack of evidence implicating a single infection has caused widespread interest in the Hygiene Hypothesis.

GRAVES' DISEASE AND THE HYGIENE HYPOTHESIS

The hygiene hypothesis implies that the immune system is educated by multiple exposures to different infections allowing it to better control autoimmune responses. Thus, improved living standards have been associated with decreased exposure to infections and an increased risk of autoimmune diseases including allergy and Type 1 diabetes mellitus (*99, 100*). BCG infection in an immunized mouse model of Graves' disease impaired the development of hyperthyroidism (*101*), agreeing with a variety of studies where infection has prevented, rather than accelerated, the development in animal models of type 1 diabetes, collagen-induced arthritis, and autoimmune encephalitis (*99*). Kondrashova et al. (*100*) have reported two childhood populations which they considered to have similar genetic backgrounds – one Finnish and wealthy and the other Russian with a much lower economic status – and which were geographically close. These investigators had previously reported a much higher rate of microbial infections in the lower economic population and with this a much reduced prevalence of type 1 diabetes mellitus, celiac disease, and allergies (*100*). They also reported a much reduced prevalence of thyroid autoantibodies in the lower economic population, using thyroid antibodies as a marker of future AITD. Their data agree with the hypothesis that multiple infections prevent the development of thyroid autoimmunity by exposing children to a wide variety of external antigens. Data from these types of analyses do agree with the hygiene hypothesis, suggesting that lack of infections dilutes the capacity of the immune system to avoid autoimmune responses. We may need such multiple exposures to infection to train our immune system to perform well. However, some infections may still be able, in susceptible individuals, to break tolerance and allow autoimmune disease to develop. Here, the role of innate immunity and the toll-like receptors appears to be important (*102*).

INFECTIONS AND GRAVES' DISEASE

Although the Coxsackie B4 virus has been shown to induce type I diabetes in mice and the encephalomyocarditis virus can induce autoimmune myositis (*99*), the data for autoimmune thyroid disease are surprisingly sparse, dated and related to thyroiditis rather than Graves' disease for which spontaneous animal models do not exist. For example, avian leukosis virus has been used to induce chicken thyroiditis with a heavy lymphocytic infiltrate (*103*), and almost 20 years ago, Penhale used a rat thymectomy model of autoimmune thyroiditis to show that keeping the animals clean made them much less susceptible to developing thyroiditis (*103*).

As far as human data are concerned, retroviral HTLV-1 infection has been reported to be associated with GD (*104*). In cocultures of T cells with HTLV-1 and rat thyrocytes (FRTL-5), the virus efficiently infected thyrocytes and induced IL-6 mRNA (*104*). Hepatitis C virus (HCV) and *Toxoplasma gondii* have also been associated with thyroid autoimmunity (*105, 106*). HCV binds to the CD81 receptor expressed on thyrocytes and induces IL-8 cytokine, suggesting that HCV may trigger autoimmunity by a bystander activation mechanism. Using proteomic technology, Tozzoli et al. detected antibodies to a series of viral and protozoal antigens and only antibodies to *Toxoplasma* were significantly increased in Italian patients with GD (*106*). These findings together with earlier observations again raise strong possibilities that infections either directly or indirectly may initiate and/or perpetuate GD. Such information, however, does not fit with the Hygiene Hypothesis discussed earlier (*99*). Furthermore, lack of the direct presence of microbial products at the site of inflammation or in the blood has caused infection to be thought unlikely as a direct cause of the disease although it remains possible, as discussed, that variable infections may induce the same clinical phenotype.

INFECTIOUS MECHANISMS IN GRAVES' DISEASE

The mechanisms by which infection may induce an autoimmune response are many (Table 28.2). The molecular mimicry hypothesis proposes that the immune system recognizes homologies between antigens in infectious agents and host tissues. The best evidence so far that infections can induce autoimmune diseases comes from animal models. Mimic peptides recognized as T-cell epitopes, which induce autoimmune disease, highlights the functional aspect of the pathogenic nature of T cells rather than the presence of cross-reactive antibodies. Newly diagnosed GD

Table 28.2
Some Potential Mechanisms by Which Infection May Influence AITD

Molecular mimicry
Polyclonal T-cell activation – the superantigens
Toll-like receptor activation and heat shock proteins
Enhanced thyroid expression of HLA molecules

patients have been shown to be more frequently seropositive for a recent infection of either virus or bacteria, indicating that infections may be associated with the disease (*107*). *Yersinia enterocolitica* has often been claimed to play a role in the pathogenesis of GD (*108, 109*). Antibodies to *Yersinia* isolated from patients with GD inhibited TSH binding (*110*), and animals immunized with *Yersinia* antigens produced antibodies that reacted with the TSHR (*108*). A TSHR cross-reactive lipoprotein from *Yersinia* has been suggested as the target antigen, which has the ability to stimulate B cells and to induce cytokine production, particularly IL-6 and IL-8 (*111, 112*). These effects possibly activate Th17 cells and downmodulate Tregs that can aid in triggering an autoimmune response against the TSHR causing TSHR antibody production and thyroid inflammation. Clearly, *Yersinia* could potentially induce autoimmunity in GD via molecular mimicry. Subsequent amino acid analyses have revealed that *Yersinia* and another bacterium, *Borrelia*, share similar homology that includes binding motifs to HLA-DR molecules and the T-cell receptor (*113*). The problem is that *Yersinia* and *Borrelia* infections do not precipitate Graves' disease, so these appear to be unimportant associations (*109*).

In addition to molecular mimicry, there are several possibilities that may render activation of autoreactive B and T cells (Table 28.2). Tissue damage caused by infection may expose autoreactive T cells to cryptic self-antigen. Local inflammation can enhance expression of MHC and costimulatory molecules on cells of target organ and Graves' ophthalmopathy and dermopathy precipitated by direct injury. Infectious agents may bind to the target self-antigen and then activate autoreactive B cells via the B-cell receptor (BCR) to receive inappropriate T-cell help. Polyclonal T-cell induction by bacterial superantigen may activate autoreactive T cells overcoming anergy or deletion. As discussed above, TLR activation via infectious products is yet another potential mechanism for the induction of autoimmunity.

A NOTE ON THE FEMALE SEX AND SUSCEPTIBILITY TO GRAVES' DISEASE

Although the genetic association of GD with loci on the X chromosome has been reported, such findings have not been consistent (*114, 115*). In contrast, the association with skewed X chromosome inactivation has been very consistent (*116*), although its physiological mechanism is poorly understood and may relate to early development. The strongest link between the female sex and GD is via pregnancy. Here, the data are strong and demonstrate immune suppression of GD during pregnancy with exacerbation or new onset in the postpartum (*117*). The immune changes of pregnancy are beyond the scope of this review, but the onset of postpartum autoimmune thyroid disease in 8–10% of all women is well documented and includes GD (*10, 117*). Nevertheless, these observations prove that pregnancy-induced changes in the control of the immune response can precipitate autoimmune thyroid disease. The role of fetal microchimerism in this precipitation remains uncertain (*118*).

DRUGS PRECIPITATING GRAVES' DISEASE

Iodine

It has long been known that the introduction of iodination in developing countries precipitates hyperthyroidism in some of the populations (*119, 120*). These outbreaks include cases of both Hashimoto's thyroiditis and Graves' disease, as well as other causes. The hypothesis has been that iodination of thyroglobulin increases its immunogenicity, as shown in vitro and in animal models (*121, 122*), which would help explain the thyroiditis, but it is more difficult to explain the Graves' disease. Most likely, it is just a matter of being able to synthesize more thyroid hormone under TSHR-Ab stimulation rather than immune changes. Cases of Graves' disease are often seen precipitated by iodine-containing drugs such amiodarone (*123*) and contrast media (for CT scanning) or other forms of iodine excess (such as seaweed tablets), and these may occur in iodine-sufficient areas.

Anti–viral Therapy

As used, for example, in HIV patients, antiretroviral therapy induces regeneration of the thymus, and the negative selection process may be impaired, causing excessive circulation of autoreactive cells in the periphery, and many cases of Graves' disease have been precipitated by such treatment (*124*). Similarly, interferon-alpha in HCV infection too frequently precipitates thyroiditis or Graves' disease by an unclear mechanism (*125*).

Immunomodulation

The consequences of immunosuppression have been most well documented after hematopoietic stem cell transplantation. The onset of Graves' disease has been widely reported as with other autoimmune diseases most likely secondary to suppression of regulatory cells (71) as discussed earlier. Recently, the role of Rituximab in calming GD and GD ophthalmopathy, by suppressing activated B cell function, has been explored, and early results suggest efficacy (126). Hence, any immunomodulatory therapy which exaggerates B-cell function may precipitate GD.

CONCLUDING REMARKS AND FUTURE DIRECTIONS

Autoimmunity represents a collection of heterogeneous disorders often controlled by complex genetic and environmental factors and stochastic contributions. A common view of GD is that TSHR-Abs promote the disease by enhancing thyroid antigen expression. However, T-cell activation and subsequent thyroid infiltration in GD patients are difficult to explain entirely via a direct autoantibody-induced mechanism. The pathogenesis of GD is more likely the result of a breakdown in the mechanisms controlling tolerance at different levels (central and peripheral) and involving different cellular subsets (mainly B and T cells). The likely scenario for T-cell activation and recruitment of inflammatory cells in the gland may be due to the production of certain cytokines and chemokines released via bystander T cells along with antibody-mediated activation of thyrocytes and/or damaged thyrocytes. The released TSHR from thyrocytes then stimulates T, B, and antigen-presenting (dendritic) cells, further activating cellular subsets to perpetuate the disease process.

There is a need to study innate and adaptive immunity in the context of TSHR autoantigen in GD. This would provide the basis for the description of the roles that different subsets of T and B cells, and their cytokine and autoantibody production, play in disease pathogenesis. A possible framework may emerge that allow immunologists to probe models of how the immune system orchestrates inflammation and how inappropriate immune responses can lead to GD. In addition, our understanding of IL-2 cytokine biology continues to grow as its role in developing both Tregs and B cells in humans becomes clear. Although the Th17 subset and their association with various diseases has attracted unprecedented levels of interest, there are already signs that Th17 cells are not the only cause of all autoimmune pathology and that Th1-like cells still play a role in many diseases. Their role in GD clearly requires clarification. It is also now obvious that the activities of individual cytokines are going to be context specific, varying between target sites, and playing distinct roles in different inflammatory conditions. Hence, detailed studies of B cells, Tregs, Th1, Th2, and Th17 cells in GD will provide potential therapeutic opportunity for active immune regulation and long-term tolerance induction.

REFERENCES

1. Adams DD, Purves HD. Abnormal responses in the assay of thyrotropin. Proc Univ Otago Med Sch 1956;34:11–12.
2. Vanderpump MP, Tunbridge WM, French JM, et al. The incidence of thyroid disorders in the community: a twenty-year follow-up of the Whickham Survey. Clin Endocrinol (Oxf) 1995;43:55–68.
3. McIver B, Morris JC. The pathogenesis of Graves' disease. Endocrinol Metab Clin North Am 1998;27:73–89.
4. Bahn RS, Heufelder AE. Pathogenesis of Graves' ophthalmopathy. N Engl J Med 1993;329:1468–1475.
5. LiVolsi VA. The pathology of autoimmune thyroid disease: a review. Thyroid 1994;4:333–339.
6. Martin A, Goldsmith NK, Friedman EW, Schwartz AE, Davies TF, Roman SH. Intrathyroidal accumulation of T cell phenotypes in autoimmune thyroid disease. Autoimmunity 1990;6:269–281.
7. McKenzie JM, Zakarija M. Fetal and neonatal hyperthyroidism and hypothyroidism due to maternal TSH receptor antibodies. Thyroid 1992;2:155–159.
8. Volpe R. Thyrotropin receptor autoantibodies. In: Peter JB, Shoenfeld Y, eds. Autoantibodies. Amsterdam: Elsevier, 1996:822–829.
9. Rees SB, McLachlan SM, Furmaniak J. Autoantibodies to the thyrotropin receptor. Endocr Rev 1988;9:106–121.
10. Davies TF. Infection and autoimmune thyroid disease. J Clin Endocrinol Metab 2008;93:674–676.
11. Bahn RS, Dutton CM, Natt N, Joba W, Spitzweg C, Heufelder AE. Thyrotropin receptor expression in Graves' orbital adipose/connective tissues: potential autoantigen in Graves' ophthalmopathy. J Clin Endocrinol Metab 1998;83:998–1002.
12. Latif R, Morshed SA, Zaidi M, Davies TF. Impact of TSH and TSH receptor antibodies on multimerization, cleavage, and signaling. Endocrinol Metab Clin North Am 2009;38(2):319–341.
13. Davies TF, Ando T, Lin RY, Tomer Y, Latif R. Thyrotropin receptor-associated diseases: from adenomata to Graves disease. J Clin Invest 2005;115:1972–1983.
14. Misrahi M, Ghinea N, Sar S, et al. Processing of the precursors of the human thyroid-stimulating hormone receptor in various eukaryotic cells (human thyrocytes, transfected L cells and baculovirus-infected insect cells). Eur J Biochem 1994;222:711–719.
15. Chazenbalk GD, Pichurin P, Chen CR, et al. Thyroid-stimulating autoantibodies in Graves disease preferentially recognize the free A subunit, not the thyrotropin holoreceptor. J Clin Invest 2002;110:209–217.
16. Kajita Y, Rickards CR, Buckland PR, Howells RD, Rees SB. Analysis of thyrotropin receptors by photoaffinity labelling. Orientation of receptor subunits in the cell membrane. Biochem J 1985;227:413–420.
17. Loosfelt H, Pichon C, Jolivet A, et al. Two-subunit structure of the human thyrotropin receptor. Proc Natl Acad Sci USA 1992;89:3765–3769.
18. Vlase H, Davies TF. Insights into the molecular mechanisms of the autoimmune thyroid diseases. In: Eisenbarth GS, ed. Endocrine and Organ Specific Autoimmunity. California: R.G. Landes Co., 1999:98–132.
19. Lipsky PE. Systemic lupus erythematosus: an autoimmune disease of B cell hyperactivity. Nat Immunol 2001;2:764–766.
20. Caturegli P, Kimura H, Rocchi R, Rose NR. Autoimmune thyroid disease. Curr Opin Rheumatol 2007;19:44–48.
21. Meffre E, Wardemann H. B-cell tolerance checkpoints in health and autoimmunity. Curr Opin Immunol 2008;20(6):632–638.
22. Ando T, Latif R, Pritsker A, Moran T, Nagayama Y, Davies TF. A monoclonal thyroid-stimulating antibody. J Clin Invest 2002;110:1667–1674.
23. Ando T, Davies TF. Monoclonal antibodies to the thyrotropin receptor. Clin Dev Immunol 2005;12:137–143.
24. Ando T, Latif R, Davies TF. Antibody-induced modulation of TSH receptor post-translational processing. J Endocrinol 2007;195:179–186.
25. Morshed SA, Latif R, Davies TF. Characterization of thyrotropin receptor

25. antibody-induced signaling cascades. Endocrinology 2009;150:519–529.
26. Gilbert JA, Kalled SL, Moorhead J, et al. Treatment of autoimmune hyperthyroidism in a murine model of Graves' disease with tumor necrosis factor-family ligand inhibitors suggests a key role for B cell activating factor in disease pathology. Endocrinology 2006;147:4561–4568.
27. Lai Kwan LQ, King Hung KO, Zheng BJ, Lu L. Local BAFF gene silencing suppresses Th17-cell generation and ameliorates autoimmune arthritis. Proc Natl Acad Sci USA 2008;105:14993–14998.
28. Salvi M, Vannucchi G, Campi I, et al. Efficacy of rituximab treatment for thyroid-associated ophthalmopathy as a result of intraorbital B-cell depletion in one patient unresponsive to steroid immunosuppression. Eur J Endocrinol 2006;154:511–517.
29. Davies TF, Bobovnikova Y, Weiss M, Vlase H, Moran T, Graves PN. Development and characterization of monoclonal antibodies specific for the murine thyrotropin receptor. Thyroid 1998;8:693–701.
30. Sanders J, Jeffreys J, Depraetere H, et al. Characteristics of a human monoclonal autoantibody to the thyrotropin receptor: sequence structure and function. Thyroid 2004;14:560–570.
31. Nagy EV, Burch HB, Mahoney K, Lukes YG, Morris JC, III, Burman KD. Graves' IgG recognizes linear epitopes in the human thyrotropin receptor. Biochem Biophys Res Commun 1992;188:28–33.
32. Sanders J, Allen F, Jeffreys J, et al. Characteristics of a monoclonal antibody to the thyrotropin receptor that acts as a powerful thyroid-stimulating autoantibody antagonist. Thyroid 2005;15:672–682.
33. Sanders J, Chirgadze DY, Sanders P, et al. Crystal structure of the TSH receptor in complex with a thyroid-stimulating autoantibody. Thyroid 2007;17:395–410.
34. Sanders J, Bolton J, Sanders P, et al. Effects of TSH receptor mutations on binding and biological activity of monoclonal antibodies and TSH. Thyroid 2006;16:1195–1206.
35. Minich WB, Lenzner C, Morgenthaler NG. Antibodies to TSH-receptor in thyroid autoimmune disease interact with monoclonal antibodies whose epitopes are broadly distributed on the receptor. Clin Exp Immunol 2004;136:129–136.
36. Sanders J, Jeffreys J, Depraetere H, et al. Thyroid-stimulating monoclonal antibodies. Thyroid 2002;12:1043–1050.
37. Schwarz-Lauer L, Pichurin PN, Chen CR, et al. The cysteine-rich amino terminus of the thyrotropin receptor is the immunodominant linear antibody epitope in mice immunized using naked deoxyribonucleic acid or adenovirus vectors. Endocrinology 2003;144:1718–1725.
38. Ando T, Latif R, Davies TF. Concentration-dependent regulation of thyrotropin receptor function by thyroid-stimulating antibody. J Clin Invest 2004;113:1589–1595.
39. Ando T, Latif R, Daniel S, Eguchi K, Davies TF. Dissecting linear and conformational epitopes on the native thyrotropin receptor. Endocrinology 2004;145:5185–5193.
40. Minich WB, Loos U. Detection of functionally different types of pathological autoantibodies against thyrotropin receptor in Graves' patients sera by luminescent immunoprecipitation analysis. Exp Clin Endocrinol Diabetes 2000;108:110–119.
41. Kakinuma A, Chazenbalk GD, Tanaka K, Nagayama Y, McLachlan SM, Rapoport B. An N-linked glycosylation motif from the noncleaving luteinizing hormone receptor substituted for the homologous region (Gly367 to Glu369) of the thyrotropin receptor prevents cleavage at its second, downstream site. J Biol Chem 1997;272:28296–28300.
42. Costagliola S, Rodien P, Many MC, Ludgate M, Vassart G. Genetic immunization against the human thyrotropin receptor causes thyroiditis and allows production of monoclonal antibodies recognizing the native receptor. J Immunol 1998;160:1458–1465.
43. Nagayama Y, Kita-Furuyama M, Ando T, et al. A novel murine model of Graves' hyperthyroidism with intramuscular injection of adenovirus expressing the thyrotropin receptor. J Immunol 2002;168:2789–2794.
44. Jeffreys J, Depraetere H, Sanders J, et al. Characterization of the thyrotropin binding pocket. Thyroid 2002;12:1051–1061.
45. Chen CR, McLachlan SM, Rapoport B. Suppression of thyrotropin receptor constitutive activity by a monoclonal antibody with inverse agonist activity. Endocrinology 2007;148:2375–2382.
46. Nakamura H, Usa T, Motomura M, et al. Prevalence of interrelated autoantibodies in thyroid diseases and autoimmune disorders. J Endocrinol Invest 2008;31:861–865.
47. Endo T, Kogai T, Nakazato M, Saito T, Kaneshige M, Onaya T. Autoantibody against Na+/I- symporter in the sera of patients with autoimmune thyroid disease. Biochem Biophys Res Commun 1996;224:92–95.

48. Yoshida A, Hisatome I, Taniguchi S, et al. Pendrin is a novel autoantigen recognized by patients with autoimmune thyroid diseases. J Clin Endocrinol Metab 2009;94(2):442–448.
49. Pritchard J, Horst N, Cruikshank W, Smith TJ. Igs from patients with Graves' disease induce the expression of T cell chemoattractants in their fibroblasts. J Immunol 2002;168:942–950.
50. Pritchard J, Han R, Horst N, Cruikshank WW, Smith TJ. Immunoglobulin activation of T cell chemoattractant expression in fibroblasts from patients with Graves' disease is mediated through the insulin-like growth factor I receptor pathway. J Immunol 2003;170:6348–6354.
51. Douglas RS, Naik V, Hwang CJ, et al. B cells from patients with Graves' disease aberrantly express the IGF-1 receptor: implications for disease pathogenesis. J Immunol 2008;181:5768–5774.
52. Davies TF, Martin A, Concepcion ES, Graves P, Cohen L, Ben-Nun A. Evidence of limited variability of antigen receptors on intrathyroidal T cells in autoimmune thyroid disease. N Engl J Med 1991;325:238–244.
53. Davies TF, Martin A, Concepcion ES, et al. Evidence for selective accumulation of intrathyroidal T lymphocytes in human autoimmune thyroid disease based on T cell receptor V gene usage. J Clin Invest 1992;89:157–162.
54. Dayan CM, Londei M, Corcoran AE, et al. Autoantigen recognition by thyroid-infiltrating T cells in Graves disease. Proc Natl Acad Sci USA 1991;88:7415–7419.
55. Jackson RA, Haynes BF, Burch WM, Shimizu K, Bowring MA, Eisenbarth GS. Ia+ T cells in new onset Graves' disease. J Clin Endocrinol Metab 1984;59:187–190.
56. Wall JR, Baur R, Schleusener H, Bandy-Dafoe P. Peripheral blood and intrathyroidal mononuclear cell populations in patients with autoimmune thyroid disorders enumerated using monoclonal antibodies. J Clin Endocrinol Metab 1983;56:164–169.
57. Martin A, Nakashima M, Zhou A, Aronson D, Werner AJ, Davies TF. Detection of major T cell epitopes on human thyroid stimulating hormone receptor by overriding immune heterogeneity in patients with Graves' disease. J Clin Endocrinol Metab 1997;82:3361–3366.
58. Martin A, Barbesino G, Davies TF. T-cell receptors and autoimmune thyroid disease – signposts for T-cell-antigen driven diseases. Int Rev Immunol 1999;18:111–140.
59. Ziegler SF. FOXP3: of mice and men. Annu Rev Immunol 2006;24:209–226.
60. Sakaguchi S. Naturally arising Foxp3-expressing CD25+CD4+ regulatory T cells in immunological tolerance to self and non-self. Nat Immunol 2005;6:345–352.
61. McLachlan SM, Nagayama Y, Pichurin PN, et al. The link between Graves' disease and Hashimoto's thyroiditis: a role for regulatory T cells. Endocrinology 2007;148:5724–5733.
62. Saitoh O, Nagayama Y. Regulation of Graves' hyperthyroidism with naturally occurring CD4+CD25+ regulatory T cells in a mouse model. Endocrinology 2006;147:2417–2422.
63. Saitoh O, Abiru N, Nakahara M, Nagayama Y. CD8+CD122+ T cells, a newly identified regulatory T subset, negatively regulate Graves' hyperthyroidism in a murine model. Endocrinology 2007;148:6040–6046.
64. Marazuela M, Garcia-Lopez MA, Figueroa-Vega N, et al. Regulatory T cells in human autoimmune thyroid disease. J Clin Endocrinol Metab 2006;91:3639–3646.
65. Owen CJ, Eden JA, Jennings CE, Wilson V, Cheetham TD, Pearce SH. Genetic association studies of the FOXP3 gene in Graves' disease and autoimmune Addison's disease in the United Kingdom population. J Mol Endocrinol 2006;37:97–104.
66. Bettelli E, Carrier Y, Gao W, et al. Reciprocal developmental pathways for the generation of pathogenic effector TH17 and regulatory T cells. Nature 2006;441:235–238.
67. Fossiez F, Djossou O, Chomarat P, et al. T cell interleukin-17 induces stromal cells to produce proinflammatory and hematopoietic cytokines. J Exp Med 1996;183:2593–2603.
68. Lubberts E, Joosten LA, van de Loo FA, Schwarzenberger P, Kolls J, Van Den Berg WB. Overexpression of IL-17 in the knee joint of collagen type II immunized mice promotes collagen arthritis and aggravates joint destruction. Inflamm Res 2002;51:102–104.
69. Afzali B, Lombardi G, Lechler RI, Lord GM. The role of T helper 17 (Th17) and regulatory T cells (Treg) in human organ transplantation and autoimmune disease. Clin Exp Immunol 2007;148:32–46.
70. Bohgaki T, Atsumi T, Koike T. Multiple autoimmune diseases after autologous stem-cell transplantation. N Engl J Med 2007;357:2734–2736.
71. Bohgaki T, Atsumi T, Koike T. Autoimmune disease after autologous hematopoietic stem

72. Baker JR, Jr. The nature of apoptosis in the thyroid and the role it may play in autoimmune thyroid disease. Thyroid 2001;11: 245–247.
73. Giordano C, Richiusa P, Bagnasco M, et al. Differential regulation of Fas-mediated apoptosis in both thyrocyte and lymphocyte cellular compartments correlates with opposite phenotypic manifestations of autoimmune thyroid disease. Thyroid 2001;11:233–244.
74. Stassi G, De MR. Autoimmune thyroid disease: new models of cell death in autoimmunity. Nat Rev Immunol 2002;2:195–204.
75. Hamilton F, Black M, Farquharson MA, Stewart C, Foulis AK. Spatial correlation between thyroid epithelial cells expressing class II MHC molecules and interferon-gamma-containing lymphocytes in human thyroid autoimmune disease. Clin Exp Immunol 1991;83:64–68.
76. Blanchard N, Shastri N. Coping with loss of perfection in the MHC class I peptide repertoire. Curr Opin Immunol 2008;20:82–88.
77. Sawai Y, DeGroot LJ. Binding of human thyrotropin receptor peptides to a Graves' disease-predisposing human leukocyte antigen class II molecule. J Clin Endocrinol Metab 2000;85:1176–1179.
78. Mackenzie WA, Davies TF. An intrathyroidal T-cell clone specifically cytotoxic for human thyroid cells. Immunology 1987;61:101–103.
79. Lira SA, Martin AP, Marinkovic T, Furtado GC. Mechanisms regulating lymphocytic infiltration of the thyroid in murine models of thyroiditis. Crit Rev Immunol 2005;25:251–262.
80. Martin AP, Coronel EC, Sano G, et al. A novel model for lymphocytic infiltration of the thyroid gland generated by transgenic expression of the CC chemokine CCL21. J Immunol 2004;173:4791–4798.
81. Kita-Furuyama M, Nagayama Y, Pichurin P, McLachlan SM, Rapoport B, Eguchi K. Dendritic cells infected with adenovirus expressing the thyrotrophin receptor induce Graves' hyperthyroidism in BALB/c mice. Clin Exp Immunol 2003;131:234–240.
82. Kabel PJ, Voorbij HA, De HM, van der Gaag RD, Drexhage HA. Intrathyroidal dendritic cells. J Clin Endocrinol Metab 1988;66: 199–207.
83. Quadbeck B, Eckstein AK, Tews S, et al. Maturation of thyroidal dendritic cells in Graves' disease. Scand J Immunol 2002;55: 612–620.
84. Brigl M, Brenner MB. CD1: antigen presentation and T cell function. Annu Rev Immunol 2004;22:817–890.
85. Roura-Mir C, Catalfamo M, Cheng TY, et al. CD1a and CD1c activate intrathyroidal T cells during Graves' disease and Hashimoto's thyroiditis. J Immunol 2005;174: 3773–3780.
86. Moody DB. TLR gateways to CD1 function. Nat Immunol 2006;7:811–817.
87. Hutchings P, Rayner DC, Champion BR, et al. High efficiency antigen presentation by thyroglobulin-primed murine splenic B cells. Eur J Immunol 1987;17:393–398.
88. Brix TH, Christensen K, Holm NV, Harvald B, Hegedus L. A population-based study of Graves' disease in Danish twins. Clin Endocrinol (Oxf) 1998;48:397–400.
89. Redondo MJ, Jeffrey J, Fain PR, Eisenbarth GS, Orban T. Concordance for islet autoimmunity among monozygotic twins. N Engl J Med 2008;359:2849–2850.
90. Tomer Y, Menconi F, Davies TF, et al. Dissecting genetic heterogeneity in autoimmune thyroid diseases by subset analysis. J Autoimmun 2007;29:69–77.
91. Hansen PS, Brix TH, Iachine I, Sorensen TI, Kyvik KO, Hegedus L. Genetic and environmental interrelations between measurements of thyroid function in a healthy Danish twin population. Am J Physiol Endocrinol Metab 2007;292:E765–E770.
92. Prummel MF, Strieder T, Wiersinga WM. The environment and autoimmune thyroid diseases. Eur J Endocrinol 2004;150: 605–618.
93. Pacini F, Vorontsova T, Molinaro E, et al. Prevalence of thyroid autoantibodies in children and adolescents from Belarus exposed to the Chernobyl radioactive fallout. Lancet 1998;352:763–766.
94. DeGroot LJ. Radioiodine and the immune system. Thyroid 1997;7:259–264.
95. Braverman LE. The physiology and pathophysiology of iodine and the thyroid. Thyroid 2001;11:405.
96. Stanbury JB, Ermans AE, Bourdoux P, et al. Iodine-induced hyperthyroidism: occurrence and epidemiology. Thyroid 1998;8:83–100.
97. Bartalena L, Martino E, Marcocci C, et al. More on smoking habits and Graves' ophthalmopathy. J Endocrinol Invest 1989;12:733–737.
98. Chiovato L, Pinchera A. Stressful life events and Graves' disease. Eur J Endocrinol 1996;134:680–682.

99. Bach JF. The protective effect of infections on immune disorders. J Pediatr Gastroenterol Nutr 2005;40 Suppl 1:S8.
100. Kondrashova A, Reunanen A, Romanov A, et al. A six-fold gradient in the incidence of type 1 diabetes at the eastern border of Finland. Ann Med 2005;37:67–72.
101. Nagayama Y, McLachlan SM, Rapoport B, Oishi K. Graves' hyperthyroidism and the hygiene hypothesis in a mouse model. Endocrinology 2004;145:5075–5079.
102. Salaun B, Romero P, Lebecque S. Toll-like receptors' two-edged sword: when immunity meets apoptosis. Eur J Immunol 2007;37: 3311–3318.
103. Penhale WJ, Young PR. The influence of the normal microbial flora on the susceptibility of rats to experimental autoimmune thyroiditis. Clin Exp Immunol 1988;72:288–292.
104. Matsuda T, Tomita M, Uchihara JN, et al. Human T cell leukemia virus type I-infected patients with Hashimoto's thyroiditis and Graves' disease. J Clin Endocrinol Metab 2005;90:5704–5710.
105. Akeno N, Blackard JT, Tomer Y. HCV E2 protein binds directly to thyroid cells and induces IL-8 production: a new mechanism for HCV induced thyroid autoimmunity. J Autoimmun 2008;31(4):339–344.
106. Tozzoli R, Barzilai O, Ram M, et al. Infections and autoimmune thyroid diseases: parallel detection of antibodies against pathogens with proteomic technology. Autoimmun Rev 2008;8:112–115.
107. Valtonen VV, Ruutu P, Varis K, Ranki M, Malkamaki M, Makela PH. Serological evidence for the role of bacterial infections in the pathogenesis of thyroid diseases. Acta Med Scand 1986;219:105–111.
108. Luo G, Fan JL, Seetharamaiah GS, et al. Immunization of mice with Yersinia enterocolitica leads to the induction of antithyrotropin receptor antibodies. J Immunol 1993;151:922–928.
109. Tomer Y, Davies TF. Infection, thyroid disease, and autoimmunity. Endocr Rev 1993;14:107–120.
110. Heyma P, Harrison LC, Robins-Browne R. Thyrotrophin (TSH) binding sites on Yersinia enterocolitica recognized by immunoglobulins from humans with Graves' disease. Clin Exp Immunol 1986;64:249–254.
111. Gangi E, Kapatral V, El-Azami El-Idrissi M, Martinez O, Prabhakar BS. Characterization of a recombinant Yersinia enterocolitica lipoprotein; implications for its role in autoimmune response against thyrotropin receptor. Autoimmunity 2004;37:515–520.
112. Zhang H, Kaur I, Niesel DW, et al. Lipoprotein from Yersinia enterocolitica contains epitopes that cross-react with the human thyrotropin receptor. J Immunol 1997;158: 1976–1983.
113. Benvenga S, Santarpia L, Trimarchi F, Guarneri F. Human thyroid autoantigens and proteins of Yersinia and Borrelia share amino acid sequence homology that includes binding motifs to HLA-DR molecules and T-cell receptor. Thyroid 2006;16:225–236.
114. Barbesino G, Tomer Y, Concepcion ES, Davies TF, Greenberg DA. Linkage analysis of candidate genes in autoimmune thyroid disease. II. Selected gender-related genes and the X-chromosome. International Consortium for the Genetics of Autoimmune Thyroid Disease. J Clin Endocrinol Metab 1998;83:3290–3295.
115. Barbesino G, Tomer Y, Concepcion E, Davies TF, Greenberg DA. Linkage analysis of candidate genes in autoimmune thyroid disease: 1. Selected immunoregulatory genes. International Consortium for the Genetics of Autoimmune Thyroid Disease. J Clin Endocrinol Metab 1998;83:1580–1584.
116. Brix TH, Knudsen GP, Kristiansen M, Kyvik KO, Orstavik KH, Hegedus L. High frequency of skewed X-chromosome inactivation in females with autoimmune thyroid disease: a possible explanation for the female predisposition to thyroid autoimmunity. J Clin Endocrinol Metab 2005;90: 5949–5953.
117. Benhaim RD, Davies TF. Increased risk of Graves' disease after pregnancy. Thyroid 2005;15:1287–1290.
118. Ando T, Imaizumi M, Graves PN, Unger P, Davies TF. Intrathyroidal fetal microchimerism in Graves' disease. J Clin Endocrinol Metab 2002;87:3315–3320.
119. Bülow Pedersen I, Laurberg P, Knudsen N, et al. Increase in incidence of hyperthyroidism predominantly occurs in young people after iodine fortification of salt in Denmark. J Clin Endocrinol Metab 2006;91: 3830–3834.
120. Laurberg P, Pedersen KM, Hreidarsson A, Sigfusson N, Iversen E, Knudsen PR. Iodine intake and the pattern of thyroid disorders: a comparative epidemiological study of thyroid abnormalities in the elderly in Iceland and in Jutland, Denmark. J Clin Endocrinol Metab 1998;83:765–769.
121. Li HS, Jiang HY, Carayanniotis G. Modifying effects of iodine on the immunogenicity of thyroglobulin peptides. J Autoimmun 2007;28:171–176.

122. Ruwhof C, Drexhage HA. Iodine and thyroid autoimmune disease in animal models. Thyroid 2001;11:427–436.
123. O'Sullivan AJ, Lewis M, Diamond T. Amiodarone-induced thyrotoxicosis: left ventricular dysfunction is associated with increased mortality. Eur J Endocrinol 2006;154:533–536.
124. Knysz B, Bolanowski M, Klimczak M, Gladysz A, Zwolinska K. Graves' disease as an immune reconstitution syndrome in an HIV-1-positive patient commencing effective antiretroviral therapy: case report and literature review. Viral Immunol 2006;19:102–107.
125. Prummel MF, Laurberg P. Interferon-alpha and autoimmune thyroid disease. Thyroid 2003;13:547–551.
126. El Fassi D, Banga JP, Gilbert JA, Padoa C, Hegedus L, Nielsen CH. Treatment of Graves' disease with rituximab specifically reduces the production of thyroid stimulating autoantibodies. Clin Immunol 2008;130(3):252–258.

Chapter 29

Graves' Ophthalmopathy

Wilmar M. Wiersinga

Summary

Graves' orbitopathy (GO) is one of the extrathyroidal manifestations of Graves' disease. The incidence of GO apparently is declining in the last few decades, likely as a result of a decreased prevalence of smoking and earlier diagnosis and treatment of hyperthyroidism. Clinical presentation is typically that of a bilateral symmetric eye disease, but why GO is unilateral or occurs in the absence of hyperthyroidism in some patients is not understood. Considerable progress has been made in unraveling the immunopathogenesis of GO. Orbital fibroblasts have been identified as the prime target cells of the autoimmune attack as they are recognized by T lymphocytes, express TSH receptors, and may undergo differentiation into adipocytes. Infiltrating T-cells rather than TSH receptor autoantibodies are likely involved in initiating orbital autoimmunity, via release of cytokines and activation of fibroblasts. Some Graves' IgG stimulate the IGF-1 receptor on orbital fibroblasts, which raises intriguing questions.

The management of GO is based on three lines of intervention: (a) to stop smoking, (b) to restore euthyroidism, and (c) to restore visual functions and appearance. In mild GO, a wait-and-see policy is recommended. In moderate-to-severe GO, intravenous pulses of methylprednisolone is the preferred treatment if the disease is active; if it is inactive, rehabilitative surgery can be done. Dysthyroid optic neuropathy requires urgent medical or surgical treatment.

Key Words: Graves' ophthalmopathy, Immunopathogenesis, Thyroid autoimmunity, TSH receptor, cytokines, Diagnosis, Hyperthyroidism, Treatment, Immunosuppression, Orbital irradiation

INTRODUCTION

Graves' ophthalmopathy (GO), also known as Graves' orbitopathy, thyroid-associated ophthalmopathy, or thyroid eye disease, is one of the extrathyroidal manifestations of Graves' disease. A basic feature of GO is swelling of extraocular muscles and orbital fat. The increased volume of muscles and fat contained within the bony surroundings of the orbital cavity gives rise to an increase of retrobulbar pressure (1). Consequently, venous drainage is impaired, and orbital fat herniates through the orbital septum (causing swelling and redness of eyelids, conjunctiva and caruncle), and the globe is pushed forwards (causing exophthalmos and overexposure of the cornea with the risk of keratitis). Impaired relaxation of the enlarged extraocular muscles causes restricted eye-muscle motility and double vision. If the development of exophthalmos (sometimes aptly referred to as nature's own decompression) is insufficient to relieve the high intraorbital pressure, optic neuropathy may develop due to direct compression of the optic nerve. The disease frequently results in marked changes of appearance (which are cosmetically disfiguring) and loss of visual functions (which can be invalidating) (Fig. 29.1). Thus, it comes as no surprise that quality of life (QoL) is markedly decreased in GO patients. GO patients score low on general health-related QoL questionnaires, even lower than patients with diabetes, emphysema, or heart failure (*2*).

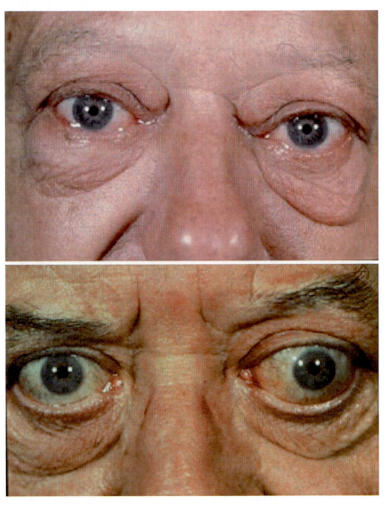

Fig. 29.1 Appearance of a patient with active (*top panel*) and inactive (*bottom panel*) Graves' orbitopathy.

Whereas eye signs and symptoms in GO are understood reasonably well from a mechanistic point of view, the immunopathogenesis of GO remains one of the unresolved enigmas of autoimmune thyroid disease. Management of GO patients can be difficult: it requires fine-tuning between thyroid-specific and eye-specific treatment modalities, and outcomes are often unsatisfactory. This review focuses both on issues that have been resolved in the last decade and unresolved issues, which unfortunately are still too many.

EPIDEMIOLOGY

A population-based cohort study in Olmsted County, Minnesota, reports an overall age-adjusted incidence rate of GO of 16.0 women and 2.9 men per 100,000 inhabitants per year, with peaks in the fifth and seventh decade of life (3). Minor eye changes not requiring specific treatment other than supportive measures occur in 74% of the cases. Smoking greatly increases the risk for GO (odds ratio 7.7, 95% CI 4.3–13.7), and smokers have more severe eye disease than nonsmokers (4). There seems to be a secular trend towards a lower incidence rate of GO. In a large U.K. clinic, the proportion of GO patients among all referred patients with Graves' hyperthyroidism declined from 57% in 1960 to 35% in 1990; there was also a decline in the prevalence of severe GO (diplopia or optic neuropathy) from 30 to 21% (5). Likewise, a European questionnaire study in 1998 indicated that 43% of respondents thought GO was decreasing in frequency, 42% thought it unchanged, and 12% thought it to be increasing (6). Interestingly, respondents reporting increased incidence of GO originated mostly from countries in which the proportion of smokers in the general population had increased since 1990. Apart from changes in smoking behavior, an alternative explanation for the declining incidence of GO could be the introduction of sensitive TSH assays in the late 1980s, allowing earlier diagnosis and treatment of Graves' hyperthyroidism (7). Passive smoking may be a risk factor for GO as well but has hardly been studied. In a recent European questionnaire study on childhood GO, about 20% of all GO cases were <10 years old and 80% were 11–18 years in countries with a smoking prevalence of <25% among teenagers; in countries with a smoking prevalence of >25% among teenagers, the distribution among the two age groups was about 50 and 50%, respectively, suggesting an effect of passive smoking because children younger than 10 years are unlikely to be smokers themselves (8). A further decline in the incidence of GO can be expected with the recent ban on smoking in public spaces in many countries, but data substantiating this view are lacking.

Age, gender, and ethnicity all affect the expression of GO for reasons incompletely understood (9). GO in children and adolescents is usually mild, whereas old age is associated with more severe GO. GO-like Graves' hyperthyroidism is more common in women than in men. However, the female to male ratio in GO decreases from 9.3 in mild GO to 3.2 in moderate GO and 1.4 in severe GO, indicating more severe GO in males. One may hypothesize that differences in characteristics of connective tissue (like the strength of the orbital septum) are involved. Asians due to shallower orbits have more frequently exophthalmos. The average age of GO patients is 49 years; 14% have other eye diseases (like cataract, glaucoma), and 9% have diabetes mellitus (10).

CLINICAL PRESENTATION

GO typically presents as a bilateral symmetric eye disease in a patient with Graves' hyperthyroidism, complaining from photophobia, swollen or red eyes, lacrimation, grittiness, protruding eyes, double vision, or loss of visual acuity and disturbed color vision. Eye changes can be classified according to the NO SPECS system (Table 29.1), which serves as a nice mnemonic in assessing the severity of GO. The relative frequency of the various eye signs varies, being highest for soft-tissue involvement (swelling and/or

Table 29.1
Assessment of GO Severity Using NO SPECS Classes as a mnemonic

	Class description	Assessment	Frequency[a]
0	No signs or symptoms		
1	Only signs, no symptoms	Lid retraction in mm	59%
2	Soft tissue involvement	Swelling and redness of eyelids and conjunctiva[b]	75%
3	Proptosis	Exophthalmos in mm[c]	63%
4	Extraocular muscle involvement	Restricted eye-muscle motility[d] Diplopia[e]	49%
5	Corneal involvement	Keratitis, corneal ulcer	16%
6	Sight loss due to optic nerve involvement	Decreased visual activity, disturbed color vision, visual field defects	21%

[a] Relative frequency in 152 newly referred patients with GO (ref. (10))
[b] A very useful detailed protocol with comparative photographs for objective assessment has been published (ref. (11))
[c] Upper normal limit is 18 mm in Asians, 20 mm in Caucasians, and 22 mm in Blacks
[d] Impairment of elevation in 49%, of abduction in 32%, and of depression in 17%
[e] Intermittent diplopia (i.e., at awakening or when tired) in 15%, inconstant diplopia (i.e., only at extremes of gaze) in 20%, constant diplopia (i.e., in primary gaze or reading position) in 14%

redness of conjunctiva and eyelids) and lowest for optic-nerve involvement (20). Most patients (40%) have mild ophthalmopathy, whereas 33% have moderate and 28% severe eye disease. Assessment of GO activity is helpful in decision making on immunosuppressive treatment. In the early active inflammatory stages of GO, immunosuppression will likely have a beneficial effect, whereas immunosuppression applied in the late inactive fibrotic stage of the disease in all likelihood will have no or only a small effect. Activity of GO is easily and rapidly assessed by the clinical activity score (CAS) (Table 29.2). Despite its subjective nature, the CAS has proven its clinical usefulness in day-to-day practice (11–13). More sophisticated methods have been developed to assess GO activity. A decreased internal reflectivity on A-mode ultrasonography of eye muscles (14), a prolonged T2-relaxation time in orbital tissues on MRI (15), and a high orbital uptake on octreoscan (16) have all been associated with a high CAS and a higher likelihood of a good response to immunosuppression. However, these techniques are demanding and require ample expertise; they are operative in a few referral centers.

The diagnosis of GO is usually straightforward, but unusual presentations do occur. Unilateral GO occurs in about 5% of all GO patients (10). Indeed, Graves' disease is the most common cause (20–30%) of unilateral exophthalmos. Patients with unilateral GO as compared to patients with bilateral GO tend to be older (54 vs. 44 years) and more often euthyroid (29% vs. 2%) (17). A large number of unilateral GO patients develop bilateral eye disease after an unpredictable time interval. Unilateral GO probably represents an early stage of GO, but the reason why the disease initially is restricted to one eye remains elusive. One may suspect involvement of local anatomical factors, but a plausible hypothesis has so far not even been formulated. It is clear that all patients with unilateral eye disease suspected to be GO should undergo orbital imaging to exclude an alternative diagnosis.

Table 29.2
Assessment of GO Activity Using the CAS (Clinical Activity Score)[a]

Inflammatory sign	Assessment	Score if present
Pain	Spontaneous retrobulbar pain	1
	Pain on attempted up, side or down gaze	1
Redness	Redness of eyelids	1
	Redness of conjunctiva	1
Swelling	Swelling of eyelids	1
	Swelling of caruncle and/or plica	1
	Chemosis	1

[a]The CAS is the sum of all items present with a maximum value of 7; a CAS of 3 or higher indicates active GO

Orbital imaging by CT-scan or MRI should also be performed if dysthyroid optic neuropathy (DON) is suspected. Effacement of the fat surrounding the optic nerve at the apex of the orbit by encroachment of severe muscle swelling (called apical crowding) is a clear risk factor for DON. DON may develop rapidly in days or weeks, but may have also an insidious onset. Delayed diagnosis of DON might be related to the fact that not all DON patients have decreased visual acuity or disturbed color vision (Table 29.3) (18). In this respect, the physician should be alert if the patient complains about blurred vision. Blurred vision that disappears after blinking is due to a disrupted tear film. Blurred vision that disappears after covering one eye is due to double vision. Blurred vision that does not disappear after these two maneuvers should raise suspicion for DON, and further examination is urgently required.

Orbital imaging shows enlarged extraocular muscles in the vast majority of GO patients, but a sizable subset of about 10–15% of all GO patients have only enlargement of the fat/connective tissue compartment (19). The reasons behind differential involvement of muscle and fat compartments are essentially unknown; maybe, smoking is involved. Equally unresolved is the question why the various extraocular muscles in GO are not affected to the same extent. Inferior rectus muscles are most frequently enlarged (in about 60%, indeed elevation is most often impaired), followed by the medial rectus muscle (~50%) and the superior rectus muscle

Table 29.3
Frequency of Abnormal Findings in 47 Patients Considered to Have Features Suspicious of Dysthyroid Optic Neuropathy (DON)[a]

	Eyes with definite DON (%)	Eyes with equivocal DON (%)	Eyes with no DON (%)
Visual acuity 0.67 or lower	80	59	32
Reduced color vision	77	56	7
Visual field defects	71	71	13
Apical crowding	95	64	43
Optic nerve stretch	33	0	43
Optic disc swelling	56	18	5
Optic disc pallor	4	12	0
Abnormal VEP latency	73	86	0
Abnormal VEP amplitude	55	57	0

VEP visual evoked potential
[a]Derived from ref. (18)

(~40%) and the lateral rectus muscle (~22%) (9). Macrophages are very abundant in all rectus muscles but relatively less in the lateral rectus (20), probably related to the greater distance between the lateral rectus and the paranasal sinuses. In view of the capacity of macrophages to act as antigen-presenting cells, it can be hypothesized that the lower density of macrophages in the lateral rectus muscle is related to the less frequent enlargement of this muscle.

Schematically, the diagnosis of GO is based on three pillars:

1. Assessment of eye changes in terms of severity (NO SPECS) and activity (CAS)
   (a) It should be remembered that none of the eye changes is really specific for the diagnosis of GO. Even bilateral symmetric eye changes can be caused by another disease, like arteriovenous fistula or Wegener's granulomatosis.
2. Evidence of coexisting thyroid autoimmunity
   (a) The setting of eye changes in a patient with Graves' hyperthyroidism is of course an important clue. In euthyroid patients, the finding of TSH receptor antibodies increases very much the likelihood that the eye changes are due to GO.
3. Orbital imaging to exclude an alternative diagnosis
   (a) CT scanning or MRI of the orbit is not routinely required to make a diagnosis of GO but is indicated in unilateral eye changes in euthyroid patients and suspected optic neuropathy. Imaging may reveal local tumors (especially meningioma, non-Hodgkin lymphoma, or metastases), orbital myositis (in which the muscle tendons are thickened as well, in contrast to GO where the swelling is typically most prominent at the muscle belly sparing the tendons), and a specific inflammatory orbital disease (formerly called pseudotumor orbitae, with ill-defined space-occupying lesions).

RELATIONSHIP WITH THYROID DISEASE

Several studies have indicated a close temporal relationship between the development of Graves' hyperthyroidism and Graves' orbitopathy: a simultaneous onset is observed in 40% of all GO patients; in 40%, the onset of GO is after that of Graves' hyperthyroidism, and in 20%, the eye disease precedes the onset of Graves' hyperthyroidism (9). Why this is so remains elusive. Although the vast majority of GO patients present themselves with a past or present history of Graves' hyperthyroidism, a minority of GO patients are hypothyroid (3%) or euthyroid (5–10%) upon presentation (*10*). In the hypothyroid GO cases, it is not unusual to observe a progressive decrease in the required l-thyroxine replacement dose, with eventual development of overt thyrotoxicosis. This course of events has been explained by a switch from TSH receptor-blocking to TSH receptor-stimulating antibodies. In the euthyroid GO cases, TSH receptor-stimulating antibodies can be found in nearly all patients using sensitive assays (*21*). Euthyroid GO is relatively often unilateral; about 25% of these patients will progress to hyperthyroidism with time, but it is not understood why most remain euthyroid.

One may conclude that in most, if not all, GO patients, evidence can be found for coexisting thyroid autoimmunity, specifically by the presence of TSH receptor antibodies in serum (assayed as TBII, TSH-binding inhibitory immunoglobulins). Conversely, it has also been found that subclinical orbital involvement exists in Graves' hyperthyroid patients without the clinical phenotype of GO (as evident from slightly enlarged muscles on CT scan or ultrasonography). Why not all Graves' hyperthyroid patients develop overt GO is only partly understood: particular polymorphisms in thyroid-specific and immunoregulatory genes and especially smoking may increase the risk of GO.

GO patients have generally much higher serum TBII concentrations than Graves' hyperthyroid patients without GO (*22*). Serum TBII is directly associated with the activity of GO as measured by the CAS, and also, but less strongly, with the severity of GO as measured by proptosis (*23, 24*). Serum TBII rises substantially for a long period of time after 131I therapy of Graves' hyperthyroidism (*25*), a treatment modality associated with a risk of worsening or developing GO (*26, 27*). Lastly, the degree of TBII elevation has prognostic value for the subsequent course of GO: the higher the TBII, the worse the course of GO (*28*). These findings provide circumstantial evidence that autoimmunity against the TSH receptor is of prime importance in the pathogenesis of GO, a view strengthened by the detection of TSH receptors on orbital fibroblasts (vide infra). However, one should keep in mind the possibility that the observed relationships between TBII and GO simply indicate that the severity of the autoimmune attack in GO patients is greater (as reflected by higher TBII levels) than in Graves' patients without GO: the associations may not necessarily indicate a causal relationship.

IMMUNOPATHO-GENESIS

The characteristic swelling of extraocular muscles and orbital fat/connective tissue is due to inflammatory edema and accumulation of glycosaminoglycans (GAGs). GAGs are large hydrophilic compounds, which osmotically attract and bind large amounts of water. Orbital GAG contents in GO (predominantly chondroitin sulfate and hyaluronic acid) are about 70% higher than in controls (*29*) and contribute greatly to volume expansion. GAGs are synthesized and secreted by orbital fibroblasts (OF), which renders these cells likely targets of the autoimmune attack. Evidence supporting OF as the prime target cells is provided by several studies. First, retrobulbar CD8+ T-cells from GO patients recognize autologous OF (but not eye-muscle extracts) in a MHC-class I-restricted manner (*30*). Secondly, retrobulbar T cells from GO patients proliferate in response to autologous proteins from OF (but not from orbital myoblasts) (*31*). Thirdly, OF proliferate in response to autologous T cells dependent on MHC class II and CD40–CD40L signaling (*32*). And, fourthly, HLA-DR expression is observed on interstitial cells including OF, but not on eye muscle fibers (*33*). Consequently, most experts in the field agree that the autoimmune reaction in GO is directed primarily against OF, and not against eye muscle cells (*34*). This view is in line with histopathological findings showing intact muscle fibers widely separated by edema; only in late stages of the disease, the extraocular muscles may become fibrotic. Autoimmunity against eye-muscle antigens (e.g., the occurrence of calsequestrin antibodies) is likely the secondary response to tissue destruction and release of sequestered proteins (*35*).

The next obvious question is about the nature of the autoantigen on OF. It could well be the TSH receptor (TSH-R). Indeed, the detection of a full-length functional TSH-R on OF was met with great enthusiasm as it provided a pathogenetic link between thyroid and orbital autoimmunity (*34, 36, 37*). Expression of the TSH-R is higher in the active than in the inactive stages of GO (*38*). Most interesting, it was found that a subset of OF (called preadipocytes and characterized by the absence of the surface marker Thy-1) may differentiate into mature adipocytes associated with upregulation of TSH-R expression (*39, 40*). This process of adipogenesis will increase volume expansion in the orbit. However, recent studies have identified the IGF-1 receptor (IGF-1-R) as another autoantigen involved in GO, as Graves' IgG recognize and activate the IGF-1-R on OF, inducing synthesis of hyaluronan; these effects can be abolished by steroids and IGF-1-R monoclonal antibodies, and are not observed in dermal fibroblasts or orbital fibroblasts from patients without GO (*41*). Although the IGF-1-R studies need to be confirmed by other groups, it raises many intriguing questions. It remains to be seen what the relative contributions are of Graves' IgG acting either via TSH-R or via IGF-1-R in the induction of GAGs. The latest study by the group of Terry Smith (*42*) reports in situ association of the TSH-R and the IGF-1-R in OF, together comprising a functional complex, suggesting that IGF-1-R may mediate some TSH-provoked signaling.

Activation of OF may occur upon binding of Graves' IgG, but this is unlikely the initiating event of GO. The earliest stages of GO more likely involves infiltration of the orbit by T cells. The lymphocytic infiltrate in orbital tissues of early GO is predominantly composed of helper/inducer and suppressor cytotoxic T cells and macrophages, with relatively few B cells (*33, 43, 44, 45, 46*). Many of these immunocompetent cells are activated memory cells (CD45RO), frequently found adjacent to blood vessels; these cells have been activated by previous exposure to (thyroid) antigen and migrate to sites of inflammation. Another argument against a major initial role of Graves' IgG is that the cytokine profile in orbital tissues of early GO which is largely derived from T helper-1 subset (indicating cell-mediated immunity), whereas cytokines in late stages of GO are predominantly Th2-derived (indicating humoral immunity) (*47*). Infiltrating T cells activate OF, mediated through costimulatory molecules, adhesion molecules, and cytokines including IFNγ, IL-1β, and TNFα (*48*). OF respond to immune stimulation by proliferating and synthesizing cytokines and lipid mediators, thereby aggravating inflammation, and by differentiation into adipocytes (derived from Thy-1 negative OF under PPARγ activation) or myofibroblasts (or scar-forming cells derived from Thy-1 positive OF triggered by TGFβ). Graves' IgG induce OF to secrete IL-16 and RANTES, very potent chemoattractants that initiate T cell migration (*49*). OF can also function as antigen-presenting cells, thereby further activating lymphocytes. Thus, OF play a central role in the immunopathogenesis of GO.

Major effector molecules in the orbital immune response are the numerous immunoregulatory agents (like adhesion molecules, chemokines, cytokines), which can be synthesized and secreted by both infiltrating immunocompetent cells and orbital fibroblasts. Cytokine mRNA profiles have been established in orbital fat/connective tissue of GO patients (*38*): expression of IL-1β, IL-2, IL-6, IL-8, and IL-10 was higher in active than in inactive GO, whereas no difference in expression between both stages was found for IL-3, IL-4, IL-5, IL-12, IL-13, IL-18, IFNγ, TNFα, and IL-1RA. It is difficult to disentangle the origin of these cytokines (whether derived from immune cells or fibroblasts) or the precise functional role of each cytokine. Studies with cultured OF have shown the capacity of various cytokines – at least in vitro – to stimulate cell proliferation, GAG synthesis, prostaglandin E2, adipogenesis, and expression of class II molecules, adhesion molecules, and CD40 (*50*); IL-1 apparently is able to induce most of these effects.

Cultured OF secrete CXCL10 in response to IFNγ and TNFα, effects attenuated by PPARγ agonists (*51*). CXCR3, the receptor for CXCL10, is highly expressed on lymphocytes and endothelial cells, providing another mechanism for homing of lymphocytes to the orbit. Indeed, high serum CXCL10 concentrations are observed especially in the active stage of GO. Recent findings also indicate activation of OF by interaction between IFN-γ induced expression of CD40 receptor on its surface with the ligand CD 154 on T cells, resulting in increased synthesis of IL-6, IL-8, Cox-2, PGE2, and hyaluronan (52). Further elucidation of the intricate cytokine network in GO is warranted, as it may give clues for potential therapeutic targets (53).

Considerable progress has been made in understanding better the immunopathogenesis of GO, but it is also immediately clear that many issues remain unresolved. Bahn (54) has aptly described the cycle of disease in GO: it starts with accumulation of immune cells in the orbit resulting in cytokine release and upregulation of TSH-R expression, subsequently leading to a cellular response of orbital fibroblasts resulting in GAG production, adipogenesis, and enhanced inflammation (PGE2 production); this will increase local trauma and orbital pressure, thereby aggravating the mechanical problem and the immune response by which the cycle is closed (Fig. 29.2).

Further progress has been made in the identification of genetic and environmental factors that could explain why not all Graves' hyperthyroid patients develop the phenotypic appearance of GO. Among the whole population of Graves' patients, particular single nucleotide polymorphisms (SNPs) in susceptibility genes differ in frequency between those without and with GO (namely ICAM-1, IFNγ, TNF, IL-23R, and PTPN12 (55–57), implying involve-

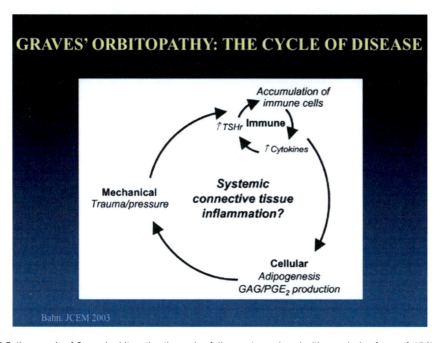

Fig. 29.2 Pathogenesis of Graves' orbitopathy: the cycle of disease (reproduced with permission from ref. (54)).

ment of these SNPs in the expression of GO. Observed polymorphisms that do not differ in frequency between Graves' patients without and with GO are in genes encoding for the TSH-R, HLA classes A, B, C, and DR3, CTLA4, PTPN22, CD40, FRCL3, IL-1α, IL-1β, IL-1RA, IL-6, IL-12B, IL-13, IL-18, and PPARγ (*55*). Finally, the biologic mechanism behind the well-known risk of smoking for the development of GO has been clarified further by exposing cultured human OF to cigarette smoke extract: smoke exposure caused a dose-dependent increase in hyaluronic acid production and in adipogenesis (*58*).

MANAGEMENT

The management of GO as recently proposed by EUGOGO (*59*) is schematically depicted in Fig. 29.3. It consists of three types of intervention:

1. *To stop smoking.* About 40% of GO patients smoke. Arguments to convince patients to stop smoking now are: (a) smokers suffer more severe GO than nonsmokers, (b) smokers have less

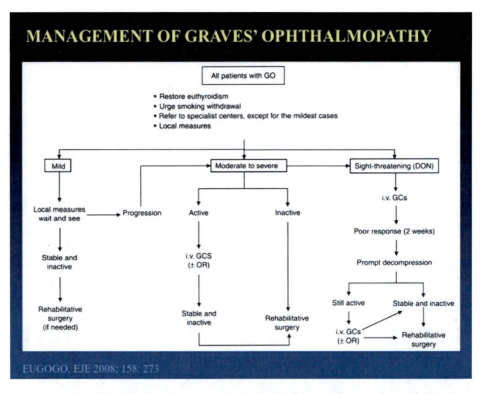

Fig. 29.3 Management of Graves' orbitopathy as recommended by the European Group on Graves' Orbitopathy (reproduced with permission from ref. (*59*)).

favorable response to treatment with steroids or retrobulbar irradiation than nonsmokers (*60*), (c) smokers are four times more likely to experience progression of GO after 131I therapy for Graves' hyperthyroidism than nonsmokers (*27*), and (d) smokers are more likely to get recurrent Graves' hyperthyroidism after a course of antithyroid drugs than nonsmokers.

2. *To restore euthyroidism.* According to a recent systematic review, 131I therapy for Graves' hyperthyroidism is associated with an increased risk of GO compared with antithyroid drugs (RR 4.23, 95% CI 2.04–8.77) (*61*). Prednisone prophylaxis was highly effective in preventing progression of GO induced by 131I therapy in patients with preexisting GO (RR 0.03, 95% CI 0.00–0.24). The most appropriate time of initiation, dose, and duration of prednisone prophylaxis are not well established (*62*). Glucocorticoid prophylaxis can probably be avoided if 131I therapy is applied in inactive GO patients (*63*) and if other risk factors like smoking and high TBII are absent. Antithyroid drugs and thyroidectomy are apparently neutral with respect to the course of GO. Subtotal thyroidectomy has no advantage over total thyroidectomy for the eye changes in moderately severe GO (*64*). Total thyroid ablation (i.e., near-total thyroidectomy followed by 131I ablation) is slightly better than near-total thyroidectomy alone for proptosis and lid aperture, but not for CAS and diplopia (*65*). In view of the limited improvements it remains to be seen whether these invasive procedures are of real benefit to the patient.

3. *To restore visual functions and appearance.* Simple local measures can be very helpful in relieving symptoms. These include sunglasses, artificial tears, lubricant ointments, and prisms. Further treatment depends on the severity and activity of the eye disease. Immunosuppression can be considered in active GO. When the disease has become inactive, rehabilitative surgery can be done as needed but always in the sequence of first orbital decompression, followed by squint surgery, and finally eyelid surgery.

    (a) *Mild GO.* In general, a wait-and-see policy is recommended in view of the tendency to spontaneous improvement during the natural course of GO. Eye changes indeed improve in about 30% of mild GO patients within 12 months (*66*). If the eye changes despite their mild nature have a profound negative impact on quality of life, orbital irradiation might be considered, which is effective in about half of the patients (*66*). The usual scheme is 20 Gy divided in ten doses of 2 Gy each given in a 2-week period, but lower doses might be equally effective. Most improvement upon radiotherapy is observed in muscle motility and diplopia (*67*). Data on long-term safety of radiotherapy are reassuring (no increased risk on secondary malignancy or premature death), but it seems prudent to restrict orbital irradiation to patients older than 35 years. There is a small risk on radiation retinopathy, mostly in patients with diabetes or hypertension in whom orbital irradiation is contraindicated (*68*).

(b) *Moderate to severe GO.* Immunosuppressive treatment is indicated if the disease is active. Steroids remain the treatment of choice, but several randomized clinical trials have indicated superiority of intravenous pulses of methylprednisolone over oral prednisone: pulse therapy has greater efficacy and fewer side effects (*69, 70*). The recommended scheme is 500 mg methylprednisolone iv weekly for 6 weeks, followed by 250 mg iv weekly for another 6 weeks. In doing so, one avoids the risk of life-threatening liver failure reported in some cases in association with higher steroid doses (*71, 72*). Oral prednisone in combination with orbital irradiation is more effective than prednisone alone, but it is unknown if combining iv steroids with radiotherapy increases the efficacy of iv pulse therapy. Unfortunately, GO frequently flares up after termination of high-dose steroids. Under these circumstances one may consider to continue with low-dose oral prednisone (20 mg daily) in combination with either cyclosporin or orbital irradiation until the disease has become inactive (which may last 6–12 months). It has not been studied if early treatment with several immunosuppressive drugs (triple therapy like in rheumatoid arthritis) is more beneficial than the currently recommended scheme.

(c) *Very severe, sight-threatening GO.* Dysthyroid optic neuropathy (DON) requires prompt medical attention. The only available randomized clinical trial (albeit with a very low sample size) indicates a preference to start with steroids: 1 g methylprednisolone intravenously on three successive days in the first week, to be repeated in the second week (total dose 6 g) (*73*). If visual functions improve after 2 weeks, continuation with oral prednisone is indicated; if not, an urgent surgical decompression is necessary.

FURTHER DEVELOPMENTS

A suitable animal model of GO is urgently needed for better understanding of the immunopathogenesis of the disease. This will also allow identification of potential therapeutic targets. A survey of putative effective treatment modalities is depicted in Fig. 29.4. Whereas somatostatin analogs so far have shown no or

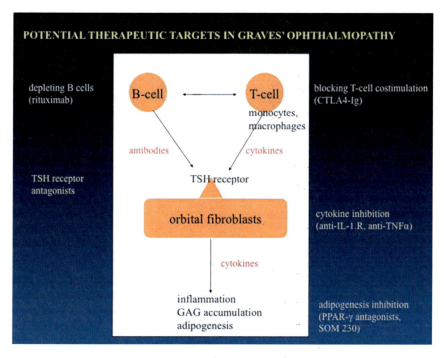

Fig. 29.4 Potential targets for new treatment modalities in Graves' orbitopathy.

little efficacy, the expectation is that the newly developed drug SOM 239 will have greater potency. Promising are the beneficial effects of rituximab and Cox-2 inhibitors observed in open trials (*74, 75*). Anticytokine therapy (especially directed against IL-1β) should be investigated (*76*). In view of the natural history of GO, the efficacy of each of these new treatment modalities should be tested in randomized clinical trials. This requires a large number of patients. For speedy progress, multicenter studies are thus necessary, which can be performed by multidisciplinary international groups like EUGOGO.

REFERENCES

1. Otto AJ, Koornneef L, Mourits MP, Deen-van Leeuwen L. Retrobular pressures measured during surgical decompression of the orbit. Br J Ophthalmol 1996;80:1042–1045.
2. Gerding MN, Terwee CB, Dekker FW, Koornneef L, Prummel MF, Wiersinga WM. Quality of life in patients with Graves' ophthalmopathy is markedly decreased: measurements by the Medical Outcomes Study Instrument. Thyroid 1997;7:885–889.
3. Bartley GB. The incidence of Graves' ophthalmopathy in Olmsted County, Minnesota. Am J Ophthalmol 1995;120:511–517.
4. Prummel MF, Wiersinga WM. Smoking and risk of Graves' disease. JAMA 1993;269:479–482.
5. Perros P, Kendall-Taylor P. Natural history of thyroid eye disease. Thyroid 1998;8:423–425.
6. Weetman AP, Wiersinga WM. Current management of thyroid-associated ophthalmopathy in Europe: results of an international survey. Clin Endocrinol 1998;49:21–28.
7. Wiersinga WM, Bartalena L. Preventing Graves' ophthalmopathy. Thyroid 2002;12:855–860.

8. Krassas GE, Segni M, Wiersinga WM. Childhood Graves' ophthalmopathy: results of a European questionnaire study. Eur J Endocrinol 2005;153:515–520.
9. Bartalena L, Pinchera A, Marcocci C. Management of Graves' ophthalmopathy: reality and perspectives. Endocr Rev 2002;21:168–199.
10. Prummel MF, Bakker A, Wiersinga WM, et al. Multi-center study on the characteristics and treatment strategies of patients with Graves' orbitopathy: the first European Group on Graves' Orbitopathy experience. Eur J Endocrinol 2003;148:491–495
11. Dickinson AJ, Perros P. Controversies in the clinical evaluation of active thyroid-associated orbitopathy: use of a detailed protocol with comparative photographs for objective assessment. Clin Endocrinol 2001;55:283–303.
12. Mourits MP, Koornneef L, Wiersinga WM, Prummel MF, Berghout A, van der Gaag R. Clinical criteria for the assessment of disease activity in Graves' ophthalmopathy: a novel approach. Br J Ophthalmol 1989;73:639–644.
13. Mourits MP, Prummel MF, Wiersinga WM, Koornneef L. Clinical activity score as a guide in the management of patients with Graves' ophthalmopathy. Clin Endocrinol 1997;47:9–14.
14. Gerding MN, Prummel MF, Wiersinga WM. Assessment of disease activity in Graves' ophthalmopathy by orbital ultrasonography and clinical parameters. Clin Endocrinol 2000;52: 641–646.
15. Prummel MF, Gerding MN, Zonneveld FW, Wiersinga WM. The usefulness of quantitative orbital magnetic resonance imaging in Graves' ophthalmopathy. Clin Endocrinol 2001;54:205–209.
16. Gerding MN, van der Zant FM, van Royen EA, et al. Octreotide-scintigraphy is a disease-activity parameter in Graves' ophthalmopathy. Clin Endocrinol 1999;50:373–379.
17. von Arx G. Atypical manifestations. In: Wiersinga WM, Kahaly GJ, eds. Graves' Orbitopathy. A multidisciplinary Approach. Switzerland: S. Karger AG Basel, 2007:212–220.
18. McKeag D, Lane C, Lazarus JH, et al. Clinical features of dysthyroid optic neuropathy: a European Group on Graves' Orbitopathy (EUGOGO) survey. Br J Ophthalmol 2007;91:455–458.
19. Forbes G, Gorman CA, Brennan MD, Gehring DG, Hstrup DM, Earnest F. Ophthalmopathy of Graves' disease: computerized volume measurements of the orbital fat and muscle. Am J Neuroradiol 1986;7:651–656.
20. Schmidt ED, Hogerwou G van, Gaag R van der, Wiersinga WM, Asmussen G, Koornneef L. Site-dependent effects of experimental hypo- and hyperthyroidism on resident macrophages in extraocular muscles of rats: a quantitative immunohistochemical study. J Endocrinol 1992;135:485–493.
21. Khoo DH, Eng PH, Ho SC. Graves' ophthalmopathy in the absence of elevated free thyroxine and triiodothyronine levels: prevalence, natural history, and thyrotropin receptor antibody levels. Thyroid 2000;10:1093–1100.
22. Vos XG, Smit N, Endert E, Tijssen JG, Wiersinga WM. Frequency and characteristics of TBII-seronegative patients in a population with untreated Graves' hyperthyroidism: a prospective study. Clin Endocrinol 2008;69: 311–317.
23. Gerding MN, Meer JWC van der, Broenink M, et al. Association of thyrotropin receptor antibodies with the clinical features of Graves' ophthalmopathy. Clin Endocrinol 2000;52:267–271.
24. Eckstein AK, Plicht M, Lax H, et al. Clinical results of anti-inflammatory therapy in Graves' ophthalmopathy and association with thyroidal autoantibodies. Clin Endocrinol 2004; 61:612–618.
25. Laurberg P, Wallin G, Tallstedt L, Abraham-Nordling M, Lundell G, Torring O. TSH receptor autoimmunity in Graves' disease after therapy with antithyroid drugs, surgery, or radioactive iodine: a 5-yr prospective randomized study. Eur J Endocrinol 2008;158: 69–75.
26. Tallstedt L, Lundell G, Torring O, et al. Occurrence of ophthalmopathy after treatment for Graves' hyperthyroidism. N Eng J Med 1992;326:1733–1738.
27. Bartalena L, Marcocci C, Bogazzi F, et al. Relation between therapy for hyperthyroidism and the course of Graves' ophthalmopathy. N Eng J Med 1998;338:73–78.
28. Eckstein AK, Plicht M, Hildegard L, et al. TSH-receptor autoantibodies are independent risk factors for Graves' ophthalmopathy and help to predict severity and outcome of the disease. J Clin Endocrinol Metab 2006;91:3463–3470.
29. Hansen C, Rouhi R, Förster G, Kahaly GJ. Increased sulfatation of orbital glycosaminoglycans in Graves' ophthalmopathy. J Clin Endocrinol Metab 1999;84:1409–1413.
30. Grubeck-Loebenstein B, Trieb K, Sztankay A, Holter W, Anderl H, Wick G. Retrobular T cells from patients with Graves' ophthalmopathy are CD8+ and specifically recognize autologous fibroblasts. J Clin Invest 1994; 93:2738–2743.
31. Otto EA, Ochs K, Hansen C, Wall JR, Kahaly GJ. Orbital tissue-derived T lymphocytes from patients with Graves' ophthalmopathy recog-

nize autologous orbital antigens. J Clin Endocrinol Metab 1996;81:3045–3050.
32. Feldon SE, Park DJJ, O'Loughlin CW, et al. Autologous T-lymphocytes stimulate proliferation of orbital fibroblasts derived from patients with Graves' ophthalmopathy. Invest Ophthalmol Vis Sci 2005;46:3913–3921.
33. Pappa A, Lawson JM, Calder V, Fells P, Lightman S. T cells and fibroblasts in affected extraocular muscles in early and late thyroid associated ophthalmopathy. Br J Opthalmol 2000;84:517–522.
34. Prabhakar BS, Bahn RS, Smith TJ. Current perspective on the pathogenesis of Graves' disease and ophthalmopathy. Endocr Rev 2003;24:802–835.
35. Gopinath B, Musselman R, Beard N, et al. Antibodies targeting the calcium binding skeletal muscle protein calsequestrin are specific markers of ophthalmopathy and sensitive indicators of ocular myopathy in patients with Graves' disease. Clin Exp Immunol 2006;145:56–62
36. Feliciello A, Porcellini A, Ciullo C, Bonavolonta G, Avvedimento EV, Fenzi G. Expression of thyrotropin-receptor mRNA in healthy and Graves' retro-orbital tissue. Lancet 1993;342:337–338.
37. Bahn RS, Dutton CM, Natt N, Joba W, Spitzweg C, Heufelder AE. Thyrotropin receptor expression in Graves' orbital adipose/connective tissues: potential autoantigen in Graves' ophthalmopathy. J Clin Endocrinol Metab 1998;83:998–1002.
38. Wakelkamp IMMJ, Bakker O, Baldeschi L, Wiersinga WM, Prummel MF. TSH-R expression and cytokine profile in orbital tissue of active vs inactive Graves' ophthalmopathy patients. Clin Endocrinol 2003;58:280–287.
39. Valyasevi RW, Erickson DZ, Harteneck DA, et al. Differentiation of human orbital preadipocyte fibroblasts induces expression of functional thyrotropin receptor. J Clin Endocrinol Metab 1999;84:2557–2562.
40. Smith TJ, Koumas L, Gagnon A, et al. Orbital fibroblast heterogeneity may determine the clinical presentation of thyroid-associated ophthalmopathy. J Clin Endocrinol Metab 2002;87:385–392.
41. Smith TJ, Hoa N. Immunoglobulins from patients with Graves' disease induce hyaluronan synthesis in their orbital fibroblasts through the self-antigen, insulin-like growth factor-1 receptor. J Clin Endocrinol Metab 2004;89:5076–5080.
42. Tsui S, Naik V, Hoa N, et al. Evidence for an association between thyroid-stimulating hormone and insulin-like growth factor 1 receptors: a tale of two antigens implicated in Graves' disease. J Immunol 2008;181: 4397–4405.
43. Eckstein AK, Quadbeck B, Tews S, et al. Thyroid-associated ophthalmopathy: evidence for CD4+ γδ T cells: de novo differentiation of RED7+ macrophages, but not of RFD1+ dendritic cells; and loss of γδ and αβ T cell receptor expression. Br J Ophthalmol 2004;88:803–808.
44. Avanduk AM, Avanduk MC, Pazarli H, et al. Immunohistochemical analysis of orbital connective tissue specimens of patients with active Graves' ophthalmopathy. Curr Eye Res 2005;70:631–638.
45. Boschi A, Daumerie Ch, Spiritus M, et al. Quantification of cells expressing the thyrotropin receptor in extraocular muscles in thyroid associated ophthalmopathy. Br J Ophthalmol 2005;89:724–729.
46. Chen M-H, Chen M-H, Liao S-Z, Chang T-C, Chuang L-M. Role of macrophage infiltration in the orbital fat of patients with Graves' ophthalmopathy. Clin Endocrinol 2008;69:332–337.
47. Aniszewski JP, Valyasevi RW, Bahn RS. Relationship between disease duration and predominant orbital T cell subset in Graves' ophthalmopathy. J Clin Endocrinol Metab 2000;85:776–780.
48. Lehmann GM, Feldon S, Smith TJ, Phipps RP. Immune mechanisms in thyroid eye disease. Thyroid 2008;18:959–965.
49. Pritchard J, Horst N, Cruikshank W, Smith TJ. IgGs from patients with Graves' disease induce the expression of T cell chemoattractants in their fibroblasts. J Immunol 2002;168:942–950.
50. Ajjan RA, Weetman AP. New understanding of the role of cytokines in the pathogenesis of Graves' ophthalmopathy. J Endocrinol Invest 2004;27:237–245.
51. Antonelli A, Rotondi M, Ferrari SM, et al. IFN-gamma-inducible alpha-chemokine CXCL10 involvement in Graves' ophthalmopathy: modulation by peroxisome proliferator-activated receptor-gamma agonists. J Clin Endocrinol Metab 2006;91:614–620.
52. Sempowski G, Rozenblat J, Smith T, Phipps R. Human orbital fibroblasts are activated through CD40 to induce proinflammatory cytokine production. Am J Physiol 1998;274:C707–C714.
53. Gianoukakis AG, Khadavi N, Smith TJ. Cytokines, Graves' disease, and thyroid-associated ophthalmopathy. Thyroid 2008;18: 953–958.
54. Bahn RS. Pathophysiology of Graves' ophthalmopathy: the cycle of disease. J Clin Endocrinol Metab 2003;88:1939–1946.

55. Bednarczuk T, Gopinath B, Ploski R, Wall JR. Susceptibility genes in Graves' ophthalmopathy: searching for a needle in a haystack? Clin Endocrinol 2007;67:3–19.
56. Huber AK, Jacobson EM, Jazdzewski K, Concepcion ES, Tomer Y. Interleukin (IL)-23 receptor is a major susceptibility gene for Graves' ophthalmopathy: the IL-23/T-helper axis extends to thyroid autoimmunity. J Clin Endocrinol Metab 2008;93:1077–1081.
57. Syed AA, Simmonds MJ, Brand OJ, Franklyn JA, Gough SC. Preliminary evidence for interaction of PTPN12 polymorphism with TSHR genotype and association with Graves' ophthalmopathy. Clin Endocrinol 2007;67:663–667.
58. Cawood TJ, Moriarty P, O'Farrelly C, O'Shea D. Smoking and thyroid-associated ophthalmopathy: a novel explanation of the biological link. J Clin Endocrinol Metab 2007;92:59–64.
59. Bartalena L, Baldeschi L, Dickinson A, et al. Consensus statement of the European Group on Graves' Orbitopathy (EUGOGO) on management of GO. Eur J Endocrinol 2008;158:273–285.
60. Eckstein A, Quadbeck B, Mueller G, et al. Impact of smoking on the response to treatment of thyroid associated ophthalmopathy. Br J Ophthalmol 2004;87:773–776.
61. Acharya SH, Avenell A, Philip S, Burr J, Bevan JS, Abraham P. Radioiodine therapy (RAI) for Graves' disease (GD) and the effect on ophthalmopathy: a systematic review. Clin Endocrinol 2008;69:943–950.
62. Tanda ML, Lai A, Bartalena L. Relation between Graves' orbitopathy and radioiodine therapy for hyperthyroidism: facts and unresolved questions. Clin Endocrinol 2008;69:845–847.
63. Perros P, Kendall-Taylor P, Neoh C, Frewins S, Dickinson J. A prospective study of the effects of radioiodine therapy for hyperthyroidism in patients with minimally active Graves' ophthalmopathy. J Clin Endocrinol Metab 2005;90:5321–5323.
64. Jarhult J, Rudberg C, Larsson E, et al. Graves' disease with moderate-severe endocrine ophthalmopathy: long-term results of a prospective randomised study of total or subtotal thyroid resection. Thyroid 2005;15:1157–1164.
65. Menconi F, Marino M, Pinchera A, et al. Effects of total thyroid ablation vs total thyroidectomy alone on the short term outcome of mild to moderate Graves' orbitopathy treated with intravenous glucocorticoids. J Clin Endocrinol Metab 2007;92:1653–1658.
66. Prummel MF, Terwee CB, Gerding MN, et al. A randomised controlled trial of orbital radiotherapy versus sham irradiation in patients with mild Graves' ophthalmopathy. J Clin Endocrinol Metab 2004;89:15–20.
67. Bradley EA, Gower EW, Bradley DJ, et al. Orbital irradiation for Graves' ophthalmopathy: a report by the American Academy of Ophthalmology. Ophthalmology 2008;115:398–409.
68. Wakelkamp IMMJ, Tan H, Saeed P, et al. Orbital irradiation for Graves' ophthalmopathy. Is it safe? A long-term follow-up study. Ophthalmology 2004;111:1557–1562.
69. Kahaly GJ, Pitz S, Hommel G, Dittmar M. Randomised, single-blind trial of intravenous versus oral steroid monotherapy in Graves' orbitopathy. J Clin Endocrinol Metab 2005;90:5234–5240.
70. Aktaran S, Akarsu E, Erbagai I, Araz M, Okumus S, Kartal M. Comparison of intravenous methylprednisolone therapy vs oral methylprednisolone therapy in patients with Graves' ophthalmopathy. Int J Clin Pract 2007;61:45–51.
71. Marino M, Morabito E, Brunetto MR, et al. Acute and severe liver damage associated with intravenous glucocorticoid pulse therapy in patients with Graves' ophthalmopathy. Thyroid 2004;14:403–406.
72. LeMoli R, Baldeschi L, Saeed P, Regensburg N, Mourits MP, Wiersinga WM. Determinants of liver damage associated with intravenous methylprednisolone pulse therapy in Graves' ophthalmopathy. Thyroid 2007;17:357–362.
73. Wakelkamp IMMJ, Baldeschi L, Saeed P, Mourits MP, Prummel MF, Wiersinga WM. Surgical or medical compression as a first-line treatment of optic neuropathy in Graves' ophthalmopathy? A randomised clinical trial. Clin Endocrinol 2005;63:323–328.
74. Salvi M, Vanuchi G, Campi I, et al. Treatment of Graves' disease and associated ophthalmopathy with the anti-CD20 monoclonal antibody rituximab: an open study. Eur J Endocrinol 2007;156:33–40.
75. Kuriyan AE, Phipps RP, O'Loughlin CW, Feldon SE. Improvement of thyroid eye disease following treatment with the cyclooxygenase-2 selective inhibitor Celecoxib. Thyroid 2008;18:911–914.
76. Paridaens D, Bosch WA van der, Loos TL van der, Krenning EP, Hagen PM van. The effect of etanercept on Graves' ophthalmopathy: a pilot study. Eye 2005;19:1286–1289.

Chapter 30

Hypoparathyroidism

Ogo I. Egbuna and Edward M. Brown

Key Words: Hypoparathyroidism, Autoimmune hypoparathyroidism, Hypercalciuria, Hypocalcemia, Calcium-sensing receptor, Parathyroid gland, Parathyroid hormone, Anticalcium sensing receptor antibodies, Hyperphosphatemia

INTRODUCTION

Hypoparathyroidism is an important component of the differential diagnosis of hypocalcemia. It refers to a heterogeneous group of disorders that have in common a relative or absolute deficiency in the quantity of secreted parathyroid hormone (PTH) or in its peripheral actions. The disorder may be due to iatrogenic, infiltrative, developmental, signaling, autoimmune, or genetic abnormalities, which make etiological differentiation important as this has implications for diagnosis, therapy, counseling, and prevention of complications. Autoimmunity is an important cause of hypoparathyroidism, either as an isolated endocrinopathy or as a component of autoimmune polyglandular syndromes (e.g., APS1 and 2, and in some classifications, 3 and 4) (*1, 2*) with a prevalence ranging from 1:600 to 1:90,000 (*2, 3*).

Over the last half-century, there has been a growing body of information describing the targets of antibodies in autoimmune disorders involving the parathyroid gland. In addition to cytosolic antigens, an increasingly recognized target of parathyroid autoimmunity is the calcium-sensing receptor (CaSR) for which activating and inactivating antibodies have been identified.

This chapter summarizes the history of antiparathyroid antibodies and the subsequent elucidation of the CaSR as a target for at least some of these antibodies, including those that can directly activate the receptor and cause autoimmune hypoparathyroidism (AH). Finally, we discuss the diagnosis and treatment of the various causes of hypoparathyroidism, including those with immunity-mediated alterations in parathyroid function.

CAUSES OF HYPOPARATHY-ROIDISM

Antibody-Mediated Inhibition/Destruction of Parathyroid Function/Anatomy

General Overview

There has been increasing clarity in the understanding of immunological perturbations involving the parathyroid gland and resultant abnormalities of calcium homeostasis, with observations suggesting that antibodies could be both the cause and result of parathyroid gland disease/destruction. The earliest and more widely recognized mechanisms of antibody-mediated hypoparathyroidism involve destructive/cytopathic antibodies targeted to cellular organelles of the parathyroid and other glands as seen in the autoimmune polyglandular syndrome 1 or 2 (APS-1 or -2). Patients with endocrinopathies linked to APS-1 or -2 often have a higher prevalence of organ-specific autoantibodies with specificities to autoantigens such as small-sized mitochondrial specific epitopes (*4, 5*) or to cell surface antigens (*6*), which are cytotoxic in culture (*7*) but are also nonspecific, as they are adsorbed onto the surface of endothelial cells (*8*). More recently, NALP 5 (NACHT leucine-rich-repeat protein 5) (*9*) has been identified as a target for antibodies in the pathogenesis of autoimmune parathyroid disease. This is in contrast to antibodies that are directed against otherwise unique epitopes in patients with isolated hypoparathyroidism without the other components of APS as will be discussed later in this chapter. The pathophysiology of APS is covered elsewhere in this book and will not be emphasized further except insofar as how these antibodies have assisted in understanding more recently described noncytolytic antibodies that modulate parathyroid secretory function. Namely, recent important observations have identified noncytotoxic antibodies that are specific for the CaSR and exert functional actions on the parathyroid (*10–12*) as opposed to destructive cytotoxic antibodies directed to autoantigens in the parathyroid cell as mentioned above.

Historical Perspective of Anti-Parathyroid Antibodies

As early as the 1940s, autoimmune destructive parathyroid disease was recognized as evidenced by fatty infiltration, lymphocytic infiltration, and atrophy (*13–15*). The first description of autoantibodies involving the parathyroid gland dates back to 1966 when Blizzard and colleagues, using indirect immunofluorescence techniques, identified autoantibodies to the parathyroid gland in 33% of patients with idiopathic hypoparathyroidism, 26% of patients with idiopathic Addison's disease, 12% of patients with

Hashimoto's thyroiditis, and 6% of normal controls (*16*). Several years later, however, Swana (*17*) and later Betterle (*5*), using similar methods, identified antimitochondrial antibodies to the oxyphil cells of the parathyroid. They suggested that these antibodies could explain the seropositivity seen by Blizzard but were not specific for the parathyroid per se. Brandi et al. in two publications in the late 1980s further investigated the potential role of antiparathyroid antibodies in the pathogenesis of AH. They first identified antibodies that reacted with bovine parathyroid cells and elicited complement-dependent cytotoxicity (*7*). In the second study, however, these antibodies were shown to be directed predominantly at bovine parathyroid endothelial cells, raising the possibility of a novel paradigm; whereby, damage to parathyroid endothelial cells serves as the basis for parathyroid gland damage and destruction (*8*). There have been no follow-up investigations, however, related to these two studies.

The CaSR as an Antigenic Target in Autoimmune Hypoparathyroidism

In 1996, soon after the cloning of the CaSR, Li and colleagues identified the CaSR as an autoantigen in a cohort of patients with AH (*18*). Those patients with AH for <5 years were more likely to harbor anti-CaSR antibodies (72%) than those with the condition for >5 years (14%), presumably because of loss of the antigen with ongoing destruction of the parathyroid glands. In retrospect, a study carried out almost a decade earlier had described autoantibodies recognizing 200 and 130 kDa autoantigens in the parathyroid glands of patients with idiopathic hypoparathyroidism results consistent with interaction of these antibodies with the dimeric and monomeric forms of the CaSR, respectively (*8*). More recently, Mayer (*19*) and Gavalas (*20*) have also shown that the serum of patients with isolated hypoparathyroidism as well as those with APS-1 contained antibodies to the extracellular domain of the CaSR, the detection of which appeared to be influenced by the assay system used. The variety of techniques used in these studies to identify anti-CaSR antibodies makes it difficult to compare the results directly, and some techniques likely underestimate the prevalence of anti-CaSR antibodies. However, it appears that a substantial proportion of patients with either APS-1 or adult-onset IH harbor anti-CaSR antibodies. Based on the studies reviewed to this point, however, it is not possible to determine whether the antibodies played any direct role in the pathogenesis of the disorder or were simply a marker of the disease process, perhaps owing to destruction of the parathyroid glands and associated production of antibodies to self-antigen. Anti-CaSR antibodies have been identified in some (*11*) but not all (*21, 22*) of the additional studies investigating the presence of these antibodies in various forms of IH.

Kifor et al. reported in 2004 (*10*) that anti-CaSR antibodies occurring in AH could exert direct functional actions on the

CaSR and, in turn, the parathyroid gland. In this report, CaSR-specific antibodies activating the receptor were shown to increase intracellular inositol phosphate concentrations through activation of phospholipase C, activate the extracellular signal-regulated kinases 1 and 2, and inhibit PTH secretion, consistent with the ability of these antibodies, in contrast to cytotoxic antibodies, to alter parathyroid cell function while permitting continued cell viability (*10*). In this report, they described two patients with idiopathic hypoparathyroidism. In one, transient hypoparathyroidism developed in a patient with Addison's disease, as manifested by hypocalcemia with an inappropriately low-normal PTH level. Over several weeks, the serum calcium and PTH levels normalized, and long-term therapy was not needed to maintain normocalcemia. In the second, a patient had coexistent hypoparathyroidism – causing seizures and requiring therapy with oral calcium and vitamin D – and difficult-to-treat Graves' disease that eventually necessitated subtotal thyroidectomy. During surgery, a parathyroid gland, normal in both size and histological criteria, was identified, demonstrating that the patient's AH had not destroyed the parathyroid glands. Both the patients harbored anti-CaSR antibodies as assessed by immunoblotting of CaSR extracted from parathyroid glands or CaSR-transfected HEK cells, immunoprecipitation utilizing the patients' sera, and an ELISA using peptides from within the CaSR's extracellular domain. In the first case, the antibody titer decreased as the hypoparathyroidism remitted. Furthermore, the anti-CaSR antibodies in both patients activated the CaSR, as documented by stimulation of PLC and MAPK in CaSR-transfected HEK293 cells and inhibition of PTH release from dispersed cells from parathyroid adenomas. Thus, in both the cases, the hypoparathyroidism may have resulted from a functional effect of the antibodies on the CaSR in the parathyroid glands and not from irreversible parathyroid damage (*10*).

Inactivating Antibodies to the CaSR- A Cause of Autoimmune Hyperparathyroidism or Hypocalciuric Hypercalcemia

As an interesting counterpoint to the activating antibodies just described, inactivating antibodies of the CaSR, acting in a predictable manner on intracellular signaling pathways, can produce PTH-dependent hypercalcemia and hypocalciuria. Kifor and colleagues described four patients, two sisters as well as a mother and her daughter, with PTH-dependent hypercalcemia, three of whom exhibited hypocalciuria (*12*). In contrast to the other three patients, the daughter had hypercalciuria, pointing out that the biochemical presentation of this condition can be similar to that of primary hyperparathyroidism. The mother had coexistent sprue, while her daughter and the two sisters had Hashimoto's thyroiditis. A genetic cause of PTH-dependent, hypocalciuric hypercalcemia is the autosomal dominant syndrome, familial hypocalciuric hypercalcemia (FHH), which results from heterozygous inactivating CaSR mutations (*23, 24*). Kifor et al., however, ruled out FHH in these patients by mutational analysis of the CaSR gene (*12*), and their other autoimmune manifestations prompted a search for an autoimmune basis for their hypocalciuric hypercalcemia. All four patients, in fact, harbored inactivating anti-CaSR antibodies that mitigated high Ca_o^{2+}-stimulated activation of PLC and MAPK and stimulated PTH secretion. This condition has been termed acquired or autoimmune hypocalciuric hypercalcemia (AHH) (*25*).

A subsequent report from the same group (*26*) described a 66-year-old hypercalcemic woman with multiple autoimmune manifestations (psoriasis, adult-onset asthma, Coomb's positive hemolytic anemia, rheumatoid arthritis, uveitis, bullous pemphigoid, sclerosing pancreatitis, and autoimmune hypophysitis with hypothyroidism and diabetes insipidus). Her hypercalcemia (as high as 13.4 mg/dl) was accompanied by elevated intact PTH levels (75–175 pg/ml) and hypocalciuria. A diagnosis of primary hyperparathyroidism had been made earlier, but a subtotal parathyroidectomy was followed within 3 weeks by recrudescence of her hypercalcemia. Remarkably, her hypercalcemia subsequently resolved during treatment with glucocorticoids for her bullous pemphigoid, and her intact PTH level decreased concomitantly to the upper limit of normal. While hypercalcemic, her serum harbored anti-CaSR antibodies, but there was a substantial drop in the titer of these antibodies during glucocorticoid therapy. To date, therapy with glucocorticoids has only been undertaken in this AHH patient and might be expected to be associated with long-term complications (e.g., osteoporosis and diabetes) if used chronically. As in the earlier four cases of AHH (*12*), the persistence of PTH-dependent hypercalcemia proves unequivocally that the anti-CaSR antibodies had not destroyed the patients' parathyroid glands. Another study (*25*) described a 74-year-old male patient who developed AHH and was found to harbor anti-CaSR antibodies. Interestingly, in this case, the antibodies mitigated the stimulatory effect of high Ca_o^{2+} on MAPK activation in CaSR-transfected HEK293 cells, while at the same time sensitizing the HEK cells to the activation of PLC by high Ca_o^{2+}, the latter effect being more consistent with an activating action of the antibody(ies). The authors interpreted these findings as evidence that the anti-CaSR antibodies stabilized a novel conformation of the receptor that activates one heterotrimeric G protein, G_q, which is responsible for activating PLC, while at the same time reducing the receptor's coupling to G_i, the G protein responsible for activating MAPK in this experimental system. Such a mechanism may make it possible for physiological agonists of the CaSR and other GPCRs to couple preferentially to one or another G protein and, in turn, signalling pathway. A provocative finding, worthy of follow-up, was the identification of anti-parathyroid antibodies in a very substantial proportion of patients with parathyroid adenomas (*27*), raising the possibility that autoimmunity to the parathyroid, and perhaps the CaSR, could participate in the pathogenesis of primary hyperparathyroidism.

Anti-CaSR Antibodies and Human Leukocyte Antigen Associations

Of equal interest are the observations of associations of CaSR-specific seropositivity in patients with sporadic idiopathic hypoparathyroidism (SIH) with major histocompatibility complex human leukocyte antigen (HLA) class II DR loci. The HLA-DR loci are involved in antigen processing by antigen-presenting cells and have been associated with several well-known autoimmune diseases, such as systemic lupus, psoriasis, and rheumatoid arthritis. The frequency of HLA-DRB1*09 or DRB1*10 was found to be higher in CaSR seropositive patients with an odds ratio of 5.2 (*11*). Like other autoimmune diseases, the genetic basis of sporadic idiopathic hypoparathyroidism due to CaSR-specific antibodies is likely polygenic in nature with a likely role for environmental risk factors in the clinical manifestation of the disease, as one patient with these antibodies has been described to have had a spontaneous remission of disease (*10*). Fluctuations in the severity of AH has also been reported (*6*), where the magnitude of the in vitro inhibitory effect of the antibodies on PTH secretion from acutely dispersed human parathyroid cells temporally correlated with the clinical course of the hypoparathyroidism and likely represented a concomitant fluctuation in antibody titers.

Finally, in studies by Blizzard (*16*) and Goswami (*11*), 6% and 13% of healthy controls were positive for parathyroid and CaSR autoantibodies, respectively. These observations raise the question of the requirement for other pathological triggers/processes that remain unidentified in the development of autoimmune parathyroid disease.

Other Causes of Hypoparathyroidism

Abnormal Development of the Parathyroid Gland

Hypoparathyroidism may result from agenesis or dysgenesis of the parathyroid glands. The most well-described examples of parathyroid gland dysembryogenesis are the DiGeorge and velocardiofacial syndromes in which maldevelopment of the third and fourth branchial pouches is frequently associated with congenital absence of not only the parathyroids but also the thymus. Despite the emphasis on thymic dysgenesis in these syndromes, clinically significant immune defects occur in very few patients. Most cases of DiGeorge syndrome are sporadic, but familial occurrence with apparent autosomal dominant inheritance has been described (*28, 29*). X-linked recessive hypoparathyroidism has also been reported in the literature (*30, 31*) and is the result of an isolated congenital defect of parathyroid gland development. Females are not affected and linkage studies have mapped the responsible gene to Xq26-q27 (*32*). More recently identified, genetic forms of abnormal development of the parathyroid glands have been reviewed in detail (*33*).

More recently, an autosomal dominant form of hypoparathyroidism due to novel, heterozygous, dominant-negative mutations in the last of the five exons of the Glial cells missing B (GCMB) gene – a key transcription factor directing parathyroid gland development – has been identified that is believed to have an impact on parathyroid gland development or the secretion of a fully functional PTH molecule (*34*). This report follows earlier cases of autosomal recessive hypoparathyroidism due to homozygous mutation of the GCMB gene (*35, 36*). It is, however, unclear if the effect of these mutations has a primary effect on PTH secretion. Of note, a recent report has shown that the GCMB gene transactivates the CaSR gene and may, therefore, play an important role in the high level, tissue-specific expression of the CaSR in the parathyroid gland (*37*).

Hypoparathyroidism Due to Abnormalities of the PTH Gene Product

The human PTH gene contains three exons located on the short arm of chromosome 11. Patients presenting with isolated hypoparathyroidism due to mutations involving the PTH gene often present with infantile-onset epilepsy and hypocalcemia. Abnormalities reported to date involve the signal peptide of the preproPTH molecule and have been described in cases of isolated hypoparathyroidism in both autosomal dominant and recessive forms. The mutations identified in these conditions have been mapped to different parts of the PTH gene [exon 2 (autosomal recessive) and exon 2-intron 2 boundary (autosomal recessive)] (*38, 40*). Mutations in the signal peptide interfere with cotranslational translocation and release of the proPTH molecule into the lumen of the rough endoplasmic reticulum and, as such, interfere with the formation of mature, fully functional PTH molecule.

Hypoparathyroidism Related to Disorders of Magnesium Homeostasis

Extracellular magnesium is a direct (type I) agonist of the CaSR with a potency 2–3 times less than that of calcium (*41*) and in vitro has been shown to inhibit PTH secretion in acutely dispersed parathyroid cells. Hypoparathyroidism is observed clinically in hypermagnesemic peritoneal dialysis patients (*42, 43*) as well as in obstetrical practice when high-dose magnesium infusions are used for the treatment of toxemia or premature labor (*44*) and likely reflects the ability of elevated serum levels of magnesium to stimulate calcium-sensing receptors expressed by parathyroid cells and thereby inhibit PTH secretion.

Interestingly, the paradoxical block of PTH secretion with severe hypomagnesemia has also been known for more than 30 years and occurs in patients with chronic alcoholism, burn injury, Gitelmans syndrome, and other forms of hereditary renal or intestinal hypomagnesemia, as well as in patients on several medications such as cisplatin, proton-pump inhibitors, and more recently, anti-EGFR monoclonal therapy such as cetuximab. In these circumstances, the inhibition of PTH secretion under magnesium deficiency seems to be mediated through a novel mechanism involving an increase in the activity of the G alpha subunits of heterotrimeric G-proteins coupled to the CaSR (45). Interestingly, the magnesium binding site responsible for inhibition of PTH secretion is not identical with the extracellular binding site of the CaSR because the magnesium deficiency-dependent signal enhancement was not altered by use of CaSR mutants with increased or decreased affinity for calcium or magnesium.

Iatrogenic and Infiltrating Causes of Hypoparathyroidism

Surgery is the most common cause of acquired hypoparathyroidism and may occur after any deep tissue neck surgery. The resulting hypoparathyroidism can be transient or permanent, and sometimes may not develop for many years (46). A chronic state of "decreased parathyroid reserve" may exist in some patients who manifest hypocalcemia only when mineral homeostasis is stressed further by other factors such as pregnancy, lactation, or illness (46). Permanent hypoparathyroidism is unusual after an initial neck exploration for primary hyperparathyroidism and develops in less than 1–2% of patients. The incidence is substantially increased with repeated neck surgery or in patients operated upon by an inexperienced surgeon.

In contrast to many other endocrine tissues, the parathyroid glands are particularly resistant to damage by many toxic agents. The administration of radioactive iodine for the treatment of thyroid disease has only rarely caused permanent, symptomatic hypoparathyroidism (47). Similarly, external beam radiation appears to have little or no effect on parathyroid gland function. Parathyroid tissue is remarkably resistant to most chemotherapeutic or cytotoxic agents, with the notable exceptions of asparaginase (48), which causes parathyroid necrosis, and ethiofos, a radio- and chemoprotector that causes reversible inhibition of PTH secretion (49). An unusual, albeit common, agent to affect parathyroid function is alcohol. Transient or permanent hypoparathyroidism has been associated with percutaneous injection of ethanol for treatment of hyperparathyroidism in dialysis patients (50) or ingestion of large quantities of alcohol and may be related to either direct effects of alcohol on the parathyroids or through induction of hypomagnesemia (51, 52).

Infiltrative processes that affect the parathyroid gland can diminish the ability of the gland to secrete PTH. Idiopathic hemochromatosis and chronic transfusion therapy are often associated with significant deposition of iron in the parathyroid glands (53). A similar pathophysiological process has been described in one patient with Wilson's disease and increased copper storage in the parathyroid glands, who developed symptomatic hypoparathyroidism (54). Pathologic involvement of the parathyroid glands can also occur in metastatic neoplasia, miliary tuberculosis, amyloidosis, and sarcoid, but clinical hypoparathyroidism rarely occurs in these conditions.

Autosomal Dominant Hypoparathyroidism (OMIM) (601298)

Autosomal dominant hypoparathyroidism (ADH) clinically mimics autoimmune hypoparathyroidism caused by activating autoantibodies of the CaSR and, although rare, may comprise a sizable fraction of cases of idiopathic hypoparathyroidism, perhaps representing as many as a third of such cases (55). Patients with this inherited form of hypoparathyroidism are commonly asymptomatic, but some patients, especially children during febrile episodes, can exhibit neuromuscular irritability, seizures, and basal ganglia calcification. Patients generally exhibit mild to moderate hypocalcemia, with serum PTH levels that are inappropriately low given the hypocalcemia (56). Affected individuals often exhibit relative or absolute hypercalciuria, with normal or frankly elevated urinary calcium excretion, respectively, in spite of their low-serum calcium concentration.

Patients with this condition harbor an activating mutation of the CaSR gene that resets the set point of Ca_o^{2+}-regulated PTH secretion leftward and lowers renal calcium reabsorption. Soon after the cloning of the CaSR, investigators (57) showed linkage of ADH to a locus on chromosome 3 q13 – the same locus containing the gene for the CaSR. Shortly afterward, a heterozygous missense mutation, Q127A, was shown to be the cause of ADH in an unrelated family (56). Since these first reports, about 40 mutations have been characterized causing ADH. The majority are missense mutations within the CaSR's extracellular domain and transmembrane domain. In addition, two deletion mutations have been described. Most ADH patients are heterozygous for the activating mutation. In one family, a homozygous mutation was described, but it was not associated with a more severe phenotype (58), and although there is a spectrum of phenotypic severity for a given genotype, the symptoms present in affected members of the same family tend to be similar.

Pseudohypoparathyroidism

Pseudohypoparathyroidism (PHP) is a term used to describe a group of disorders reflecting tissue resistance to PTH action and is characterized by hypocalcemia, hyperphosphatemia, and high plasma PTH levels in the absence of renal insufficiency or magnesium deficiency. Mutations in the GNAS1 gene located on chromosome 20q13.2-20q13.3 result in abnormalities in heterotrimeric G protein (specifically, the $G\alpha_s$ subunit)-mediated adenylate cyclase activation and thereby cyclic adenosine monophosphate mediated signaling, which is crucial in mediating the effects of PTH in various tissues, including kidney and bone.

The first description of PHP by Albright was made over 50 years ago in patients with hypocalcemia resistant to injection with extracts of parathyroid tissue, as well as hyperphosphatemia, rounded facies, short stature, obesity, brachydactyly, short and low-set nasal bridge, strabismus, and ectopic calcifications (59). There have been subsequent descriptions of other key features of this condition, including elevated serum PTH levels (*60*), low urinary cyclic adenosine monophosphate (cAMP) levels (*61, 62*), and autosomal dominant, heterozygous germline inactivation mutations of the GNAS1 gene (*63, 65*), providing important insights into the molecular basis of the pathogenesis, symptoms, signs, and treatment options for the disease.

Recent studies confirm that the GNAS1 gene normally exhibits the imprinting phenomenon observed in PHP (*66*), which explains the variations in phenotype depending upon the origin (maternal or paternal) of the mutation. Genomic imprinting results from a gamete-of-origin-specific marking of the genome that ultimately produces a functional difference between the genetic information contributed by each parent. *GNAS* is a complex locus that generates multiple gene products through the use of four alternative first exons that splice onto a common set of downstream exons (exons 2–13) (*67, 70*). Mutations involving any of these alternative first exons in the GNAS gene have been reported and explain the heterogeneity of presentations possible in PHP.

Variants of PHP: Based on the abnormalities of the various components of the transduction of the cell membrane PTHR1 signal, the pseudohypoparathyroidism may be divided into distinct forms.

PHP type 1a: Clinical features include the Albright's hereditary osteodystrophy (AHO) phenotype described above. Hypocalcaemia and hyperphosphatemia are not typically present until 5 years of age, but PTH elevations may be documented much earlier and sometimes are associated with slight hypercalcemia (*71*). Gonadal dysfunction can occur, especially in women (*72*), both disorders resulting from the associated defect in signaling via $G\alpha_s$. A majority of patients have heterozygous inactivating mutations in the gene encoding the Gs-α subunit protein. There is considerable variability in relation to tissue responsiveness to G_s protein deficiency, which may also be explained by the differences in the quantity of cAMP necessary to activate kinases and generate physiological responses in each tissue. The absence of imprinting in other target tissues would be an explanation for patients with PHP1a who do not develop resistance to other hormones (*73, 74*).

PHP type 1b: There are no features of AHO since defective imprinting does not have an effect on $G_s\alpha$ expression in the majority of the tissues where it is expressed biallelically (i.e., the $G\alpha_s$ genes from both chromosomes are expressed). PHP-Ib is caused by heterozygous deletions within STX16, the gene encoding syntaxin 16, upstream of GNAS, or by deletions within GNAS involving exon NESP55 and two of the antisense exons (*75*). However, there are the same biochemical features as PHP 1a, including blunted urinary cAMP response to administration of

PTH, associated with selective resistance to PTH and not to other hormones.

PHP type 1c: These patients present with the AHO phenotype and resistance to multiple hormones (PTH, thyroid stimulating hormone, gonadotropins, and glucagon). Gα_s activity is normal and so is G$_i$ activity. Studies show reduced activity of the membrane's adenyl cyclase catalytic subunit, and the molecular defect responsible for this is yet to be identified (*76*).

PHP type 2: Patients present with a normal phenotype, normal cAMP urinary excretion but no phosphaturic responses to PTH. It is probably associated with signaling defects distal to cAMP formation because Gα_s activity is normal. The associated molecular defect is yet to be identified, but there are suggestions that it may be an acquired rather than familial defect.

Pseudo-PHP (PPHP): Describes patients with the AHO phenotype, but without the usual laboratory findings. AHO patients who inherit Gα_s mutations from their fathers develop only PPHP. This is due to the fact that the Gα_s gene is expressed primarily from the maternal allele in target tissues for several hormones (renal proximal tubules, thyroid, and ovaries). Mutations in the active maternal allele lead to Gα_s expression deficiency and resistance to these hormones (PHP 1b), while mutations of the paternal allele have little or no effect on genetic expression or hormonal signaling. The presence of a Gα_s allele, however, is not sufficient in all tissues, and different phenotypes probably result from tissue-specific combinations of haploinsufficiency due to paternal imprinting.

DIAGNOSIS OF HYPOPARA-THYROID SYNDROMES

Hypoparathyroidism is an important part of the differential diagnosis of hypocalcemia. Other differentials include vitamin D deficiency or resistance, renal failure, tumor lysis syndrome, rhabdomyolysis, drugs such as bisphosphonates and gadolinium chelates, postparathyroidectomy "hungry bone" syndrome, acute pancreatitis, and the use of calcium chelators, such as citrate used in preservation of blood. Review of the patient's medical and family histories including all medications may suggest the cause of hypoparathyroidism. The presence of other autoimmune endocrinopathies (e.g., adrenal insufficiency) or candidiasis should prompt consideration of APS type 1. Immunodeficiency and other congenital defects point to the DiGeorge syndrome. Physical examination should include an assessment for Chvostek's and Trousseau's signs, skin signs such as neck scars, bronzing, vitiligo or candidiasis, or signs of liver disease, suggesting infiltrative disease. After surgical parathyroidectomy, hypocalcemia may reflect the hungry bone syndrome or transient or permanent hypoparathyroidism and needs to be carefully evaluated. Laboratory testing should include measurements of serum total (albumin corrected) and ionized calcium, albumin, phosphorus, magnesium, creatinine, intact PTH, and 25-hydroxyvitamin D_3 levels. Since levels of 1,25-dihydroxyvitamin D_3 in hypoparathyroidism may be high, normal or low, measurement of this metabolite of vitamin D is not of significant diagnostic utility.

In cases of hypomagnesemia, an assessment of 24-h urinary magnesium excretion or a spot magnesium/creatinine ratio may be useful in defining the etiology of hypoparathyroidism possibly related to hypomagnesemia. Elevated or even detectable urinary levels of magnesium suggest renal losses as the cause of magnesium depletion, since the kidney should conserve magnesium avidly when body stores are depleted.

PTH infusion/subcutaneous injection and subsequent blood and urinary testing are the most consistent and readily available clinical tests for the distinction of the diverse variants of PHP.

Specialized testing in reference laboratories for fluorescence in situ hybridization, mutational analysis of potential culprit genes, or novel protein/hormone assays and referral to an endocrinologist/geneticist may be warranted to establish the cause of hypoparathyroidism and appropriately treat/counsel patients when the diagnosis/etiology is not clear from routine evaluation.

TREATMENT OF HYPOPARATHYROIDISM

The treatment of hypoparathyroidism ideally should be guided by the implicated etiological process(es). This may involve correction of serum levels of magnesium, treatment of infiltrative disease, or identification of iatrogenic causes to name a few. More generic treatment with a goal of symptom control usually involves administration of active metabolites of vitamin D, such as $1,25(OH)_2D_3$ (®Rocaltrol), in the order of 0.5–1.5 µg/day, as well as calcium supplementation of about 1–3 g of elemental calcium in 2–4 divided doses (2, 77). The desired therapeutic result is to maintain the serum calcium close to the lower limit of normal (8–8.5 mg/dl) while at the same time avoiding the hypercalciuria (>4 mg/kg/day) and hyperphosphatemia that results from increased gastrointestinal absorption of calcium and phosphate in the absence of the renal Ca^{2+} conservation and phosphaturia normally promoted by PTH. If the desired serum calcium concentration cannot be achieved without overt hypercalciuria, treatment with a thiazide diuretic may reduce renal calcium excretion to an acceptable level. For overt hyperphosphatemia, a low phosphate diet and/or the use of phosphate binders may be necessary, although this is seldom needed in adults. This can become an important consideration in children, however, where the intake of dietary phosphate is closely linked with protein intake that is critical for growth.

Another approach to the same problem of excessive renal calcium excretion during treatment with calcium and vitamin D is once, or preferably twice, daily subcutaneous injection of PTH(1-34) also known Teriparitide (Forteo®), which utilizes the renal calcium-conserving action of PTH to achieve the desired level of serum calcium without excessive hypercalciuria while minimizing the likelihood of hyperphosphatemia (78).

The identification of patients with activating antibodies to the CaSR raises the possibility of treatment with pharmacological antagonists (calcilytics) of the receptor (79). Antagonizing the antibody-mediated activation of the CaSR could stimulate PTH secretion and promote reduced renal calcium excretion due to the actions of the drug in parathyroid and kidney, respectively, thereby returning serum calcium toward normal. Even in patients with AH and irreversible loss of parathyroid function, it might be possible to develop a calcilytic that would increase renal tubular calcium reabsorption at any given level of serum calcium by antagonizing the renal CaSR, thereby facilitating maintenance of the desired level of serum calcium without hypercalciuria.

ACKNOWLEDGMENTS

Ogo Egbuna is supported by an NIH career development award DK076733, and Edward Brown is supported by NIH grant, DK078331.

REFERENCES

1. Betterle C. Parathyroid and autoimmunity. Ann Endocrinol (Paris). 2006;67:147–154.
2. Whyte MP. Autoimmune hypoparathyroidism. In: Bilezikian JP, Marcus R, Levine MA, eds. The Parathyroids. 2nd ed. San Diego: Academic Press. 2001;791–805.
3. Myhre AG, Halonen M, Eskelin P, Ekwall O, Hedstrand H, Rorsman F, et al. Autoimmune polyendocrine syndrome type 1 (APS I) in Norway. Clin Endocrinol (Oxf). 2001;54: 211–217.
4. Irvine WJ, Scarth L. Antibody to the oxyphil cells of the human parathyroid in idiopathic hypoparathyroidism. Clin Exp Immunol. 1969;4:505–510.
5. Betterle C, Caretto A, Zeviani M, Pedini B, Salviati C. Demonstration and characterization of anti-human mitochondria autoantibodies in idiopathic hypoparathyroidism and in other conditions. Clin Exp Immunol. 1985;62:353–360.
6. Posillico JT, Wortsman J, Srikanta S, Eisenbarth GS, Mallette LE, Brown EM. Parathyroid cell surface autoantibodies that inhibit parathyroid hormone secretion from dispersed human parathyroid cells. J Bone Miner Res. 1986;1:475–483.
7. Brandi ML, Aurbach GD, Fattorossi A, Quarto R, Marx SJ, Fitzpatrick LA. Antibodies cytotoxic to bovine parathyroid cells in

autoimmune hypoparathyroidism. Proc Natl Acad Sci U S A. 1986;83:8366–8369.
8. Fattorossi A, Aurbach GD, Sakaguchi K, Cama A, Marx SJ, Streeten EA, et al. Anti-endothelial cell antibodies: detection and characterization in sera from patients with autoimmune hypoparathyroidism. Proc Natl Acad Sci U S A. 1988;85:4015–4019.
9. Alimohammadi M, Bjorklund P, Hallgren A, Pontynen N, Szinnai G, Shikama N, et al. Autoimmune polyendocrine syndrome type 1 and NALP5, a parathyroid autoantigen. N Engl J Med. 2008;358:1018–1028.
10. Kifor O, McElduff A, LeBoff MS, Moore FD, Jr., Butters R, Gao P, et al. Activating antibodies to the calcium-sensing receptor in two patients with autoimmune hypoparathyroidism. J Clin Endocrinol Metab. 2004;89:548–556.
11. Goswami R, Brown EM, Kochupillai N, Gupta N, Rani R, Kifor O, et al. Prevalence of calcium sensing receptor autoantibodies in patients with sporadic idiopathic hypoparathyroidism. Eur J Endocrinol. 2004;150:9–18.
12. Kifor O, Moore FD, Jr., Delaney M, Garber J, Hendy GN, Butters R, et al. A syndrome of hypocalciuric hypercalcemia caused by autoantibodies directed at the calcium-sensing receptor. J Clin Endocrinol Metab. 2003;88:60–72.
13. Leonard M. Chronic Idiopathic hypoparathyroidism with superimposed Addison's disease in a child. J Clin Endocrinol Metab. 1946;6:493–506.
14. Craig J, Schiff L, Boone J. Chronic Moniliasis associated with Addison's disease. Am J Dis Child. 1955;89:669–684.
15. Whitaker L, Landing B, Esselborn V, Williams R. The syndrome of familial juvenile hypoadrenocorticism and superficial moniliasis. J Clin Endocrinol Metab. 1956;16:1374–1387.
16. Blizzard RM, Chee D, Davis W. The incidence of parathyroid and other antibodies in the sera of patients with idiopathic hypoparathyroidism. Clin Exp Immunol. 1966;1:119–128.
17. Swana GT, Swana MR, Bottazzo GF, Doniach D. A human-specific mitochondrial antibody its importance in the identification of organ-specific reactions. Clin Exp Immunol. 1977;28:517–525.
18. Li Y, Song YH, Rais N, Connor E, Schatz D, Muir A, et al. Autoantibodies to the extracellular domain of the calcium sensing receptor in patients with acquired hypoparathyroidism. J Clin Invest. 1996;97:910–914.
19. Mayer A, Ploix C, Orgiazzi J, Desbos A, Moreira A, Vidal H, et al. Calcium-sensing receptor autoantibodies are relevant markers of acquired hypoparathyroidism. J Clin Endocrinol Metab. 2004;89:4484–4488.
20. Gavalas NG, Kemp EH, Krohn KJ, Brown EM, Watson PF, Weetman AP. The calcium-sensing receptor is a target of autoantibodies in patients with autoimmune polyendocrine syndrome type 1. J Clin Endocrinol Metab. 2007;92:2107–2114.
21. Soderbergh A, Myhre AG, Ekwall O, Gebre-Medhin G, Hedstrand H, Landgren E, et al. Prevalence and clinical associations of 10 defined autoantibodies in autoimmune polyendocrine syndrome type I. J Clin Endocrinol Metab. 2004;89:557–562.
22. Gylling M, Kaariainen E, Vaisanen R, Kerosuo L, Solin ML, Halme L, et al. The hypoparathyroidism of autoimmune polyendocrinopathy-candidiasis-ectodermal dystrophy protective effect of male sex. J Clin Endocrinol Metab. 2003;88:4602–4608.
23. Hauache OM. Extracellular calcium-sensing receptor: structural and functional features and association with diseases. Braz J Med Biol Res. 2001;34:577–584.
24. Egbuna OI, Brown EM. Hypercalcaemic and hypocalcaemic conditions due to calcium-sensing receptor mutations. Best Pract Res Clin Rheumatol. 2008;22:129–148.
25. Makita N, Sato J, Manaka K, Shoji Y, Oishi A, Hashimoto M, et al. An acquired hypocalciuric hypercalcemia autoantibody induces allosteric transition among active human Ca-sensing receptor conformations. Proc Natl Acad Sci U S A. 2007;104:5443–5448.
26. Pallais JC, Kifor O, Chen YB, Slovik D, Brown EM. Acquired hypocalciuric hypercalcemia due to autoantibodies against the calcium-sensing receptor. N Engl J Med. 2004;351:362–369.
27. Bjerneroth G, Juhlin C, Gudmundsson S, Rastad J, Akerstrom G, Klareskog L. Major histocompatibility complex class II expression and parathyroid autoantibodies in primary hyperparathyroidism. Surgery. 1998;124:503–509.
28. Campbell JM, Knutsen AP, Becker BA. A 39-year-old father is diagnosed in adulthood as having partial DiGeorge anomaly with a combined T- and B-cell immunodeficiency after diagnosis of the condition in his daughter. Ann Allergy Asthma Immunol. 2008;100:620–621.
29. Keppen LD, Fasules JW, Burks AW, Gollin SM, Sawyer JR, Miller CH. Confirmation of autosomal dominant transmission of the

DiGeorge malformation complex. J Pediatr. 1988;113:506–508.
30. Bowl MR, Nesbit MA, Harding B, Levy E, Jefferson A, Volpi E, et al. An interstitial deletion-insertion involving chromosomes 2p25.3 and Xq27.1, near SOX3, causes X-linked recessive hypoparathyroidism. J Clin Invest. 2005;115:2822–2831.
31. AndrewNesbit M, Bowl MR, Harding B, Schlessinger D, Whyte MP, Thakker RV. X-linked hypoparathyroidism region on Xq27 is evolutionarily conserved with regions on 3q26 and 13q34 and contains a novel P-type ATPase. Genomics. 2004;84:1060–1070.
32. Trump D, Dixon PH, Mumm S, Wooding C, Davies KE, Schlessinger D, et al. Localisation of X linked recessive idiopathic hypoparathyroidism to a 1.5 Mb region on Xq26-q27. J Med Genet. 1998;35:905–909.
33. Shoback D. Clinical practice. Hypoparathyroidism. N Engl J Med. 2008;359:391–403.
34. Mannstadt M, Bertrand G, Muresan M, Weryha G, Leheup B, Pulusani SR, et al. Dominant-negative GCMB mutations cause an autosomal dominant form of hypoparathyroidism. J Clin Endocrinol Metab. 2008;93: 3568–3576.
35. Thomee C, Schubert SW, Parma J, Le PQ, Hashemolhosseini S, Wegner M, et al. GCMB mutation in familial isolated hypoparathyroidism with residual secretion of parathyroid hormone. J Clin Endocrinol Metab. 2005;90: 2487–2492.
36. Ding C, Buckingham B, Levine MA. Familial isolated hypoparathyroidism caused by a mutation in the gene for the transcription factor GCMB. J Clin Invest. 2001;108: 1215–1220.
37. Canaff L, Zhou X, Mosesova I, Cole DE, Hendy GN. Glial Cells Missing-2 (GCM2) transactivates the calcium-sensing receptor gene: effect of a dominant-negative GCM2 mutant associated with autosomal dominant hypoparathyroidism. Hum Mutat. 2009; 30(1):85–92.
38. Sunthornthepvarakul T, Churesigaew S, Ngowngarmratana S. A novel mutation of the signal peptide of the preproparathyroid hormone gene associated with autosomal recessive familial isolated hypoparathyroidism. J Clin Endocrinol Metab. 1999;84: 3792–3796.
39. Arnold A, Horst SA, Gardella TJ, Baba H, Levine MA, Kronenberg HM. Mutation of the signal peptide-encoding region of the preproparathyroid hormone gene in familial isolated hypoparathyroidism. J Clin Invest. 1990;86:1084–1087.

40. Parkinson DB, Thakker RV. A donor splice site mutation in the parathyroid hormone gene is associated with autosomal recessive hypoparathyroidism. Nat Genet. 1992;1: 149–152.
41. Chen CJ, Anast CS, Posillico JT, Brown EM. Effects of extracellular calcium and magnesium on cytosolic calcium concentration in fura-2-loaded bovine parathyroid cells. J Bone Miner Res. 1987;2:319–327.
42. Wei M, Esbaei K, Bargman JM, Oreopoulos DG. Inverse correlation between serum magnesium and parathyroid hormone in peritoneal dialysis patients: a contributing factor to adynamic bone disease? Int Urol Nephrol. 2006;38:317–322.
43. Navarro JF, Mora C, Macia M, Garcia J. Serum magnesium concentration is an independent predictor of parathyroid hormone levels in peritoneal dialysis patients. Perit Dial Int. 1999;19:455–461.
44. Donovan EF, Tsang RC, Steichen JJ, Strub RJ, Chen IW, Chen M. Neonatal hypermagnesemia: effect on parathyroid hormone and calcium homeostasis. J Pediatr. 1980;96: 305–310.
45. Quitterer U, Hoffmann M, Freichel M, Lohse MJ. Paradoxical block of parathormone secretion is mediated by increased activity of G alpha subunits. J Biol Chem. 2001;276:6763–6769.
46. Wade JS, Fourman P, Deane L. Recovery of parathyroid function in patients with "transient" hypoparathyroidism after thyroidectomy. Br J Surg. 1965;52:493–496.
47. Mora-Fernandez C, Navarro JF. PTH decrease after radioiodine treatment in a patient with end-stage renal disease. Clin Nephrol. 1999;52(5): 337–338.
48. O'Regan S, Carson S, Chesney RW, Drummond KN. Electrolyte and acid-base disturbances in the management of leukemia. Blood. 1977;49(3):345–353.
49. Wadler S, Haynes H, Beitler JJ, Goldberg G, Holland JF, Hochster H, et al. Management of hypocalcemic effects of WR2721 administered on a daily times five schedule with cisplatin and radiation therapy. The New York Gynecologic Oncology Group. J Clin Oncol. 1993;11(8):1517–1522.
50. Koiwa F, Kakuta T, Tanaka R, Yumita S. Efficacy of percutaneous ethanol injection therapy (PEIT) is related to the number of parathyroid glands in haemodialysis patients with secondary hyperparathyroidism. Nephrol Dial Transplant. 2007;22(2):522–528.
51. Vamvakas S, Teschner M, Bahner U, Heidland A. Alcohol abuse: potential role in electrolyte

disturbances and kidney diseases. Clin Nephrol. 1998;49(4):205–213.
52. Laitinen K, Lamberg-Allardt C, Tunninen R, Karonen SL, Tahtela R, Ylikahri R, et al. Transient hypoparathyroidism during acute alcohol intoxication. N Engl J Med. 1991;324(11):721–727.
53. Multicentre study on prevalence of endocrine complications in thalassaemia major. Italian Working Group on Endocrine Complications in Non-endocrine Diseases. Clin Endocrinol (Oxf). 1995;42(6):581–586.
54. Carpenter TO, Carnes DL, Jr., Anast CS. Hypoparathyroidism in Wilson's disease. N Engl J Med. 1983;309(15):873–877.
55. Lienhardt A, Bai M, Lagarde JP, Rigaud M, Zhang Z, Jiang Y, et al. Activating mutations of the calcium-sensing receptor: management of hypocalcemia. J Clin Endocrinol Metab. 2001;86(11):5313–5323.
56. Pollak MR, Brown EM, Estep HL, McLaine PN, Kifor O, Park J, et al. Autosomal dominant hypocalcaemia caused by a Ca(2+)-sensing receptor gene mutation. Nat Genet 1994;8(3):303–307.
57. Finegold DN, Armitage MM, Galiani M, Matise TC, Pandian MR, Perry YM, et al. Preliminary localization of a gene for autosomal dominant hypoparathyroidism to chromosome 3q13. Pediatr Res. 1994;36(3):414–417.
58. Lienhardt A, Garabedian M, Bai M, Sinding C, Zhang Z, Lagarde JP, et al. A large homozygous or heterozygous in-frame deletion within the calcium-sensing receptor's carboxylterminal cytoplasmic tail that causes autosomal dominant hypocalcemia. J Clin Endocrinol Metab. 2000;85(4):1695–1702.
59. Albright F, Burnett C, Smith P. Pseudohypoparathyroidism: an example of 'Seabright-Bantamsyndrome'. Endocrinology. 1942;30:922–932.
60. Tashjian AH, Jr., Frantz AG, Lee JB. Pseudohypoparathyroidism: assays of parathyroid hormone and thyrocalcitonin. Proc Natl Acad Sci U S A. 1966;56(4):1138–1142.
61. Chase LR, Melson GL, Aurbach GD. Pseudohypoparathyroidism: defective excretion of 3′,5′-AMP in response to parathyroid hormone. J Clin Invest. 1969;48(10):1832–1844.
62. Spiegel AM, Levine MA, Aurbach GD, Downs RW, Jr., Marx SJ, Lasker RD, et al. Deficiency of hormone receptor-adenylate cyclase coupling protein: basis for hormone resistance in pseudohypoparathyroidism. Am J Physiol. 1982;243(1):E37–E42.

63. Levine MA, Ahn TG, Klupt SF, Kaufman KD, Smallwood PM, Bourne HR, et al. Genetic deficiency of the alpha subunit of the guanine nucleotide-binding protein Gs as the molecular basis for Albright hereditary osteodystrophy. Proc Natl Acad Sci U S A. 1988;85(2):617–621.
64. Schwindinger WF, Miric A, Zimmerman D, Levine MA. A novel Gs alpha mutant in a patient with Albright hereditary osteodystrophy uncouples cell surface receptors from adenylyl cyclase. J Biol Chem. 1994;269(41):25387–25391.
65. Carter A, Bardin C, Collins R, Simons C, Bray P, Spiegel A. Reduced expression of multiple forms of the alpha subunit of the stimulatory GTP-binding protein in pseudohypoparathyroidism type Ia. Proc Natl Acad Sci USA. 1987;84(20):7266–7269.
66. Davies SJ, Hughes HE. Imprinting in Albright's hereditary osteodystrophy. J Med Genet. 1993;30(2):101–103.
67. Liu J, Nealon JG, Weinstein LS. Distinct patterns of abnormal GNAS imprinting in familial and sporadic pseudohypoparathyroidism type IB. Hum Mol Genet. 2005;14(1):95–102.
68. Yu S, Yu D, Lee E, Eckhaus M, Lee R, Corria Z, et al. Variable and tissue-specific hormone resistance in heterotrimeric Gs protein alpha-subunit (Gsalpha) knockout mice is due to tissue-specific imprinting of the gsalpha gene. Proc Natl Acad Sci USA. 1998;95(15):8715–8720.
69. Hayward BE, Kamiya M, Strain L, Moran V, Campbell R, Hayashizaki Y, et al. The human GNAS1 gene is imprinted and encodes distinct paternally and biallelically expressed G proteins. Proc Natl Acad Sci USA. 1998;95(17):10038–10043.
70. Wroe SF, Kelsey G, Skinner JA, Bodle D, Ball ST, Beechey CV, et al. An imprinted transcript, antisense to Nesp, adds complexity to the cluster of imprinted genes at the mouse Gnas locus. Proc Natl Acad Sci USA. 2000;97(7):3342–3346.
71. Shalitin S, Davidovits M, Lazar L, Weintrob N. Clinical heterogeneity of pseudohypoparathyroidism: from hyper- to hypocalcemia. Horm Res. 2008;70(3):137–144.
72. Levine MA. Pseudohypoparathyroidism: from bedside to bench and back. J Bone Miner Res. 1999;14(8):1255–1260.
73. Weinstein LS, Yu S, Warner DR, Liu J. Endocrine manifestations of stimulatory G protein alpha-subunit mutations and the role of genomic imprinting. Endocr Rev. 2001;22(5):675–705.

74. Weinstein LS, Liu J, Sakamoto A, Xie T, Chen M. Minireview: GNAS: normal and abnormal functions. Endocrinology. 2004;145(12):5459–5464.
75. Juppner H, Bastepe M. Different mutations within or upstream of the GNAS locus cause distinct forms of pseudohypoparathyroidism. J Pediatr Endocrinol Metab. 2006;19(Suppl 2):641–646.
76. Lania A, Mantovani G, Spada A. G protein mutations in endocrine diseases. Eur J Endocrinol. 2001;145(5):543–559.
77. Bringhurst FR, Demay MB, Kronenberg HM. Hormones and disorders of mineral metabolism. In: Wilson JD, Foster DW, Kronenberg HM, Larsen PR, eds. Williams Textbook of Endocrinology. 9th ed. Philadelphia: W.B. Saunders. 1998;1155–1209.
78. Winer KK, Ko CW, Reynolds JC, Dowdy K, Keil M, Peterson D, et al. Long-term treatment of hypoparathyroidism: a randomized controlled study comparing parathyroid hormone-(1-34) versus calcitriol and calcium. J Clin Endocrinol Metab. 2003;88(9):4214–4220.
79. Nemeth EF. Calcimimetic and calcilytic drugs: just for parathyroid cells? Cell Calcium. 2004;35(3):283–289.

Chapter 31

Premature Gonadal Insufficiency

Janice Huang, Micol S. Rothman, and Margaret E. Wierman

Summary

Early gonadal failure, if left untreated, results in sex hormone deficiency with infertility and ultimately, long-term health consequences. Research in clinical detection, treatment, and mechanism of action has primarily focused on the female with premature ovarian insufficiency (POI); few data are available concerning the male with early testicular failure. In addition to iatrogenic causes, the differential diagnosis of premature gonadal dysfunction includes genetic and autoimmune etiologies. Although the majority of cases are still termed "sporadic" or "idiopathic," research is underway to identify the pathways important for gonadal development and function to characterize the potential genetic and environmental factors that predispose patients to early gonadal dysfunction. This chapter reviews the current state of knowledge concerning these processes and available treatment options.

Key Words: Premature ovarian insufficiency, Early menopause, Estrogen deficiency, Autoimmune ovarian failure, Gonadal dysgenesis

INTRODUCTION

During embryonic development of the female, germ cells migrate to the urogenital ridge to form the primordial gonads. A series of processes are necessary to ensure normal oocyte number and function. It is estimated that approximately seven million oocytes are initially contained within both ovaries (1–3). Over the course of a woman's reproductive life span, only approximately 500 of the oocytes are released, and the other progenitor cells degenerate (1, 4). Various processes may underlie the defects observed in women with premature ovarian insufficiency (POI), including a lower complement of oocytes at baseline, a more rapid rate of apoptosis of the oocytes, or a mechanism that results in an increased consumption of the oocytes through an autoimmune process (5). Research over the later part of the twentieth century has been focused on pinpointing the etiology of POI with only limited success. In addition to the obvious risks of iatrogenic ovarian failure from surgery, radiation, and/or chemotherapy, investigators have described genetic, autoimmune, and metabolic causes of POI that will be further outlined below. A similar differential diagnostic approach can be outlined in the male with early testicular failure, and the data supporting this diagnosis will be reviewed, although data are more limited and mechanistic studies are lacking.

PREMATURE OVARIAN INSUFFICIENCY: OVERVIEW

Premature ovarian insufficiency (POI) was recognized in the 1930s in women with amenorrhea and elevated urinary gonadotropins (6) and in conjunction with adrenal insufficiency by Fuller Albright in 1942 (7). He described a process in which histologic abnormalities of the ovaries consistent with menopause, including fibrosis and scarring, in addition to oocyte depletion, were observed in amenorrheic young women. The term premature ovarian failure (POF) was coined and defined as 4–6 months of amenorrhea associated with elevated follicle-stimulating hormone (FSH) levels in a woman under the age of 40 (8). This somewhat absolute definition tends to exclude a number of women who have clinically significant ovarian dysfunction, but do not meet these criteria. Furthermore, the clinical course of early ovarian failure is often long and unpredictable (9, 10). Thus, the term POI has returned to more accurately reflect the clinical spectrum of primary ovarian dysfunction (5).

Women with POI generally present with signs and symptoms of estrogen deficiency including hot flashes, irregular menses or amenorrhea, and frequent mood changes beginning more than a decade prior to when their healthy cohorts experience these symptoms correlating with decline of ovarian function (10–12). Estimates suggest that approximately 1% of all women meet the criteria for having POI (11, 13). There is often a long delay in the diagnosis of the ovarian dysfunction as providers may fail to measure hormone levels to confirm or refute the clinical impression. During the evolution of the process, however, 20% of women with POI diagnosis experience spontaneous ovulation, and 50% of women experience intermittent ovarian function, making the strict definition of POF less clinically useful (9).

Etiology of Premature Ovarian Failure

Iatrogenic Including Surgical, Post Chemotherapy or Radiotherapy

Women who have had a unilateral oophorectomy have higher baseline follicle-stimulating hormone (FSH) levels due to loss of gonadal inhibin production (14). Some investigators have suggested a decreased responsiveness to exogenous gonadotropins in these patients, but few prospective studies on rates of fertility are available (14). These women have been reported to have an earlier onset of menopause (14), but this could be due to multiple factors including

Surgical

genetic or autoimmune predisposition, vascular compromise, postoperative adhesions, the underlying process for which the ovary was removed etc. Obviously, bilateral oophorectomy results in a dramatic and acute loss of sex hormone production.

Radiation and Chemotherapy-Induced Ovarian Dysfunction

Both radiation and chemotherapy administration to women are associated with early ovarian failure (15–17). In childhood cancer survivors, 6.3% never had completion of a normal pubertal development with functioning hypothalamic-pituitary-ovarian axis and 8.1% developed POI (18). The type of chemotherapy, including alkyating agents, and the extent of the exposure are predictors of risk (18, 19). Combination of chemotherapeutic drugs together with radiation exposure increased the risk of POI (20). Rates increased to over 50% in adult women treated with alkylating agents and to 100% in those receiving high-dose chemotherapy for bone-marrow transplantation (21).

Since only a few cells in the adult ovary divide in each cycle, the ovaries are less sensitive to radiation than the testes; however, since they are in the pelvis, the radiation dose exposure is often higher (22). The dose of radiation and age of the patient at the time of radiation treatment correlate with the risk of ovarian failure (22). Haukvik et al. evaluated 99 women with Hodgkin's disease; of whom, 63 received chemotherapy (23). They reported a 56% rate of POI in women who were treated with alkylating agents. The prevalence was 13%, however, in those who had not received chemotherapy, suggesting the effects of the disease itself or other therapeutic interventions, such as radiotherapy, impacted on the risk of gonadal insufficiency. Some have advocated the use of Gonadtropin-releasing hormone (GnRH) agonist administration to induce a reversible medical castration prior to chemotherapy or radiation to try and preserve ovarian function (24). This is theoretically feasible, but no prospective controlled studies are available. Others have suggested the use of ovarian hyperstimulation and preservation of oocytes or fertilized embryos before administration of chemotherapy (25). Oocyte cryopreservation is less successful than embryo cryopreservation due to the damage to the meiotic spindle from ice crystals (25). Again, no prospective studies are available to evaluate overall efficaciousness of this approach, which deserves further investigation.

Genetic

Turner's Syndrome

The observation that up to 30% of women with "idiopathic" POI have a family history of POI supports the importance of underlying genetic etiology (26). Turner's Syndrome, or gonadal dysgenesis, (X) was one of the earliest disorders to be linked with POI (reviewed in (27)). Clinically, Turner's syndrome is characterized by the absence of a normal second X chromosome in females, denoted X (monosomy). There are a variety of phenotypes that are seen with this syndrome, but common clinical findings include short stature, chronic lymphedema, gonadal dysgenesis, and cardiac malformations (including coarctation of the aorta and hypoplasic left ventricle) (*27*).

Mosaicism, the population of two genotypes within an individual, results in a spectrum of clinical phenotypes observed with Turner's syndrome (denoted 45X/XX, X/XXX, X/XY) and is observed in 15% of patients (*27*). When the mosaic form of Turner's syndrome is diagnosed in utero, 90% of infants will have no abnormal clinical features. However, if testing is done after birth due to noticeable clinical abnormalities, patients with mosaic Turner's will have prognoses that are similar to the monosomic disorder. If the mosaicism includes a portion of the Y chromosome, the individual is at risk for gonadalblastoma (7–30%) (*28*). Thus, karyotyping of all young women with POI is suggested. Whereas only 10% of patients with classical Turner's syndrome patients (X) will have menarche, menses will occur in 40% of those with mosaicisms (e.g., X/XX) (*27*). The variability of the extent of gonadal dysgenesis in the mosaic population is not well understood. In those cases identified prenatally, gonadotropin levels were initially normal 3 months postnatally, reflecting the retention of normal hypothalamic-pituitary-ovarian axis function (*29*). However, as Turner's syndrome is associated with increased rates of oocyte apoptosis (*30*), the long-term protective effects of mosaicism are variable and incomplete, and all these girls or women ultimately develop POI.

Fragile X Syndrome

Fragile X is an X-linked form of mental retardation due to abnormalities in the FRM1 and 2 genes and is associated with a risk of POI from 13 to 26% (*31–34*). These genes code for a protein that plays a critical role in the proper development of synapses in the central and peripheral nervous systems. The severity of the Fragile X syndrome mental retardation phenotype increases with higher numbers of repeated triplet nucleic acids on the X chromosome called permutations. Dysregulation of the FMR genes also plays a role in development of POI (*33, 34*). Women with familial POI have a risk of permutations in the FRM1 gene of 14%, whereas in women with sporadic POI, mutations are documented in only 2%, supporting the role of the gene defect. The trinucleotide repeated gene sequences result in increased concentrations of FMR mRNA, but not protein within intraovarian lymphocytes, which, in turn, are toxic to the gonadal tissue. The exact mechanism by which increased FMR mRNA leads to premature ovarian senescence is not well understood. Women with Fragile X syndrome have higher FSH and decreased inhibin B levels despite normal ovarian function that reflects early ovarian compromise (*34*). The American College of Obstetrics and Gynecology (ACOG) has recommended that all women with POI be screened for Fragile X (*33, 35*). The carriers appear to also be at risk for the development of a neurological disorder called fragile X-associated tremor/ataxia syndrome (FRAX) with ataxia, dementia, tremor, and Parkinsonian features (36).

Genetic Metabolic Disorders Resulting in POI

In addition to mutations on the X chromosome, autosomal genetic abnormalities may also result in POI. Best studied is the mutation of the galactose 1-phosphate uridyl transferase (GALT) enzyme that converts galactose to glucose causes galactosemia (37, 38). These subjects present with mental retardation, liver, and renal insufficiency. Early gonadal failure is a risk in this syndrome. The high levels of galactose metabolites are toxic to a number of cell lineages including ovarian oocytes. Of interest, the destruction of the ovarian tissue by these toxic metabolites occurs postnatally (39). Within 2 months after birth, infants with undiagnosed galactosemia have irrevocable damage to ovarian tissue. However, those infants diagnosed at birth and treated appropriately were spared ovarian damage. These data support the early screening for galactosemia in affected families. Recently, patients with a mild form of the disease with 50% activity were documented to have an increased rate of infertility and earlier menopause; however, subsequent screening of heterozygote women did not show increased incidence of POI (40, 41).

AUTOIMMUNE POI

Support for an Autoimmune Etiology in POI

The observation of an increased incidence of gonadal failure in subjects with other autoimmune disorders such as primary adrenal insufficiency (Addison's disease) or autoimmune thyroid disease (Hashimoto's or Graves' disease) spurred research on the potential autoimmune etiologies of POI in the 1960–1970s (reviewed in (42)). Estimates vary, but approximately 5–30% of women who present with ovarian failure have an autoimmune etiology (13, 43).

Investigators have attempted to use animal models to replicate the autoimmune destruction of the gonad observed in women with autoimmune POI. In studies involving thymectomized neonatal mice, a model in which suppressor T cells are inhibited with loss of self-tolerance, a severe lymphocytic infiltration of the maturing ovarian follicle was observed, suggesting an underlying autoimmune process (44). This was further confirmed in studies where normal mouse ovaries were transplanted into a thymectomized mouse, and these heterologous ovaries were destroyed via the same lymphocytic infiltrative mechanism (45). Antioocyte antigen (AOA) autoantibody titers correlated with the degree and progression of oophritis in thymectomized mice at different stages of development (46). A decline in the AOA titers correlated with the decline in ovarian function. Mice thymectomized during a sensitive period of postnatal growth (generally day 3), developed these autoantibodies against maturing follicles and thecal cells with sparing of the oocyte and this process correlated with increasing AOA titers (*44*). Titers were the highest during sexual maturation (days 50–90) when follicular turnover rates were the highest. The titers decreased substantially in older mice as the ovary was becoming quiescent and atrophic (days 150–360). AOA themselves, however, were not shown to have a direct cytotoxic effect on the ovary or oocyte, making the intial trigger and underlying mechanism of gonadal destruction in this model unclear. More recent studies have identified antibodies against an oocyte cytoplasmic protein called MATER, which is under investigation (*47, 48*).

Attempts to use AOA titers as a diagnostic tool to screen women with POI for autoimmune etiologies have been disappointing (*49*). Antiovarian antibody tests are commercially available using an indirect immunonofluorescence with Cynomolgus monkey ovary as well as enzyme-linked immunosorbent assay (ELISA) techniques. In a study of 30 idiopathic POI subjects compared with 38 control subjects, ovarian antibodies were detected in 27% of those with idiopathic POI by ELISA, but only 7% using the immunofluorescence technique. Conversely, in selected subjects with autoimmune POI with ovarian antibodies detected using immunofluorescence, only 53% had positive antibodies by ELISA (*49*). In a study of women with POI compared to normal women, 13 of 26 of POI women and 8 of 26 normal women had positive ovarian antibodies (*50*). The inconsistency of the results as well as the high false positive rate makes these commercially available ovarian antibody tests not useful clinically to evaluate women at the risk of autoimmune POI.

Immune System Errors   Beyond attempts to identify the specific autoantibody associated with the autoimmune gonadal destruction, additional studies have postulated defects in the immune system contributing to the risk of POI development. Studies have attempted to confirm altered cellular and/or humoral immunity with variable consistency. The detection of a particular major histocompatibility compex (MHC) class II molecule in ovarian tissue of women with POI did not correlate with disease progression (*51*). The major histocompatibility complex (MHC) class II is thought to be the cornerstone in regulating self-immunity as it is involved in antigen presentation. Genetic abnormalities that regulate the DR3 subclass expression of the MHC II are associated with a higher rate of POI in some, but not all, studies.

Reports of increased activated T cells, decrease in natural killer cells, decrease in macrophage migration inhibition factor, and increase in leukocyte migration inhibition factor have all been reported in women with POI and other autoimmune diseases (reviewed in (*42*)). The cytokine IL-12 has multiple roles in the development of the immune system including a shift of the predominance of helper cell types. Two types of helper CD4 cells include Th-1 and Th-2 that are important cell and humoral immune mediators. In the murine model, the Th-2 type predominates in neonatal life; postnatally, Th-1 dominates. Maity et al. reported that the postthymectomy murine model of autoimmune oophritis was associated with a failure of the Th-1 shift in helper cell dominance postnatally (*45*). Administration of IL-12 immediately postnatally to the mice, shifted the dominant immune response back to Th-1 and lessened the extent of the oophritis. Whether these abnormalities occur in human ovaries with POI is unknown.

Association of POI with Other Autoimmune Disorders

Autoimmune POI is associated with other endocrine autoimmune disorders in approximately 30% of cases (*43*). Autoimmune polyglandular syndrome type I and II (APS-I and APS-II) represent the two classically defined syndromes (reviewed in (*12, 42*)). APS-I presents in childhood with hypoparathyroidism, chronic mucocutaneous candidiasis, and primary adrenal insufficiency. APS-II includes primary adrenal insufficiency, autoimmune thyroid disease, type I diabetes mellitus, and a mix of other autoimmune disorders.

APS-I is defined as the clustering of hypoparathyroidism, chronic mucocutaneous candidiasis (although this can be absent in some adolescent patients), and primary adrenal insufficiency (*52*). POI develops in 45–60% of the subjects with APS-I, with testicular failure reported less commonly (2% of 365 patients) (*42, 53–55*). This genetic syndrome is an autosomal recessive disease with sporadic penetrance. Overall, it is a rare disease with an incidence of 1 in 25,000 in Finland but with higher rates documented in some ethnic populations such as Sardinians and Iranian Jews (*53, 55*). Early research suggested that development of antibodies to the 21-hydroxylase enzyme destroys the adrenal cortex with potential concomitant cross-reaction in the ovary (*56–59*). The molecular defect for APS-I has been localized to chromosome 21 to mutations in the AIRE gene, which is a transcriptional regulator of T cells (*53*). More recently, some groups have reported an increased incidence of HLA associations including A28 and A3 in APS-I although the significance of these haplotypes has not been confirmed yet (*60*).

APS-II is a much more common autoimmune disorder affecting between 14 and 20 million people with a prominent female predominance (*61*). Although the classic disorder includes Addison's disease, autoimmune thyroid disease, and type 1 diabetes mellitus, other autoimmune disorders such as myasthenia gravis and celiac disease are observed as well. Five to fifty percent of these subjects have either early ovarian or testicular failure (*55*). Whereas APS-II may target genetically susceptible individuals, some postulate that it may be initiated by an environmental trigger (*55*). The underlying genetic defect in this cluster of autoimmune disorders is unknown. Again, women with POI and APS-II often have antibodies to 21-OH (*58, 62*).

Intensive investigation has explored the autoimmune etiology of adrenal and gonadal insufficiency in these complex disorders as well as in sporadic cases to identify markers of those at risk. Initial studies showed that the enzyme, 21-hydroxylase, was shown to be highly immunogenic, whereas more recent studies have suggested that 17-hydroxylase and cytochrome P450 side-chain cleavage enzymes are also immunogenic and may cross-react with gonadal as well as adrenal tissue (*63, 64*). Chen et al. devised 35S-labeled assays to measure antibodies to 21-hydroxylase and 17-hydroxylase in subjects with Addison's disease with or without APS-I or APS-II (*65*). The majority of patients with autoimmune primary adrenal insufficiency had antibodies to 21-OH (68–96%). Immunofluorescence studies documented the presence of both 21-OH and 17-hydroxylase antibodies in human gonadal tissue (*65*). Whether these antibodies play an integral role in the pathogenesis or will serve as clinical predictors of which patients with other autoimmune disorders such as type 1 diabetes will develop primary adrenal insufficiency or gonadal insufficiency, respectively, is under active investigation. Of interest, women who develop POI in the absence of adrenal insufficiency do not usually have antibodies to the adrenal enzymes, and the pathogenesis of their gonadal failure is unknown.

Autoimmune POI and Ovarian Cysts

A small subset of women with autoimmune POI present clinically with large luteinized follicular cysts, similar to what has been reported in patients with 17–20 desmolase deficiency (*66*). In describing three women with this process, Welt and coworkers documented increased postmenopausal luteinizing hormone (LH) levels together with high normal premenopausal FSH levels (*66*). Concomitant estradiol and androstenedione levels were low, but inhibin B concentrations were high. These data suggested to the authors that theca cell destruction with preservation of granulosa cell function is characteristic of human oophoritis, which would be in contrast to established animal models. Additional research is necessary to clarify the similarities and differences between the pathophysiology of the process in the human compared to animal model systems.

TREATMENT CONSIDERATIONS WITH POI

Hormonal Therapy

If contraception is of concern, barrier methods have been recommended because of a theoretical possibility that hormonal contraceptives might not be as effective in women with elevated

Fertility Issues

gonadotropin levels (5, 67). However, there are no controlled studies to support this hypothesis. Since many of these women are young and estrogen deficient, oral contraceptives are a safe, convenient mode of hormonal therapy (68). With aging, considerations of the pros and cons of long-term low-dose hormone therapy must be individualized (69).

Case reports of intermittent success with ovarian hyperstimulation protocols or high dose glucocorticoid suppression of the autoimmune process in an attempt to restore or maintain fertility are limited (10, 70). There are no clinical trials available. Estradiol therapy alone was not shown to improve menstrual cyclicity. Taylor and coworkers randomly assigned a group of 37 women with POI to receive estradiol (2 mg/day) or placebo for 3 months with weekly ultrasound monitoring of ovarian morphology (71). Over 75% of subjects showed evidence of follicular development and a few ovulated and conceived, but it was independent of estrogen treatment. In vitro fertilization with donor oocytes is often employed for fertility in women with POI (25). The theoretical idea of developing ovarian regeneration with stem cells is intriguing, but at present, this is a hope for the future.

Prevention of or Treatment of Osteoporosis

Estrogen repletion in young women who are estrogen deficient has been shown to prevent bone loss (72). Adequate calcium and vitamin D intake as well as regular weight-bearing exercise should be encouraged. Screening with a dual-energy X-ray absorptiometry (DXA) to assess the bone density can be done; however, pharmacological therapy is not usually indicated unless there are secondary causes of osteoporosis. Referral to a metabolic bone specialist should be considered, as the benefits of using bisphophonates in young women must be carefully balanced against the risks of potential long-term retention in the skeleton (73).

PREMATURE TESTICULAR FAILURE

Overview of Early Testicular Failure

Testicular failure refers to the inability of the testes to produce adequate number of sperms and diminished steroidogenic capacity as assessed by testosterone production (74). Testicular failure can be observed in males who had postpubertal mumps and associated orchitis (74). In addition to these observations relating early gonadal failure in the male to viral infection and infiltrative processes, other etiologies include genetic abnormalities, autoimmune causes, and iatrogenic causes. In comparison with POI, there is a paucity of literature describing the exact incidence or underlying mechanisms of testicular failure. Some have suggested that it is a lack of clinical detection because men do not have the clear-cut signs of gonadal failure as do reproductively aged women who lose their menses (75). Others have suggested that the organizational structure of the male testis compared with the female ovary explains the difference in frequency of reported autoimmune testicular failure (75).

Germ cell migration to the genital ridge occurs similarly in males as in females during early development; however, cues from the Y chromosome allows for further differentiation of the parenchymal cells to develop into Sertoli and Leydig cells while the Wolffian ducts differentiate into the vas deferens and epididymis (74). In the XY male, the SRY (sex-determining region Y) leads to the differentiation of the gonad into a testis (76). Testosterone and anti-Mullerian hormone are produced by week 9 of gestation. Descent of the testicles is mediated by Leydig cell secretion of insulin like 3 (INSL3) as well as testosterone. Local conversion of testosterone to dihyrdrotestosterone (DHT) then leads to the further differentiation of the external male genitalia.

Etiology of Testicular Failure

Early Testicular Failure from Surgery, Chemotherapy or Radiotherapy

Of interest, the male gonad appears to be somewhat more protected from iatrogenic toxins than the ovary. Whereas girls or women receiving chemotherapy or radiation in childhood or adolescence have a high incidence of complete gonadal failure, the incidence is lower in men (17, 21). Incidence of oligo- or azospermia is related to the dose and duration of chemotherapy (17, 77). Spermatogenesis is usually initially impaired, but, because of the recycling of progenitors during spermatogenic development, recovery can occur. The Leydig cell population responsible for androgen biosynthesis is more resistant to chemotherapy or radiation (78), and thus, testosterone production is often maintained even with sperrmatogenic defects.

Genetic

Klinefelter's syndrome (47-XXY) is a common genetic abnormality (1 in 500–800 male births) causing male hypogonadism (79). The clinical abnormalities are often missed at birth unless an astute clinician notes smaller testes; most present with delayed or stuttering pubertal development with eventual hypogonadism. In patients with Klinefelter's syndrome, there is a lack of germ cells, causing the small testicular size at any age of development (79, 80). The seminiferous tubules are replaced with progressive fibrosis, and ultimately, the Leydig cells are unable to produce adequate amounts of testosterone. Some patients have low normal testosterone levels to adulthood; others need supplementation to complete pubertal development. Initially subjects have elevated FSH levels due to the lack of inhibin and normal or high normal LH and low normal testosterone levels. With progressive Leydig cell failure, the testosterone levels drop and the LH levels rise. Androgen replacement is needed only once hypogonadism develops. Other common clinical manifestations include taller height due to the lack of epiphyseal fusion in some individuals, eunichoid body habitus related to the disordered testosterone to estradiol ratio, and gynecomastia.

Klinefelter's syndrome has variability of both genotype and phenotype. Approximately, one-third of patients with Klinefelter's syndrome have genotypic variation. Whereas the 47-XXY genotype is most common, 48-XXXY and 46-XX males (translocation of the testis-determining factor) are rare but are associated with more severe clinical features (*81*). Phenotype is also influenced by a polymorphism in the androgen receptor gene. As seen in Fragile X syndrome, this polymorphism is a trinucleotide repeat error in the translational activity of this gene thereby worsening physical abnormalities. Mosiacism is also common in males with Klinefelter's syndrome (46-XY/47-XXY) (*81*). These individuals have a less severe phenotype with presentations ranging from mild hypogonadism to full loss of testicular steroidogenesis. These men usually do not exhibit gynecomastia (*81*).

Turner's syndrome: A variation of Turner's syndrome in the male is the mosaic form: 45-X/46-XY (*82*).

Premature Testicular Failure and Other Autoimmune Disorders

Males with either of the two classic APS disorders are at risk for autoimmune testicular failure (*52, 53*). Whereas the incidence of POI in APS-I ranges from 35 to 69%, premature testicular failure is reported at a significantly lower rate of 2–28% (*83*). Similar to the models used to study autoimmune oophoritis, the thymectomized mouse model has been used to examine epididymoorchitis (*84*). Some investigators found that tumor necrosis factor (TNF) was a particularly important cytokine in this process (*85*). When TNF was neutralized in vivo, the inflammatory reaction was significantly attenuated. In thymectomized murine models, an autoimmune epididymitis/orchitis occurred at a frequency of 80–90%, and the pathology consistently was antibody mediated.

A number of autoantigens have been identified including the testes-expressed protein (TSGA-10). Reimand et al. amplified TSGA-10 proteins from the sera of patients with APS1 (*86*). These experiments used radioimmunoprecipitation (RIPA) to identify antibody development to the specific protein. More than 7.5% of the patients with APS-I had antibodies to TSGA-10 proteins compared with healthy sera-negative cohorts. The clinical importance of this protein in the pathogenesis of early testicular failure has yet to be determined. Roper et al. searched for genetic evidence of distinct autoimmunity to each of the male gonad components using the mouse model (*87*). This group used whole-genome exclusion mapping to find specific unique chromosomal loci. Three discreet loci were identified: Chromosome 8 for orchitis, chromosome 16 for epididmitis, chromosome 1 for vastitis. The search for the underlying loci responsible is under active investigation. Similar work in the human testis has not been performed.

TREATMENT OPTIONS FOR EARLY TESTICULAR FAILURE

Androgen Replacement for Early Hypogonadism

In testicular failure, there is eventual need for testosterone replacement therapy, but there remains the question exactly when the therapy should be started (88). In men with hypogonadism from a variety of causes, testosterone therapy has been shown to decrease fat mass and increase muscle strength (88). There are data emerging that testosterone may help reduce cardiovascular and favorably impact the metabolic syndrome (89–91). The gynecomastia of Klinefelter's may, in part, respond to treatment with testosterone therapy; more definitively, surgery can be done for removal (92).

Fertility

There are recent developments in fertility options in the male with testicular failure. In Klinefelter's syndrome, although most men are born with spermatogonia, there is massive germ-cell apoptosis by the time of puberty (93). Gonadotrophin elevation generally occurs by that time. There has been some recent success reported with testicular sperm extraction (TESE) followed by in vitro fertilization. In a specialized center, where men were pretreated with an aromatase inhibitor to inhibit local estrogen production to optimize intratesticular testosterone concentrations and spermatogenesis, sperm were retrieved 72% of the time (39 of 54 subjects), and there were 18 pregnancies with a success rate of 46% (18/39) (78). These are exciting observations, but the techniques are difficult and often expensive and therefore should be performed in specialized centers. After chemotherapy, there is a temporary but often protracted period of oligospermia which may return to normal after several years (94).

Osteoporosis

Both testosterone and estrogen play a role in bone density and maintenance of the skeleton in the male (95). Men with hypogonadism are at risk for osteoporosis. We recommend the performance of bone-density measurements if other risk factors are present or as a baseline measurement to get a sense of peak bone mass attained, although in the otherwise healthy young man with early gonadal failure, as in the female, routine treatment of low bone density other than sex-steroid replacement is generally not indicated. Although treatment with testosterone can improve bone mass in hypogonadal men (88), large trials showing decrease in rates of fracture are not available (95). Calcium, Vitamin D, and weight-bearing exercise should be optimized. If osteoporosis develops later in life, there are consistent data to support the use of bisphophonates as effective therapy in men with hypogonadism and osteoporosis (96).

SUMMARY

Premature ovarian or testicular failure is uncommon, but detection and treatment may prevent adverse long-term health outcomes. In addition to iatrogenic causes of surgery and chemotherapy and radiation, the differential diagnosis includes an ever expanding list of genetic causes that predispose to early gonadal failure. Autoimmune etiologies have been explored for many years, but still, there are no diagnostic tests that predict an autoimmune etiology and no specific treatment approaches available. Replacement of sex-hormone deficiencies, where possible, and treatment of the consequences of early sex-hormone deficiencies on other target organs when hormone replacement is not advised should be the goals of treatment after appropriate diagnosis. Future research will define the molecular mechanisms of early gonadal demise and hopefully develop markers of the processes early in their course to more appropriately target disease-specific therapies.

REFERENCES

1. Faddy MJ. Follicle dynamics during ovarian ageing. Mol Cell Endocrinol. 2000;163(1–2):43–48.
2. Nikolaou D, Templeton A. Early ovarian ageing: a hypothesis. Detection and clinical relevance. Hum Reprod. 2003;18(6):1137–1139.
3. Baker TG. A quantitative and cytological study of germ cells in human ovaries. Proc R Soc Lond B Biol Sci. 1963;158:417–433.
4. Faddy MJ, Gosden RG, Gougeon A, Richardson SJ, Nelson JF. Accelerated disappearance of ovarian follicles in mid-life: implications for forecasting menopause. Hum Reprod. 1992;7(10):1342–1346.
5. Welt CK. Primary ovarian insufficiency: a more accurate term for premature ovarian failure. Clin Endocrinol (Oxf). 2008;68(4):499–509.
6. Heller CG, Heller EJ. Gonadotropic hormone: urine assays of normally cycling, menopausal, castrated, and estrin treated human females. J Clin Invest. 1939;18(2):171–178.
7. Leaf A. Fuller Albright 1900–1969. Natl Acad Sci. 1976;5–6.
8. de Moraes-Ruehsen M, Jones GS. Premature ovarian failure. Fertil Steril. 1967;18(4):440–461.
9. Nelson LM, Anasti JN, Kimzey LM, et al. Development of luteinized graafian follicles in patients with karyotypically normal spontaneous premature ovarian failure. J Clin Endocrinol Metab. 1994;79(5):1470–1475.
10. Rebar RW, Erickson GF, Yen SS. Idiopathic premature ovarian failure: clinical and endocrine characteristics. Fertil Steril. 1982;37(1):35–41.
11. Coulam CB, Adamson SC, Annegers JF. Incidence of premature ovarian failure. Obstet Gynecol. 1986;67(4):604–606.
12. Goswami D, Conway GS. Premature ovarian failure. Hum Reprod Update. 2005;11(4):391–410.
13. Nelson LM, Bakalov VK. Mechanisms of follicular dysfunction in 46,XX spontaneous premature ovarian failure. Endocrinol Metab Clin North Am. 2003;32(3):613–637.
14. Lass A. The fertility potential of women with a single ovary. Hum Reprod Update. 1999;5(5):546–550.
15. Warne GL, Fairley KF, Hobbs JB, Martin FI. Cyclophosphamide-induced ovarian failure. N Engl J Med. 1973;289(22):1159–1162.
16. Whitehead E, Shalet SM, Blackledge G, Todd I, Crowther D, Beardwell CG. The effect of combination chemotherapy on ovarian function in women treated for Hodgkin's disease. Cancer. 1983;52(6):988–993.

17. Byrne J, Mulvihill JJ, Myers MH, et al. Effects of treatment on fertility in long-term survivors of childhood or adolescent cancer. N Engl J Med. 1987;317(21):1315–1321.
18. Chemaitilly W, Mertens AC, Mitby P, et al. Acute ovarian failure in the childhood cancer survivor study. J Clin Endocrinol Metab 2006;91(5):1723–1728.
19. Horning SJ, Hoppe RT, Kaplan HS, Rosenberg SA. Female reproductive potential after treatment for Hodgkin's disease. N Engl J Med. 1981;304(23):1377–1382.
20. Wallace WH, Kelsey TW. Ovarian reserve and reproductive age may be determined from measurement of ovarian volume by transvaginal sonography. Hum Reprod. 2004;19(7):1612–1617.
21. Meirow D. Reproduction post-chemotherapy in young cancer patients. Mol Cell Endocrinol. 2000;169(1–2):123–131.
22. Giuseppe L, Attilio G, Edoardo DN, Loredana G, Cristina L, Vincenzo L. Ovarian function after cancer treatment in young women affected by Hodgkin disease (HD). Hematology. 2007;12(2):141–147.
23. Haukvik UK, Dieset I, Bjoro T, Holte H, Fossa SD. Treatment-related premature ovarian failure as a long-term complication after Hodgkin's lymphoma. Ann Oncol. 2006;17(9):1428–1433.
24. Blumenfeld Z, Avivi I, Eckman A, Epelbaum R, Rowe JM, Dann EJ. Gonadotropin-releasing hormone agonist decreases chemotherapy-induced gonadotoxicity and premature ovarian failure in young female patients with Hodgkin lymphoma. Fertil Steril. 2008;89(1):166–173.
25. Boldt J, Tidswell N, Sayers A, Kilani R, Cline D. Human oocyte cryopreservation: 5-year experience with a sodium-depleted slow freezing method. Reprod Biomed Online. 2006;13(1):96–100.
26. Coulam CB, Stringfellow S, Hoefnagel D. Evidence for a genetic factor in the etiology of premature ovarian failure. Fertil Steril. 1983;40(5):693–695.
27. Sybert VP, McCauley E. Turner's syndrome. N Engl J Med. 2004;351(12):1227–1238.
28. Gravholt CH, Fedder J, Naeraa RW, Muller J. Occurrence of gonadoblastoma in females with Turner syndrome and Y chromosome material: a population study. J Clin Endocrinol Metab. 2000;85(9):3199–3202.
29. Koeberl DD, McGillivray B, Sybert VP. Prenatal diagnosis of 45,X/46,XX mosaicism and 45,X: implications for postnatal outcome. Am J Hum Genet. 1995;57(3):661–666.
30. Modi DN, Sane S, Bhartiya D. Accelerated germ cell apoptosis in sex chromosome aneuploid fetal human gonads. Mol Hum Reprod. 2003;9(4):219–225.
31. Oberle I, Rousseau F, Heitz D, et al. Instability of a 550-base pair DNA segment and abnormal methylation in fragile X syndrome. Science. 1991;252(5009):1097–1102.
32. Pieretti M, Zhang FP, Fu YH, et al. Absence of expression of the FMR-1 gene in fragile X syndrome. Cell. 1991;66(4):817–822.
33. Sullivan AK, Marcus M, Epstein MP, et al. Association of FMR1 repeat size with ovarian dysfunction. Hum Reprod. 2005;20(2):402–412.
34. Welt CK, Smith PC, Taylor AE. Evidence of early ovarian aging in fragile X premutation carriers. J Clin Endocrinol Metab. 2004;89(9):4569–4574.
35. Wittenberger MD, Hagerman RJ, Sherman SL, et al. The FMR1 premutation and reproduction. Fertil Steril. 2007;87(3):456–465.
36. Ennis S, Murray A, Youings S, et al. An investigation of FRAXA intermediate allele phenotype in a longitudinal sample. Ann Hum Genet. 2006;70(Pt 2):170–180.
37. Kaufman FR, Kogut MD, Donnell GN, Goebelsmann U, March C, Koch R. Hypergonadotropic hypogonadism in female patients with galactosemia. N Engl J Med. 1981;304(17):994–998.
38. Levy HL, Driscoll SG, Porensky RS, Wender DF. Ovarian failure in galactosemia. N Engl J Med. 1984;310(1):50.
39. Forges T, Monnier-Barbarino P, Leheup B, Jouvet P. Pathophysiology of impaired ovarian function in galactosaemia. Hum Reprod Update. 2006;12(5):573–584.
40. Cramer DW, Harlow BL, Barbieri RL, Ng WG. Galactose-1-phosphate uridyl transferase activity associated with age at menopause and reproductive history. Fertil Steril. 1989;51(4):609–615.
41. Knauff EA, Richardus R, Eijkemans MJ, et al. Heterozygosity for the classical galactosemia mutation does not affect ovarian reserve and menopausal age. Reprod Sci. 2007;14(8):780–785.
42. Hoek A, Schoemaker J, Drexhage HA. Premature ovarian failure and ovarian autoimmunity. Endocr Rev. 1997;18(1):107–134.
43. Conway GS. Clinical manifestations of genetic defects affecting gonadotrophins and their receptors. Clin Endocrinol (Oxf). 1996;45(6):657–663.
44. Nair S, Mastorakos G, Raj S, Nelson LM. Murine experimental autoimmune oophoritis develops independently of gonadotropin stimulation and is primarily localized in the stroma and theca. Am J Reprod Immunol. 1995;34(2):132–139.

45. Maity R, Caspi RR, Nair S, Rizzo LV, Nelson LM. Murine postthymectomy autoimmune oophoritis develops in association with a persistent neonatal-like Th2 response. Clin Immunol Immunopathol. 1997;83(3):230–236.
46. Taguchi O, Nishizuka Y, Sakakura T, Kojima A. Autoimmune oophoritis in thymectomized mice: detection of circulating antibodies against oocytes. Clin Exp Immunol. 1980;40(3):540–553.
47. Tong ZB, Nelson LM. A mouse gene encoding an oocyte antigen associated with autoimmune premature ovarian failure. Endocrinology. 1999;140(8):3720–3726.
48. Tong ZB, Gold L, Pfeifer KE, et al. Mater, a maternal effect gene required for early embryonic development in mice. Nat Genet. 2000;26(3):267–268.
49. Wheatcroft NJ, Salt C, Milford-Ward A, Cooke ID, Weetman AP. Identification of ovarian antibodies by immunofluorescence, enzyme-linked immunosorbent assay or immunoblotting in premature ovarian failure. Hum Reprod. 1997;12(12):2617–2622.
50. Wheatcroft NJ, Toogood AA, Li TC, Cooke ID, Weetman AP. Detection of antibodies to ovarian antigens in women with premature ovarian failure. Clin Exp Immunol. 1994;96(1):122–128.
51. Anasti JN, Adams S, Kimzey LM, Defensor RA, Zachary AA, Nelson LM. Karyotypically normal spontaneous premature ovarian failure: evaluation of association with the class II major histocompatibility complex. J Clin Endocrinol Metab. 1994;78(3):722–723.
52. Nagamine K, Peterson P, Scott HS, et al. Positional cloning of the APECED gene. Nat Genet. 1997;17(4):393–398.
53. An autoimmune disease, APECED, caused by mutations in a novel gene featuring two PHD-type zinc-finger domains. Nat Genet. 1997;17(4):399–403.
54. Kim TJ, Anasti JN, Flack MR, Kimzey LM, Defensor RA, Nelson LM. Routine endocrine screening for patients with karyotypically normal spontaneous premature ovarian failure. Obstet Gynecol. 1997;89(5 Pt 1):777–779.
55. Ahonen P, Myllarniemi S, Sipila I, Perheentupa J. Clinical variation of autoimmune polyendocrinopathy-candidiasis-ectodermal dystrophy (APECED) in a series of 68 patients. N Engl J Med. 1990;322(26):1829–1836.
56. Goudie RB, McDonald E, Anderson JR, Gray K. Immunological features of idiopathic Addison's disease: characterization of the adrenocortical antigens. Clin Exp Immunol. 1968;3(2):119–131.
57. Irvine WJ, Chan MM, Scarth L, et al. Immunological aspects of premature ovarian failure associated with idiopathic Addison's disease. Lancet. 1968;2(7574):883–887.
58. Rabinowe SL, Ravnikar VA, Dib SA, George KL, Dluhy RG. Premature menopause: monoclonal antibody defined T lymphocyte abnormalities and antiovarian antibodies. Fertil Steril. 1989;51(3):450–454.
59. Luborsky JL, Visintin I, Boyers S, Asari T, Caldwell B, DeCherney A. Ovarian antibodies detected by immobilized antigen immunoassay in patients with premature ovarian failure. J Clin Endocrinol Metab. 1990;70(1):69–75.
60. Cervato S, Mariniello B, Lazzarotto F, et al. Evaluation of the AIRE gene mutations in a cohort of Italian patients with autoimmune-polyendocrinopathy-candidiasis-ectodermal-dystrophy (APECED) and in their relatives. Clin Endocrinol (Oxf). 2009;70(3):421–428.
61. Meyerson J, Lechuga-Gomez EE, Bigazzi PE, Walfish PG. Polyglandular autoimmune syndrome: current concepts. CMAJ. 1988;138(7):605–612.
62. Winqvist O, Gebre-Medhin G, Gustafsson J, et al. Identification of the main gonadal autoantigens in patients with adrenal insufficiency and associated ovarian failure. J Clin Endocrinol Metab. 1995;80(5):1717–1723.
63. Falorni A, Laureti S, Candeloro P, et al. Steroid-cell autoantibodies are preferentially expressed in women with premature ovarian failure who have adrenal autoimmunity. Fertil Steril. 2002;78(2):270–279.
64. Dal Pra C, Chen S, Furmaniak J, et al. Autoantibodies to steroidogenic enzymes in patients with premature ovarian failure with and without Addison's disease. Eur J Endocrinol. 2003;148(5):565–570.
65. Chen S, Sawicka J, Betterle C, et al. Autoantibodies to steroidogenic enzymes in autoimmune polyglandular syndrome, Addison's disease, and premature ovarian failure. J Clin Endocrinol Metab. 1996;81(5):1871–1876.
66. Welt CK, Falorni A, Taylor AE, Martin KA, Hall JE. Selective theca cell dysfunction in autoimmune oophoritis results in multifollicular development, decreased estradiol, and elevated inhibin B levels. J Clin Endocrinol Metab. 2005;90(5):3069–3076.
67. Kalantaridou SN, Nelson LM. Autoimmune premature ovarian failure: of mice and women. J Am Med Womens Assoc. 1998;53(1):18–20.
68. Christin-Maitre S. The role of hormone replacement therapy in the management of premature ovarian failure. Nat Clin Pract Endocrinol Metab. 2008;4(2):60–61.
69. Martin KA, Freeman MW. Postmenopausal hormone-replacement therapy. N Engl J Med. 1993;328(15):1115–1117.

70. Kalantaridou SN, Braddock DT, Patronas NJ, Nelson LM. Treatment of autoimmune premature ovarian failure. Hum Reprod. 1999;14(7):1777–1782.
71. Taylor AE, Adams JM, Mulder JE, Martin KA, Sluss PM, Crowley WF, Jr. A randomized, controlled trial of estradiol replacement therapy in women with hypergonadotropic amenorrhea. J Clin Endocrinol Metab. 1996;81(10):3615–3621.
72. Khan A. Premenopausal women and low bone density. Can Fam Physician. 2006;52:743–747.
73. Gourlay ML, Brown SA. Clinical considerations in premenopausal osteoporosis. Arch Intern Med. 2004;164(6):603–614.
74. Lee PA, O'Dea LS. Primary and secondary testicular insufficiency. Pediatr Clin North Am. 1990;37(6):1359–1387.
75. Tung KS, Lu CY. Immunologic basis of reproductive failure. Monogr Pathol. 1991;(33):308–333.
76. Lee PA. Precocious, Early and Delayed Female Pubertal Development. 3rd ed. Philadelphia: Lippincott Williams and Wilkins. 2002.
77. Brydoy M, Fossa SD, Dahl O, Bjoro T. Gonadal dysfunction and fertility problems in cancer survivors. Acta Oncol. 2007;46(4):480–489.
78. Schiff JD, Palermo GD, Veeck LL, Goldstein M, Rosenwaks Z, Schlegel PN. Success of testicular sperm injection and intracytoplasmic sperm injection in men with Klinefelter syndrome. J Clin Endocrinol Metab. 2005;90(11):6263–6267.
79. Lanfranco F, Kamischke A, Zitzmann M, Nieschlag E. Klinefelter's syndrome. Lancet. 2004;364(9430):273–283.
80. Hargreave TB. Genetics and male infertility. Curr Opin Obstet Gynecol. 2000;12(3):207–219.
81. Mandoki MW, Sumner GS, Hoffman RP, Riconda DL. A review of Klinefelter's syndrome in children and adolescents. J Am Acad Child Adolesc Psychiatry. 1991;30(2):167–172.
82. Fraccaro M, Ikkos D, Lindsten J, Luft R, Tillinger KG. Testicular germinal dysgenesis (male Turner's syndrome). Report of a case with chromosomal studies and review of the literature. Acta Endocrinol (Copenh). 1961;36:98–114.
83. Tung K, Taguchi O, Teuscher C. Testicular and Ovarian Autoimmune Diseases in Autoimmune Disease Models: A Guidebook. New York: Academic Press. 1995.
84. Tung KS, Smith S, Matzner P, et al. Murine autoimmune oophoritis, epididymoorchitis, and gastritis induced by day 3 thymectomy. Autoantibodies. Am J Pathol. 1987;126(2):303–14.
85. Yule TD, Tung KS. Experimental autoimmune orchitis induced by testis and sperm antigen-specific T cell clones: an important pathogenic cytokine is tumor necrosis factor. Endocrinology. 1993;133(3):1098–1107.
86. Reimand K, Perheentupa J, Link M, Krohn K, Peterson P, Uibo R. Testis-expressed protein TSGA10 an auto-antigen in autoimmune polyendocrine syndrome type I. Int Immunol. 2008;20(1):39–44.
87. Roper RJ, Doerge RW, Call SB, Tung KS, Hickey WF, Teuscher C. Autoimmune orchitis, epididymitis, and vasitis are immunogenetically distinct lesions. Am J Pathol. 1998;152(5):1337–1345.
88. Bhasin S, Cunningham GR, Hayes FJ, et al. Testosterone therapy in adult men with androgen deficiency syndromes: an endocrine society clinical practice guideline. J Clin Endocrinol Metab. 2006;91(6):1995–2010.
89. Allan CA, Strauss BJ, Burger HG, Forbes EA, McLachlan RI. Testosterone therapy prevents gain in visceral adipose tissue and loss of skeletal muscle in nonobese aging men. J Clin Endocrinol Metab. 2008;93(1):139–146.
90. Saad F, Gooren L, Haider A, Yassin A. An exploratory study of the effects of 12 month administration of the novel long-acting testosterone undecanoate on measures of sexual function and the metabolic syndrome. Arch Androl. 2007;53(6):353–357.
91. Kapoor D, Goodwin E, Channer KS, Jones TH. Testosterone replacement therapy improves insulin resistance, glycaemic control, visceral adiposity and hypercholesterolaemia in hypogonadal men with type 2 diabetes. Eur J Endocrinol. 2006;154(6):899–906.
92. Bojesen A, Gravholt CH. Klinefelter syndrome in clinical practice. Nat Clin Pract Urol. 2007;4(4):192–204.
93. Paduch DA, Fine RG, Bolyakov A, Kiper J. New concepts in Klinefelter syndrome. Curr Opin Urol. 2008;18(6):621–627.
94. Tsatsoulis A, Whitehead E, St John J, Shalet SM, Robertson WR. The pituitary-Leydig cell axis in men with severe damage to the germinal epithelium. Clin Endocrinol (Oxf). 1987;27(6):683–689.
95. Khosla S, Amin S, Orwoll E. Osteoporosis in men. Endocr Rev. 2008;29(4):441–464.
96. Smith MR. Androgen deprivation therapy for prostate cancer: new concepts and concerns. Curr Opin Endocrinol Diabetes Obes. 2007;14(3):247–254.

Chapter 32

Celiac Disease and Intestinal Endocrine Autoimmunity

Leonardo Mereiles, Marcella Li, Danielle Loo, and Edwin Liu

Key Words: Transglutaminase autoantibodies, HLA, HLA-DR3, Gliadin, Gluten-free diet, Genetics

Although celiac disease (CD) is unrelated directly to the endocrine system, it still deserves mention owing to its close association with other autoimmune diseases, in particular type 1 diabetes and autoimmune thyroid disease. CD is an immune-mediated disease primarily of the small intestine but with a wide spectrum of clinical symptoms that is no longer isolated to the gastrointestinal tract. The classic presentation of CD occurs in a young child with growth failure, diarrhea, abdominal distension, and irritability shortly following the introduction of gluten in the diet. However, the clinical presentation of this disease has changed over the past decade, possibly as a result of both improved screening methods as well as the evolution of the natural disease course. Today's celiac patient is often identified through screening due to a genetic risk for CD, who otherwise would not have sought medical attention for relatively minor symptoms if present at all.

Individuals at risk for CD include children with dermatitis herpetiformis, dental enamel defects, type 1 diabetes, autoimmune thyroiditis, IgA deficiency, Down syndrome, Turner syndrome, Williams' syndrome, and first-degree relatives of patients with CD or type 1 diabetes. Children with short stature and unexplained anemia are also at risk.

Autoantibodies to tissue transglutaminase (TG) are a hallmark of CD autoimmunity. It is the single best antibody test for the screening of CD. Transglutaminase is an 85 kDa nearly ubiquitous protein that belongs to a family of calcium-dependent enzymes that cross-links protein by epsilon-gamma glutamyl lysine isopeptide bonds. Gliadin is a wheat storage protein present within gluten that carries a high proline and glutamine content and is an ideal substrate for TG. In rye, the protein is called secalin, and in barley, it is called hordein. All the three proteins are known to trigger the immune response and toxicity in CD, but gliadin is perhaps the best characterized. TG is known to play an enzymatic role in the pathogenesis of CD, through specific deamidation of glutamines into glutamic acid in gliadin. This results in the generation of negatively charged gliadin peptides that fit better into the pockets of the MHC molecules DQ2 or DQ8 and are subsequently more immunogenic to gliadin-reactive T cells. There is currently no known immunologic role for TG, although it has been debated whether or not the presence of anti-TG autoantibodies may neutralize the enzymatic activity. Furthermore, it is not understood why TG autoantibodies even appear in celiac disease. It has been hypothesized that the autoantibodies occur due to the close association of TG to gliadin peptides (forming complexes) that are subsequently taken up and processed during antigen presentation and presented to gliadin-reactive CD4 T cells. These gliadin-reactive T cells are then hypothesized to provide help TG-reactive B cells.

Antibodies against gliadin are also present in CD, but its usefulness in the diagnosis of celiac disease is doubtful, and no longer routinely used. It has been suggested that anti-gliadin antibodies are more sensitive than TG autoantibodies for CD screening in children younger than 2 years of age (*1*), but that remains a controversial topic. However, antibodies (IgA and IgG) against the deamidated form of specific gliadin peptides (deamidated gliadin peptides, DGP) are much more sensitive and specific for CD and may be more useful diagnostically than typical antigliadin antibodies, but this has not been tested comprehensively in children younger than age 2. DGP antibodies have been reported to appear earlier than TG autoantibodies in some cases and may even resolve sooner on a GFD, suggesting that it may be useful for monitoring dietary compliance.

The diagnosis of CD can be suggested by gastrointestinal symptoms such as failure to thrive, abdominal pain, diarrhea, vomiting, or constipation. IgA deficiency is more common in CD (seen in 2% of symptomatic celiacs), and therefore, when suspected, quantitative determination of IgA could be performed to facilitate interpretation of a negative TG autoantibody test. CD can be screened by the presence of transglutaminase IgA autoantibodies in the serum. Diagnosis is confirmed by small intestinal biopsy. Treatment for CD is complete dietary elimination of gluten, known as a gluten-free diet, guided by dietary education from a qualified dietician. There is evidence that even small amounts of gluten ingested on a regular basis by individuals with

CD can lead to mucosal changes on intestinal biopsy (2). Currently, a limit of 20 ppm is proposed by the Codex Alimentarius as defining gluten-free, but there is a lack of solid scientific evidence for a threshold of gluten consumption below which no harm occurs.

CD is a prime example of how genes and environment can interact to produce a clinically apparent disease. Dietary ingestion of gluten, found in wheat, rye, and barley is the trigger for the immune-mediated disease that leads to intestinal villous atrophy, crypt hyperplasia, and intestinal epithelial lymphocytes in the small bowel. Removal of gluten from the diet (in the form of a gluten-free diet) essentially reverses the disease and permits full clinical and histologic recovery. The disease occurs mainly in the presence of the permissive HLA haplotypes DQ2 [DQ A1*0501, DQB1*0201] or DQ8 [DQA1*0301, DQB1*0302] so that the absence of either molecule virtually excludes the possibility of CD. An exception to this rule is when an individual expresses the DR7 haplotype [DQA1*0201, DQB1*0202] along with DR5 [DQA1*0501 DQB1*03] such that a functional DQ2 molecule is still created in trans (in the form of DQA1*0501 and DQB1*0202, which is very similar to DQB1*0201).

Our understanding of the prime genetic risk for celiac disease (DQ2 or DQ8 molecules) allows one to screen those considered to be at highest risk for disease: those with type 1 diabetes, first-degree relatives of diabetics or celiacs, and individuals with HLA-DQ2 or DQ8 (Fig. 32.1). There are three large-scale natural history studies instituted by major universities designed to

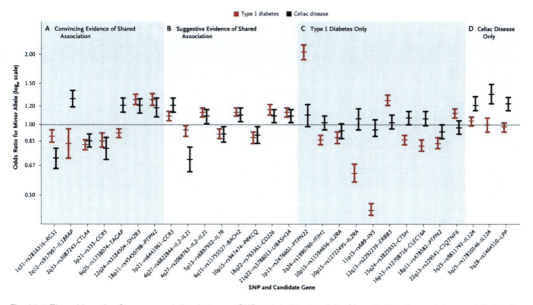

Fig. 32.1 The odds ratios for an association between SNPs related to the risk of type 1 diabetes and those related to the risk of CD. Taken with permission.

identify those at risk for both type 1 diabetes and celiac disease. In the University of Colorado, the DAISY study (Diabetes Autoimmunity Study of the Young) led by Marian Rewers, children at risk for both type 1 diabetes and celiac disease are screened prospectively for the development of both islet and celiac disease autoantibodies. Transglutaminase autoantibodies are measured in regular intervals in children with a family history of type 1 diabetes or if they have been identified at birth as having HLA-DQ2 or DQ8. At present, over 31,000 newborns have been screened for the high-risk HLA from the general population. To date, the median follow-up is 7.3 years, for a total of 18,500 person-years. By the age of 5 years, 8.4% children with DR3/3 genotype, 7.8% with DR3/x genotype, and 1.0% with other HLA-DR genotypes have developed CDA (confirmed TG antibody positive on multiple occasions). The cumulative incidence of CDA by age 10 was estimated at, respectively, 13.7%, 11.1%, and 2.7%. It is known that transglutaminase autoantibodies will continue to appear throughout childhood, but it is not known if the rate of seroconversion is stable in adulthood. In addition, the antibodies can fluctuate dramatically over a period of months to years and at times can even become negative spontaneously without dietary intervention. In fact, it has been documented by Simell et al. (*3*) and us (unpublished findings) that approximately 30% of individuals followed in such a prospective manner will have evidence of transient transglutaminase autoantibody positivity, resulting in confirmed disappearance of the antibodies at last follow-up. However, it appears that those expressing high titers of transglutaminase autoantibodies are more likely to have persistent autoantibodies and are also more likely to have biopsy confirmation of celiac disease. Besides the characterization of the development of transglutaminase autoantibodies, environmental factors have been followed closely for their potential influence on the development of autoimmunity. Evidence from Norris et al. (*4*) suggest that the timing of the first introduction of cereals in an infant's diet may affect the development of transglutaminase autoantibodies – cereals introduced before 3 months of age and possible after 7 months of age were associated with increased risk of celiac autoimmunity. Early rotavirus infection may also cause an increased risk of celiac disease (*5*).

It is well documented that treated celiac disease will result in complete normalization of the intestinal histology as well as improvement in related symptoms. Untreated individuals diagnosed with celiac disease are at increased risk of long-term complications such as iron-deficiency anemia, osteoporosis, and even small bowel lymphoma. However, individuals identified as having celiac disease through population screening are typically asymptomatic, or would not otherwise have sought medical care. It is unknown whether or not asymptomatic individuals diagnosed with celiac disease will have long-term complications as those identified clinically, but this difference between "symptomatic" and "asymptomatic" celiacs may be artificial. A Dutch study of type 1 diabetics found that those also with a diagnosis of celiac disease were significantly lower in height and weight SDS and also had more symptoms on questionnaire. Furthermore, they reported improvement in weight SDS, hemoglobin, ferritin, and mean corpuscular volume after 2 years of a gluten-free diet (6). The ROSE study (Research On gluten-Sensitive Enteropathy) in Denver has followed asymptomatic type 1 diabetics with evidence of celiac disease autoimmunity (persistent TG autoantibody positivity). When matched for age, sex, and duration of diabetes, subjects with celiac disease autoimmunity had lower weight, BMI, and midarm circumference Z scores than those without celiac disease autoimmunity, suggesting that there is a negative effect on body composition (7). Two-year follow-up data in this study do not show significant clinical benefit of gluten-free treatment in those with celiac disease autoimmunity (manuscript in preparation). In a smaller study, the presence of CD at the time of diagnosis type 1 diabetics was associated with lower BMI SDS and also HgbA1C compared to controls. Treatment with GFD resulted in an improvement in BMI in 12 months and further improvement of HgbA1C (8). Despite the lack of good data to support a clear benefit of GFD, current recommendations are to institute a GFD if celiac disease is confirmed, with aims of preventing potential long-term complications.

In guidelines supplied by the AGA (9), NASPGHAN (10), and the ADA (11), recommendations are to screen individuals at risk for CD (including those in a risk group such as type 1 diabetes) after 3 years of age provided they have been receiving a regular gluten-containing diet for at least 1 year, using transglutaminase IgA autoantibodies. The AGA maintains that routine measurement of total IgA levels is not recommended since the prevalence of IgA deficiency in CD is sufficiently low. However, the ADA recommends that patients with type 1 diabetes should be screened with transglutaminase autoantibodies or endomysial autoantibodies, with documentation of normal IgA levels and testing should occur soon after the diagnosis of diabetes and subsequently if symptoms occur. Since there is evidence that individuals with type 1 diabetes or a family history of diabetes or celiac disease could develop celiac disease in the future, periodic screening could be performed over a period of some years and also if symptoms develop.

Once a diagnosis is made of CD, treatment with GFD should be started with the guidance of a qualified dietician providing comprehensive patient education. Unfortunately, adherence to a GFD is as low as 50% in teenagers and could be even worse in an asymptomatic individual. Although detailed dietary history on clinical follow-up may reveal transgressions in the prescribed diet, there is really no good way to truly monitor the GFD. An indirect way would be to follow the serial decrease in TG autoantibody titers over time. However, it can take up to 2 years for autoantibodies to become undetectable with highly sensitive and specific radioimmunoassays, and in some cases, these antibodies may never completely resolve despite best estimates of GFD adherence. DGP antibodies might also be used to monitor dietary adherence as well and has the added attractiveness of measuring antibodies directly against the dietary antigens rather than an autoantigen such as TG. These antibodies parallel the natural fluctuations of TG autoantibodies over time but have been shown to resolve sooner than TG autoantibodies in individuals on GFD.

About 20% of individuals with CD will have other autoimmune diseases – a risk suggested to increase with the duration of gluten exposure (12) – with diabetes (5–10%) (13, 14) and thyroid (14%) disease (15) being the most common (16). In one series of subjects with CD and concurrent autoimmune disease, roughly 1/4 of subjects were diagnosed first with celiac disease, meaning 3/4 first presented with another autoimmune disease. Those diagnosed with CD at a later age (and subsequently treated with GFD) were more likely to have an associated autoimmune disease (12). In contrast, Cosnes found that younger age of diagnosis of CD was associated with increased risk of other autoimmune disease and compliance with GFD was protective (17). In a retrospective study by Bonamico, at least one diabetes or thyroid-related antibody was present in approximately 50% of subjects with undiagnosed CD but in only 20% of patients with CD on a GFD, suggesting that gluten exposure might be a risk for autoimmunity (18). Ventura followed islet autoantibodies GAD, IAA, and ICA for 2 years in newly-diagnosed CD subjects and reported that all resolved by the end of follow-up on GFD (15). In addition, TPO autoantibodies were present in 14% at diagnosis, and after 2 years had decreased to only 2% following GFD. None of the subjects had clinical diabetes or thyroiditis. However, it is important to recognize that spontaneous resolution of single islet autoantibody positivity can occur independent of treatment with gluten-free diet.

Genetic susceptibility plays an important role in CD pathogenesis as is evident from family and twin studies. First-degree relatives of patients with CD have an 8–10% disease prevalence (19), and monozygotic twins have an 83–86% concordance rate (20, 21), whereas dizygotic twins do not differ from siblings. Although CD is a complex genetic disorder, HLA-DQ genotype appears to account for 40% of the familial aggregation (22). More than 95% of the affected individuals have either the HLA-DR3-DQ2 (*DQA1*05-DQB1*02*) or DR4-DQ8 (*DQA1*03-DQB1*0302*) haplotype. These gene variants are necessary for the disease to develop, but it is not sufficient in itself. Forty percent of the general population will also have either DR3-DQ2 or DR4-DQ8, yet only 3% of individuals in the general population carrying DR3-DQ2 will develop evidence of celiac autoimmunity (23), suggesting that HLA typing alone has very low specificity to identify individuals with increased risk for developing CD. The identification of additional genetic risk factors for CD may add in the ability to stratify individuals into different risk categories, as is possible with many monogenic disorders (Table 32.1).

GENOMEWIDE ASSOCIATION STUDIES IN CD

Although the HLA-DQ and DR genes may have a strong effect on CD development, they cannot explain the entire heritable risk. A recent genomewide association study of CD in a UK population (24) (778 cases, 1422 controls) revealed eight non-HLA genes to be associated with CD after replication in an Irish (416 cases, 957 controls) and Dutch cohort (508 cases, 888 controls) at $p < 5 \times 10^{-7}$: *RGS1* on 1q31, *IL18RAP* on 2q12, *CCR3* on 3p21, *IL12A* on 3q25, *LPP* on 3q28, *IL2-IL21* on 4q27, *TAGAP* on 6q25, and *SH2B3* on 12q24 (24, 25). A substantial number of these risk factors have also been replicated in an Italian celiac cohort (26). More recently, the *TNFAIP3* locus has been identified as an additional CD locus (submitted).

The HLA-DQB1*0201 or *0302 alleles, associated with CD, also determine risk for type 1A diabetes and Addison's disease, pointing to shared genetic predisposition. Because of the parallel occurrence of CD and T1D in some patients and families,

Table 32.1

	Prevalence	Prevalence
General population	1:104–1:133	0.7–1%
Non-DQ2		0.3%
DQ2 (DQA1*0501/DQB1*0201)	1:30	3%
Symptomatic	1:33–1:56	2–3%
FDR type 1 diabetes		5%
FDR celiac disease		5%
Type 1 diabetes	1:12	8–10%
Type 1 diabetes + DQ2/DQ2		33%
Autoimmune thyroiditis		7–8%

a more comprehensive study was performed in which the known CD non-HLA loci were evaluated in patients with type 1 diabetes. The same 8 CD-susceptible loci were tested in over 8,000 samples from type 1 diabetics. Three regions, RGS1, IL18RAP, and TAGAP showed strong evidence of an association with type 1 diabetes. In addition, SH2B3 has been previously reported to be associated with type 1 diabetes. Therefore, four out of the eight CD-susceptible loci identified by GWAS are also associated with type 1 diabetes. Conversely, of the 18 type 1 diabetes-susceptible loci tested in CD, CTLA4, CCR5, and likely PTPN22 demonstrate an association, increasing the total number of non-HLA CD-susceptible loci from 8 to 11. In summary, these currently known genetic risk factors for CD explain some 50% of the genetic risk associated with disease, and there are currently seven non-HLA celiac loci that are shared with T1D. These "autoimmune genes" provide the basis for our understanding of the genetic architecture in these autoimmune diseases that tend to occur together. This figure, previously published (27), shows the odds ratios for an association between SNPs related to the risk of type 1 diabetes and those related to the risk of CD. Panel A shows SNPs having strong evidence of a shared association for both diseases. Panel B shows SNPs having evidence suggestive of a shared association for both diseases. Panel C shows SNPs with an association in type 1 diabetes, but not in CD. Panel D shows SNPs with an association in CD, but not in type 1 diabetes. Note that four alleles, *RGS1*, *CTLA4*, *SH2B3*, and *PTPN2*, show the same direction of association in the two diseases, suggesting a common biologic mechanism to both diseases. Although CCR3 and CCR5 on chromosome 3p21 are both independently associated with CD, only CCR5 is significantly associated with type 1 diabetes (CCR3 narrowly missed the cutoff for significance). Since both loci are in the same region, these results indicate that there are two or more causal variants or genes in this region, which is rich in chemokine and chemokine receptor genes. The minor alleles of the SNPs for *IL18RAP* and *TAGAP* regions were negatively associated with type 1 diabetes, but positively associated with celiac disease. Therefore, there may be opposite biologic effects of these two causal variants within the region, or the SNPs may be tagging different causal variants for each disease within the same region.

INTESTINAL ENDOCRINE AUTOIMMUNITY

Celiac disease is not the only autoimmune disease of the gastrointestinal tract associated with type 1 diabetes. Autoimmunity to the gastrointestinal neuroendocrine system is seen in Autoimmune

Polyendocrine Syndrome type 1 (APS-1), leading to evidence of malabsorption, diarrhea, or intestinal dysmotility in up to 25–30% of patients. The gastrointestinal neuroendocrine system plays an important role in the regulation of gastrointestinal motility. Most neuroendocrine cells in the gastrointestinal tract express chromogranin A (CgA), identified immunohistologically as CgA positive, and are referred to as enterochromaffin cells (EC). The main function of the EC cell is to produce peptide hormones, the most common of which is serotonin. In the stomach, there are G cells producing gastrin, EC cells producing serotonin, and D cells producing somatostatin. The small intestine contains multiple endocrine cell types, including cells producing cholecystokinin, secretin, gastric inhibitory polypeptide, motilin, enteroglucagon, substance P, and neurotensin-storing cells. In the colon, cells producing peptide YY, glicentin, serotonin, and somatostatin along with many other hormones are present. Some gastrointestinal peptides, such as somatostatin or pancreatic glucagon, were found to be abnormal in patients with severe idiopathic constipation (*28*). These observations indicate that the gastrointestinal neuroendocrine system may contribute to the pathology of altered colonic motility.

Autoantibodies against the neurotransmitter tryptophan hydroxylase and also histidine decarboxylase are present in patients with APS-1 and gastrointestinal dysfunction. Tryptophan hydroxylase is the rate-limiting step of serotonin synthesis and is found in enterochromaffin cells as well as neuronal cells in the intestine, suggesting that autoimmunity to this autoantigen may lead to intestinal dysmotility. Sera from these individuals stain enterochromaffin cells producing serotonin on duodenal biopsy (for those with autoantibodies to tryptophan hydroxylase) and histamine on gastric biopsy (for those with autoantibodies to histidine decarboxylase). Both are associated with loss of their respective serotonin- or histamine-producing EC cells (*29*). Both autoantibodies to HDC and TPH are also seen in patients having APS-1 with evidence of chronic active hepatitis (presumed to be autoimmune hepatitis) even though endocrine cells have not been described to be expressed in the liver. In a larger study of ten autoantibodies identified in APS-1, autoimmune hepatitis was associated with autoantibodies to (aromatic L-amino acid decarboxylase (AADC), TPH, and cytochrome P450 1A2 (CYP 1A2) (*30*). Radiobinding assays have been established for all of these autoantigens, and allow for molecular-based autoantibody testing in a high-throughput fashion.

Unfortunately, clinical manifestations of gastrointestinal dysfunction have been poorly described in all of these series. A case report describes the presence of fat malabsorption felt due to a deficiency in cholecystokinin and loss of CCK-producing EC in the duodenum, although autoantibodies were not identified (*31*).

However, specific symptoms related to autoantibodies such as intractable constipation or diarrhea have not been classified. It is possible that such intestinal endocrine autoantibodies may not be restricted to only APS-1. For example, a reduction in colonic endocrine cells, namely, enteroglucagon and serotonin immunoreactive cells has been implicated in idiopathic slow-transit constipation. Such abnormalities in EC cells and levels of serotonin and peptide YY have been documented to be associated with colonic inertia in presumably nonautoimmune patients (*32–34*). Therefore, as more neuroendocrine autoantigens are identified, phenotypic characterization should be performed to help identify clinical symptoms potentially associated with loss of specific cells. Furthermore, if molecular-based autoantibody assays are available, then the search for such autoantibodies in gastrointestinal disorders not previously thought to be autoimmune might be revealing.

REFERENCES

1. Lagerqvist C, Dahlbom I, Hansson T, et al. Antigliadin immunoglobulin A best in finding celiac disease in children younger than 18 months of age. J Pediatr Gastroenterol Nutr 2008;47(4):428–435.
2. Catassi C, Fabiani E, Iacono G, et al. A prospective, double-blind, placebo-controlled trial to establish a safe gluten threshold for patients with celiac disease. Am J Clin Nutr 2007;85(1):160–166.
3. Simell S, Hoppu S, Hekkala A, et al. Fate of five celiac disease-associated antibodies during normal diet in genetically at-risk children observed from birth in a natural history study. Am J Gastroenterol 2007;102(9):2026–2035.
4. Norris JM, Barriga K, Hoffenberg EJ, et al. Risk of celiac disease autoimmunity and timing of gluten introduction in the diet of infants at increased risk of disease. JAMA 2005;293(19):2343–2351.
5. Stene LC, Honeyman MC, Hoffenberg EJ, et al. Rotavirus infection frequency and risk of celiac disease autoimmunity in early childhood: a longitudinal study. Am J Gastroenterol 2006;101(10):2333–2340.
6. Hansen D, Brock-Jacobsen B, Lund E, et al. Clinical benefit of a gluten-free diet in type 1 diabetic children with screening-detected celiac disease: a population-based screening study with 2 years' follow-up. Diab care 2006;29(11):2452–2456.
7. Simmons JH, Klingensmith GJ, McFann K, et al. Impact of celiac autoimmunity on children with type 1 diabetes. J Pediatr 2007;150(5):461–466.
8. Amin R, Murphy N, Edge J, Ahmed ML, Acerini CL, Dunger DB. A longitudinal study of the effects of a gluten-free diet on glycemic control and weight gain in subjects with type 1 diabetes and celiac disease. Diabetes Care 2002;25(7):1117–1122.
9. AGA Institute. AGA Institute Medical Position Statement on the Diagnosis and Management of Celiac Disease. Gastroenterology 2006;131(6):1977–1980.
10. Hill ID, Dirks MH, Liptak GS, et al. Guideline for the diagnosis and treatment of celiac disease in children: recommendations of the North American Society for Pediatric Gastroenterology, Hepatology and Nutrition. J Pediatr Gastroenterol Nutr 2005;40(1):1–19.
11. Silverstein J, Klingensmith G, Copeland K, et al. Care of children and adolescents with type 1 diabetes: a statement of the American Diabetes Association. Diabetes Care 2005;28(1):186–212.
12. Ventura A, Magazzu G, Greco L. Duration of exposure to gluten and risk for autoimmune disorders in patients with celiac disease. SIGEP Study Group for Autoimmune Disorders in Celiac Disease. Gastroenterology 1999;117(2): 297–303.
13. Cronin CC, Feighery A, Ferriss JB, Liddy C, Shanahan F, Feighery C. High prevalence of celiac disease among patients with insulin-dependent (type I) diabetes mellitus. Am J Gastroenterol 1997;92(12):2210–2212.
14. Not T, Tommasini A, Tonini G, et al. Undiagnosed coeliac disease and risk of autoim-

mune disorders in subjects with Type I diabetes mellitus. Diabetologia 2001;44(2):151–155.
15. Ventura A, Neri E, Ughi C, Leopaldi A, Citta A, Not T. Gluten-dependent diabetes-related and thyroid-related autoantibodies in patients with celiac disease. J Pediatr 2000;137(2):263–265.
16. Neuhausen SL, Steele L, Ryan S, et al. Co-occurrence of celiac disease and other autoimmune diseases in celiacs and their first-degree relatives. J Autoimmun 2008;31(2):160–165.
17. Cosnes J, Cellier C, Viola S, et al. Incidence of autoimmune diseases in celiac disease: protective effect of the gluten-free diet. Clin Gastroenterol Hepatol 2008;6(7):753–758.
18. Toscano V, Conti FG, Anastasi E, et al. Importance of gluten in the induction of endocrine autoantibodies and organ dysfunction in adolescent celiac patients. Am J Gastroenterol 2000;95(7):1742–1748.
19. Hogberg L, Falth-Magnusson K, Grodzinsky E, Stenhammar L. Familial prevalence of coeliac disease: a twenty-year follow-up study. Scand J Gastroenterol 2003;38(1):61–65.
20. Greco L, Romino R, Coto I, et al. The first large population based twin study of coeliac disease. Gut 2002;50(5):624–628.
21. Nistico L, Fagnani C, Coto I, et al. Concordance, disease progression, and heritability of coeliac disease in Italian twins. Gut 2006;55(6):803–808.
22. Bevan S, Popat S, Braegger CP, et al. Contribution of the MHC region to the familial risk of coeliac disease. J Med Genet 1999;36(9):687–690.
23. Hoffenberg EJ, Mackenzie T, Barriga KJ, et al. A prospective study of the incidence of childhood celiac disease. J Pediatr 2003;143(3):308–314.
24. Hunt KA, Zhernakova A, Turner G, et al. Newly identified genetic risk variants for celiac disease related to the immune response. Nat Genet 2008;40(4):395–402.
25. van Heel DA, Franke L, Hunt KA, et al. A genome-wide association study for celiac disease identifies risk variants in the region harboring IL2 and IL21. Nat Genet 2007;39(7):827–829.
26. Romanos J, Barisani D, Trynka G, Zhernakova A, Bardella MT, Wijmenga C. Six new celiac disease loci replicated in an Italian population confirm association to celiac disease. J Med Genet 2009;46(1):60–63.
27. Smyth DJ, Plagnol V, Walker NM, et al. Shared and distinct genetic variants in type 1 diabetes and celiac disease. N Engl J Med 2008;359(26):2767–2777.
28. van der Sijp JR, Kamm MA, Nightingale JM, et al. Circulating gastrointestinal hormone abnormalities in patients with severe idiopathic constipation. Am J Gastroenterol 1998;93(8):1351–1356.
29. Ekwall O, Hedstrand H, Grimelius L, et al. Identification of tryptophan hydroxylase as an intestinal autoantigen. Lancet 1998;352(9124):279–283.
30. Soderbergh A, Myhre AG, Ekwall O, et al. Prevalence and clinical associations of 10 defined autoantibodies in autoimmune polyendocrine syndrome type I. J Clin Endocrinol Metab 2004;89(2):557–562.
31. Hogenauer C, Meyer RL, Netto GJ, et al. Malabsorption due to cholecystokinin deficiency in a patient with autoimmune polyglandular syndrome type I. N Engl J Med 2001;344(4):270–274.
32. Zhao RH, Baig KM, Wexner SD, et al. Abnormality of peptide YY and pancreatic polypeptide immunoreactive cells in colonic mucosa of patients with colonic inertia. Dig Dis Sci 2004;49(11–12):1786–1790.
33. Zhao R, Baig MK, Wexner SD, et al. Enterochromaffin and serotonin cells are abnormal for patients with colonic inertia. Dis Colon Rectum 2000;43(6):858–863.
34. Baig MK, Zhao RH, Woodhouse SL, et al. Variability in serotonin and enterochromaffin cells in patients with colonic inertia and idiopathic diarrhoea as compared to normal controls. Colorectal Dis 2002;4(5):348–354.

Chapter 33

Pituitary Autoimmunity

Annamaria De Bellis, Antonio Bizzarro, and Antonio Bellastella

Summary

Lymphocytic hypophysitis (LYH) is an autoimmune disease characterized by selective destruction of pituitary hormone-secreting cells due to an autoimmune aggression to pituitary gland. Moreover, the organ-specific disease of the neurohypophyseal system is characterized by selective immune attack to hypothalamic vasopressin-secreting cells often accompanied by lymphocytic-infundibulo neurohypophysitis (autoimmune inflammatory process involving the infundibulum stem and the posterior lobe). Even though LYH is still considered uncommon, its true prevalence and incidence are underestimated because it is largely misdiagnosed. With regard to criteria for autoimmunity in LYH, animal models of LYH, as indirect evidence, and presence of listing of autoimmune markers, as circumstantial evidence, have been described. Pituitary biopsy is still considered the gold diagnostic standard for LYH in symptomatic patients, but it is not always consented because it is an invasive procedure. Morphological findings on magnetic resonance imaging (MRI) of hypothalamic-pituitary region may be helpful, but sometimes they overlap those of pituitary adenoma. Thus, search for antipituitary antibodies (APA) could be considered a further tool for diagnosing LYH. However, even though organ-specific antibodies are thought to be good markers of many autoimmune endocrine diseases, the role of APA in LYH is still discussed owing to various methodological and clinical interpretative difficulties. In fact, several methods have been proposed to detect APA; immunoblotting assay and in vitro transcription–translation and immunoprecipitation of pituitary protein assay have identified a significant number of putative pituitary antigens. A recent reevaluation of APA by immunofluorescence method in patients with other autoimmune diseases and in patients with apparently idiopathic hypopituitarism allowed us to find out those with pituitary impairment (APA positive at high titers), suggesting that the occurrence of LYH in these patients is more frequent than that so far considered. Moreover, a selective staining of somatotrophs and gonadotrophs in patients with idiopathic isolated growth hormone deficiency and in patients with isolated hygonadotropic hypogonadism, respectively, has been evidenced by a four-layer fluorochrome method. The detection of APA immunostaining selectively the pituitary hormone-producing cells could be suggested as an ideal tool in diagnosing LYH in patients with hypopituitarism and normal morphological findings on hypothalamic-pituitary MRI.

With respect to the therapeutic strategy of LYH, a careful follow-up is required in patients without important adrenal impairment and symptoms and/or signs of severe compression as the visual field impairment, since a possible spontaneous remission can occur. Corticosteroid or other immunosuppressive therapies in patients with pituitary-mass symptoms have been proposed not only to reduce the pituitary mass but also to recover pituitary function. Moreover, replacement therapy of pituitary hormone deficiencies, when occurring, has to be associated. Cabergoline therapy in patients with hyperprolactinemia and hypopituitarism has been observed to induce remission of pituitary impairment in some patients with

LYH, probably interrupting the immune damage of the pituitary cells through the normalization of PRL levels and/or a direct immunosuppressive effect of the drug, but further studies are required to confirm these assumptions.

Key Words: Antipituitary antibodies, Idiopathic hypopituitarism, Lymphocytic hypophysitis, T lymphocyte infiltration

INTRODUCTION

Inflammatory processes of the pituitary gland can be classified as primary, in which the inflammation primitively affects the pituitary gland, or secondary when the inflammatory pituitary process is induced by systemic diseases or is confined around pituitary lesions as craniopharyngiomas and pituitary adenomas (1). Primary hypophysitis is classified on the histological basis into three subtypes: granulomatous hypophysitis (GHR), xanthomatous hypophysitis (XH), and lymphocytic hypophysitis (LYH) (2). It is still discussed whether these are three truly distinct entities or different expressions of the same disease, since they share some characteristics and some authors suggest a common autoimmune pathogenesis (3). Anyway, autoimmune hypophysitis is usually identified as LYH, which is characterized by an extensive infiltration of the pituitary gland by lymphoplasmacytic cells (4). The lymphocytic infiltration involving the infundibulum stem and the posterior lobe is considered as lymphocytic infudibuloneurohypophysitis. This spontaneous reversible inflammatory process sometimes occurs when an autoimmune specific disease of the neurohypophyseal system, characterized by selective immune attack to vasopressin-producing cells of the hypothalamic nuclei, involves also the infundibulum and the posterior lobe (5). The lymphocytic infudibulopanhypophysitis (LIPH) is characterized by the global involvement of the anterior lobe, the posterior one, and the infudibulum (Table 33.1) (6). In this chapter, we will discuss only about LYH.

HISTORICAL NOTES

Two cases of Addison's disease with lymphoid infiltration extended not only to the adrenal gland but also to the thyroid and the pituitary were identified from 1930 to 1937 (7, 8). Subsequently, a case of panhypopituitarism due to lymphoplasmacytic pituitary infiltration was described by Rapp and Pashkis in 1953, (9) but these authors could not classify this disorder as autoimmune

Table 33.1
Classification of Hypophysitis

Primary	Secondary
Lymphocytic hypophysitis	• Local lesions • Germinomas • Craniopharyngiomas • Pituitary adenomas
Granulomatous hypophysitis	• Systemic diseases • Crohn's disease • Sarcoidosis • Wegener's granulomatosis • Takayasu's disease • Langerhans cell histiocytosis • Infective etiology • Bacterial fungal
Xanthomatous hypophysitis	

because the concept of the endocrine autoimmunity was introduced only some years later for Hashimoto's thyroiditis (10). Goudie and Pinkerton (11) in 1962 described the occurrence of postpartum amenorrhea and hypothyroidism in a young woman who subsequently died of severe acute secondary adrenal insufficiency after appendicectomy. Autoptical findings showed infiltration of lymphocytes and plasma cells in pituitary other than in thyroid and adrenal gland, suggesting for the first time that autoimmunity could play a role also in affecting pituitary gland.

EPIDEMIOLOGY

Few information is available on the incidence and prevalence of hypophysitis, and the population-based data are scarce (12). Very few cases of LYH were described in the literature after the first description and before the introduction of pituitary biopsy and magnetic resonance imaging (MRI) as diagnostic procedures (13–15); then, in subsequent years, the number of diagnosed cases of this autoimmune disease was considerably increased, probably due to improved imaging criteria (16). In particular, about 500 cases of LYH have been diagnosed until March 2008, only taking into account the cases in which the marked inflammatory process of the pituitary gland is able to determine the symptoms and signs related to pituitary enlargement (*17–19*). At present, LYH is still considered uncommon, but its true prevalence and incidence are underestimated because this disease is largely misdiagnosed (*20, 21*). In fact, histopathological observation by transsphenoidal pituitary biopsy is the gold diagnostic standard for LYH in patients with hypopituitarism symptoms and signs of an expanding pituitary mass (*22*). MRI observation is an important tool in diagnosis of LYH, but despite the recent development of sophisticated diagnostic imaging techniques, the diagnosis of LYH on MRI remains problematic. In particular, in many cases of suspected LYH with pituitary enlargement on MRI, the pituitary biopsy is not consented, and frequently in these patients, morphological findings of LYH on MRI can overlap those of pituitary adenoma (*23–26*). Moreover, in other cases, in spite of normal MRI characteristics of the pituitary gland, varying degrees of pituitary failure may be also present; for this reason, in these cases, LYH may be misdiagnosed, and patients are considered to present with idiopathic hypopituitarism (*27, 28*). Finally, specific characteristics of possible LYH may be observed also in patients in late phase of complete or selective hypopituitarism, as in patients with Sheehan's syndrome or with empty sella syndrome or with hypopituitarism occurring some years after a brain injury (*17, 29–31*). Recently, we observed in some patients with idiopathic hyperprolactinemia the presence of antipituitary antibodies (APA) at high titers associated to ACTH or GH deficiency (GHD), suggesting the occurrence of a possible LYH in these patients (*32–34*). LYH is more frequent in women during their reproductive age, and in particular, it is strongly correlated with pregnancy or postpartum period; instead, it is very rare in the pediatric and in the senior population (*35, 36*).

CRITERIA OF AUTOIMMUNITY

For a long time, on the basis of the criteria designed by Witebsky and Rose to define a disease as autoimmune, some endocrine diseases, previously considered as idiopathic, have been recognized as autoimmune (*37*). These criteria have been revised by Rose and Bona who described the direct, indirect, or circumstantial evidence (*38*). Direct evidence requires the transmissibility of the disease from human to human or from human to animal, mediated by autoantibodies, as evidenced in some neonatal autoimmune diseases such as Graves' disease, myasthenia gravis, pemphigus vulgaris; however, this transfer is not yet demonstrated in LYH; in fact, APA are not able to transfer the disease from mother to newborn (*18*). LYH fulfills indirect and circumstantial evidence of autoimmunity. As indirect evidence, studies of animal models with experimental LYH have been described (see after). Lymphoplasmacytic nature of the histological lesions, presence of APA, association with other autoimmune diseases and/or presence of other autoantibodies, improvement of symptoms and reduction of pituitary mass in response to immunosuppressive drugs, and sometimes, cycles of spontaneous remission and relapse could be present as circumstantial evidence (*27*). Studies performed to evidence a correlation between LYH and genes influencing autoimmunity are lacking. Recent reports observed that patients with melanoma and other carcinomas developed LYH and other autoimmune diseases during therapy with cytotoxic T-lymphocyte-associated antigen-4 (CTLA4) – blocking antibodies, suggesting a possible correlation between CTLA4 and LYH (*39–41*). In this context, future studies could evidence that a microsatellite polymorphism on CTLA4 gene, as evidenced for other autoimmune diseases, could be associated with the development of LYH. Finally, it has been shown that the pregnancy influences the course of many autoimmune diseases, and the strong temporal association between pregnancy and LYH suggests that the frequent onset of this disease in pregnancy could be included in circumstantial evidence of LYH (Table 33.2).

Table 33.2
Evidence for Autoimmunity in Lymphocytic Hypophysitis

Evidence	Present in LYH
Direct	*Absent*
Indirect	*Present*
Animal models	
Circumstantial	*Present*
Listing of autoimmune markers	
• Lymphoplasmacytic nature of the histological lesions	
• Presence of antipituitary autoantibodies	
• Association with other autoimmune diseases and/or presence of other autoantibodies	
• Improvement of symptoms and reduction of pituitary mass and/or remission of pituitary failure in response to immunosuppressive drugs	
Close association with pregnancy	
Onset of lymphocytic hypophysitis during therapy with CTLA-4 blocked antibodies in cancer	

ANIMAL MODELS

Some studies on animal models performed in recent years open the way to understand the pathogenesis and the natural history of human LYH. Experimental subcutaneous injection of human pituitary gland homogenates with Freund's adjuvant into rats and rabbit induced a disease hystologically similar to LYH (42, 43); on the other hand, even though the induction of LYH in hamsters is associated to the development of pituitary antibodies, the passive transfer of these antibodies does not spread the disease (44). Some studies suggest that influenza virus could induce pituitary autoimmunity. Onodera et al. infected with reovirus type 1 SJZ mice that developed diabetes, gastritis, and delayed growth; they observed viral particles within growth-hormone-producing cells and antibodies against pituitary cells (45). In 2002, De Jersey et al. created transgenic mice that expressed a nucleoprotein of influenza-A virus (strain A/N/T/60/1968) specifically in growth-hormone-producing cells; this protein determined an activation of monoclonal CD8 cells that infiltrated the pituitary gland with subsequent anterior panhypophysitis and dwarfism (46). These studies support the theory that viral infections can trigger an autoimmune hypophysitis; in fact, a benign meningo-encephalitis associated with LYH in human patients may occur. Recently, in Caturegli's laboratory, it has been observed that female SJL/J mice immunized with mouse pituitary extract developed an autoimmune pituitary disease closely mimicking the human LYH (47). In particular, in the early phase of this experimental LYH, a small lymphoid infiltration appeared in the pituitary gland with normal anterior pituitary function and without APA; in the subsequent florid phase of LYH, a greater abundance of lymphocytic infiltration in the enlarged pituitary gland appeared with subsequent ACTH deficiency and the appearance of APA; this was in strong correlation with lymphocytic infiltration. Finally, in the late phase, the pituitary gland became atrophic with subsequent appearance of secondary hypothyroidism.

ANTIPITUITARY ANTIBODIES

In the last 20 years, a fairly good progress has been achieved in identifying specific antigens in autoimmune-specific diseases. With regard to endocrine autoimmunity, the thyroid, adrenals, gonads, parathyroids, and pancreatic islet cells can be subject to autoimmune attacks, and most of the autoantigens involved have been identified and studied in detail, to use them not only for pathogenetic studies but also for specific autoantibody assay (48, 49).

In most cases, organ-specific autoantigens are proteins with function and activity well defined such as enzymes or receptors, but the expression of these antigens in the affected organs is often not specific. For example, thyroglobulin and thyroid peroxidase are truly organ-specific thyroid antigens not expressed in other organs; by contrast, glutamic-acid-decarboxylase (GAD-65), insulin antibodies (IA-2 and IA-2b), or the calcium-sensing receptor (Ca-SR) are expressed and functional in other tissues as well as in those affected by autoimmunity (*50*). For this reason, endocrine autoimmune diseases could be classified as organ-specific autoimmune diseases when antibodies directed to truly specific antigens or antibodies against specific impaired hormone-producing cells are identified. Although T cells play a pivotal role in the pathogenesis of the majority of organ-specific autoimmune diseases, some organ-specific antibodies are not only good diagnostic markers of the disease but also good predictive markers of future onset of clinical phase of the disease (*51–53*). Lymphocytic hyphophysitis is classified as an organ-specific autoimmune disease because it is caused by selective destruction of pituitary hormonal secreting-cells in the anterior pituitary gland by immune cells. Even if APA are frequently present in patients with LYH, they cannot be considered as having a pathogenetic role because they are unable to transfer the disease from humans to humans or from humans to animals (*3*). In order to consider APA good diagnostic markers of LYH, the detection methods of these antibodies need at least one of these two requirements: first, the methods for the detection of antibodies directed to known antigens have to be able to identify specific pituitary antigens; second, the methods for the detection of antibodies directed to pituitary cells have to be able to identify selectively pituitary hormone-producing cells in impaired functional state. The methods so far used to detect APA have been well studied in recent years but, at this time their diagnostic role in LYH is still discussed for some problems (*27*). To detect APA, mostly used methods are the indirect immunofluorescence (IF), the immunoblotting assay, and the in vitro transcription and translation assay (*12*).

INDIRECT IMMUNOFLUORE-SCENCE METHOD

Using the immunofluorescence method, APA react with cytoplasmic antigens distinct from pituitary hormones, but the target antigens are still unknown (*54*). The main problem of this method is the use of pituitary sections as substrate obtained from a variety of species and under a variety of conditions (*55, 56*). The ideal substrate was considered the fetal human pituitary gland (*57*), but for practical and ethical issues, subsequently, the detection of

APA by these substrates was not yet performed. At present, in our immunoendocrinology laboratory, young pituitary baboon sections have been used as substrate for detection of APA with satisfactory results (28). The second problem for the detection of APA by indirect immunofluorescence is that this method is subjective and not quantitative. In particular, the immunostaining of pituitary gland is very difficult with respect to the immunostaining of other endocrine glands. In fact, two distinct patterns of immunofluorescence are present: the first, characterized by a granular cytoplasmatic staining confined to some pituitary cells, the second, characterized by a diffused staining trough the acini involving the majority of the pituitary cells (multiple pattern) (58, 59). The latter staining may be frequently observed in sera of patients with autoimmune diseases, as autoimmune polyendocrine syndromes (APS) apparently positive for APA (multiple pattern) and with normal pituitary function (57). In this connection, we suggest that multiple pattern of the pituitary cells seems to be nonspecific while the pattern of immunostaining of single cell-types may be considered positive for APA. The third problem in the detection of APA by immunofluorescence is that they can be present not only in patients with suspected autoimmune pituitary diseases but also in those with pituitary diseases secondary to other nonautoimmune-specific causes, such as pituitary adenoma and in some healthy subjects (28). However, in these cases, APA are usually present at low titers (<1:8) and they can be considered negative; on the contrary, in the sera of patients with LYH, only when they are present at high titer (>1:8), they are considered positive, as already observed for other autoantibodies (60).

Another problem in the detection of APA is that the pituitary contains at least five different hormone-secreting cells; therefore, if APA are cell-specific APA, it is possible that APA present in sera of patients with autoimmune isolated GHD may be different with respect to those of patients with autoimmune isolated gonadotropin or ACTH deficiency or with panhypopituitarism. In this view, a four-layer double fluorochrome method, after the simple indirect immunofluorescence, is needed to further identify APA (55, 61). Bottazzo et al. showed that in sera of patients with single or associated autoimmune endocrine diseases and normal pituitary function, APA immunostained only prolactin (PRL)-secreting cells in most sera and, sometimes, all pituitary hormone-secreting cells (62). Recently, we reintroduced the four-layer fluorochrome method to detect APA in adult patients with isolated idiopathic GHD and in autoimmune endocrine patients and, subsequently, in children with idiopathic GHD and in patients with idiopathic hypogonadotropic hypogonadism (63–65). Specific staining of somatotrophs and gonadotrops alone was typical of isolated GHD or isolated gonadotropic deficiency, respectively. However, sera of patients with GHD associated with autoimmune thyroid diseases immunostained not only GH-producing cells but also other pituitary hormone-secreting cells, showing a different pattern of immunostaining (multiple pituitary cell types) as evidenced for cytoplasmatic components of islet cell antibodies (ICA). In fact, in type 1 diabetes mellitus, ICA detected by immunofluorescence have been considered good markers of the specific impairment of beta cells, even though they immunostain not only β- but also α- and δ-cells (*66, 67*).

OTHER METHODS TO DETECT ANTIBODIES DIRECTED TO PUTATIVE PITUITARY ANTIGENS

As previously described, another technique for APA detection is the immunoblotting, based on the recognition of some cytosolic proteins by their molecular weight in sera of patients with putative LYH (*68*). An important problem of this method is that unlike the immunofluorescence method, the sera of these patients react with antigens with linear epitopes without a natural structure rather than with antigens with a tridimensional structure (*12*). Moreover, it is also possible that some antigens present in vivo could disappear during the long and sophisticated preparation of the immunoblotting (*27*). The ideal goal of this method is to identify the molecular weight of the specific pituitary proteins, but this is very difficult because the pituitary enzymes may be also present in other tissues, such as thyroid, hypothalamus, and neuroendocrine tissues including the placenta (*69–71*). The first pituitary antigen reported was a pituitary cytosolic protein of 22 kDa recognized in the sera of patients with LYH and isolated ACTH or GHD (*72*). This protein was then identified as a nonapeptide fragment corresponding to the pituitary GH1 or the placental GH2 (*73*), suggesting that GH could be the target of the antibodies of patients with LYH, as insulin in type 1 diabetes mellitus. In particular, APA by immunofluorescence recognize unknown cytoplasmatic antigens, but not GH, as ICA recognize intracytoplasmatic antigens, but not insulin. Bensing et al. detected in patients with isolated ACTH deficiency, APA against a not well identified pituitary cytosolic autoantigen of 36 kDa (*74*); Crock et al. identified APA directed to a protein a 49 kDa by immunoblotting not only in 70% patients with biopsy-proven hypophysitis and in 50% with suspected disease but also in patients with other autoimmune diseases, with pituitary adenoma and sometimes in normal controls (*75*). Subsequently, this protein was identified as α-enolase, an enzyme ubiquitously expressed (*76*). Using in vitro transcription–translation assay, the prevalence of antibodies to α-enolase was even higher (46%) in patients with adenoma, suggesting that these antibodies are not useful in diagnosis of LYH (*77*). Recently, Lupi et al. evidenced by immunoblotting that the antibodies of the sera of patients with LYH recognized two new candidate autoantigens, one of them identified as chorionic somathomammotropin (78). Moreover, APA have been detected by in vitro transcription–translation and immunoprecipitation of pituitary proteins method. Using this method, Tanaka et al. demonstrated the presence of antibodies against pituitary-specific protein called PGSF1a and PGSF2 (pituitary gland-specific factor) in few patients with proven LYH and also in 77% of patients with rheumatoid arthritis (73, 79).

HISTOPATHOLOGICAL OBSERVATIONS

Histopathological findings by transsphenoidal pituitary biopsy evidence a diffuse infiltration of lymphocytes and plasma-cells (2). These infiltrates are in concordance with the composition of inflammatory infiltrates of other endocrine autoimmune diseases, such as Hashimoto's thyroiditis and type 1 diabetes mellitus (21). Independent from the histopathological observations, T-cell subsets (CD4+ and CD8+), B-cells, and macrophages contribute significantly to the inflammatory infiltrate (22). Moreover, the high expression of MHC-Class II epitope and co-stimulatory molecules B7-1 and B7-2 on macrophages in hypophysitis seems to be important in initial phase of LYH. Lymphocytes are sometimes arranged in lymphoid follicles with a germinal centre, which are associated with focal or diffuse areas of atrophic pituitary cells surrounded by lymphoplasmacytic aggregates whereas areas of reactive fibrosis can be observed in the remaining pituitary tissue.

ASSOCIATION WITH OTHER AUTOIMMUNE DISEASES AND WITH OTHER ORGAN-SPECIFIC ANTIBODIES

Autoimmune endocrine diseases are characterized by their frequent association in the same patient not only with other autoimmune endocrine diseases but also with nonendocrine autoimmune diseases. This autoimmune overlapping condition in the same individual indicates an APS (48, 80). Also, LYH is frequently associated with other endocrine and nonendocrine autoimmune disease (Table 33.3); the most common association of LYH is with autoimmune thyroid diseases (28, 81, 82). Moreover, the association with central diabetes insipidus, type 1 diabetes mellitus, Addison's disease, hypoparathyroidism, chronic atrophic gastritis, pernicious anemia, and celiac disease has been described (56, 75, 83–87). Less frequently, LYH can be associated with systemic lupus erythematosus, Sjögren's syndrome, rheumathoid arthritis, autoimmune hepatitis, and primary biliary cirrhosis (88–91). Moreover, in patients affected by LYH, some organ-specific antibodies can be detected in spite of normal functional state or subclinical impairment of the respective glands (21) (Table 33.4). The coexistence of LYH with one or more organ- and/or nonorgan-specific autoimmune diseases indicates an APS (27). In particular, when LYH is associated with hypoparathyroidism, mucocutaneous candidiasis, and Addison's disease, it could be included among the autoimmune diseases of type 1 APS (92). Few cases of LYH could fall within the complete type 2 APS when associated with Addison's disease, autoimmune thyroid disease, and/or type 1

Table 33.3

Organ-specific autoimmune diseases

Endocrine	Non endocrine	Intermediated	Systemic autoimmune diseases
Type-1 diabetes mellitus	Celiac disease	Primary biliary cirrhosis	Systemic lupus erythematosus (LES)
Hashimoto's thyroiditis	Chronic atrohic gastritis	Autoimmune hepatitis	Sjogren's syndrome (SS)
Graves' disease	Multiple sclerosis		Rheumatoid arthritis (AR)
Addison's disease			

Table 33.4
Organ-Specific Antibodies in Lymphocytic Hypophysitis

Thyroperoxidase antibodies (TPOAbs)
Thyroglobulin antibodies (TgAbs)
Vasopressin-cell antibodies (AVPcAbs)
Islet-cell antibodies (ICAs)
Glutamic acid decarboxylase antibodies (GADAbs)
Adrenocortical antibodies (ACAs)
21-Hydroxylase antibodies (21-OHAbs)
Parietal-cell antibodies (PCAs)
Tissue transglutaminase antibodies (TTGAs)

diabetes mellitus; in other cases, LYH is included in incomplete type 2 APS when associated with chronic autoimmune thyroiditis and presence of adrenal antibodies (ACA), 21-hydroxylase antibodies (21-OHAb), and ICA (*20, 21, 27*). Most cases of LYH show characteristics of complete type-3 APS (autoimmune thyroid disease with or without other autoimmune disease, but not Addison's disease and hypoparathyroidism) (*82*). Finally, when LYH does not belong to the above mentioned combinations, it can be included in type 4 APS, e.g., coexistence of LYH with autoimmune central diabetes insipidus and/or presence of vasopressin-cell antibodies (AVPcAb) (*93*).

LYH AND PREGNANCY

A complex interaction between the maternal endocrine system and immune system could influence the course of autoimmune diseases in pregnancy. Some autoimmune diseases, such as rheumatoid arthritis and multiple sclerosis, may improve, others, such as systemic lupus erythematosus, can worsen during pregnancy (*94, 95*). LYH is the only autoimmune disease that shows a close temporal relationship with pregnancy (*14*). In particular, LYH may be present in young pregnant women in the second or third trimester rather than in the first one with frequent subsequent spontaneous remission of pituitary/mass symptoms, hypopituitarism, and disappearance of APA in a more or less long period after delivery (*96–98*). Currently, the reason for this particular relationship between LYH and pregnancy is not well known; even though, during pregnancy, the hypertrophy and hyperplasia of pituitary cells usually occur, and the hyperestrogenism increases the pituitary blood flow (*29*). In this connection, it is possible that pituitary cryptic antigens, becoming much more accessible to the immune system, can trigger autoimmune pituitary process in pregnancy (*30*). However, some putative pituitary antigens have the same epitope of placental antigens as observed by O'Dwjer et al. (*69*) who showed that pituitary autoantibodies from patients with peripartum LYH recognize enolase in the pituitary as well as in the placenta. Moreover, as described above, pituitary GH-1 sharing with placental GH-2 and chorionic somatomammotropin was recently identified (*73, 78*). In conclusion, the sharing of placental and pituitary antigens (molecular mimicry) could explain the association of LYH with pregnancy. Another possible cause of the close association between LYH and pregnancy, in particular, could be the presence of high PRL levels in this condition. With regard to PRL, many studies evidenced its immunostimulatory role; in particular, we recently observed that high PRL levels could have a role in perpetuating the immune process in LYH (*32, 33*).

DIAGNOSIS

The diagnosis of LYH is very difficult, as previously described in epidemiological section; taking into account that at onset, this autoimmune disease can present with two different phases, its natural history is very variable (26). In fact, during the natural history of the disease an endless series of reversible changes in morphological, clinical, and functional findings of the disease can be observed, and the rise and fall of APA were frequently noted (27). For this reason, we suggest that the changes of characteristics of LYH could be due to the metamorphosis of pituitary autoimmunity. At the onset of the disease, the first phase of LYH is characterized by pituitary mass/effect-related symptoms and signs frequently accompanied by symptoms of pituitary failure (99, 100); the second face of LYH is characterized by normal characteristics on MRI and varying degrees of pituitary failure. Even though the pituitary biopsy is still considered the diagnostic gold standard for LYH when symptoms of mass effect are present, it is an invasive procedure not always consented by the patients (20). In these cases, a presumptive diagnosis of LYH with pituitary enlargement could be made on the basis of clinical features and imaging and laboratory findings (4). In particular, with regard to the symptoms of mass effect, headache develops frequently and occurs in a dramatic fashion and then other symptoms, such as visual impairment, nausea, and vomiting, could also be present (17). Moreover, with regard to symptoms due to isolated/multiple pituitary hormone deficiencies, ACTH is the most frequent as the earliest pituitary hormone deficiency followed by LH, FSH, GH, TSH, and PRL deficiency (35, 99, 100). These symptoms and signs usually are not correlated with the magnitude of the changes of MRI findings, suggesting that pituitary hormone deficiencies could be due to the direct attack of the autoimmune process on the pituitary acini cells (101). Finally, hyperprolactinemia may be frequently observed in patients with LYH and enlargement of the pituitary gland on MRI (20). A multifactorial etiology has been suggested for the hyperprolactinemia: in some cases, it can be due to a decrease in the dopamine delivery to the anterior pituitary due to stalk compression by a pituitary suprasellar inflammatory mass or in other ones due to an alteration of dopamine receptors. Hyperprolactinemia can be also present in patients with LYH with normal findings of the pituitary region on MRI (32). In these cases, the diffuse lymphocyte infiltration of the pituitary gland could determine an increase of PRL release by both lactotrophs and immune cells infiltrating the gland, taking into account the relationship between the immune system and PRL (102). Anyway, the PRL increase in LYH could be secondary to the inflammatory process of the pituitary gland; on the other hand, high levels of PRL could have a role in perpetuating the immune process in LYH, taking into account their endocrine, paracrine, and autocrine effects. Finally, in some patients with only LYH without presence of radiological findings of lymphocytic infundibulo neurohypophysitis, central diabetes insipidus can be present (*103*). In our personal experience, we demonstrated that all patients with LYH and central diabetes insipidus showed the presence of AVPcAb. This evidence suggests that central diabetes insipidus could not be attributed to compression of the posterior lobe and the infundibulum stem but to the direct immune attack on vasopressin-producing cells of the hypothalamic nuclei of the neurohypophyseal system. Presumptive diagnostic criteria for diagnosis of LYH with pituitary enlargement are summarized in Table 33.5. The diagnosis of this form of LYH requires the coexistence of at least four of the described

Table 33.5
Diagnostic Criteria of Lymphocytic Hypophysitis with Pituitary Enlargement

Criteria	Notes
Women in peripartum period	
Young patients	
Isolated/multiple/total hypopituitarism	– Early ACTH deficiency followed by TSH(47%), LH/FSH(42%), and GH(36.7%), PRL(33%) deficiencies – Not associated with changes of pituitary on MRI
Acute onset of headache with mass effect symptoms (ophthalmoplegia, visual field defects, nausea, or vomiting)	
Characteristic MRI findings	– Intense and homogeneous enhancement of pituitary mass – Suprasellar expansion especially "tongue-like" extension – Delay of complete enhancement time in dynamic MRI (>50 s)
Acute improvement pituitary MRI findings after corticosteroid therapy	– Accompanied sometimes with remission of hypopituitarism
Presence of antibodies to pituitary hormone-producing cells in impairment state with or without presence of antibodies to pituitary antigens	
Presence of other autoimmune diseases or other antibodies	
Acute onset of central diabetes insipidus	
Lymphomonocytic pleocytosis in the CSF	

criteria. In particular, the presence of APA is only one of the criteria for diagnosis of probable LYH; on the other hand, the presence of APA is a very important criterion for diagnosis of LYH in patients with hypopituitarism but with normal characteristics of the pituitary region on MRI. Future studies to compare detection of APA by different methods are necessary to use these antibodies in routine clinical practice for the diagnosis of LYH. However, we hypothesize that the detection of APA immunostaining selectively the hormone-producing cells in impaired functional state could be an ideal tool in the diagnosis of LYH (Fig. 33.1).

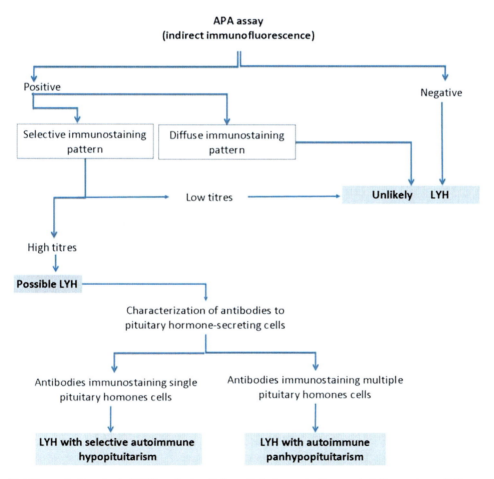

Fig. 33.1 Diagnostic flow chart of LYH in patients with hypopituitarism and with normal pituitary region on MRI.

THERAPEUTIC STRATEGIES

Before the beginning of the therapy of LYH, two important considerations may be made: first, the different expressions of this autoimmune disease require different therapeutic strategies; second, since a possible spontaneous remission during the natural history of LYH can be observed, the improvement occurring after surgical or medical treatment could be related to spontaneous resolution rather than to the treatment itself (20, 27). However, the remission of LYH after therapy quickly occurs while the spontaneous resolution may be more delayed overtime. In patients with LYH when pituitary mass/symptoms and signs are present without severe visual fields impairment the ideal gold therapy is the corticosteroid treatment (104). It has been reported that high dose of methylprednisolone determines not only a reduction of pituitary mass, but also an improvement of hypopituitarism and disappearance of hyperprolactinemia or central diabetes insipidus if present (105, 106). The remission of hypopituitarism, normalization of PRL levels with disappearance of APA could be due to reduction of the diffuse infiltration of the pituitary gland; in addition, the remission of central diabetes insipidus with disappearance of AVPcAb could be due to the reduction of lymphocytic infiltration of the neurohypophyseal system (83). Subsequently, in patients with LYH with persisting hypopituitarism despite corticosteroid therapy, an adequate hormone replacement therapy should be made. In patients with symptoms and/or signs of severe compression and visual field impairment, a prompt decompression of pituitary mass by endoscopic trans-sphenoidal surgery is necessary. Moreover, in patients with hypopituitarism, hormonal replacement therapy has to be performed. The possible resolution of the pituitary impairment after a short-term hormone replacement is frequently observed. This remission could be attributed to spontaneous resolution of the immune process; on the other hand, hormone replacement therapy, as reported for other autoimmune disease, could also act as isohormonal therapy in determining the turning off of the immune process and subsequently a recovery of the pituitary function in LYH (83). With regard to the putative effect of dopamine agonists on LYH with hypopituitarism, cabergoline therapy, when hyperprolactinemia is present, seems to be able to induce the disappearance of APA and recovery of a normal anterior pituitary function, probably by interrupting the pituitary cell damage through the normalization of PRL levels or by a direct immunosuppressive effect of the drug (34, 102).

REFERENCES

1. Sautner D, Saeger W, Lüdecke DK, Jansen V, Puchner MJ. Hypophysitis in surgical and autoptical specimens. Acta Neuropathol 1995;90:637–644.
2. Tashiro T, Sano T, Xu B, Wakatsuki S, Kagawa N, Nishioka H, Yamada S, Kovacs K. Spectrum of different types of hypophysitis: a clinicopathologic study of hypophysitis in 31 cases. Endocr Pathol 2002;13:183–195.
3. Caturegli P, Newschaffer C, Olivi A, Pomper MG, Burger PC, Rose NR. Autoimmune hypophysitis. Endocr Rev 2005;26:599–614.
4. Hashimoto K, Takao T, Makino S. Lymphocytic adenohypophysitis and lymphocytic infundibuloneurohypophysitis. Endocr J 1997;44:1–10.
5. Pivonello R, De Bellis A, Faggiano A, Di Salle F, Petretta M, Di Somma C, Perrino S, Altucci P, Bizzarro A, Bellastella A, Lombardi G, Colao A. Central diabetes insipidus and autoimmunity: relationship between the occurrence of antibodies to arginine vasopressin-secreting cells and clinical, immunological, and radiological features in a large cohort of patients with central diabetes insipidus of known and unknown etiology. J Clin Endocrinol Metab 2003;88:1629–1636.
6. Maghnie M, Genovese E, Sommaruga MG, Arico M, Locatelli D, Arbustini E, Pezzotta S, Severi F. Evolution of childhood central diabetes insipidus into panhypopituitarism with a large hypothalamic mass: is 'lymphocytic infundibuloneurohypophysitis' in children a different entity? Eur J Endocrinol 1998;139:635–640
7. Susman W. Atrophy of the adrenals associated with Addison's disease. J Pathol Bacteriol 1930;33:749–760.
8. Duff GL, Berstein C. Five cases of Addison's disease with so-called atrophy of the adrenal gland. Bull Johns Hopkins Hosp 1933;52:67–83.
9. Rapp JJ, Pashkis KE. Panhypopituitarism with idiopathic hypoparathyroidism. Ann Intern Med 1953;39:1103–1107.
10. Roitt IM, Doniach D, Campbell PN, Hudson RV. Autoantibodies in Hashimoto's disease. Lancet 1956;2:820–822.
11. Goudie EB, Pinkerton PH. Anterior hypophysitis and Hashimoto's disease in a young woman. J Pathol Bacteriol 1962;83:584–585.
12. Crock PA, Bensing S, Smith CJA, Burns C, Robinson PJ. Autoimmune hypophysitis. In: Weetman AP, ed. Autoimmune Diseases in Endocrinology. Totowa, NJ: Humana Press, 2008:357–392.
13. Cosman F, Post KD, Holub DA, Wardlaw SL. Lymphocytic hypophysitis. Report of 3 new cases and review of the literature. Medicine 1989;68:240–256.
14. Asa SL, Bilbao JM, Kovacs K, Josse RG, Kreines K. Lymphocytic hypophysitis of pregnancy resulting in hypopituitarism: a distinct clinicopathologic entity. Ann Intern Med 1981;95:166–171.
15. Quencer RM. Lymphocytic adenohypophysitis: autoimmune disorder of the pituitary gland. AJNR Am J Neuroradiol 1980;1:343–345.
16. Ahmadi J, Scott Myers G, Segall HD, Sharma OP, Hinton DR. Lymphocytic adenohypophysitis: contras-enhanced MR imaging in five cases. Radiology 1995;195:30–34.
17. Beressi N, Beressi JP, Cohen R, Modigliani E. Lymphocytic hypophysitis. A review of 145 cases. Ann Intern Med 1999;150:327–341.
18. Caturegli P, Lupi I, Landek-Salgado M, Kimura H, Rose NR. Pituitary autoimmunity: 30 years later. Autoimmun Rev 2008;7:631–637.
19. Thodou E, Asa SL, Kontogeorgos G, Kovacs K, Horvath E, Ezzat S. Lymphocytic hypophysitis: clinicopathological findings. J Clin Endocrinol Metab 1995;80:2302–2311.
20. Bellastella A, Bizzarro A, Coronella C, Bellastella G, Sinisi AA, De Bellis A. Lymphocytic hypophysitis: a rare or underestimated disease? Eur J Endocrinol 2003;149:363–376.
21. De Bellis A, Ruocco G, Battaglia M, Conte M, Coronella C, Tirelli G, Bellastella A, Pane E, Sinisi AA, Bizzarro A, Bellastella G. Immunological and clinical aspects of lymphocytic hypophysitis. Clin Sci 2008;114:413–421.
22. Gutenberg A, Buslei R, Fahlbusch R, Buchfelder M, Brück W. Immunopathology of primary hypophysitis: implications for pathogenesis. Am J Surg Pathol 2005;29:329–338.
23. Riedl M, Czech T, Slootweg J, Czernin S, Hainfellner JA, Schima W, Vierhapper H, Luger A. Lymphocytic hypophysitis presenting

as a pituitary tumor in a 63-year-old man. Endocr Pathol 1995;6:159–166.
24. Chelaïfa K, Bouzaïdi K, Harzallah F, Menif E, Ben Messaoud M, Turki I, Slim R. Lymphocytic hypophysitis. J Neuroradiol 2002;29:57–60.
25. Nakamura Y, Okada H, Wada Y, Kajiyama K, Koshiyama H. Lymphocytic hypophysitis: its expanding features. J Endocrinol Invest 2001;24:262–267.
26. Levine SN, Benzel EC, Fowler MR, et al. Lymphocytic adenohypophysitis: clinical, radiological, and magnetic resonance imaging characterization. Neurosurgery 1988;22: 937–941.
27. De Bellis A, Bizzarro A, Bellastella A. Pituitary antibodies and lymphocytic hypophysitis. Best Pract Res Clin Endocrinol Metab 2005;19:67–84.
28. De Bellis A, Bizzarro A, Conte M, Perrrino S, Coronella C, Solimeno S, Sinisi AM, Stile LA, Pisano G, Bellastella A. Antipituitary antibodies in adults with apparently idiopathic growth hormone deficiency and in adults with autoimmune endocrine diseases. J Clin Endocrinol Metab 2003;88:650–654.
29. Goswami R, Kochupillai N, Crock PA, Jaleel A, Gupta N. Pitutary autoimmunity in patients with Sheehan's syndrome. J Clin Endocrinol Metab 2002;87:4137–4141.
30. De Bellis A, Kelestimur F, Sinisi AA, Ruocco G, Tirelli G, Battaglia M, Bellastella G, Conzo G, Tanriverdi F, Unluhizarci K, Bizzarro A, Bellastella A. Anti-hypothalamus and anti-pituitary antibodies may contribute to perpetuate the hypopituitarism in patients with Sheehan's syndrome. Eur J Endocrinol 2008;158:147–152.
31. Tanriverdi F, De Bellis A, Bizzarro A, Sinisi AA, Bellastella G, Pane E, Bellastella A, Unluhizarci K, Selcuklu A, Casanueva FF, Kelestimur F. Antipituitary antibodies after traumatic brain injury: is head trauma-induced pituitary dysfunction associated with autoimmunity? Eur J Endocrinol 2008;159:7–13.
32. De Bellis A, Bizzarro A, Pivonello R, Lombardi G, Bellastella A. Prolactin and autoimmunity. Pituitary 2005;8:25–30.
33. De Bellis A, Colao A, Pivonello R, Savoia A, Battaglia M, Ruocco G, Tirelli G, Lombardi G, Bellastella A, Bizzarro A. Antipituitary antibodies in idiopathic hyperprolactinemic patients. Ann N Y Acad Sci 2007;1107: 129–135.
34. De Bellis A, Colao A, Savoia A, Coronella C, Pasquali D, Conte M, Pivonello R, Bellastella A, Sinisi AA, Bizzarro A, Lombardi G, Bellastella G. Effect of long-term cabergoline therapy on the immunological pattern and pituitary function of patients with idiopathic hyperprolactinaemia positive for antipituitary antibodies. Clin Endocrinol 2008;69: 285–291.
35. Ezzat S, Josse R. Autoimmune hypophysitis. In: Volpè R, ed. Autoimmune Endocrinopathies. Totowa, NJ: Humana Press, 1999:337–348.
36. Gellner V, Kurschel S, Scarpatetti M, Mokry M. Lymphocytic hypophysitis in the pediatric population. Childs Nerv Syst 2008;24:785–792.
37. Witebsky E, Rose NR, Terplan K, Paine JR, Egan RW. Chronic thyroiditis and autoimmunization. JAMA 1957;164:1439–1447.
38. Rose NR, Bona C. Defining criteria for autoimmune diseases (Witebsky's postulates revisited). Immunol Today 1993;14: 426–430.
39. Blansfield JA, Beck KE, Tran K, Yang JC, Hughes MS, Kammula US, Royal RE, Topalian SL, Haworth LR, Levy C, Rosenberg SA, Sherry RM. Cytotoxic T-lymphocyte-associated antigen-4 blockage can induce autoimmune hypophysitis in patients with metastatic melanoma and renal cancer. J Immunother 2005;28:593–598.
40. Beck KE, Blansfield JA, Tran KQ, Feldman AL, Hughes MS, Royal RE, Kammula US, Topalian SL, Sherry RM, Kleiner D, Quezado M, Lowy I, Yellin M, Rosenberg SA, Yang JC. Enterocolitis in patients with cancer after antibody blockade of cytotoxic T-lymphocyte-associated antigen 4. J Clin Oncol 2006;20:2283–2289.
41. Yang JC, Hughes M, Kammula U, Royal R, Sherry RM, Topalian SL, Suri KB, Levy C, Allen T, Mavroukakis S, Lowy I, White DE, Rosenberg SA. Ipilimumab (anti-CTLA4 antibody) causes regression of metastatic renal cell cancer associated with enteritis and hypophysitis. J Immunother 2007;30: 825–830.
42. Levine S. Allergic adrenalitis and adenohypophysitis: further observations on production and passive transfer. Endocrinology 1969;84:469–475.
43. Klein I, Kraus KE, Martines AJ, Weber S. Evidence for cellular mediated immunity in an animal model of autoimmune pituitary disease. Endocr Res Commun 1982;9: 145–153.
44. Yoon JW, Choi DS, Liang HC, Baek HS, Ko IY, Jun HS, Gillam S. Induction of an organ-specific autoimmune disease, lymphocytic hypophysitis, in hamsters by recombinant rubella virus glycoprotein and prevention of disease by neonatal thymectomy. J Virol 1992;66:1210–1214.

45. Onodera T, Toniolo A, Ray UR, Jenson AB, Knazek RA, Notkins AL. Virus-induced diabetes mellitus. XX. Polyendocrinopathy and autoimmunity. J Exp Med 1981;1:1457–1473.
46. De Jersey J, Carmignac D, Le Tissier P. Factors affecting the susceptibility of the mouse pituitary gland to CD8 T-cell-mediated autoimmunity. Immunology 2004;111:254–261.
47. Tzou SC, Lupi I, Landek M, Gutenberg A, Tzou YM, Kimura H, Pinna G, Rose NR, Caturegli P. Autoimmune hypophysitis of SJL mice: clinical insights from a new animal model. Endocrinology 2008;149:3461–3469.
48. Betterle C, Dal Pra C, Mantero F, Zanchetta R. Autoimmune adrenal insufficiency and autoimmune polyendocrine syndromes: autoantibodies, autoantigens, and their applicability in diagnosis and disease prediction. Endocr Rev 2002;23:327–364.
49. Leslie RD, Atkinson MA, Notkins AL. Autoantigens IA-2 and GAD in Type I (insulin-dependent) diabetes. Diabetologia 1999;42:3–14.
50. Nowak EJ, Lernmark A. Immunological markers and disease prediction. In: Gill RG, Harmon JT, Maclaren NK, eds. Immunologically Mediated Endocrine Diseases. Philadelphia: Lippincott Williams & Wilkins, 2002:529–548.
51. De Bellis A, Bizzarro A, Rossi R, Amoresano Paglionico V, Criscuolo T, Lombardi G, Bellastella A. Remission of subclinical adrenocortical failure in subjects with adrenal autoantibodies. J Clin Endocrinol Metab 1993;76:1002–1007.
52. De Bellis A, Bizzarro A, Amoresano Paglionico V, Di Martino S, Criscuolo T, Sinisi AA, Lombardi G, Bellastella A. Detection of vasopressin cell antibodies in some patients with autoimmune endocrine disease without overt diabetes insipidus. Clin Endocrinol 1994;40:173–177.
53. Laureti S, De Bellis A, Muccitelli VI, Calcinaro F, Bizzarro A, Rossi R, Bellastella A, Santeusanio F, Falorni A. Levels of adrenocortical autoantibodies correlate with the degree of adrenal dysfunction in subjects with preclinical Addison's disease. J Clin Endocrinol Metab 1998;83:3507–3511.
54. Bottazzo GF, Doniach D. Pituitary autoimmunity: a review. J R Soc Med 1978;71:433–436.
55. Pouplard A. Pituitary autoimmunity. Horm Res 1982;16:289–297.
56. Mauerhoff T, Mirakian R, Bottazzo GF. Autoimmunity and the pituitary. In Doniach D, Bottazzo GF, eds. Endocrine and Other Organ-Oriented Autoimmune Disorders. Bailliere's Clin Immunol and Allergy, vol 1. London: WB Saunders, 1987:217–235.
57. Gluck M, Scherbaumm WA. Substrate specificity for the detection of autoantibodies to anterior pituitary cells in human sera. Horm Metab Res 1990;22:541–545.
58. Mirakian R, Cudworth AG, Bottazzo GF, Richardson CA, Doniach D. Autoimmunity to anterior pituitary cells and the pathogenesis of insulin-dependent diabetes mellitus. Lancet 1982;1:755–759.
59. Iughetti L, De Bellis A, Predieri B, Bizzarro A, De Simone M, Balli F, Bellastella A, Bernasconi S. Growth hormone impaired secretion and antipituitary antibodies in patients with coeliac disease and poor catch-up growth after a long gluten-free diet period: a causal association? Eur J Pediat 2006;165:897–903.
60. Falorni A, Laureti S, De Bellis A, Zanchetta R, Tiberti C, Arnaldi G, Bini V, Beck-Peccoz P, Bizzarro A, Dotta F, Mantero F, Bellastella A, Betterle C, Santeusanio F, SIE Addison Study Group. Italian Addison network study: update of diagnostic criteria for the etiological classification of primary adrenal insufficiency. J Clin Endocrinol Metab 2004;89:1598–1604.
61. Bottazzo GF, McIntosh C, Stanford W, Preece M. Growth hormone cell antibodies and partial growth hormone deficiency in a girl with Turner's syndrome. Clin Endocrinol 1980;12:1–9.
62. Bottazzo GF, Pouplard A, Florin-Christensen A, Doniach D. Autoantibodies to prolactin-secreting cells of human pituitary. Lancet 1975;2:97–101.
63. De Bellis A, Bizzarro A, Perrino S, Coronella C, Conte M, Pasquali D, Sinisi AA, Betterle C, Bellastella A. Characterization of antipituitary antibodies targeting pituitary hormone-secreting cells in idiopathic growth hormone deficiency and autoimmune endocrine disease. Clin Endocrinol 2005;63:45–49.
64. De Bellis A, Salerno M, Conte M, Coronella C, Tirelli G, Battaglia M, Esposito V, Ruocco G, Bellastella G, Bizzarro A, Bellastella A. Antipituitary antibodies recognized GH-producing cells in children with idiopathic growth hormone deficiency and in children with idiopathic short stature. J Clin Endocrinol Metab 2006;91:2484–2489.
65. De Bellis A, Sinisi AA, Conte M, Coronella C, Bellastella G, Esposito D, Pasquali D, Ruocco G, Bizzarro A, Bellastella A. Antipituitary antibodies against gonadotropin-secreting cells in adult male patients with apparently idiopathic hypogonadotropic hypogonadism. J Clin Endocrinol Metab 2007;92:604–607.

66. Bottazzo GF, Florin-Christensen A, Doniach D. Islet-cell antibodies in diabetes mellitus with autoimmune polyendocrine deficiencies. Lancet 1974;2:1279–1283.
67. Lendrum R, Walker G, Gamble DR. Islet-cell antibodies in juvenile diabetes mellitus of recent onset. Lancet 1975;1:880–882.
68. Crock P, Salvi M, Miller A, Wall J, Guyda H. Detection of anti-pituitary autoantibodies by immunoblotting. J Immunol Methods 1993;162:31–40.
69. O'Dwyer DT, Clifton V, Hall A, Smith R, Robinson PJ, Crock PA. Pituitary autoantibodies in lymphocytic hypophysitis target both gamma- and alpha-enolase – a link with pregnancy? Arch Physiol Biochem 2002;110(1–2):94–98.
70. Nakahara R, Tsunekawa K, Yabe S, Nara M, Seki K, Kasahara T, Ogiwara T, Nishino M, Kobayashi I, Muratami M. Association of pituitary antibody and type 2 iodothyronine deiodinase antibody in patients with autoimmune thyroid disease. Endocr J 2005;52:691–699.
71. Bensing S, Hulting AL, Höög A, Ericson K, Kämpe O. Lymphocytic hypophysitis: report of two biopsy-proven cases and one suspected case with pituitary autoantibodies. J Endocrinol Invest 2007;30:153–162.
72. Takao T, Nanamiya W, Matsumoto R, Asaba K, Okabayasi T, Hashimoto, K. Antipituitary antibodies in patients with lymphocytic hypophysitis. Horm Res 2001;55:288–292.
73. Tanaka S, Tatsumi KI, Kimura M, Takano T, Murakami Y, Takao T, Hashimoto K, Kato Y, Amino N. Detection of autoantibodies against the pituitary-specific proteins in patients with lymphocytic hypophysitis. Eur J Endocrinol 2002;147:767–775.
74. Bensing S, Kasperlik-Zaluska AA, Czarnocka B, Crock PA, Hulting A. Autoantibodies against pituitary proteins in patients with adrenocorticotropin-deficiency. Eur J Clin Invest 2005;35:126–132.
75. Crock P. Cytosolic autoantigens in lymphocytic hypophysitis. J Clin Endocrinol Metab 1998;83:609–618.
76. O'Dwyer DT, Smith AI, Matthew ML, Andronicos NM, Ranson M, Robinson PJ, Crock, P.A. Identification of the 49-kDa auoantigen associated with lymphocytic hypophysitis as a-enolase. J Clinl Endocrinol Metab 2002;87:752–757.
77. Tanaka S, Tatsumi KI, Takano T, Murakami Y, Takao T, Yamakita N, Tahara S, Teramoto A, Hashimoto K, Kato Y, Amino N. Anti-alpha-enolase antibodies in pituitary disease. Endocr J 2003;50:697–702.
78. Lupi I, Broman KW, Tzou SC, Gutenberg A, Martino E, Caturegli P. Novel autoantigens in autoimmune hypophysitis. Clin Endocrinol 2008;69:269–278.
79. Tanaka S. Novel autoantibodies to pituitary gland specific factor 1a in patients with rheumatoid arthritis. Rheumatology 2003;42:353–356.
80. Betterle C, Greggio NA, Volpato M. Clinical review 93: autoimmune polyglandular syndrome type 1. J Clin Endocrinol Metab 1998;83:1049–1055.
81. Barbaro D, Loni, G. Lymphocytic hypophysitis and autoimmune thyroid disease. J Endocrinol Invest 2000;23:339–340.
82. Manetti L, Lupi I, Morselli LL, Albertini S, Casottini M, Grasso L, Genovesi M, Pinna G, Mariotti S, Bogazzi F, Bartalena L, Martino E. Prevalence and functional significance of antipituitary antibodies in patients with autoimmune and non-autoimmune thyroid diseases. J Clin Endocrinol Metab 2007;92:2176–2181.
83. De Bellis A, Colao A, Di Salle F, Muccitelli VI, Iorio S, Perrino S, Pivonello R, Coronella C, Bizzarro A, Lombardi G, Bellastella A. A longitudinal study of vasopressin cell antibodies, posterior pituitary function, and magnetic resonance imaging evaluations in subclinical autoimmune central diabetes insipidus. J Clin Endocrinol Metab 1999;84:3047–3051.
84. De Bellis A, Colao A, Bizzarro A, Di Salle F, Coronella C, Solimeno S, Vetrano A, Pivonello R, Pisano G, Lombardi G, Bellastella A. Longitudinal study of vasopressin-cell antibodies and of hypothalamic-pituitary region on magnetic resonance imaging in patients with autoimmune and idiopathic complete central diabetes insipidus. J Clin Endocrinol Metab 2002;87:3825–3829.
85. Sobrinho-Simões M, Brandão A, Paiva ME, Vilela B, Fernandes E, Carneiro-Chaves F. Lymphoid hypophysitis in a patient with lymphoid thyroiditis, lymphoid adrenalitis, and idiopathic retroperitoneal fibrosis. Arch Pathol Lab Med 1985;109:230–233.
86. Mazzone T, Kelly W, Ensinck J. Lymphocytic hypophysitis. Associated with antiparietal cell antibodies and vitamin B12 deficiency. Arch Intern Med 1983;143:1794–1795.
87. Collin P, Kaukinen K, Välimäki M, Salmi J. Endocrinological disorders and celiac diseases. Endocr Rev 2002;23:464–483.
88. Ji JD, Lee SY, Choi SJ, Lee YH, Song GG. Lymphocytic hypophysitis in a patient with systemic lupus erythematosus. Clin Exper Rheumatol 2000;18:78–80.

89. Li JY, Lai PH, Lam HC, Lu LY, Cheng HH, Lee JK, Lo YK. Hypertrophic cranial pachymeningitis and lymphocytic hypophysitis in Sjögren's syndrome. Neurology 1999;15: 420–423.
90. Piñol V, Cubiella J, Navasa M, Fernández J, Halperin I, Bruguera M, Rodés J. Autoimmune hepatitis associated with thyroiditis and hypophysitis. A case report. Gastroenterol Hepatol 2000;23:123–125.
91. Nishiki M, Murakami Y, Koshimura K, Sohmiya M, Tanaka J, Yabe S, Kobayashi I, Kato Y. A case of autoimmune hypophysitis associated with asymptomatic primary biliary cirrhosis. Endocr J 1998;45:697–700.
92. Bensing S, Fetissov SO, Mulder J, Perheentupa J, Gustafsson J, Husebye ES, Oscarson M, Ekwall O, Crock PA, Hokfelt T, Hulting AL, Kampe O. Pituitary autoantibodies in autoimmune polyendocrine syndrome type 1. Proc Natl Acad Sci USA 2007;104:949–954.
93. De Bellis A, Bizzarro A, Bellastella A. Autoimmune central diabetes insipidus. In: Vincent G, George C, eds. Immunoendocrinology in Health Disease. New York, NY: Marcel Dekker, 2004:439–459.
94. Ostensen M, Villiger PM. Immunology of pregnancy-pregnancy as a remission inducing agent in rheumatoid arthritis. Transpl Immunol 2002;9:155–160.
95. Lockshin MD, Sammaritano LR. Lupus pregnancy. Autoimmunity 2003;36:33–40.
96. Hayes FJ, McKenna TJ. The occurrence of lymphocytic hypophysitis in a first but not subsequent pregnancy. J Clin Endocrinol Metab 1996;81:3131–3132.
97. Tsur A, Leibowitz G, Samueloff A, Gross DJ. Successful pregnancy in a patient with pre-existing lymphocytic hypophysitis. Acta Obstet Gynecol Scand 1996;75:772–774.
98. Gagneja H, Arafah B, Taylor HC. Histologically proven lymphocytic hypophysitis: spontaneous resolution and subsequent pregnancy. Mayo Clin Proc 1999;74:150–154.
99. Cheung CC, Ezzat S, Smyth HS, Asa SL. The spectrum and significance of primary hypophysitis. J Clin Endocrinol Metab 2001;86:1048–1053.
100. Ezza S, Josse RG. Autoimmue hypophysitis trends. Endocrinol Metab 1997;8:74–80.
101. Levy MJ, Jäger HR, Powell M, Matharu MS, Meeran K, Goadsby PJ. Pituitary volume and headache: size is not everything. Arch Neurol 2004;61:721–725.
102. De Bellis A, Bizzarro A, Bellastella A. Role of prolactin in autoimmune diseases. In: Walker S, Jara LJ, eds. Endocrine Manifestations of Systemic Autoimmune Disease. Vol. 4. Handbook of Systemic Autoimmune Diseases, vol. 9. Amsterdam: Elsevier, 2008:29–43.
103. Rivera JA. Lymphocytic hypophysitis: disease spectrum and approach to diagnosis and therapy. Pituitary 2006;9:35–45.
104. Beressi N, Cohen R, Beressi JP, Dumas JL, Legrand M, Iba-Zizen MT, Modigliani E. Pseudotumoral lymphocytic hypophysitis successfully treated by corticosteroid alone: first case report. Neurosurgery 1994;35:505–508.
105. Kristof RA, Van Roost D, Klingmüller D, Springer W, Schramm J. Lymphocytic hypophysitis: non-invasive diagnosis and treatment by high dose methylprednisolone pulse therapy? J Neurol Neurosurg Psychiatry 1999;67:398–402.
106. Uyama A, Sasaki M, Ikeda M, Asada M, Teramura K, Tachibana M. A case of lymphocytic hypophysitis successfully treated with steroid pulse therapy. No Shinkei Geka 2007;35:1115–1119.
107. Stern BJ, Krumholz A, Johns C, Scott P, Nissim J. Sarcoidosis and its neurological manifestations. Arch Neurol 1985;42:909–917.
108. Ng WH, Gonzales M, Kaye AH. Lymphocytic hypophysitis. J Clin Neurosci 2003;10: 409–413.

Index

A

Acanthosis nigricans 371
Accelerator hypothesis 285
Activation-induced cell death (AICD) 10, 62
Adaptive immunity
    B lymphocyte and autoantibodies 202
    CD4 and CD8 T lymphocytes 203–204
Addison's disease 144, 147, 149–151, 548
    AAD and cellular autoimmunity 407–408
        autoimmune POF diagnosis 405
        identification 402
        21OHAb, AAD immune marker 404
        PAI etiological classification 403–404
        placental barrier detection 402
    APS-2 associated ADD, genetics
        AAD genetics 407
        chromosome 6, genetic marker 405
        HLA-DRB1'04 subtypes 405–406
        MHC class I chain-related A (MICA) 406–407
        T1DM, endocrine autoimmune diseases 406
    causes of 400
    PAI diagnosis and clinical managment
        Addisonian crisis 401
        clinical signs and symptoms 400–401
        substitutive therapy 401
    primary adrenal insuffciency (PAI) 399
    sublinical AAD
        ACTH stimulation test 409
        adrenal dysfunction classification 408–409
        estimation 409–410
        risk factors 410
Adrenocorticotropic hormone (ACTH) 118
Agonistic antithyrotropin receptor 416–417
AICD. *See* Activation-induced cell death
AITD. *See* Autoimmune thyroid diseases
Amiodarone 171
Anticytokine therapy 497
Antigen-presenting cells (APCs) 4–6, 10, 184–186
Antigen-specific autoreactive T cells
    AICD 62
    down-modulate antigen-presenting cells 62

experimental models 61–62
LADA 63
therapeutics 62
Antigen specific immunomodulation
    diapep 277, 301–302
    glutamic acid decarboxylase 65 (GAD65) 300–301
    insulin 299–300
    mechanisms 298
Anti-insulin receptor autoantibodies
    associated diseases 370, 371
    cell surface insulin receptor 370
    hyperglycemia and hypoglycemia
        antireceptor antibodies 377
        IgG antireceptor antibodies 378
        murine fatty fibroblasts 377–378
        titers, antagonist effect 378
    type B insulin resistance (*See* Type B insulin resistance)
Antioocyte antigen (AOA) 523
Antipituitary antibodies (APA)
    disappearance 558, 562
    histological lesions 551
    hormone-secreting cells 554
    immunofluorescence method 547, 555
    immunoprecipitation 556
    LYH 553
    rise and fall 559
    transcription–translation 556
APA. *See* Antipituitary antibodies
APECED. *See* Autoimmune polyendocrinopathy-
        candidiasis-ectodermal dystrophy
APS-1. *See* Autoimmune polyendocrine syndrome type 1
APS-2. *See* Autoimmune polyendocrine syndrome type 2
Atherogenic dyslipidemia 70
Autoimmune animal model 199
Autoimmune diabetes 254
Autoimmune polyendocrine syndrome type 1 (APS-1)
    AIRE
        autosomal dominant 108–109
        cellular mechanisms 106–107
        extrathymic expression 109–110
        molecular mechanism 103–105
        mutations 95–97

Index

Autoimmune polyendocrine syndrome type 1 (APS-1) (*Continued*)
  Candida 100
  diagnosis 116–117
  disease-relevant autoantigens 107–108
  ectodermal manifestations
    autoantibodies 123
    clinical details 124–126
    diagnosis 122
    enamel dysplasia 121–122
    eye 121
    hypoplasia /aplasia 122
    skin 121
  endocrine manifestations
    adrenal failure 118–119
    hypoparathyroidism 117–118
    ovarian/gonadal insufficiency 119
    thyroid disease 119
    type 1 diabetes 119
  gastro-intestinal manifestations
    autoimmune hepatitis 120
    symptoms 120–121
  heterogeneity 99
  lymphocytic infiltration 97–98
  mucocutaneous candidiasis
    chronic 119
    treatment 120
  overlapping models 98
  thymic epithelial cells
    HEL 102
    IGRP 103
    peripheral self expression 102
    T-cell precursors 103
  thymus
    antigen-presenting cells 101
    CD4⁺ and CD8⁺ T cells 100
    tissue-specific antigens (TSAs) 100
Autoimmune polyendocrinopathy-candidiasis-ectodermal dystrophy (APECED) 115
Autoimmune polyendocrine syndrome type 2 (APS-2)
  autoimmune diseases 143
  diagnosis and treatment 151–152
  disease components 146
  overlapping components 144
  pathophysiology
    clinical presentation 150–151
    environmental factors 148
    genetic risk 145
    immunologic tolerance 145
    markers, autoimmune process 148–149
    markers, gland failure 149–150
  type 1A diabetes, development stage 144–145
Autoimmune regulator (*AIRE*) gene
  autosomal dominant 108–109
  cellular mechanisms 106–107

  extrathymic expression 109–110
  molecular mechanism 103–105
  mutations 95–97
Autoimmune thyroid disease, animal models
  agonistic antithyrotropin receptor (TSHR) 416–417
  central tolerance 421–423
  environmental factors
    Bacillus Calmette-Guerin 419
    Graves' disease 419
    infectious agents 418–419
  Freund's adjuvant 416
  genetic factors
    experimetal autoimmune thyroid diseases 418
    MHC haplotypes 417
    TPO immunization 417
  Graves' hyperthyroidism 416
  immune response characterization
    antigens phagocytosis 419
    B cells, pathogenesis 420–421
    Hashimoto's thyroiditis 420
    Th17 cells 419–420
  peripheral tolerance 421
  thyroglobulin (Tg) 416
  thyroid peroxidase (TPO) 416
Autoimmune thyroid diseases (AITD)
  epidemiology 428
  gene mapping
    costimulatory molecules 435
    Crohn's disease 434
    FOXP3 gene 435
  regulator genes and susceptibility
    CD40 431–432
    CTLA-4 429–431
    HLA-DR 429
    protein tyrosine phosphatase-22 gene 432–433
  thyroid-specific genes
    thyroglobulin 433–434
    TSH receptor 434
Autosomal dominant hypoparathyroidism (ADH) 509

B

Bayes' theory 45
β cell 337
  CTLA-4 gene polymorphisms 336
  death mechanism 335
  DR4-DQ4 homozygote analysis 335–336
  environmental factor 336–337
  genetic factors 334
  T-cell immunoreactivity 337–339
  type 1A diabetes 337
  viral infection 337
β-cell apoptosis 285
B cell autoantigen
  B lymphocytes 23
  candidate B cell gene 24–26

fusion peptide libraries... 22
ganglioside ELISAs... 23
ICA reaction preabsorption 22–23
λ gt-11 libraries 20–22
mAbs... 26–27
NAAPAs.. 23–24
T1D sera... 22
B-cell receptor (BCRs).. 460
Biological immunomodulators
abatacept (CTLA4-Ig) 305–306
anti-CD3 mabs 303–305
rituximab (anti-CD20) 305
B lymphocytes 202

C

Calcium-sensing receptor (CaSR)
anti-CaSR antibodies 506
autoantigen.. 503
autoimmune hypoparathyroidism 509
extracellular domain.. 503
heterotrimeric G-proteins 508
monomeric forms 503
mutants... 508
noncytotoxic antibodies 502
target... 501
Candidate B cell gene.. 24–26
CaSR. *See* Calcium-sensing receptor
Celiac disease (CD)
complications... 539
DAISY study... 538
diagnosis...536, 539–540
genetic susceptibility.......................................540–541
genomewide association studies......................541–542
GFD adherence.. 540
gliadin.. 536
HLA haplotypes.. 537
intestinal endocrine autoimmunity
APS-1... 543
enterochromaffin cells (EC) 543
radiobinding assays 543
serotonin and peptide YY 544
tryptophan hydroxylase.................................. 543
long-term complications..................................... 538
MHC molecules 536
tissue transglutaminase 535
transglutaminase autoantibodies.............................. 538
Class II-associated haplotypes............................... 253
Clinical activity score (CAS) 487, 490
Cognate autoantigen 43–44
C-reactive protein... 76–78
Crohn's disease 434
CTLA-4 gene polymorphisms................................ 336
Cyclosporine A.. 187

D

Dendritic cells 468–469
Diabetes control and complication trial (DCCT) 294
Diabetes development
B lymphocyte and autoantibodies............................ 202
CD4 and CD8 T lymphocytes........................203–204
Diabetes-prone BioBreeding (BBDP)
antigen presenting cells...................................185–186
beta cells 184–185
insulitis 184
leukocytes 190
T cells
cyclosporine A inhibition................................. 187
diabetogenic effect... 189
Iddm4 gene... 189
lymphopenia.. 187
memory/effector cell characteristics............187–188
MHC interactions 189
self-peptide-MHC bearing cells....................... 188
transcription factor Foxp3............................189–190
type 1 diabetes (T1D).. 183
Diabetic ketoacidosis (DKA) 150
DR4-DQ4 homozygote analysis.........................335–336
Drug-induced endocrine autoimmunity
amiodarone 171
Campath-1H alemtuzumab.................................... 171
epidemiology 165–166
genetic factors 161–162
granulocyte-macrophage colony-stimulating
factor (GM-CSF)....................................170–171
Graves' disease 160–161
highly active antiretroviral therapy (HAART) 172
hypothyroidism...159–160
IFNα-induced thyroiditis..................................... 159
interferon alpha (IFNα)
drugs association 158
hepatitis C virus (HCV) infection..................... 158
interleukin 2 169–170
ipilimumab (anti-CTLA4 antibody) 170
nonauto-immune interferon-induced thyroiditis
glutamic acid decarboxylase (GAD)
antibodies... 165
insulin autoantibodies (IAAs)........................... 165
thyroid dysfunction....................................... 164
TSH-receptor antibodies (TRAb).................... 164
type 1 diabetes (T1D)..................................... 165
nongenetic factors
baseline TAbs presence 163
IFNα direct effects.. 163
pthogenesis 163
Ribavirin (Riba).. 162
viral genotype.. 162
pathogenesis 166–167

Drug-induced endocrine autoimmunity (*Continued*)
    sulfhydryl compound and insulin autoimmune syndrome (IAS)
        diabetic neuropathy treatment 173
        drugs exposure 173
        Japanese population, disease risk........................ 172
    T1D, IFNα treatment
        adrenal dysfunction... 169
        disease clinical presentation 167–168
        pituitary dysfunction.. 169
        therapy effects.............................168–169, 1168
        thyroid dysfunction.. 159
Dyslipidemia 74
Dystrophia myotonica kinase 29

E

ELISPOT assay.. 28
Enamel dysplasia 121–122
Enterochromaffin cells (EC) 543
Escherichia coli... 221, 419
European Nicotinamide Diabetes Intervention Trial (ENDIT) 282, 284, 286

F

Fas expression 239
First phase insulin response (FPIR)
    calculation.. 284
    islet autoantibodies 280
    type 1 diabetes 287
Forkhead box p3 (FOXP3)... 129
    structure and function
        expression 135–136
        nTreg cell 134–135
        pathway.. 137
        transcription factors 134
FoxP3 gene 252
FPIR. *See* First phase insulin response
Fragile X-associated tremor/ataxia syndrome (FRAX).. 523
Fulminant type 1 diabetes mellitus
    β–cell
        CTLA-4 gene polymorphisms 336
        death mechanism 335
        DR4-DQ4 homozygote analysis 335–336
        environmental factor..................................336–337
        genetic factors 334
        T-cell immunoreactivity..............................337–339
        type 1A diabetes 337
        viral infection 337
    diagnostic criteria 332
    epidemiology 333–334
    therapy and prognosis.................................339–340
    type 1A diabetes 332

G

Galactose 1-phosphate uridyl transferase (GALT).. 523
Genomewide association studies, celiac disease 541–542
Gliadin 536
Glucocorticoid prophylaxis.. 495
Glucose tolerance test (GTT) 362–363
Glutamic acid decarboxylase autoantibodies (GADA) 16–18, 25, 26, 33
Glycemic control theraphy 379
Glycosaminoglycans (GAGs)..............................490–491
Gonadtropin-releasing hormone (GnRH) 521
Graves' disease (GD)...41, 427–430
    autoimmunity 458
    environmental precipitators
        hygiene hypothesis 471
        infections 472–473
        initiating factors...470–471
    environment *vs.* genetic susceptibility...............469–470
    heterogeneous disorders....................................... 475
    humoral immunity..458–460
    IFNα, hepatitis B virus (HBV) and HCV infections 160
    intrathyroidal antigen presentation
        B cells 469
        dendritic cells... 468–469
        thyrocytes.. 468
    precipitating drugs
        anti–viral therapy 474
        immunomodulation 475
        iodine... 474
    T cells
        antigen-specific.. 466
        regulatory..466–477
        Th17 cells 467
    thyroid disease pattern 161
    TSHR
        autoimmune arthritis 462
        B-cell repertoire... 461
        epitope geography.. 460
        female sex and susceptibility 474
        humoral immunity... 465
        monoclonal antibodies..................................... 462
        signal transduction....................................464–465
        stimulating epitopes...................................462–464
Graves' model 416
Graves' ophthalmopathy/orbitopathy (GO)
    clinical presentation
        abnormal findings......................................488–489
        CAS.. 487
        DON 488
        no specs system 486

epidemiology
    connective tissue characteristics 486
    hyperthyroidism 485
extraocular muscles 483
immunopathogenesis
    biologic mechanism 494
    CD45RO cells 492
    cytokine release 493
    GAGs 490–491
    immunoregulatory agents 492
    orbital fibroblasts (OF) 491
    SNPs 493
management 485
    immunopathogenesis 496–497
    moderate to severe condition 496
    restore euthyroidism 495
    stop smoking 494
    visual functions and appearance 495–496
quality of life (QoL) 484
thyroid disease
    hypothyroid / euthyroid 489
    TSH receptor-stimulating antibodies 490
GTT. *See* Glucose tolerance test

H

Harmonisation programme 46–47
Hashimoto's thyroiditis (HT) 420, 427–429, 433, 549
Hematopoietic stem cell transplantation
    (HSCT) 138–139
Hen egg lysozyme (HEL) 102–103
Highly active antiretroviral therapy (HAART) 172
High sensitivity/specificity autoantibody assays
    autoantibodies 42–43
    cognate autoantigen 43–44
    detection assay 44–45
    detection systems 49
    high quality standardised assays 46–47
    specificity and disease relevance 45–46
    thresholds 47–49
HSCT. *See* Hematopoietic stem cell transplantation
Hyperadiponectinemia 374
Hyperglycemia 298
Hypoparathyroidism 117–118
causes
    abnormal development 506–507
    ADH 509
    antibodies inactivation 504–506
    anti-CaSR antibodies 506
    anti-parathyroid antibodies 502–503
    CaSR 503–504
    Iatrogenic and infiltrating 508
    magnesium homeostasis 507–508
    pseudohypoparathyroidism 509–511
    PTH gene product 507
diagnosis
    Chvostek's and Trousseau's signs 511
    PTH infusion/subcutaneous injection 512
parathyroid hormone 501
treatment 512–513
Hypoplasia/aplasia 122

I

IAS. *See* Insulin autoimmune syndrome/hirata disease
Immune dysregulation, polyendocrinopathy, enteropathy, X-linked (IPEX)
clinical manifestations
    genetic autoimmune syndromes and primary immunodeficiencies 132–133
    milder forms 131
    triad symptoms 131
    type-1 diabetes (T1D) 130
FOXP3 structure and function
    nTreg cell 134–135
    transcription factors 134
regulatory T cells
    CD4⁺CD25⁺FOXP3⁺ T cells 135
    FOXP3 expression 135–136
    FOXP3 pathway 137
    key pathogenics 135
therapies
    corticosteroids, immunosuppressive drugs 137–138
    hematopoietic stem cell transplantation (HSCT) 138–139
Immunodominant epitopes 31–32
Immunologic homunculus hypothesis 206–207
Immunopathogenesis
adaptive immunity
    B lymphocyte and autoantibodies 202
    CD4 and CD8 T lymphocytes 203–204
autoimmune animal model 199
genetics
    CTLA4 gene, type 1A diabetes 201
    diabetes prevention 200
    islet autoimmunity association 200
    multiple gene polymorphism 200–201
    type 1A diabetes 201
humanized mice 205–206
immunologic homunculus hypothesis 206–207
innate immunity 202
preclinical model 207
regulatory T cells 204–205
Innate immunity
    dendritic cells 81
    TLR4 receptor 82

Index

Insulin 299–300
Insulin autoantibodies (IAA) 281
Insulin autoimmune syndrome
    (IAS)/Hirata disease
  amino acids role DRβ chain
    DRB1-chain, monoclonal responders 360
    DR4 susceptibility 359
    X-ray crystallography 359, 361
  clinical features 347–349
  clonality 351–355
  control 356, 357
  DRB1-chain 361–362
  drug exposure 345–346
  glucose tolerance test (GTT) 362–363
  hypoglycemia distribution 344–345
  insulin and autoantibody 350–351
  Japanese patients distribution 345
  monoclonal responder 358–359
  polyclonal responder 358
  spontaneous hypoglycemia 344
  T-cell receptor interaction 361
  treatment 363, 364
  type VII hypersensitivity 363
Insulin resistance and metabolic syndrome
  markers 323
  pathophysiology 322
Interleukin 2 169–170
Intestinal endocrine autoimmunity
  APS-1 543
  enterochromaffin cells (EC) 543
  radiobinding assays 543
  serotonin and peptide YY 544
  tryptophan hydroxylase 543
Intrathyroidal antigen presentation
  B cells 469
  dendritic cells 468–469
  thyrocytes 468
Intravenous glucose tolerance test (IVGTT) 280
IPEX. *See* Immune dysregulation, polyendocrinopathy,
    enteropathy, X-linked
Islet autoantibodies 46
Islet cell antibodies 279, 281
Islet cell autoantibodies (ICAs) 18–19, 149
Islet reactive T cells
  beta-cell lesion 321
  immunological mechanisms 319
  tolerance /protection 320
Islet-specific glucose-6-phosphatase-related protein
    (IGRP) 28, 103
Islet transplantation (ITX)
  cell based approach, diabetes treatment 385–386
  challenges
    kidney graft function protection 389
    pancreas transplant programs 388

    post-Edmonton protocol 388
    tolerogenic strategies 390
  exenatide 388
  future perspectives and challenges
    allosensitization 388
    cytoprotective treatments 388–389
    immunosuppression-related side
      effects 389
    islet autografts 389–390
  glucose metabolism normalization 386
  infusion and isolation procedures 386–387
  outcomes 387–388
  type 1 diabetes (T1D) treatment 385

K

Kilham rat parvovirus
  genes 224–225
  Parvoviridea 216
  proinflammatory pathways 222–224
  susceptibility 218
  T-cell-mediation 219
  TLR pathways 220–222
  Treg downmodulation 220

L

Latent autoimmune diabetes of adults
    (LADA) 63
  autoantibodies
    GAD65 318
    HLA haplotype 317
    nonautoimmune type 2 318
    vs. type 1 diabetes 317
  genetics
    childhood type 1 diabetes 322
    CTLA-4 321
    pathogenesis 322
  insulin resistance and metabolic syndrome
    markers 323
    pathophysiology 322
  islet reactive T cells
    beta-cell lesion 321
    immunological mechanisms 319
    tolerance /protection 320
  patient history 323
  treatment
    antigen-specific immunomodulation 323
    diamyd 324
    thiazoledinedione 323
Lymphocytic hypophysitis (LYH)
  APA 547
  pregnancy 558
Lymphoid tyrosine phosphatase (LYP) 432
Lymphopenia 254

M

Magnetic resonance imaging (MRI) 547, 549, 561
Major histocompatibility complex (MHC) genes....... 444–445
    classification 5
    haplotype 7
    polymorphisms and mutations....................................... 6
Metabolic syndrome and inflammation
    abdominal obesity.. 70
    atherogenic dyslipidemia 70
    ATP III clinical identification 72
    cardiovascular disease.. 69
    drugs
        hyperglycemia 85
        TZDs 84
    elevated blood pressure 71
    inflammasome
        β-cell function 83
        NALP and PYCARD 82
    innate immunity
        dendritic cells... 81
        TLR4 receptor 82
    insulin resistance.. 70–71
    oxidative stress
        adipocytes 73
        dyslipidemia... 74
        obesity... 72–73
        TNFα... 73
        vasodilatory agents... 75
    proinflammatory cytokines
        IL-6 80
        nitric oxide 80
        plasminogen-activator inhibitor 1 81
        resistin... 81
        TNFα and IL-1β.. 78–80
    proinflammatory state 71
    prothrombotic state 71
    type 2 diabetes
        C-reactive protein 76–78
        interleukin-β... 76
        NF-κB activation.. 75
        NHANES 76
        WHO 71
Methylprednisolone.. 496
Mucocutaneous candidiasis
    chronic... 119
    treatment 120
Myasthenia gravis (MG) 56
Mycobacterium bovi 419
Myeloperoxidase activity 446

N

National Institute of Health (NIH) 371
Network for Pancreatic Organ Donors
    with Diabetes (nPOD) 235

Nucleic acid programmable protein arrays
    (NAAPAs)... 23–24

O

Orbital fibroblasts (OF)... 491
Ovarian insufficiency
    autoimmunity
        endocrine disorders......................................525–526
        immune system errors..................................524–525
        ovarian cysts.. 526
        support..523–524
    etiology
        chemotherapy/radiotherapy 520–521
        ovarian dysfunction.. 521
    FSH... 520
    genetics
        fragile X syndrome 522
        metabolic disorders 523
        Turner's syndrome 521–522
Oxidative stress
    adipocytes 73
    dyslipidemia.. 74
    obesity.. 72–73
    TNFα... 73
    vasodilatory agents.. 75

P

Pancreas
    beta cells conservation 235
    pathology study 235–236
    regeneration 244–245
    transplantation... 393
        alemtuzumab induction 393–394
        daclizumab induction... 393
        euglycemia restoration 390, 394
        exocrine drainage 392
        immunosuppression 392–393
        renal function improvement............................... 394
        T1D/ESRD hypercoaguable
            state...391–392
        venous drianage 392
Pancreatic beta cells... 268
Parathyroid hormone (PTH) 501
Parvoviridea 216
Pattern-recognition receptors
    (PRRs) 4
peri-islet Schwann cells
    (pSCs) 25
Peripheral autoreactivity
    autoimmune diseases 59–60
    neoepitopes... 61
    posttranslational modification 60–61
Persistent hyperinsulinemic hypoglycemia
    of infancy (PHHI).. 246

Pituitary autoimmunity
    Addison's disease 548
    animal models 552
    antipituitary antibodies 552–553
    autoimmune and organ-specific
        antibodies 556–558
    autopsy findings 549
    criteria 550–551
    epidemiology
        GHD 550
        MRI 549
    Hashimoto's thyroiditis 549
    histopathology 556
    immunofluorescence method 553–555
    LIPH 548
    LYH
        APA 547
        pregnancy 558
    putative pituitary antigens 555–556
Plasminogen-activator inhibitor 1 81
Premature gonadal insufficiency
    autoimmunity
        endocrine disorders 525–526
        immune system errors 524–525
        ovarian cysts 526
        support 523–524
    etiology
        chemotherapy/radiotherapy 520–521
        ovarian dysfunction 521
    FSH 520
    genetics
        fragile X syndrome 522
        metabolic disorders 523
        Turner's syndrome 521–522
    testicular failure
        androgen replacement 530
        autoimmune disorders 529
        chemotherapy / radiotherapy 528
        fertility 530
        genetics 528–529
        osteoporosis 530
    treatment
        fertility 527
        hormonal therapy 526–527
        osteoporosis 527
Primary adrenal insufficiency (PAI) 399
Primers
    APCs 4
    central and peripheral tolerance 9–10
    MHC genes
        classification 5
        haplotype 7
        polymorphisms and mutations 6
    PRRs 4
    TCR gene rearrangement 7–9

Proinflammatory cytokines
    IL-6 80
    nitric oxide 80
    plasminogen-activator inhibitor 1 81
    resistin 81
    TNFα and IL-1β 78–80
Proteomics 27
PRRs. *See* Pattern-recognition receptors
pSCs. *See* peri-islet Schwann cells
Pseudohypoparathyroidism 509–511
Psychosocial stress 275
PTH. *See* Parathyroid hormone

R

Receiver operating characteristic (ROC) 49
Regulatory T (Treg) cells
    CD4⁺CD25⁺FOXP3⁺ T cells detection 135
    FOXP3
        expression 135–136
        pathway 137
    key pathogenics 135
Ribavirin (Riba) 162
Rituximab (anti-CD20) 305
ROC. *See* Receiver operating characteristic

S

Saccharomyces cerevisiae zymosan 419
Schistosoma mansoni 419
Single nucleotide polymorphisms
    (SNPs) 254, 493–494
Sodium-iodide symporter (NIS) 433
Staphylococcus aureus 221
Stress proteins 25

T

T cell antigen
    dystrophia myotonica kinase 29
    IGRP 28
    responses 28
T-cell autoimmunity
    antigen-specific autoreactive T cells
        AICD 62
        down-modulate antigen-presenting cells 62
        experimental models 61–62
        LADA 63
        therapeutics 62
    peripheral autoreactivity
        autoimmune diseases 59–60
        neoepitopes 61
        posttranslational modification 60–61
    self-antigens
        AIRE gene mutation 54–55
        associations 57–58
        Hassall's corpuscles 54

insulin transcription polymorphisms 61
myasthenia gravis (MG) 56
T-cell selection 53
VNTR genotype 56
T-cell lymphopenia 187
T-cell precursors 103
T-cell receptor (TCR) 145
T cells
antigen-specific 466
regulatory 466–477
Th17 cells 467
TECs. *See* Thymic epithelial cells
TEDDY study 287
Testicular failure
androgen replacement 530
autoimmune disorders 529
chemotherapy / radiotherapy 528
fertility 530
genetics 528–529
osteoporosis 530
Thiazolidinediones (TZDs) 84
Thymic epithelial cells (TECs)
HEL 102
IGRP 103
peripheral self expression 102
T-cell precursors 103
Thyroglobulin (TG) 149, 433–434
Thyroid disease 119
Thyroiditis
apoptosis 450
CD4+CD25+ cells
defect 449
Th1 cytokines 449
Treg cells 448
iodine and autoimmunity
APCs 446
CD8+ 447
hormones T3 and T4 445
mechanisms 446
reactive oxygen species 446
major histocompatibility complex 444–445
T and B cells
B-cell depletion 448
experiments 447
intrathyroidal APCs 447
Thyroid peroxidase (TPO) 149, 433
Thyroid stimulating antibody (TSAb) 415
Thyroid-stimulating hormone receptor (TSHR)
autoimmune arthritis 462
B-cell repertoire 461
epitope geography 460
female sex and susceptibility 474
humoral immunity 465
monoclonal antibodies 462

signal transduction 464–465
stimulating epitopes 462–464
Thyroid stimulating immunoglobulin
(TSI) 149
Tissue transglutaminase (TTG) 149
T lymphocytes 203–204
TNF-R receptor (TNFR) 431
Toll-like receptor (TLR) pathways 220–222
Topoisomerase I (TOPI) 24
Topoisomerase II 24
Tryptophan hydroxylase 543
Tryptophan hydroxylase (TPH) 116
TSHR. *See* Thyroid-stimulating hormone receptor
TSH-receptor antibodies (TRAb) 164
TSI. *See* Thyroid stimulating immunoglobulin
Turner's syndrome 521–522
Type 1A diabetes 332, 337
Type 1 autoimmune diabetes (T1D)
antigen-specific immune therapy 18
B cell autoantigen
B lymphocytes 23
candidate B cell gene 24–26
fusion peptide libraries 22
ganglioside ELISAs 23
ICA reaction preabsorption 22–23
λ gt-11 libraries 20–22
mAbs 26–27
NAAPAs 23–24
T1D sera 22
β cell islets
apoptosis 239
cells composing insulitis lesion 237, 239
Fas expression 239
immunohistochemical review 238–239
interferon α 243
MHC class I 242–243
MHC class II 239–241
pancreas sections 240–241
type 1 diabetes 241
insulin autoantibodies 16
insulitis
islet forms 234–235
morphological factors 234
islet cell autoantibody 18–19
non-autoimmune forms
monogenic 246–247
secondary, (PHHI) 246
T2D clinical history 245–246
non-obese diabetics 17
pancreas
beta cells conservation 235
pathology study 235–236
regeneration 244–245
serum C-peptide analysis 232

Type 1 autoimmune diabetes (T1D) (*Continued*)
   T cell antigen
      dystrophia myotonica kinase 29
      IGRP 28
      responses 28
   T2D patient clinical history 232
   ZnT8
      autoantibody detection 30–31
      biomarkers 29
      immunodominant epitopes 31–32
      rs13266634 SNP genotype 33
Type B insulin resistance
   anti-insulin receptor autoantibody characteristics
      binding inhibition 376
      biological activity 377
      ^{125}I-labeled cell surface insulin receptors
         degradation 376
      polyclonal IgGs 375
      type 1 insulin-like growth factor
         (IGF) receptors 375–376
   clinical characteristics
      Acanthosis nigricans 371
      autoimmune disorder 371–372
      hematologic abnormalities 372
      ovarian enlargement
         and hyperandrogenism 371
      proteinuric renal disease 372
   metabolic characteristics
      clinical effects 373
      glucosuria and polyuria 373
      glycemic status 374
      hyperadiponectinemia 374
      hypoglycemia development 373
   treatment
      glycemic control theraphy 379
      immunosuppression 378–379
      lupus nephritis association 379
Type 1 diabetes 119
   additional loci 259–261
   animal models
      class II-associated haplotypes 253
      diabetogenic loci 254
      insulin genes 253
      lymphopenia and autoimmune diabetes 254
      SNP 254
   antigen specific immunomodulation
      diapep277 301–302
      glutamic acid decarboxylase 65
         (GAD65) 300–301
      insulin 299–300
      mechanisms 298
   β-cell
      autoimmunity 279
      destruction and dysfunction 283–285
   beta-cell loss 268

   biological immunomodulators
      abatacept (CTLA4-Ig) 305–306
      anti-CD3 mabs 303–305
      rituximab (anti-CD20) 305
   combination therapies 306–307
   combinatorial analysis 261
   CTLA4 259
   DCCT 294
   environment 261
   etiology
      childhood obesity and rapid growth rate 275
      environmental risk factors 272–273
      genetic risk factors 271–272
      nutrition 274–275
      perinatal factors 275–276
      psychosocial stress 275
      viruses 273–274
   GAD65 268
   genetic profile 280–281
   genetics 254–255
   glucose tolerance 287–288
   IL2RA 259
   immunomodulation
      hyperglycemia 298
      residual C-peptide 297
   immunopathogenesis 294–296
   insulin gene 258
   insulin resistance 285–287
   islet cell antibodies (ICAs) 279, 281
   MHC 255–258
   nonantigen specific immunomodulation 302
   nonmajor histocompatibility complex genes 258
   predictors 281–282
   prevalence and incidence 269–271
   PTPN22 259
   T lymphocytes 252
   zinc transporter 282–283
Type 2 diabetes
   C-reactive protein 76–78
   interleukin-β 76
   NF-κB activation 75
   NHANES 76
Type VII hypersensitivity 363

V

Variable nucleotide tandem repeat (VNTR) 145, 201
Virus-induced type 1 diabetes
   autoimmunity 219
   humoral and cellular immunity 219–220
   Kilham rat parvovirus
      genes 224–225
      Parvoviridea 216
      proinflammatory pathways 222–224
      susceptibility 218
      T-cell-mediation 219

TLR pathways 220–222
Treg downregulation 220
LEW1.WR1 rats 216

X

X-ray crystallography 359, 361

Z

Zinc transporter 8 (ZnT8)
  autoantibody detection 30–31
  biomarkers 29
  immunodominant epitopes 31–32
  rs13266634 SNP genotype 33